Radiology in Forensic Medicine

Giuseppe Lo Re • Antonina Argo
Massimo Midiri • Cristina Cattaneo
Editors

Radiology in Forensic Medicine

From Identification to Post-mortem Imaging

Springer

Editors
Giuseppe Lo Re
Policlinico Paolo Giaccone Radiology Department
Palermo
Italy

Massimo Midiri
Institute of Radiology University Hospital
Palermo
Italy

Antonina Argo
Department of Health Promotion, Maternal and Child Care
Policlinico Giaccone
Palermo
Italy

Cristina Cattaneo
Department of Biomedical Sciences
University of Milan
Milan
Italy

ISBN 978-3-319-96736-3 ISBN 978-3-319-96737-0 (eBook)
https://doi.org/10.1007/978-3-319-96737-0

This Springer imprint is published by the registered company Springer Nature Switzerland AG
The registered company address is: Gewerbestrasse 11, 6330 Cham, Switzerland

Foreword

Forensic medicine is a growing scientific field in our time, due to the latest researches in the understanding of the causes of death and the increasing number of mass disasters.

In fact, we all have assisted a large number of victims of mass disasters such as terrorist attacks and environmental disasters, which carry the necessity of a fast and secure way of reporting the causes of body lesions or death.

Forensic radiology plays a pivotal role in this new scenario thanks to its faster and accurate detection possibility of body injuries, sometimes in the same place where the disasters occurred, with different techniques: X-ray, computed tomography. Sometimes, magnetic resonance could also be useful in the forensic field, especially in neurological lesions.

The use of radiological examinations together with conventional autopsy has increased the diagnostic accuracy of causes of death, shortening the execution time of forensic studies.

Consequently, in the last years, the term "virtual autopsy" was coined, which refers to a new diagnostic radiological tool that is helpful especially in the examination of burned corpse, shot bodies, orthopedic fractures, or in case of massive emphysema.

3D images also help in court discussion for forensic cases, and the recorded radiological data can also be used for many years after first evaluation, unlike conventional autopsy.

The Italian Society of Medical and Interventional Radiology (SIMR) looks at this new field of radiological studies with great interest; altogether with forensic medicine, it is sure that forensic radiology will have a large visibility in the near future.

I've read the chapters written by all the authors of this book, and I think that it is an important knowledge tool in forensic science, both for forensic and radiological specialists, primarily as a result of a complete and simple description of different forensic aspects and of the high iconographic quality of images.

Corrado Bibbolino
Ethical and Forensic Section
Italian Society of Medical and
Interventional Radiology (SIMR)
Genoa, Italy

Preface

To date, medical examiners have relied primarily on cadaveric inspection, as well as the conclusions drawn from conventional autopsy and laboratory methods, in order to define a decedent's cause of death and contextualize it in terms of corresponding judicial findings. Only in particular cases—such as those in which the decedent had sustained multiple traumas or had lesions which were caused by a firearm—was imaging used as additional evidentiary support. In fact, the possibility to obtain a direct view of the body has permitted, and continues to permit, medical examiners the power to approach the state of the cadaver and its present lesions in a more holistic way.

There are, however, instances in which the work of medical examiners appears to be especially difficult. For example, when it comes to the identification of traumatic bone lesions (like those which occur in the ribs, spine, splanchnocranium, or at the base of the skull) and the establishment of these specific aspects in correlation to the eventual presence of collected areas (subcutaneous, respiratory, abdominal, cerebral); the study of lungs in drowning victims; or the evaluation of vascular lesions. Under no circumstances do these scenarios present an insurmountable level of difficulty, but here, the use of imaging methods improves the quality of and speed at which diagnoses can be reached by medical examiners.

In this sense, forensic radiology plays an important role that should be well defined with respect to radiology as it is used in living patients. Recently, forensic radiology has made its way from the margins of conventional practices to now becoming a more structured, widely used method. Perhaps this resulted after the introduced concept of virtual autopsy, sometimes a "substitute" for physical autopsy, which allows for a single diagnostic application for the photographic documentation of the corpse, the study of computed tomography (CT) scans either with or without the injection of contrast, the RM of the SSN study, and histological evaluation by automated guided biopsy. Finally, with the frequency of mass disasters that occur worldwide, the topics on the ways in which we can scientifically address these crises are prevalently discussed.

Over the years, the medical-legal community have had the opportunity to witness the growing interest in the comparison of imaging methods as they apply to the forensic sciences, both by forensic doctors and those within the judicial system.

The use of simple and low-cost radiological methods, such as CT/MRI scans of the body, could significantly help medical examiners to obtain more accurate results when used in conjunction with autopsy findings. This, of course, is possible without being disruptive to the normal radiological or medical routine, and/or without causing a significant increase to labor and material costs.

For members of both the medical and legal professions, there are undeniable advantages to the possibility of obtaining images of cadavers that could continuously be re-visited and re-evaluated. Namely, it relieves some of the burden of this work by speeding up processing time.

It is already common for radiologists and forensic physician, in the spirit of collaboration, to share experiences and diagnostic information with each other. We therefore find that, in fact, we have a shared purpose which allows both medical subspecialties to support, rather than replace, one another.

In this text, the authors addressed these questions and shared their own operational experiences hoping that they can garner the interest of the broader scientific community and medical-legal environment.

Palermo, Italy Giuseppe Lo Re
Palermo, Italy Antonina Argo
Palermo, Italy Massimo Midiri
Milan, Italy Cristina Cattaneo

Contents

1 A Brief History of Forensic Radiology

Roberto Lagalla

Since its discovery in 1845, thanks to the Nobel Prize William Conrad Roentgen, radiology was used not just for medical-diagnostic purposes on the living but also in lawsuits and for the evaluation of cadaveric remains.

Among the first applications of forensic radiology, in 1896, a unique use of radiology is reported for the evaluation of an Egyptian mummy at the Natural History Museum in Vienna. Indeed, the museum had purchased an Alexandrian mummy as a human mummy; however, the bandages covering the mummy referred to an animal. Thus, the mummy, which was not violated to avoid the corruption of the content, underwent an X-ray study that depicted the beautiful radiological image of a big bird mummy.

Many cases of application of radiology purposes with "paleoradiological" purposes have been reported and the introduction of CT, especially of the newer multislice CT scanners, has further widened the applicability and usefulness of radiologic techniques in the study of corpses preserved over the millennia.

Indeed, the possibility of studying the corpses without any alteration of their integrity represents the greater radiological inspection advantage compared to human direct corpse inspection, so that it is reported as nondestructive examination (NDE) technique.

Many diagnostic possibilities in the identification of the mummies have been demonstrated by radiology, as the possibility to define the age, presence of preexisting diseases, and the causes of death of the mummy itself, as well as the mummification process.

Concerning this matter, the English Heritage published in 2006 the guidelines of the X-radiography of archaeological metalwork.

Over the years, forensic radiology applications have also addressed to the evaluation of the artifacts, and it demonstrated to be particularly suited for the definition of their historical period and the methods used for their production.

Important mingling between forensic and radiological applications have been demonstrated not just for paleoradiological purposes.

Since the beginning, in fact, the important role of radiology in the assessment of the causes of responsibility in criminal cases has been understood. Indeed, radiology methods offer the coroner and the magistrate, the possibility to "fossilize the time" in the identification of pathological processes caused by third parties, so that they can be always evaluated by the magistrate and the experts/appraisers who follow one another over the years during a legal process.

Moreover, the forensic radiological findings are not just re-evaluable over the years

R. Lagalla (✉)
Department of Pathobiology and Medical Biotechnologies, University of Palermo, Palermo, Italy
e-mail: roberto.lagalla@unipa.it

G. Lo Re et al. (eds.), *Radiology in Forensic Medicine*,
https://doi.org/10.1007/978-3-319-96737-0_1

with the same diagnostic accuracy, but also easily disclosed and shareable, conversely to conventional autopsy findings that is intrinsically a unique procedure that cannot be entirely re-performed.

In addition, forensic radiology provides new real points of interpretation of detrimental events, being able to provide an overview of the body without compromising its integrity; this last point finds its practical manifestation when radiology is required for the detection of the causes of death. This is why forensic radiology is actually routinely referred in the scientific literature and forensic clinical practice, with the term "Virtopsy."

The term Virtopsy, neologism composed by the fusion of the words virtual and autopsy, summarizes the ability to perform a minimally invasive preliminary assessment of bodies that must, inevitably, be followed in most of the cases by an assessment through conventional forensic autopsy. According to the writer and to the most recent and prestigious scientific publications, the two procedures cannot and should not be considered as alternatives to each other, but as two distinct moments, the forensic and the radiological one, of a single overall diagnostic procedure which has as its ultimate goal the identification of the deceased, determine causes of death, and distinguish premortem and postmortem structural alterations in cases of dubious criminal responsibility.

Italy has been one of the forerunners nations in autopsy studies. It is important to remember the pioneering autopsy forensic research performed by Andrea Vesalius, who worked in the XVI century at the University of Padua.

However, forensic radiology finds its application not just in the study of the deceased; indeed, immediately after the discovery of X-rays, these have been used to assist particularly difficult legal and forensic investigations in criminal cases.

The first court case involving the conventional radiography was reported in North America where, on Christmas Eve of 1895, Mr. Tolson Cunning was shot in the legs by Mr. George Holder. Given the failed first attempt of the surgeon to find the bullet and being Mr. Cunning symptomatic, despite the healed wound, the surgeon asked the advice of a professor of physics at McGill University, John Cox, to take a wounded limb radiography. After an exposure of 45 min, the radiograph obtained showed the bullet flattened between the tibia and fibula enabling the surgeon to remove the bullet and to Mr. Cunning to bring proof of attempted murder. To date, radiology is still used in cases needing age estimation of people without documents. This aspect is particularly useful in those border nations, as Italy, in which a significant number of migrants leaving the African and Eastern countries hoping to reach Europe and improve their quality of life arrives every year. It would be really impossible in some cases for forensic scientists to determine with reasonable certainty the age of subjects, sometimes even accused of particularly heinous crimes such as smuggling of migrants.

However, as in a singular and sad carousel, the different aspects of forensic radiology outlined so far are gathered each other. It is well known all over the world, the high number of deaths in the Mediterranean routes of this human migration. Radiology section of the Department of Palermo has recently been involved in an important and fundamental assessment procedure involving both autopsy and virtopsy in a large number of dead bodies recovered from a navy shipwrecked off the coast of Libya, and that I want to remember as "Melilli's forensic radiology hope operation." Melilli is the name of the Sicilian military base where the forensic operations were performed.

To date, there are many applications in which radiology and forensic medicine have melted their interests and applications, but further developments are predictable. Thus, we can imagine a future in which the two medical specialties, although maintaining their intrinsic specific characteristics, are considered essential to each other in the evaluation necropsy cases and in some medical-legal lawsuits.

2 Strength and Limits of Conventional Forensic Medicine

Burkhard Madea

2.1 Introduction

Since about 20 years Forensic postmortem imaging was developed systematically at first in Bern, then whole Switzerland and now worldwide [1–5]. Richard Dirnhofer, the father of "Virtopsy",[1] summarizes the scientific development of postmortem imaging techniques as follows [1]:

> *It was against the background of rapid technological advances in various imaging techniques, that at the turn of the century, the academic concept of the "Virtopsy" research programme was realized at the University of Bern in Switzerland. The aim of this project has been to develop a minimally invasive autopsy procedure in which evidentially relevant findings are obtained from a corpse predominantly by means of medical imaging methods. Depending on the individual case and the specific issue involved, this leaves, the option open to perform a conventional autopsy to acquire further relevant facts, such as histological, toxicological and bacteriological examinations.*
>
> *The international impact of this idea has been reflected in an exponential increase in scientific publications around the world dealing with forensic radiology. For instance, the recently published study by M. Baglivo et al. showed a tenfold increase in the volume of publications compared to the turn of the millennium, when the "Virtopsy" project started.This academic "hype" in the field of postmortem radiology has had a very positive influence on the attractiveness of radiology for the new generation of academics in forensic medicine.*
>
> *In short, the results of these numerous publications documents that postmortem imaging is not only equal to autopsy in many respects but that this method can even achieve better results than conventional autopsy procedures. This has also called into question the status of conventional autopsy as the "gold standard" for obtaining and recording forensic medical findings.*

He questions already if the traditional autopsy is still the "gold standard" for obtaining and recording forensic medical findings.

The purpose of this chapter is not to argue for or against traditional autopsy or postmortem forensic imaging but to briefly address evolution, importance and decline of the traditional autopsy.

The importance of the different imaging techniques in solving different forensic questions has been outlined especially by Dirnhofer [1–3] and Grabherr [4, 5].

There is no doubt about the importance of forensic imaging.

2.2 Technique, History and Tasks of the Autopsy

The modern autopsy has been defined as follows [6]:

> An autopsy is the systematic external and internal examination of a body to establish the presence or

[1]The term "Virtopsy" is a neologism comprising the words "virtual" and "autopsy". It is used for imaging in Forensic Medicine, especially postmortem imaging (CT, MRT, surface scanning, Angiography).

B. Madea (✉)
Institute of Forensic Medicine, University Hospital Bonn, Bonn, Germany
e-mail: b.madea@uni-bonn.de

G. Lo Re et al. (eds.), *Radiology in Forensic Medicine*,
https://doi.org/10.1007/978-3-319-96737-0_2

absence of disease by gross and microscopic examination of body tissues. The pathologist makes a surgical incision from shoulder to shoulder and from the midpoint of the shoulder-to-shoulder incision to the pubic bone. The skin is reflected, and each organ in the chest, including the neck structures, abdomen and pelvis, is removed and carefully examined. An incision is also made from the mastoid bone on the right to the mastoid bone on the left, and the scalp is pulled forward and the bony cap removed to reveal the brain. The brain is removed and examined. The pathologist takes a small sample or biopsy of all tissues and archives them in formalin to maintain them for future references.

For hospital autopsies, depending on the list or permissions given by the person qualified to give permission, tissues and organs may be retained for study, research, or other investigations. The pathologist submits small 2 × 2 cm sections of tissue to the histology laboratory, where thin slices a few microns thick are subjected to chemical treatment to preserve them. The tissue blocks are shaved, so that a thin layer can be mounted on a glass slide and stained with dyes to differentiate cells. The pathologist can recognize diseases in the stained tissue. Medicolegal autopsies are conducted to determine the cause of death; assist with the determination of the manner of death as natural, suicide, homicide, or accident; collect medical evidence that may be useful for public health or the courts; and develop information that may be useful for reconstructing how the person received a fatal injury. [6]

Autopsies have been performed to:

- Establish the cause of death.
- Assist in determining the manner of death (i.e. homicide, suicide).
- Compare the premortem and postmortem findings.
- Produce accurate vital statistics.
- Monitor the public health.
- Assess the quality of medical practice.
- Instruct medical students and physicians.
- Identify new and changing diseases.
- Evaluate the effectiveness of therapies such as drugs, surgical techniques and prosthesis.
- Reassure family members.
- Protect against false liability claims and settle valid claims quickly and fairly [7].

Bowman and Anderson et al. also summarized the uses of autopsy [8].

Bowman (1983)	Anderson et al. (1979)
Assisting in development and quality assurance of new technologies, procedures and therapies Quality assurance for clinical diagnosis and treatment Improving accuracy and value of vital statistics Source of organs and tissues for transplantation Evaluation and distribution of insurance benefits Monitoring and identifying environmental disease Medical education Forensic pathology Disclosing the nature of an individual death Risk management Reassurance to family Explaining unknown or unanticipated complications of disease Identifying communicable diseases	Instrument of quality assessment of medical care by peer review Continuing education of physicians Provision of reliable database on causes of death and disease Recognition of harbingers of disease Grief counselling for family Identification of communicable diseases Forensic pathology Monitoring and identifying environmental disease Materials and problems for basic research Medical education

Table 2.1 Types of autopsy (according to [9])

• Anatomic autopsy
– Structure and function of human body
– Andreas Vesalius (1514–1564)
– Great progress in the sixteenth to eighteenth centuries
• Clinical autopsy
– Cause, locus, aetiology, pathogenesis of disease
– Giovanni Battista Morgagni (1682–1771)
– Marie François Xavier Bichat (1771–1802)
– Carl von Rokitansky (1804–1878)
– Rudolf Virchow (1821–1902)
• Forensic autopsy
– Cause and manner of death
– Causality of external violence for death
– Live birth or stillbirth determination
– Medical malpractice
– Johannes Bohn (1640–1718)
– Johann Ludwig Casper (1796–1864)
– Eduard von Hofmann (1837–1897)

There are three types of autopsy: the anatomic autopsy, the clinical autopsy and the forensic autopsy (Table 2.1). The anatomic autopsy studies the structure and function of the human body. The clinical autopsy studies the cause, locus, aetiology and pathogenesis of disease, and was the main method for medical research in the nineteenth and early twentieth centuries. The forensic autopsy is essential in determining the cause and manner of death and the causality of external violence for death.

The anatomic autopsy was largely developed at Italian universities, especially at the University of Padua [9–20]. Andreas Vesalius (1514–1564) published his famous series of books on human anatomy, *De Humani Corporis Fabrica Libri Septem.*

Clinical autopsy also developed at the University of Padua [14, 16, 18–20]. Giovanni Battista Morgagni (1682–1771) performed autopsies to study the cause and locus of disease and wrote his famous book *De Sedibus et Causis Morborum* based on his studies. Morgagni looked for diseases of the organs as the cause of death.

Marie Xavier Bichat (1771–1802) studied tissues ("membranes") as the cause of disease and death [21].

The history of the development of pathology at the Paris Hospital was well described by Erwin Ackerknecht in 1967 and later by Michel Foucault in his book, *The Birth of the Clinic* (1994) [10, 11, 22, 23].

Further major developments in clinical pathology were achieved in Vienna by the pathologist Carl von Rokitansky (1804–1878), who personally conducted more than 30,000 autopsies at a small morgue in the neighbourhood of the Vienna General Hospital [11, 24–29]. Rokitansky wrote famous handbooks on both general pathology and special pathology. Furthermore, he wrote a book on atrial septal defects and built a new Institute of Pathology, which still exists today.

Further developments in clinical pathology were made in Berlin by Rudolf Virchow, who studied the cell as the cause of death and disease [9, 11, 28, 30, 31].

Rudolf Virchow (1821–1902) was the founder of cellular pathology. He also founded the Museum of Pathology, which still stands in the Charité area of Berlin, and which displays specimens from Virchow's collection [31]. Virchow was not only responsible for the ongoing development of clinical pathology, but also for developing the methods of forensic autopsy. He published a book on autopsy techniques, *Die Sections-Technik im Leichenhause des Charité Krankenhauses*, which was very important for the standardization of autopsy rules in practice. Similar books were published in other German countries and in Austria. Meanwhile, the Council of Europe published recommendations for the international harmonization of autopsy rules.

Handbooks on autopsy techniques are available worldwide [24, 32–40].

Clinical autopsy was the main method of medical research in the nineteenth and early twentieth centuries [8, 28]. Many diseases have been discovered or critically clarified through autopsy. A partial list of these diseases is shown in Table 2.2.

Even in the twentieth century new diseases were discovered by the systematic analysis of autopsy results (f.i. AIDS).

The forensic autopsy was developed in the nineteenth century [9, 14, 30, 41]. However, as early as the seventeenth century professors of forensic medicine working at the University of Leipzig were requesting autopsy rather than wound inspection to determine the cause and manner of death. In Germany, Johann Ludwig Casper (1796–1874) played an essential role in the development of forensic medicine and forensic autopsy. Casper wrote his well-known handbook of forensic medicine based on his personal experiences at autopsies. The morgue at the Institute of Forensic Medicine in Berlin was modelled after the morgue at the Institute of Forensic Medicine in Paris. In Austria, Eduard von Hofmann (1837–1897), who wrote a famous handbook on forensic medicine as well as an atlas of forensic medicine, was instrumental in the further development of forensic medicine and forensic autopsy.

As in clinical pathology, forensic pathology revealed new autopsy findings and allowed critical evaluation through further systematic observations and experiments, including

- Hydrostatic lung test.
- Contrecoup lesions of the orbit in cases of falling on the back of the head.
- Simon's bleedings (haemorrhages of the intervertebral disk of the lumbar spine) in cases of hanging.
- Inner knee sign in death due to hypothermia.

Table 2.2 Partial list of diseases discovered or critically clarified through autopsy since 1950 (according to [8])

Cardiovascular lesions	Bronchopulmonary lesions	Gastrointestinal lesions
• Tricuspid valve disease due to metastasizing carcinoid tumour	• Alveolitis (diffuse alveolar damage, shock lung, respiratory distress syndrome)	Whipple's disease
• Understanding of congenital heart lesions leading to modern surgical treatment	• Oxygen toxicity	Protein-losing enteropathy
• Atheromatous embolism	• Pneumocystis pneumonia	Congenital intestinal atresia
• Asymmetric cardiac hypertrophy	• Infantile respiratory distress syndrome (hyaline membrane disease)	Pancreatic cystic fibrosis
• Dissecting aneurysm and variations thereon	• Legionnaire's disease	Vascular insufficiency syndromes and haemorrhagic enteropathy
• Primary cardiomyopathy	• Pulmonary alveolar proteinosis, desquamative pneumonia	Protein and potassium loss from villous adenoma
• Subaortic muscular stenosis	• Diseases resulting from inhalation of industrial dusts: asbestosis, berylliosis, bagassosis, silo-filler's disease	
• Rheumatoid disease of aorta and aortic valve	• Lipid pneumonia	
• Complications of cardiac surgery	• Diffuse interstitial fibrosis	
• Diseases of the cardiac conducting system		
• Idiopathic hypertrophic subaortic stenosis		
• Cardiomyopathies		
• Mitral valve prolapse		

From Hill and Anderson (1996)

– Patterned contact entrance wounds.

According to autopsy rules which were mainly developed in the nineteenth century in various countries the gross autopsy findings have to be described according to the following criteria [15, 24, 32–34, 38]:

Description of gross autopsy findings:

1. Location and form of organs, situs
2. Height and weight (of the body, of organs, etc.)
3. Surface
   (a) Organs surface
   (b) Serosa, mucosa, adhesions
4. Consistency
5. Coherence, consolidation
6. Cut surface
   (a) Structure
   (b) Colour
   (c) Fluids, congestion, smear
7. Odour

The pathologist has to use all his senses to make a complete description of autopsy results.

The gross tissue alterations are evaluated according to the following criteria:

General gross tissue alterations due to disease:

- Blood content
  - Acute anaemia
  - Chronic anaemia
  - Acute hyperaemia
  - Chronic venous congestion
- Obstruction of blood
  - Thrombosis
  - Thrombembolus
- Necrosis
  - Ischaemic necrosis
  - Haemorrhagic necrosis
  - Caseous necrosis
  - Gangrenous necrosis
- Oedema
- Haemorrhage

- Dystrophia
  - Cloudy swelling
  - Fatty degeneration
- Hyaline
- Amyloid
- Pigments
  - Anthracosis
  - Haemosiderin
  - Melanin
  - Bile pigment
  - Lipofuscin
  - Malaria pigment
  - Ochronotic pigment
  - Heavy metals
  - Iatrogenic pigment
- Inflammation
  - Serous
  - Catarrhalic
  - Fibrinous
  - Purulent
  - Haemorrhagic
  - Necrotizing
  - Gangrenous
- Reparation
- Calcification
- Tumours, neoplasms
  - Macroscopic difference benign and malign tumours
  - Primary tumour/metastasis
  - Carcinoma/sarcoma

By a traditional autopsy all these gross tissue alterations can be evaluated.

2.3 Autopsy as Quality Control of Clinical Medicine

The autopsy is still today the gold standard for clarifying the cause and manner of death and is much superior to an external examination taking into account the clinical history of the patient [24, 36, 42–49]. Autopsy-detected errors in clinical diagnosis can be classified as follows [47, 48, 50, 51]:

- **Major errors (class II)**
  Clinically missed diagnoses involving a principal underlying disease or primary cause of death
- **Class I errors**
  Major errors that, had they been detected before death, might have affected patient prognosis or outcome (at a minimum, allowed discharge from the hospital alive)

According to a study by Goldman et al. [43], class I errors have remained relatively stable over the centuries. According to a meta-analysis by Shojania et al. [48], class I errors are found today in 8–10% of autopsies. The diseases most frequently associated with major discrepancies between antemortem and postmortem diagnoses are listed in Table 2.3. In many clinical disciplines, autopsy reveals additional information that has important clinical relevance (Table 2.4).

In very specialized and well-equipped hospitals like the University Hospital Zurich class one errors are now as low as 2% [50, 51, 53]. This decrease of class one errors is to some part due to improved imaging techniques.

However, the autopsy rate has markedly declined over time in Europe and the United States [6, 49, 54–57]. The clinical autopsy rate in Germany is now below 2% and the forensic autopsy rate is stable at about 2% (Table 2.5) [54].

The autopsy is of special importance in medical malpractice cases [58–62]. Without autopsy, toxicology and histology [63] clinicians are walking in the fog as far as malpractice claims, especially adverse drug events are concerned.

Table 2.3 Diseases most frequently associated with major discrepancies between antemortem and postmortem diagnoses (according to [42])

Autopsy diagnosis	% Discrepancy
Pulmonary embolism	46.8
Peritonitis	45.1
Postoperative haemorrhage/infection	37.9
Vascular insufficiency of the intestine	37.2
Lung abscess	34.1
Renal infarct	31.6
Metastatic carcinoma	30.6
Alzheimer's disease	30.0

Adapted from ref. [42]

Table 2.4 Percentage of cases in which autopsy revealed additional information and the percentage of those cases in which the additional findings were clinically relevant (according to [52])

Discipline	Cases with additional information (%)	Diagnostic or clinical relevance (%)
Internal medicine	82.1	26.1
Surgery	68.0	64.7
Neurosurgery	66.7	40.0
Anaesthesiology/intensive care	93.8	60.0
Paediatrics	50.0	100
Neonatology	36.4	25.0
Cardiac surgery	89.1	26.0
Total	74.8	32.9

From Ref. [52]

Table 2.5 Autopsy frequency in some European countries (according to [54])

Country	Year	Total (%)	Clinical pathological (%)	Forensic (%)
Great Britain	1999	17.3	2.1	15.2
Sweden	1992	22	16	6
Finland	1992	31.1	14.2	16.9
Denmark	1992	16	13.6	2.4
Germany	1999	5.1	3.1	2.0
Germany	1994	6.1	4.2	1.9

2.4 Decline of the Clinical Autopsy

The reasons for the decline of the clinical autopsy are several [15, 32, 36, 44, 45, 49]. The famous Austrian/German pathologist Herwig Hamperl (1899–1976), who worked in Vienna, Berlin, Prague, Salzburg, Marburg and Bonn, wrote an autobiography where he published the number of autopsies performed at the different locations where he worked and the number of examined biopsies [56] (Fig. 2.1). While at the beginning of his career in Vienna there was a high autopsy rate and few biopsies were examined by the end of Hamperl's career there was a reverse picture: a low autopsy rate (about 700 per year at the Bonn University Hospital) and a high biopsy rate. Compared to the times of Hamperl the rate of clinical autopsies decreased further dramatically.

It has to be kept in mind that the decline of the autopsy rate, especially the non-forensic autopsy, started centuries before the implementation of postmortem imaging into forensic and clinical pathology practice.

Other reasons for the resistance against autopsy are [28]:

- Loss of the important role of autopsy in exploring morphological conditions of virtually every disease
- Clinical pathology vs. autopsy pathology (biopsies instead of autopsies)
- Development of individual rights
  - Consent is necessary to perform autopsy
  - Questions about who can provide consent

Furthermore, pathologists are not paid adequately for either clinical or forensic autopsies and lost interest in performing autopsies.

Furthermore clinicians are resistant against autopsies for different reasons:

- Autopsies seem not necessary in times of high tech-medicine since cause of death and underlying diseases have already been diagnosed sufficiently
- Fear for medical malpractice claims

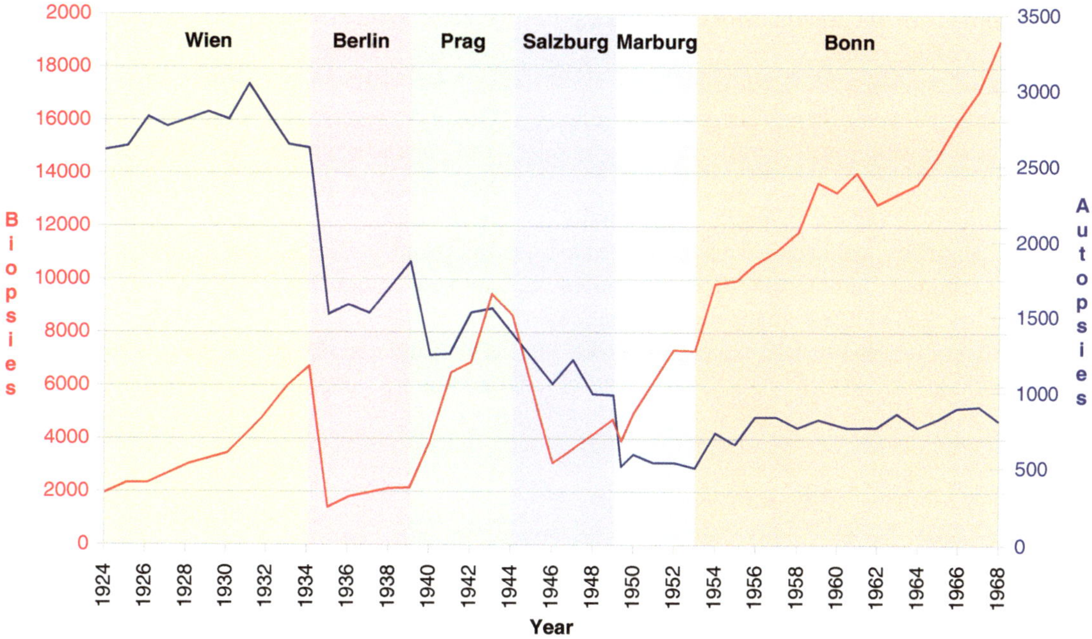

Fig. 2.1 Herwig Hamperl (1899–1976) worked in various cities (Vienna, Berlin, Prague, Salzburg, Marburg, Bonn). Number of autopsies performed and number of examined biopsies by location. The number of autopsies decreased, the number of biopsies increased considerably

- They don't want to share their DRG-claims (money for treating the patients) with the pathologist
- Too much time delay until the final report of the pathologist is finished

2.5 Limitations of Autopsy Compared to Radiology

In recent years limitations of autopsy relative to radiology have been outlined. The purposes of forensic radiology can be summarized as follows [1–3]:

- Patient identification
- Gender determination
- Body length measurement
- Discrimination of individual features (dental, intracorporeal)
- Documentation
- Revealing foreign material (bullets, inserted foreign bodies)
- Identification of injuries and organ disease (to determine cause and manner of death)
- Evaluating vitality of sustained injuries
- Forensic reconstruction
- Education
- Research

According to Dirnhofer, this method of documenting forensic findings is investigator independent, objective, and noninvasive and provides qualitative improvements in forensic pathologic investigation, because digitally stored data can be recalled at any time to provide fresh, intact topographic and anatomic-clinical information. Dirnhofer et al. described the systematic limitations of classical autopsy as follows:

- No complete autopsy from top to toe
- Destructive method—anatomy destroyed by preparation
- Preparation and documentation of findings impaired in cases of putrefaction
- Preparation results depend on lighting conditions
- No 3D presentation of results

- Contamination of specimens for further analysis (toxicology, etc.)
- "Bloody" photographic documentation
- Conventional autopsy not accepted by relatives or some religions

Advantages of the noninvasive or minimally invasive approach achieved with postmortem surface scanning and multi-slice computed tomography as well as magnetic resonance imaging over current forensic examination techniques include

- Precise, objective and clear documentation of forensic findings for the court
- Calibrated 3D documentation of findings
- Quality assurance through digital data archiving and transfer
- Reduction of psychological trauma for the next-of-kin
- Improved judicature in cultures with low autopsy acceptance [1–3]

The advantages of imaging according to Dirnhofer are summarized in Tables 2.6 and 2.7.

Table 2.6 Advantages of imaging (according to [3])

Imaging methods	Advantage of application in the justice system
Objective data collection; "Mechanized" objectivity without human influence	Independence from the specific forensic pathologist. Considerably easier to obtain second opinions
Better reproducibility	Presentation of the findings themselves as evidence—not just the expert report
"Bloodless" documentation	"Nontraumatic" presentation of findings in the courtroom
Teleforensics	Interpretation not just by two pairs of eyes but by multiple investigators
True-to-scale 3-D facsimile of the body as an item of evidence	Real-data forensic reconstructions are very accurate (e.g. road accidents, shootings, stabbings)
Postmortem angiography	Clear definition of sources of bleeding in all trauma cases and in investigations into treatment errors Clear information following cardiac and vascular interventions. 3-D record of bleeding in the soft tissues
Postmortem CT scans with simultaneous surface documentation	Possibility of making 3-D morphometric comparisons, accurate in colour and scale, between the shape and size of injuries and the alleged weapon. Independent of place and time Reconstruction of road accidents and homicides based on real data. Contamination-free 3-D comparisons, joint examination, and processing of a case by forensic scientists, police, and judiciary Introduction of the 3-D model of the deceased/injured person into the 3-D model of the crime scene
Clear detection of accumulations of gases in the body	Avoidance of gas embolisms in arteries and veins and escape of air into the chest, often overlooked because they are not visible at autopsy. These findings can be relevant to the cause of death
Cause célèbre	Clear information given to the public
Detection of foreign bodies, parts of projectiles, weapons	Clear localization of foreign bodies Reliable image-guided asservation
Non-destructive procedure	No debate over autopsy on religious grounds
Reliable recording of findings in areas difficult to dissect: head, neck, pelvis and peripheral vessel regions	Additional information from findings to establish the cause of death and forensic reconstruction
Ability to archive a "facsimile" of the corpse for use as evidence	Additional and subsequent expert opinions always possible at a later date (e.g. cremation, no need for exhumation)

Table 2.7 Documentation of findings and expert assessment using imaging (according to [1])

Allocation of responsibilities	
1. External examination—surface scan	→ 3D visualization—improved
↓	
2. Imaging of internal findings (CT, MR, …)	→ Non-destructive, whole body—improved
↓	
3. Storage of data as a true-to-scale 3D model—**signed only by radiographer (MTRA)**	→ New, most valuable element (for critical discussion as defined by K.R. Popper)
↓	
4. Capture of findings using the Schwarzacher perception method—overall view, detail, naïve, viewing, leafing through the visual memory	→ Identical to autopsy
↓	
4a. Recording of findings by radiographer	→ Identical to autopsy
↓	
4b. Multiple-investigator principle of capturing findings	→ Improved through possibility of teleradiology
↓	
5. Written documentation of findings by reading—**signed solely by radiologist**	→ Remains the same—corresponds to current autopsy report
↓	
6. Joint (forensics and radiology) preparation of forensic diagnostics from the findings—**signed jointly by radiologist and forensic specialist**	→ Improved—corresponds to the summary autopsy report or the forensic pathological diagnosis
↓	
7. Interpretation of the diagnosis and findings for expert report, taking account of all the circumstances (E. von Hofmann, premises, evidenced facts such as information pool, examination of the scene, toxicology, histology, etc.)—**signed solely by forensic specialist**	→ Remains unchanged—corresponds to the forensic report. Does, however, enable more effective critical examination based on Item 3 within the framework of the assessment of evidence, second opinions, decisive expert reports

2.6 Can Postmortem Imaging Replace the Autopsy Completely

Especially for trauma victims the value of postmortem imaging not only for the documentation of injuries but also for clarifying cause and manner of death has been shown [64–67].

In an unselected autopsy material the classical autopsy is still superior to postmortem imaging.

In a recent investigation, Roberts et al. [68] concluded: "Our findings identify important shortcomings of cross sectional imaging in the diagnosis of cause of death in adults and provide the evidence needed to refine imaging techniques and enable them to be safely introduced into autopsy services". Indeed, the major discrepancy rate between autopsy-determined and radiologically determined cause of death was 32% (26–40) for computed tomography and 43% (36–50) for magnetic resonance imaging. These findings indicate that postmortem imaging is not superior to a simple external examination. Postmortem imaging is essential for documentation, but to clarify cause and manner of death the traditional autopsy remains at least at the present moment the gold standard for unsolved cases.

The benefits of the autopsy fall into seven broad categories [15]**:**

1. Benefits to physicians and health care organizations
2. Benefits to the family of the deceased
3. Benefits to public health
4. Benefits to medical education
5. Benefits to medical discovery and applied clinical research

6. Benefits to basic biomedical research
7. Benefits to law enforcement and jurisprudence [15]

Finkbeiner et al. further elaborated the benefits of autopsy [15]:

1. Benefits to physicians and health care organizations
   (a) Establishment of final diagnoses and cause of death
   (b) Correlation of physical and laboratory findings with pathologic changes of disease
   (c) Autopsy is the gold standard for evaluating the accuracy of diagnosis and the outcome of therapy
   (d) Autopsy provides critical data for medical quality assurance
   (e) Autopsies may also reduce hospital and physician malpractice risk
   (f) Autopsy may contribute to accurate billing
2. Benefits to the family of the deceased
   (a) identification or definition of hereditary or contagious diseases
3. Benefits to public health
   (a) Detection of contagious diseases
   (b) Identification of environmental hazards
   (c) Contribution of accurate vital statistics
4. Benefits to medical education
   (a) Education of students in medicine and other health-related disciplines
5. Benefits to medical discovery and applied clinical research
   (a) Modern molecular techniques coupled with and supplementing postmortem examinations have identified diseases related to emerging and re-emerging infectious agents
6. Benefits to basic biomedical research
   (a) Provides investigators with normal and diseased human tissues for research
7. Benefits to law enforcement and jurisprudence

There is no doubt that in the future postmortem imaging will fulfil these benefits as well.

References

1. Dirnhofer R, Schick J (2016) Bildgebung in der Rechtsmedizin. Der gläserne Körper als Beweismittel. NWV Verlag GmbH, Graz
2. Dirnhofer R, Schick R (2010) Virtopsy. Obduktion neu in Bildern: gerichtsmedizinische Vorstellung und prozessrechtliche Diskussion einer neuen wissenschaftlichen Autopsiemethode. Schriftenreihe Recht der Medizin. Manz, Wien
3. Dirnhofer R (2016) Postmortem imaging: a part of forensic medicine. In: Grabherr S, Grimm JM, Heinemann A (eds) Atlas of postmortem angiography. Springer, Berlin, pp 35–43
4. Grabherr S, Baumann P, Fahrni S, Mangin P, Grimm J (2015) Virtuelle vs. reale forensische bildgebende Verfahren. Einsatzgebiete, Vorteile und Limits. Rechtsmedizin 25:493–509
5. Grabherr S, Grimm JM, Heinemann A (eds) (2016) Atlas of postmortem angiography. Springer, Berlin
6. National Research Council (2009) Strengthening forensic sciences in the United States. A path forward. National Academies Press, Washington, DC
7. Lundberg GD (1998) Low-tech autopsies in the era of high-tech medicine. Continued value for quality assurance and patient safety. JAMA 208:1273–1274
8. Hill RB, Anderson RE (1988) The autopsy—medical practice and public policy. Butterworths, Boston
9. Madea B (2014) History of forensic medicine. In: Madea B (ed) Handbook of forensic medicine. Wiley, Chichester, pp 3–14
10. Ackerknecht EH (1950/1951) Early history of legal medicine. Legal medicine in transition (16th–18th centuries). Legal medicine becomes a modern Science (19th century). Ciba Symp 7:1286–1304. Reprinted in: (1977) Legacies in Law and Medicine, 249–265
11. Brugger CM, Kühn H (1985) Sektion der menschlichen Leiche. Ferdinand Enke Verlag, Stuttgart
12. Del Negro P (ed) (2003) The University of Padova. Eight centuries of history. Offset invicta Padua
13. Dhom G (2001) Geschichte der Histopathologie. Springer, Berlin
14. Feola T (2007) Profilo storico della medicina legale. Editioni Minerva Medica, Turino
15. Finkbeiner W, Ursell P, Davis R (2004) Autopsy pathology. a manual and atlas. Churchill Livingstone, Philadelphia
16. Fischer Homberger E (1983) Medizin vor Gericht. Zur Sozialgeschichte der Gerichtsmedizin. Verlag Hans Huber, Bern
17. Madea B (2014) Handbook of forensic medicine. Wiley, Chichester
18. Wolf-Heidegger G, Cetto AM (1967) Die anatomische Sektion in bildlicher Darstellung. S. Karger, Basel
19. Zanatta A, Thiene G, Valente M, Zampieri F (2015) Text atlas of historical pathology from the Museum of Pathological Anatomy of Padua University. Antilia, Treviso

20. Universita de Studi di Padova (2004) The Palazzo del Bo. Padua
21. Bichat MFX (1800) Recherches physiologiques sur la vie et la mort (General Anatomy Applied to Physiology and Medicine). Brosson, Gabon et Cie, Paris
22. Ackerknecht EH (1967) Medicine at the Paris Hospital 1794–1848. Johns Hopkins University Press, Baltimore
23. Foucault M (1994) The birth of the clinic. An archaeology of medical perception. Vintage, London
24. Bankl H, Bankl HC (1999) Pathologisch-Morphologische Diagnostik. Angewandte pathologische Anatomie für die Praxis. Springer, Berlin
25. Hausner E (2008) Die historische Sammlung des Instituts für Gerichtliche Medizin der Universität Wien. Edition Hausner. Desktop-Publishing, Oliver Hausner, Wein
26. Lesky E (1978) Die Wiener Medizinische Schule im 19. Jahrhundert. Verlag Böhlau, Graz
27. Lesky E (1981) Meilensteine der Wiener Medizin. Große Ärzte Österreichs in drei Jahrhunderten. Wilhelm Maudrich, Wien
28. Prüll CR (ed) (1998) Pathology in the 19th and 20th century. The relationship between theory and practice. European Association for the History of Medicine and Health Publications, Ipswich Book Company, Sheffield
29. Rumpler H, Denk H, Ottner C (2005) Carl Freiherr von Rokitansky 1804–1878. Pathologe, Politiker, Philosoph, Gründer der Wiener Medizinischen Schule des 19. Jahrhunderts. Böhlau Verlag, Wien
30. Geserick G, Vendura K, Wirth E (2005) Das Institut für Rechtsmedizin der Charité in Berlin-Mitte. Ansichten und Einblicke, Berlin
31. Schnalke T, Atzl I (2010) Dem Leben auf der Spur: im Berliner Medizinhistorischen Museum der Charité. Prestel, München
32. Burton JL, Rutty GN (2010) The hospital autopsy. A manual of fundamental autopsy practice, 3rd edn. CRC Press, Taylor & Francis Group, Boca Raton, FL
33. Falk H, Pfeiffer K (1964) Praktische Sektionsdiagnostik mit Schnellmethoden: für Gerichtsmediziner und Pathologen. Edition Leipzig. Thieme, Leipzig
34. Hamperl H (1956) Leichenöffnung. Befund und Diagnose. Eine Einführung in den Pathologisch-Anatomischen Seziersaal und Demonstrationskurs. Springer, Berlin
35. Ludwig J (2002) Handbook of Autopsy Practice, 3rd edn. Humana Press, Totowa, NJ
36. Madea B (2014) Die Ärztliche Leichenschau. Rechtsgrundlagen, Praktische Durchführung, Problemlösungen, 3. Auflage. Springer, Berlin
37. Madea B (ed) (2016) Estimation of the time since death, 3rd edn. Boca Raton, FL, CRC Press, Taylor & Francis
38. Rössle R (1947) Sektionstechnik. 6. Aufl. Springer, Berlin
39. Saternus KS, Madea B (2007) Forensic autopsy–handling of the human corpse. Research in legal medicine, vol 36. Schmidt-Römhild, Lübeck
40. Sheaff MT, Hopster DJ (2005) Post mortem technique handbook, 2nd edn. Springer, London
41. Madea B (ed) (2015) Rechtsmedizin. Befunderhebung, Rekonstruktion, Begutachtung. 3. Auflage. Springer, Berlin
42. Battle RM, Pathak D, Humble CG (1987) Factors influencing discrepancies between premortem and postmortem diagnosis. JAMA 258(3):339–344
43. Goldman L et al (1983) The value of autopsy in three medical areas. N Engl J Med 308(17):1000–1005
44. Goldman L (1984) Diagnostic advances vs. the value of the autopsy 1912–1980. Arch Pathol Lab Med 108:501
45. Madea B, Rothschild M (2010) The post mortem external examination: determination of the cause and manner of death. Dtsch Ärztebl Int 107:575–588
46. Shojania KG, Burton EC, McDonald KM, Goldman L (2002) The autopsy as an outcome and performance measure. University of California at San Francisco (UCSF)-Stanford University Evidence-Based Practice Center, San Francisco
47. Shojania KG, Burton EC, McDonald KM, Goldman L (2002) The autopsy as an outcome and performance measure. Evid Rep Technol Assess (Summ) 58:1–5
48. Shojania KG, Burton EC, McDonald KM, Goldman L (2003) Changes in rates of autopsy-detected diagnostic errors over time. A systematic review. JAMA 289:2849–2856
49. Shojania KG, Burton EC (2008) The vanishing nonforensic autopsy. N Engl J Med 358:873–875
50. Moch H (2011) Dokumentation der diagnostischen Qualität im Krankenhaus. Auswertung der Autopsieberichte. Pathologe 32:282–286
51. Moch H (2013) Autopsie und moderne Medizin. In: Tag B, Mausbach J, Moch H (eds) Autopsie und Religion. Die Sektion aus medizinischer, ethischer und religiöser Sicht. VDG, Weimar
52. Nestler K, Gradistanac T, Wittekind C (2008) Evaluation des klinischen Nutzens der Obduktion. Eine Untersuchung am Institut für Pathologie des Universitätsklinikums Leipzig. Pathologe 29:449–454
53. Schwanda-Burger S, Moch H, Muntwyler J, Salomon F (2012) Diagnostic errors in the new millennium: a follow-up autopsy study. Mod Pathol 25:777–783
54. Brinkmann B et al (2002) Aktuelle Daten zur Obduktionsfrequenz in Deutschland. DMW 127:791–795
55. Groß D, Esser A, Knobloch H, Tag B (2007) Tot und toter Körper. Der Umgang mit dem Tod und der menschlichen Leiche am Beispiel der klinischen Obduktion. Kassel University Press, Kassel
56. Hamperl H (1972) Werdegang und Lebensweg eines Pathologen. Schattauer Verlag, Stuttgart
57. Timmermans S (2006) Postmortem: how medical examiners explain suspicious deaths (fieldwork encounters and discoveries). The University of Chicago Press, Chicago
58. Madea B (2008) Autoptisch bestätigte Behandlungsfehler. Z Evid Fortbild Qual Gesundhwesen (ZEFQ) 102:535–541

59. Madea B (2009) Medico-legal autopsies as a source of information to improve patient safety. Legal Med 11:S76–S79
60. Madea B, Preuß J (2009) Medical malpractice as reflected by the forensic evaluation of 4450 autopsies. Forensic Sci Int 190:58–66
61. Madea B, Musshoff F, Preuss J (2009) Medical negligence in drug associated deaths. Forensic Sci Int 190:67–73
62. Kohn LT, Corrigan JM, Donaldson MS (2000) To err is human. building a safer health system. National Academic Press, Washington, DC
63. Madea B (2012) Histology in forensic practice. Forensic Sci Med Pathol 8:64–65
64. Chevallier C, Doenz F, Vaucher P, Palmiere C, Dominguez A, Binaghi S, Mangin P, Grabherr S (2013) Postmortem computed tomography angiography vs. conventional autopsy: advantages and inconveniences of each method. Int J Legal Med 127:981–989
65. Donchin Y, Rivkind AI, Bar-Ziv J, Hiss J, Almog J, Drescher M (2011) Utility of postmortem computed tomography in trauma victims. J Trauma 37(4):552–556
66. Leth PM, Struckmann H, Lauritsen J (2013) Interobserver agreement of the injury diagnoses obtained by postmortem computed tomography of traffic fatality victims and a comparison with autopsy results. Forensic Sci Int 225:15–19
67. Weustink AC, Hunink MGM, van Dijke CF, Renken NS, Krestin GP, Oosterhuis JW (2009) Minimally invasive autopsy: an alternative to conventional autopsy? Radiology 250(3):897–904
68. Roberts IS, Benamore RE, Benbow EW, Lee SH, Harris JN, Jackson A, Mallett S, Patankar T, Peebles C, Roobottom C, Traill ZC (2012) Postmortem imaging as an alternative to autopsy in the diagnosis of adult deaths: a validation study. Lancet 379:136–142

Medicolegal Aspects of Forensic Radiology

3

Claudio Buccelli, Massimo Niola, and Pierpaolo Di Lorenzo

With increasing frequency emerges the need for the coroner to have support, in carrying out his activity, from the knowledge of colleagues specialized in other disciplines, in the vast panorama of professional figures that modern medicine offers.

Within this interpretation, the radiology has constituted and constitutes an indispensable support in all areas of forensic and insurance medicine.

In particular, the need to deal with the radiologist specialist with such frequency in the activity of the coroner to be defined almost daily, from the conduct of law civil claims (whether in the field of civil liability or private accident), to investigations carried out on the body, on cases of medical responsibility, and in these cases the need to share both competences of the coroner to that of different specialist becomes, to bear in mind, a legal and ethical obligation.

The particular synergy between the radiologist and the medical examiner is rooted in one of the cardinal principles of forensic medicine: the verification of causal link.

In a nutshell, the medical examiner is constantly having to relate a given fact, relevant under legal, insurance, or even administrative profiles, with a given pathology or lesion: this is true both for the forensic expert and for the "damage compensation" expert physician.

In this perspective the figure of the forensic radiologist fits who, more and more frequently, is expected to evaluate various aspects in the framework of the clinical and judicial events faced essentially to achieve the scientific evidence necessary to produce adequate responses the need for a truthful assessment of the facts:

- Precise diagnosis of the existing pathological picture and compatibility of the latter with the damaging event.
- Answer to questions concerning the history of injuries.
- Fair identification of residual after-effects.
- Indication of any worsening evolution.

First of all, therefore, the radiologist specialist, called to perform an ex-novo instrumental survey or to second evaluation of an already previously performed and deficient for medicolegal purposes, will have to exhibit in the most meticulous and accurate as "see" in the images obtained, using clear terms and diagnostic accuracy that can make his analysis even more complete and unambiguous.

It is useful to remember, in fact, how the medical-legal expert often has only a fragmented description of the traumatic event or of

C. Buccelli · M. Niola (✉) · P. Di Lorenzo
Department of Biomedical Advanced Sciences – Legal Section, University of Napoli Federico II, Naples, Italy
e-mail: masniola@unina.it; pierpaolo.dilorenzo@unina.it

G. Lo Re et al. (eds.), *Radiology in Forensic Medicine*,
https://doi.org/10.1007/978-3-319-96737-0_3

the clinical event, having to rely exclusively on the documentation (including diagnostic investigations) inherent to the clinical process and produced by the parties cause. However, these investigations have, by their very nature, an almost insurmountable limit: they have been performed for diagnostic and therapeutic purposes, sometimes in urgency, and certainly not for the purpose of establishing a causal or chronological link with a given traumatic event. An emblematic example is that of costal fractures, which are often described, in clinical records or radiological reports, as "multiple costal fractures" (Fig. 3.1a, b); well, this diction appears to be at least limiting for the coroner because it lacks the seat of the aforementioned lesions, often useful for reconstructing the injurious modality, and because the number and characteristics of the fractures in question are not specified, all parameters useful in the medicolegal evaluation of the case.

Once the injurious picture has been identified, it is of great interest to clarify its pathogenesis or to study its etiology (endogenous or exogenous) in order to express itself on the compatibility of the aforesaid framework with the injured event complained of.

The exact etiology of the lesion, in fact, has constant and fundamental importance in the field of forensics and insurance doctor: the traumatic nature of a lesion is intuitively relevant in criminal cases (e.g.: personal injury), in civil (e.g.: compulsory compensation for damages), in the social insurance field (e.g.: accident at work) and private (e.g.: right of the insured to indemnity). The exclusion of an exogenous pathogenesis and, therefore, the diagnosis of natural pathology solve all these problems in a clearly negative sense.

Therefore the differential diagnosis between pathological or natural modifications, made by the radiologist in the forensic field, is an indispensable part of the mosaic of data that can be used for the medicolegal evaluation.

The chronological evaluation of the identified injurious situation is of similar importance, which is able to assess the temporal compatibility of a certain alteration with a significant legal or insurance fact.

With the various instrumental imaging techniques (CT and MRI in particular), it is possible, in a good percentage of cases, to arrive at a differential diagnosis between an acute lesion, a direct consequence of the traumatic event complained of and an injury, instead, preexisting at the trauma.

A classic example of this evaluation method is the one related to the study of the knee joint, for which, in fact, it is possible to radiologically differentiate an acute meniscus lesion, established

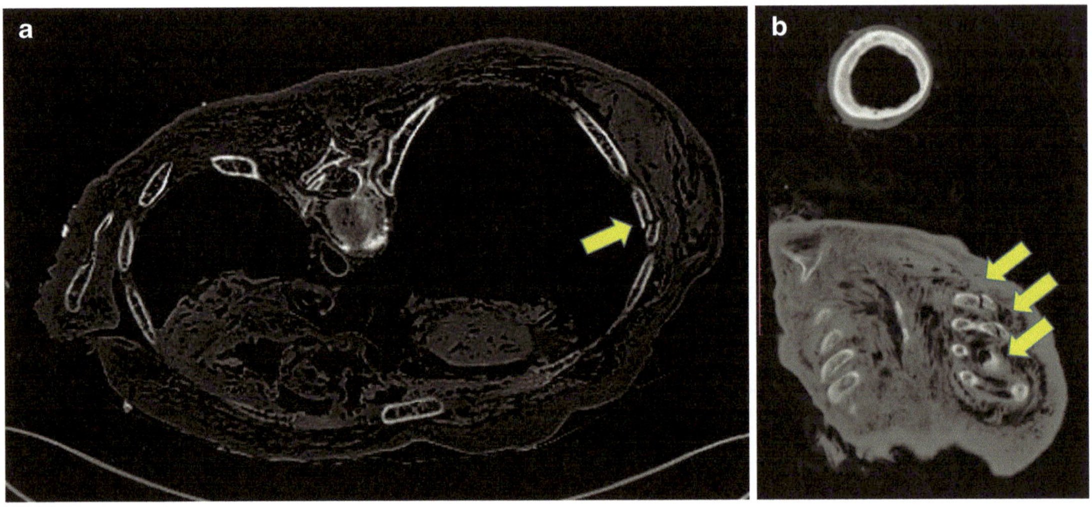

Fig. 3.1 Images of PMCT of a decomposed body, acquired in prone position, show multiple costal fractures in axial (**a**) and coronal MPR (**b**) 128 rows CT images (arrows). Courtesy of Prof. Massimo Midiri, DIBIMED, University of Palermo

on an intact meniscus, with respect to a lesion that has occurred, instead, on a meniscus that had already lost its anatomical integrity, showing degenerative structural alterations. In the first hypothesis, in fact, the lesion has sharp, rather regular contours and the contiguous meniscal tissue presents the regular intensity of the MR signal and the regular density at the CT. In the second hypothesis, however, the lesion appears rather broad, its contours are blurred and irregular with relief of inhomogeneity and hyperintensity to MRI and hypodensity to CT.

What has been said so far, therefore, responds to that inevitable and rigorous verification of the etiological relationship between the traumatic event and the injurious picture requested by the radiologist working in the forensic field. In fact, location, age and mode of production, qualitative (modal) and quantitative detrimental suitability are all aspects of an affair that the coroner addresses in every assessment and the recourse to the opinion of the radiologist specialist, as we have illustrated, becomes indispensable.

Finally, further judgment should be placed in relation to the entity of the after-effects in order to express a real medical-legal prognosis, studying the anatomical picture of the outcomes in such a way as to consider it, depending on the case, an aggravating factor of the functional limitations, detectable with semiotics. The finding, for example, of fracture-welded abutments with off-set, incipient arthrotic manifestations predictably destined to worsen in the consequences of intra-articular fractures or, also, the wound outcomes of cerebral contusive outbreaks provide further elements that, related to the objective clinical data, allow greater definition by reducing the margins of approximation and, consequently, allowing a more punctual medical-legal evaluation.

3.1 Virtual Autopsy and Identification

One of the fields of application in which forensic radiology, in the last decade, is gaining an increasingly important role is certainly that of the coronary medical-legal investigation.One of the first experiences in this field was that of the Institute of Forensic Medicine of the University of Bern that in the mid-90s gave birth to a research project, called Virtopsy Project (a term coined by the words virtual and autopsy), in order to demonstrate the advantages deriving from the use of noninvasive or minimally invasive radiological methods in the forensic field, such as TC MultiSlice, MRI, and contrastographic techniques.

These methods, in fact, offer advantages compared to the classical techniques of image acquisition (ultrasound and Rx) which are burdened by a limit represented by a certain degree of subjectivity, resulting strictly dependent on the operator in discriminating what is relevant from what is not. Computed tomography (CT) and magnetic resonance imaging (MRI), on the other hand, allow the acquisition of the entire body volume in a very short period of time with the possibility of storing the raw data, which can be transmitted remotely or used for post-processing reworking with 3D image reconstruction software. The application of the CT to the postmortem examination allows the forensic doctor a detailed study of the injuries from major traumas (deaths related to road accidents, precipitation), the trajectory of the projectiles and the distance of fire (the latter through identification with micro-TC of gunshot residues at the entrance hole level) in cases of firearm victims and also personal identification in case of mass catastrophic events or discovery of human remains that are not identifiable with other methods of recognition (investigations) such as dactyloscopy, photography, and laboratory. In these areas, in fact, the MultiSlice CT offers the possibility to study minutely complex fracture patterns with dispersion of bone fragments, the presence of hemorrhagic effusions, of gas in the context of tissues or body cavities, as well as of any radiosensitive foreign bodies providing objective data, observer-independent, archived in the perspective of revaluations at a distance of time and space, obtained in a noninvasive way and above all not vitiated by the inevitable reorganization of organs and tissues operated by the sector during the traditional necroscopic examination. However, it must be stressed that the judicial autopsy is not only necessary but also irreplaceable. This, in fact, is essential for the correct study of the macroscopic characteristics of the cadaver and of any organ lesions present, allowing the correct sampling aimed at the histological study of the organs or parts of them. The autopsy investigation, however, does not end exclusively in the external investigation of the corpse, but requires a corollary of investigations (toxicological, genetic) aimed at making the complex process of acquisition of the test as more consistent with the need for technical objectivity—scientific knowledge of forensic sciences. In this context, therefore, the virtual autopsy is inserted: decisive aid in the judicial autoptic investigation, like the other forensic investigations but not substitute of the judicial autopsy. In conclusion, there is no field of forensic medicine in which it is not useful to have recourse to the radiologist specialist whose evaluation, as we have seen, is decisive in deciding many insurance, civil law, and forensic issues in relation to implement the quality of the medical–legal investigation.

Further Reading

Du Chesne A, Benthaus S, Brinkmann B (1999) Manipulated radiographic material—capability and risk for the forensic consultant? Int J Legal Med 112:329–332

Greulich WE, Pyle SI (1966) Radiographic atlas of skeletal development of the hand and wrist. Stanford University Press, Stanford

Kahana T, Goldstein S, Kugel C, Hiss J (2002) Identification of human remains through comparison of computerized tomography and radiographic plates. J Forensic Ident 52:151–158

Kahana T, Hiss J Forensic radiology in forensic pathology reviews, vol 3. Humana Press, Totowa, NJ, pp 443–460

Olivetti L, Fileni A, De Stefano F, Cazzulani A, Battaglia G, Pescarini L (2008) The legal implications of error in radiology. Radiol Med 113:599–608

Richardson ML, Frank MS, Stern EJ (1999) Digital image manipulation: what constitutes acceptable alteration of a radiologic image? Am J Roentgenol 164:228–229

Rutty GN, Morgan B, Robinson C et al (2017) Diagnostic accuracy of post-mortem CT with targeted coronary angiography versus autopsy for coroner-requested post-mortem investigations: a prospective, masked, comparison study. Lancet (London, England) 390(10090):145–154

Smaltino F, Tamburrini O, Buccelli C, De Ferrari F (2000) Radiologia forense. Mediserve, Milano

Stewart TD (1979) Essentials in forensic anthropology. Charles C Thomas, Springfield, IL

Tanner JM, Whitehouse RH, Cameron N, Marshal WA, Healy NJR, Goldshetein H (1991) Assessment of skeletal maturity and prediction of adult height (TW2 Method), 2nd edn. Academic Press, London

Thali MJ, Vock P (2003) Role and techniques in forensic imaging. In: Payne-James J, Busuttil A, Smock W (eds) Forensic medicine: clinical and pathological aspects. Greenwich Medical Media, London, pp 731–746

Thali MJ, Yen K, Vock P et al (2003) Image-guided virtual autopsy findings of gunshot victims performed with multi-slice computed tomography and magnetic resonance imaging and subsequent correlation between radiology and autopsy findings. Forensic Sci Int 138:8–16

4 Imaging Techniques for Forensic Radiology in Living Individuals

Alfonso Reginelli, Anna Russo, Elisa Micheletti, Roberto Picascia, Antonio Pinto, Sabrina Giovine, Salvatore Cappabianca, and Roberto Grassi

The most recognized use of forensic radiology is postmortem study, in particular to define the injury that caused the death [1]; however, nowadays the radiologic technology is considered very useful to provide evidence for legal cases, to improve technology to prevent future deaths, to help the development of new legal theories and practices regarding visual evidence, to severe the difference between acquittal or conviction in a court of law and to distinguish between fraud and assault, and also to investigate accidental or non-accidental injury.

It's very important the quality of the images produced, because they have to be in high quality to be admitted as a credible evidence in court. The images have to be marked and notated to be well interpreted by radiologists and other health or science professionals.

A. Reginelli · A. Russo · E. Micheletti · R. Picascia
S. Cappabianca · R. Grassi (✉)
Department of Internal and Experimental Medicine, University of Campania "Luigi Vanvitelli", Naples, Italy
e-mail: alfonso.reginelli@unicampania.it; salvatore.cappabianca@unicampania.it; roberto.grassi@unicampania.it

A. Pinto
Department of Radiology, Cardarelli Hospital, Naples, Italy

S. Giovine
Department of Radiology, SG Moscati Hospital, Aversa, Italy

There are a lot of areas in which radiology can be used for forensic purpose such as abuse or violence against people, from children to women to elders; aspects concerning illegal practice like using or smuggling drugs and injuries caused by penetrating tools.

4.1 Forensic Radiology in Non-accidental Injuries

The importance of the radiologist consists in recognizing the elements that suggest an abuse and distinguish between violence and pathologic injuries [2]. Non-accidental injuries can be documented as fractures, injury patterns and occult injuries. The people who suffered violence refers either vague medical histories or details unrelated to the abusive injury, making it difficult for the radiologists to understand the causes of the injury and making him suspect a non-accidental one [3].

1. In the case of injured children, fractures are just secondary to cutaneous injuries [4]. For example, rib fractures are very suggestive of abuse and they are more frequently seen in adolescents than in younger children because in those ones bones are more flexible and deform before they break (Figs. 4.1 and 4.2) [2]. However, the radiologists have to consider other metabolic diseases like skeletal

G. Lo Re et al. (eds.), *Radiology in Forensic Medicine*,
https://doi.org/10.1007/978-3-319-96737-0_4

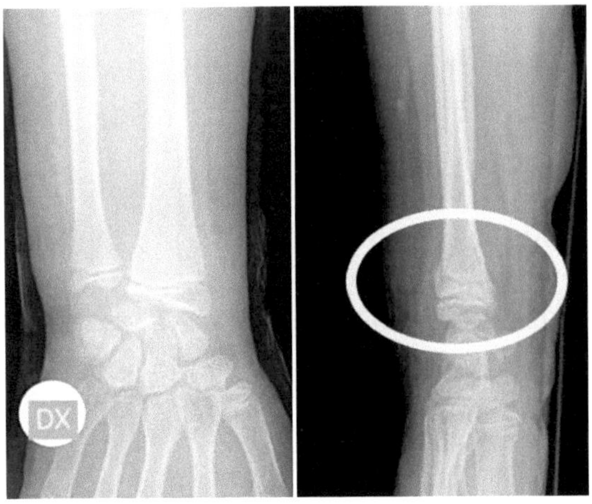

Fig. 4.1 Plain radiograph shows fracture of distal radial epiphysis in child in lateral projection (white circle)

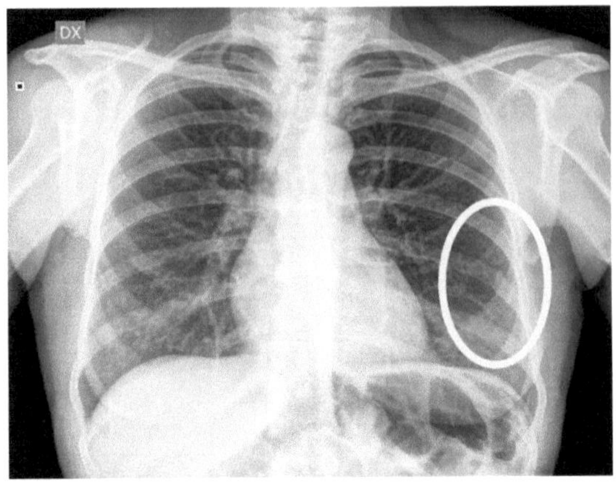

Fig. 4.3 Plain radiograph: outcome of previous left eighth rib fracture (white circle)

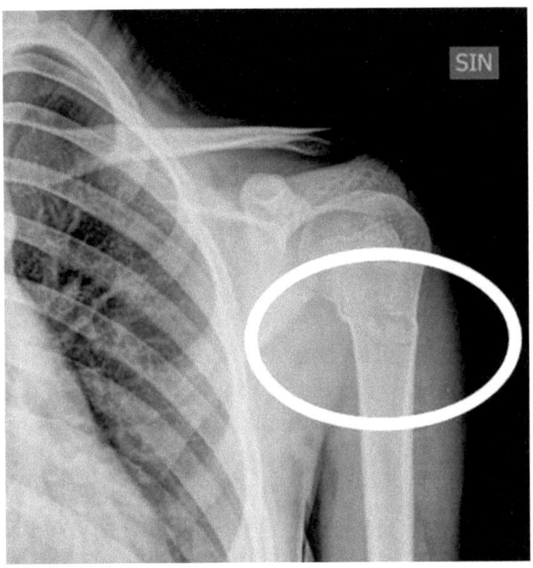

Fig. 4.2 Plain radiograph shows sub-periostal proximal metaphysis fracture in child (black circle)

dysplasia and osteogenesis imperfecta [2]. Differential diagnosis must also be made on the fractures in the other part of the body, because rib fractures are the most frequent, but there can also be metaphyseal lesion of long bones, skull fractures and pelvic fractures (Figs. 4.3 and 4.4). For the abuse cases, which can be repeated in time, the American College of Radiology (ACR) published guidelines for execution of skeletal surveys with a series of radiographic images that encompass the child's entire skeleton or the complete region indicated by symptoms and clinical sign [5]. In most cases radiography alone can detect inflicted osseous injuries [2]. It's important to establish a chronological data of the injuries, estimating the time the fracture occurred and the mechanism of injury [2], to identify a possible assailant and if there already are other healed fractures that can be suggestive of a pattern of abuse [6]. To do that we can use other exams such as skeletal scintigraphy to differentiate the older injuries and to discover subtle fractures that can be difficult to reveal with other techniques [7]. CT scanning is often used both in trauma imaging and as a proof in investigation of children who could have been abused, but introduces a higher radiation dose; even Magnetic Resonance (MR) examinations are useful to replace bone scintigraphy, but some children have trouble to remain still for a longer period of time without sedation [4]. These two type of imaging examinations are used in case of neurological injuries such as head trauma (in the suspect of shaking injuries, impact forces, subdural haematoma or skull fracture), spinal trauma and thoracoabdominal trauma [7]. Albeit CT and MRI may be useful in selected cases, right now they can't replace the radiographic skeletal survey [2].

2. In case of women violence, there is very little amount of medical imaging in literature,

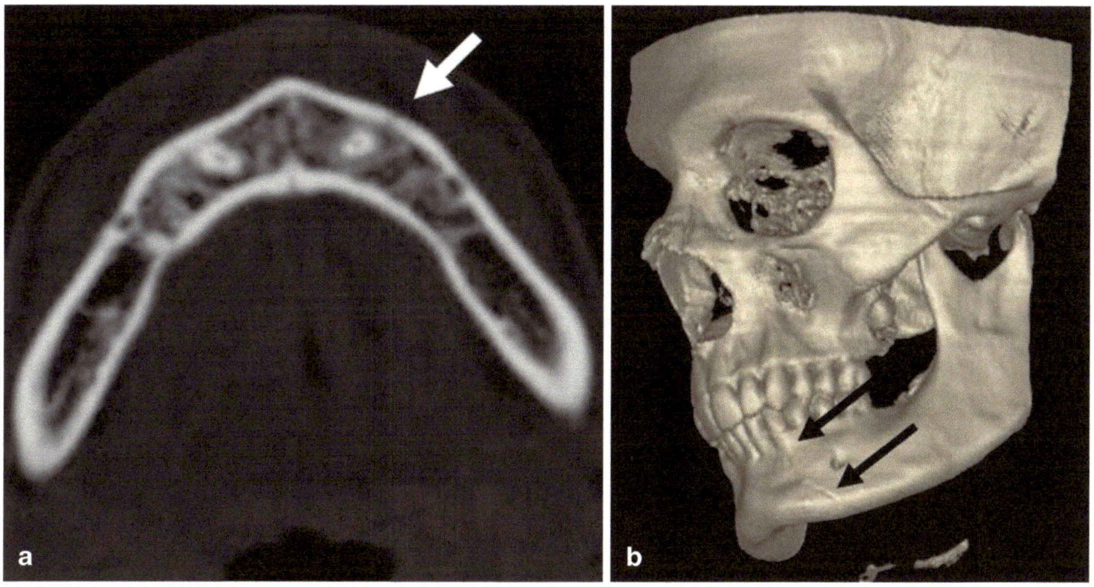

Fig. 4.4 CT axial scan (**a**, white arrow) and 3D reconstruction (**b**, black arrows): fracture of the left mandibular ramus

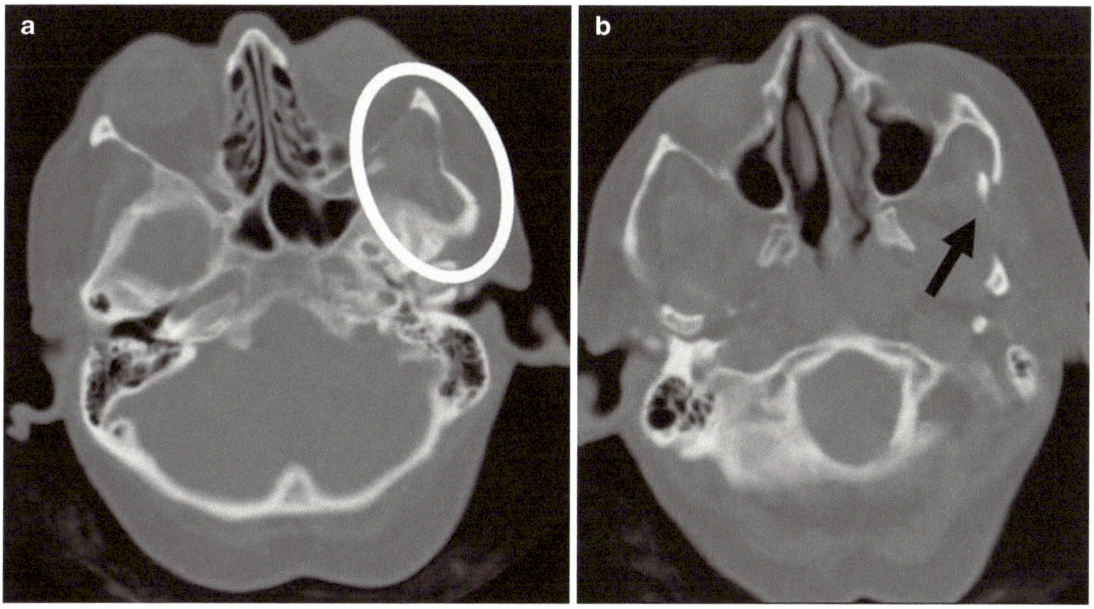

Fig. 4.5 Axial CT scan: multi-fragmentary fracture of the right maxillary bone (**a**, **b**) (white circle and black arrow)

because the signs can be very subtle and there can be few clues about what happened that could help the radiologist to perceive what happened; a signal, for example, could be the presence of older fractures [8]. Radiographic examinations can provide evidence of domestic abuse, even though the incidence of recognized and reported cases is lower than the actual one [9]. It is very important to pay attention to the patient history. The radiographic images are the most useful, and it is important to note the injuries and consider if they match up with what the patient refers (Figs. 4.5 and 4.6) [8]. The most injured sites

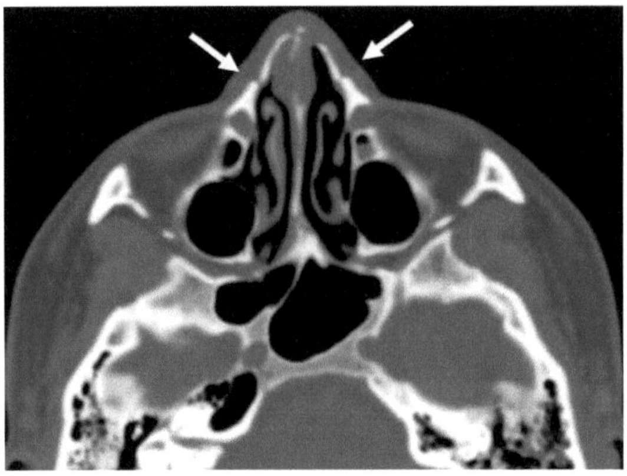

Fig. 4.6 Axial CT scan: nasal bones fracture in women (white arrows)

are head, neck and face and in general consist of fractures; they may be accidental, but the radiologists have to investigate the signals that it could be an abuse. The imaging produced in the hospital can be important evidence and they can be used as legal documentation [9].

3. The elder abuse is very common and under-recognized. There are different kinds of elder abuse like sexual abuse, emotional abuse, neglect and physical abuse, and in general the offenders are the relatives or acquaintances or other people elders trust in. In case of physical abuse, the emergency department represents a critical point to identify non-accidental injuries [10]. They may have physical or radiographic signs that don't match the history provided by the family members or the patient [9]. In this case the radiologists are in an optimal position to raise suspicion for mistreatment; for example, transverse humeral fractures most often require a high-energy mechanism of injury and it could be suspicious if the reported history by the caregivers doesn't match up [10]. The most common injuries are located in the upper extremity, associated with contusions and abrasions, especially at the arms because one of the mechanism could be the grasping of the abuser or the use of restraints, or it could be the result of attempted self-defence by the victim. The injuries of the posterior torso and of the lower extremity, or the ones on dorsal or plantar side of the foot are very suspicious of physical abuse because these areas are not so common for accidental injuries. However right now there isn't a convincing evidence that distinguish accidental from non-accidental injuries, so the radiologists have to take care of risk factors like dementia, depression and social isolation independently from the presence of a caregiver [11].

4.2 Forensic Radiology in Illegal Abuse and in Smuggling of Drugs

1. The use of recreational drugs is a new phenomenon that can be explored because there are pharmacological effects that can be seen by the use of radiological techniques. For the illicit nature of recreational drugs, the first one who can report and suggest the diagnosis is the radiologist. There are some common complications known as consequences of the use of drugs, like perforation of nasal septum induced by the use of cocaine (that provokes vasoconstriction) and sometimes it can simulate Wegener granulomatosis. The aspiration pneumonia isn't rare in users of consciousness-altering drugs and it can be seen like a consolidation in chest radiography or CT, especially involving the apical and posterior segments of the upper lobes and apical segments of the lower lobes. In case of pulmonary oedema the radiologist may help to differentiate if it is cardiogenic or noncardiogenic induced by drugs, thanks to some radiographic tricks, such as absence of pleural effusion and absence of cardiomegaly; in general the noncardiogenic oedema caused by drugs takes the form of bilateral perihilar airspace opacification and the radiographic abnormalities resolve rapidly. Also the pulmonary alveolar haemorrhage resolves rapidly and it is useful the high-resolution CT to distinguish it from pulmonary oedema. Other than pulmonary complications there are neurological complications such as intracranial haemorrhage, ischaemic stroke and diffuse

cerebral oedema. There can be other complications like infections, musculoskeletal complications, renal disorders and gastrointestinal disorders. However many of the imaging features aren't specific and in the patient history information about drug abuse may have been omitted. For this reason some pathologic conditions may remain unexplained if there isn't the suspicious for the abuse of drugs [12].

2. Body packing is the insertion or ingestion of packed illicit substances in the human body. The materials used to create the packet are condoms, latex gloves and balloons. The smuggled drugs can be found inside human body, most frequently inside the gastrointestinal tract, the vagina and the ears. The most used radiologic techniques to identify the packing are radiography and CT; even US and MRI can be used, but they don't play a great role. The radiologist has a very important medico-legal role because other than identifying the packages, he also has to provide accurate information about their quantity and localization. If these packages break, there could be pathologic issues [13]. One of the used techniques is to swallow illicit drugs, packaged. After that, constipating agents are ingested to allow several hours of waiting before the faecal expulsion. On arrival at the destination laxatives are used to get rid of their packets (Fig. 4.7) [14, 15]. The packages ingested usually are between 1 and 25, and the rupture problem usually depends on the wrapping manner and the material used. If it occurs, this

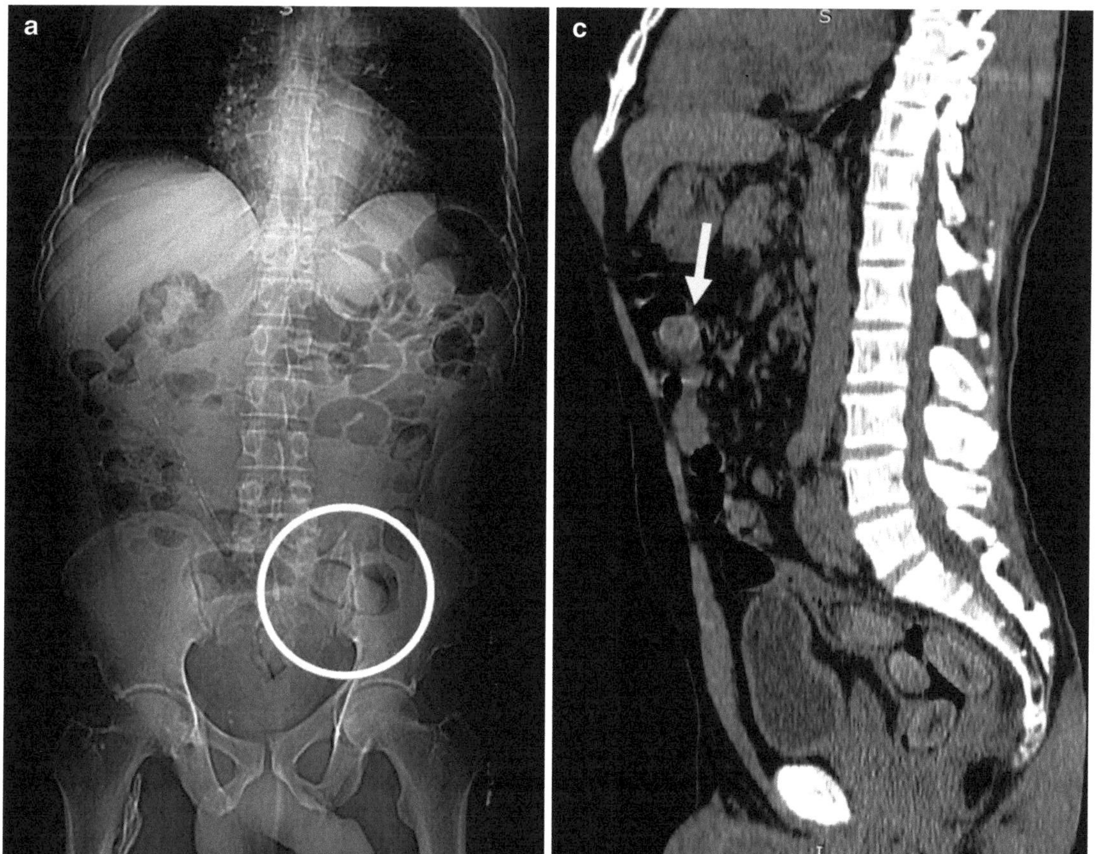

Fig. 4.7 On plain abdominal radiographs show a smooth and uniformly shaped oblong structure (**a**); on CT examination show with more detail of plain abdominal film, the ingested packets as round or oval dense foreign bodies located within the different side of gastrointestinal tract (**b**, **c**)

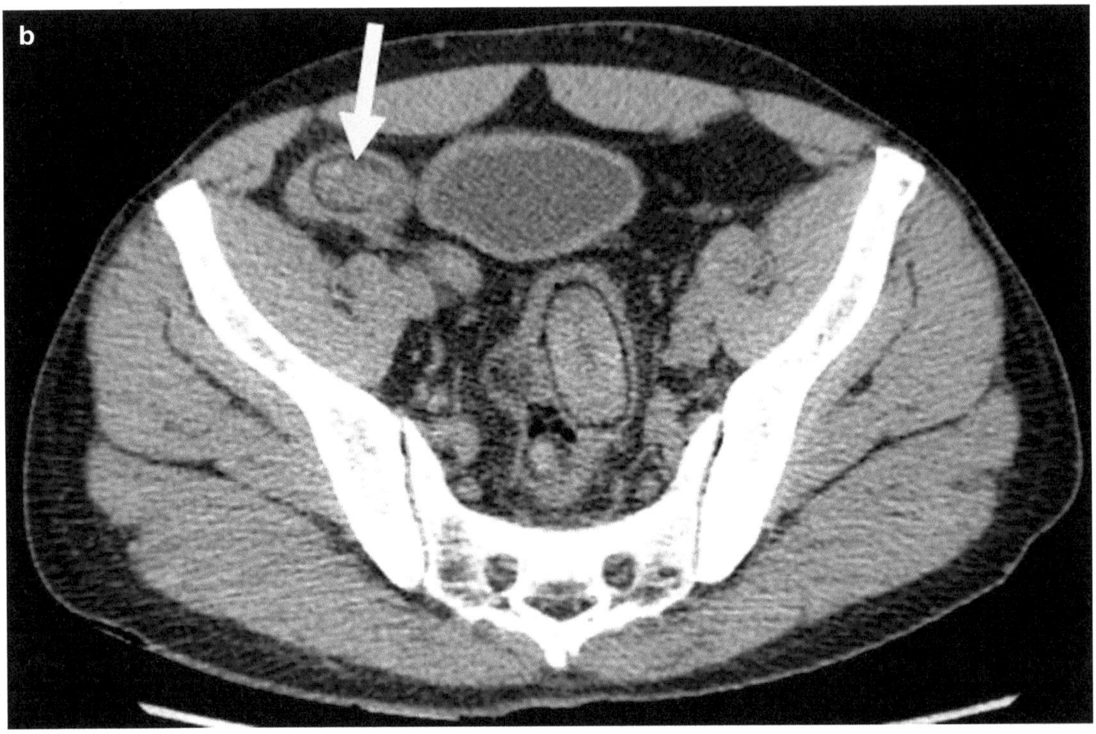

Fig. 4.7 (continued)

situation cold also bring to death [16]. The clinical manifestations are acute drug toxicity and intestinal obstruction; together they are described as "body packer syndrome" [17]. Imaging is essential to identify and diagnose body packing. Reginelli A. and Russo A. (and others) have described their "body pack" valuation protocol in asymptomatic patients. They use at first instance plain abdominal radiography, in case of unclear results, then an abdominal CT can be performed [13]. In abdominal radiography imaging it can be seen as a radio-dense strange body, defined as "tic-tac sign", "dense wrapping material", or "parallelism sign" [18]. Another sign is the "rosette-like appearance" that is formed by air trapped in the knot where a condom is tied [19]. The CT show the packages like a strange body or bodies, ovals or round. If there is insufficient air-rim around the packets and a high density with regular bowel contents are suggestive of ruptured packets [13]. In US the packages appear like hyperechogenic structures with posterior acoustic shadowing, but the problem is the failure to identify the exact number of packages [20]. The MRI is rarely used because of the lack of protons into packages and it has motion artefacts caused by the bowel loops. The best way to reveal foreign body like package is MDTC [13].

4.3 Forensic Radiology in Trauma Caused by Penetrating Tools

Within the severe civilian traumas there are the penetrating wounds that can be divided in two classes: sharp penetrating trauma like wounds caused by knife and gunshot wounds or ballistic traumas (Figs. 4.8 and 4.9) [21].

1. When a patient arrives with a knife wound it may be difficult to discover the wound track,

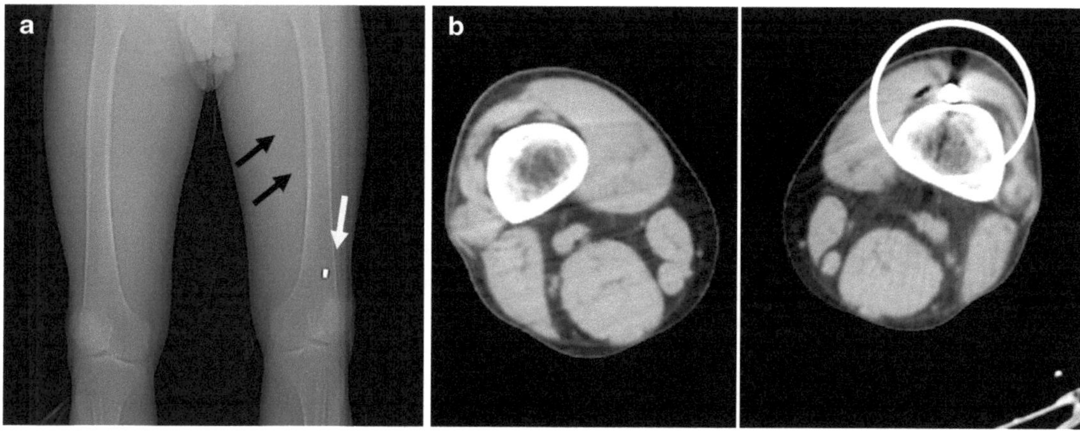

Fig. 4.8 (**a**) Scout CT view show bullet in the upper left side of the knee; (**b**) axial view of CT scan shows the bullet to be lodged deeply in the muscle to the left knee

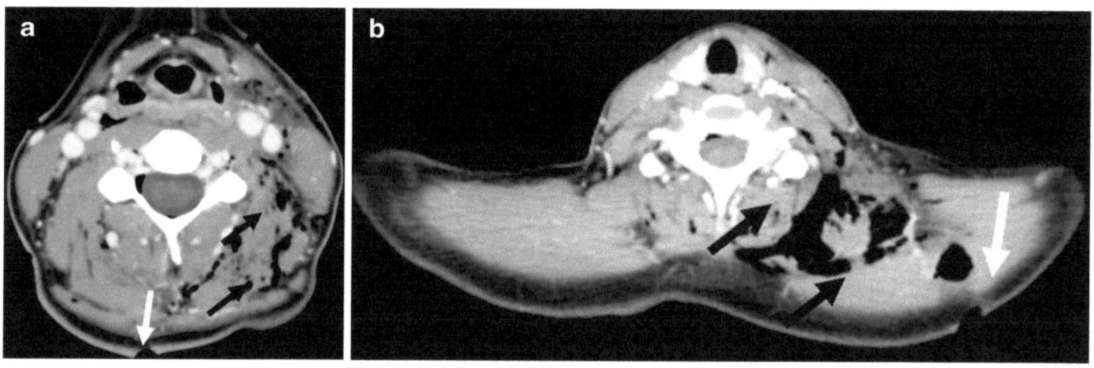

Fig. 4.9 (**a**) Axial CT scan; arrows are pointing at air and haematoma at the wound site (white arrow), delineating the wound track (black arrows). (**b**) Same patient. Axial section of CT scan inferior; arrows are pointing at muscle haematoma of the thoracic wall muscles, delineating the wound track

but it's very important to understand its extension and its relationship with the surrounding organs. MDTC is the first choice in these cases [22]. Blade head injury can be classified as non-penetrating, penetrating and perforating [23]. The last one is relatively rare thanks to efficient defence wall like the skullcap; however when a patient arrives into the emergency room with this kind of injury, the radiologist has to do an evaluation locating the whole intracranial section of the sharp tool, searching the relation with vital areas of the nervous system, such as cranial arteries and veins [24]. In case of calvarium trauma, the first thing to do is to a plain film to recognize bone lesions and if there is a foreign body. In case of penetrating head injury the primary imaging option is the MDCT, even though there could be artefacts due to the metallic foreign bodies [21]. Radiologists should identify the entry wounds, if there is fragmented and non-fragmented bone lesions, pneumoencephalus and intracerebral or intraventricular bleeding [22]. If there is no presence of metallic foreign bodies, it could be possible to use the MRI to observe secondary brain injuries like traumatic cerebral oedema, hydrocephalus, post-traumatic ischaemic stroke and so on [21]. The most frequent sharp penetrating injuries to the chest are pneumo-, haemo- or haemopneumothoraces [22]. The complications tend to appear with delay and even after

5 days after a negative first radiography, so it is important to do a proper follow-up and observation [24]. At first chest plain films are done to diagnose simple rib fractures, also considering its complications like pneumothorax, haemothorax and parenchymal contusions and/or laceration [22]. MDTC is superior in sensitivity to detect a pneumothorax [25]. Even the heart or the intra pericardial aorta and pulmonary vessels can be involved in the sharp penetrating thoracic trauma [21]. MDTC is very important in the detection of haemopericardium exposing wound paths, pericardial abnormalities and pneumopericardium [26]. It is also used for aortic damage, lesion to the airways and the oesophagus; moreover for diaphragmatics lesions, sagittal and coronal CT reconstructions can be useful. Penetrating bowel lesions can be seen on CT with signs of peritoneal damage, free intraperitoneal fluid and air [22]. In general with radiologic techniques is possible to understand the mechanical force, the shape of the weapon and the force used and the nature of the tissue injured and more important if the wound is self-inflicted or not [22].

2. In case of gunshot wounds, the most important thing is to understand if the patient is haemodynamically stable. In case of stability the doctors have to understand where is the entry and the exit wound, what kind of structure can be damaged and the trajectory. The placement and the path of projectile is important, and it can depend on the type of bullet, its velocity and mass and the physical characteristics of the penetrated tissue [27]. The head and the torso are the most vulnerable areas [28]. Normally in haemodynamically stable patients an X-ray is performed and if there is the presence of signs and symptoms of vascular damage at clinical examination a CT too. It is also used to evaluate the retroperitoneum and with IV contrast it can correctly identify hepatic, spleen, urogenital lesions, haematomas, intra-abdominal vessel injuries. CT findings can include wound track outlined by haemorrhage, bullet, free air or bone fragments that can be found into the peritoneal cavity and intraperitoneal organ injury. Contrast studies can be useful in case of damage of the oesophagus, a massive air leak indicates a major bronchial injury. Diaphragm rupture is unusual but in case of it, it's accompanied with injuries of other organs. The rupture is diagnosed by chest X-ray, CT and ultrasound [27]. Injuries to the liver and spleen are frequent and the diagnostic methods used are Ct scan, MRI, gastrointestinal contrast studies and US [29]. Moreover, in case of abdominal content herniated through the diaphragm, there is a particular sign called the "CT collar sign" [30–33]. When the injury is on the extremities the conventional radiography is useful to identify missile and ballistic fragments and the CT provides the spatial, contrast and temporal resolution required to determine the most likely trajectory and the anatomical structure at risk [27].

4.4 Conclusions

The evidence produced by radiologic techniques can be used as scientific basis for forensic investigation [6]. However it is very important to establish a defined imaging protocol to perform radiologic images forensically useful, like in the case of assault, attempted murder or abuse. Furthermore, instructing the personnel both on the legal implications (of the image product) and on the most appropriate procedure to follow is needed; and having the awareness and the suspicion that certain situations, which presented like accidental, could be not accidental, is also key. Moreover radiologists have to keep in mind that every image can have a forensic and legal implications.

References

1. Brogdon BG (1998) Scope of forensic radiology. In: Brogdon BG (ed) Forensic radiology. CRC Press LLC, Boca Raton, FL, pp 35–54
2. Offiah A, van Rijin RR, Perez-Rossello JM, Kleinman PK (2009) Skeletal imaging of child abuse. Pediatric Radiol 39(5):461–470
3. Hobbs CJ, Bilo RA (2009) Nonaccidental trauma: clinical aspects and epidemiology of child abuse. Pediatr Radiol 39(5):457–460

4. van Rijin RR (2009) How should we image skeletal injuries in child abuse? Pediatr Radiol 39(suppl 2):S226–S229
5. American College of Radiology Practice guideline for skeletal surveys in children. Revised 2006. www.acr.org/SecondaryMainMenuCategories/quality_safety/guidelines/dx/musc/skeletal_surveys.aspx. Accessed 16 Nov 2009
6. Kudlad M, Odle T, Kisner L (2010) The state of forensic radiography in the United States. American Society of Radiologic Technologists, Albuquerque, NM
7. Di Pietro MA et al (2009) Diagnostic imaging of child abuse. Pediatrics 123(5):1430–1435
8. American College of Radiology (2014) Putting together the pieces: radiologists sometimes hold the key to diagnosing inter-partner violence, but are they watching for the signs? https://acrbulletin.org/topics/quality-safety/157-putting-together-the-pieces
9. Lee NG (2001) Forensic in emergency care. In: Lee NG (ed) Legal concepts and issues in emergency care. WB Saunders Company, Philadelphia, PA, pp 102–115
10. Wong NZ, Rosen T, Sanchez AM, Bloemen EM, Mennit KW, Hentel K, Nicola R, Murphy KJ, LoFaso VM, Flomenbaum NE, Lachs MS (2017) Imaging findings in elder abuse: a role for radiologists in detection. Can Assoc Radiol J 68:16–20
11. Murphy K, Waa S, Jaffer H, Sauter A, Chan A (2013) A literature review of findings in physical elder abuse. Can Assoc Radiol J 64:10–14
12. Hagan IG, Burney K (2007) Radiology of recreational drug abuse. Radiographics 27(4):919–940
13. Reginelli A, Russo A, Urraro F, Maresca D, Martiniello C, D'Andrea A, Brunese L, Pinto A (2015) Imaging of body packing: errors and medicolegal issues. Abdom Imaging 40:2127–2142
14. Khan FY (2005) The cocaine "body-packer" syndrome: diagnosis and treatment. Indian J Med Sci 59(10):457–458
15. Wetly CV, Mittleman RE (1981) The "body packer syndrome"-toxicity following ingestion of illecit drugs packaged for transposition. J Forensic Sci 26(3):492–500
16. Arena JM (1979) Positioning: toxicology, symptoms, treatment, 4th edn. Charles C Thomas, Springfield, IL
17. Kulkarni VM, Gandhi JA, Gupta RA et al (2012) Body packer syndrome. J Postgrad Med 69:225–226
18. Sica G, Guida F, Bocchini G et al (2015) Imaging of drug smuggling by body packing. Semin Ultrasound CT MR 36(1):39–47. https://doi.org/10.1053/j.sult.2014.10.003
19. Marc B, Baud FJ, Aelion MJ et al (1990) The cocaine body-packer syndrome: evaluation of a method of contrast study of the bowel. J Forensic Sci 35(2):345–355
20. Wackerle B, Rupp N, Clarmann M et al (1986) Demonstration of narcotic packages in "body packers" by various imaging methods. In vitro and in vivo investigations. Fortschr Roentgenstr 145:274–277
21. de Vries CS, Africa M, Gebremariam FA, van Rensburg JJ, Otto SF, Potgieter HF (2010) The imaging of stab injuries. Acta Radiol 51:92–106
22. Reginelli A, Pinto A, Russo A, Fontanella G, Rossi C, Del Prete A, Zappia M, D'Andrea A, Guglielmi G, Brunese L (2015) Sharp penetrating wounds: spectrum of imaging findings and legal aspects in the emergency settings. Radiol Med 120:856–865
23. Hijiaz TA, Cento EA, Walker MT (2011) Imaging of head trauma. Radiol Clin N Am 49:81–103
24. Schatz DV, de la Pedraja J, Erbella J, Hameed M, Vail SJ (2000) Efficacy of follow-up evaluation in penetrating thoracic injuries. J Emerg Med 20:281–284
25. Trupka A, Waydhas C, Hallfeldt KK, Nast-Kolb D, Pfeifer KJ, Schweiberer L (1997) Value of computed thoracic tomography in the first assessment of severely injured patient with blunt chest trauma: results of a prospective study. J Trauma 29:502–509
26. Demetiades D, van der Veen BW (1983) Penetrating injuries to the heart: experience over two years in South Africa. J Trauma 23:1034–1041
27. Reginelli A, Russo A, Maresca D, Mertiniello C, Cappabianca S, Brunese L (2014) Imaging assessment of gunshot wounds. Semin Ultrasound CT MRI 36:57–67
28. Maiden N (2009) Ballistic review. Mechanism of bullet wound trauma. Forensic Sci Med Pathol 5(3):204–209
29. Nchimi J, Szapiro D, Ghaye B et al (2005) Helical CT of blunt diaphragm rupture. Am J Roentgenol 184:24–30
30. Navarro J, Cuesta J, Alaron J et al (2008) Traumatic rupture of the diaphragm. Arch Bronconeumol 44:197–203
31. Cirillo M, Caranci F, Tortora F, Corvino F, Pezzullo F, Conforti R, Cirillo S (2012) Structural neuroimaging in dementia. J Alzheimers Dis 29(suppl 1):16–19. https://doi.org/10.3233/JAD-2012-129000
32. Caranci F, Tedeschi E, Leone G, Reginelli A, Gatta G, Pinto A, Squillaci E, Briganti F, Brunese L (2015) Errors in neuroradiology. Radiol Med 120(9):795–801. https://doi.org/10.1007/s11547-015-0564-7
33. Muccio CF, Di Blasi A, Esposito G, Brunese L, D'Arco F, Caranci F (2013) Perfusion and spectroscopy magnetic resonance imaging in a case of lymphocytic vasculitis mimicking brain tumor. Pol J Radiol 78(3):66–69. https://doi.org/10.12659/PJR.884011

Imaging Techniques for Postmortem Forensic Radiology

5

Gaia Cartocci, Alessandro Santurro, Paola Frati, Giuseppe Guglielmi, Raffaele La Russa, and Vittorio Fineschi

5.1 Introduction

Imaging techniques are powerful tools in forensic sciences, and their importance is widely recognized. In recent years, modern imaging techniques, especially cross-sectional imaging, have become increasingly common and routinely applicable in forensic practice.

Forensic pathology aims to identify cause of death and trace evidence, pinpoint factors contributing to causes of accidents and provide information for relatives of the deceased on hereditary diseases. Postmortem forensic radiology, consequently, aims to acquisition, interpretation, and reporting of radiologic images for the purpose of forensic investigations, in the living as well as the deceased. In this context, the use of radiological imaging in the postmortem, in particular, is becoming increasingly widespread.

In late 1990s, a variety of alternative noninvasive procedures were proposed as substitute for conventional autopsy. Virtopsy project, promoted by the Institutes of Forensic Medicine, Diagnostic Radiology and Neuroradiology at the University of Bern, Switzerland, started off with the aim to apply cross-sectional imaging techniques to forensic sciences. The concept of "virtopsy" (crasis of the terms "virtual" and "autopsy"), and the project so named, was born to overcome the obstacles posed by relatives of deceased and to provide objective and indestructible documentation of postmortem evidence. In this way, correlating postmortem whole-body imaging findings obtained by CT and MRI, with findings obtained at traditional autopsy, it could be possible to assess these imaging techniques as complementary or even as alternative to postmortem examination.

Since this first step, significant amount of progress on postmortem imaging was made by working-groups around the world. The concept of using CT and MRI technology to obtain autopsy information has slowly gained popularity. Virtopsy utility has been well shown over the years with many other studies and became very useful in forensic practice routine, so postmortem radiology is going to become a distinct subspecialty of forensic medicine and radiology.

G. Cartocci (✉) · A. Santurro · P. Frati · R. La Russa
V. Fineschi
Department of Anatomical, Histological, Forensic and Orthopaedic Sciences, Sapienza University of Rome, Rome, Italy
e-mail: gaia.cartocci@uniroma1.it; alessandro.santurro@uniroma1.it; paola.frati@uniroma1.it; raffaele.larussa@uniroma1.it; vittorio.fineschi@uniroma1.it

G. Guglielmi
Department of Radiology, University of Foggia, Foggia, Italy
e-mail: giuseppe.guglielmi@unifg.it

G. Lo Re et al. (eds.), *Radiology in Forensic Medicine*,
https://doi.org/10.1007/978-3-319-96737-0_5

5.2 Forensic Radiology and Postmortem Imaging

Forensic radiology and postmortem imaging have gained increasing importance in the field of forensic sciences. Although the term forensic radiology seems quite new, first postmortem X-ray images were obtained soon after the discovery of X-rays in 1895 by Röntgen. Since then, the field of forensic radiology has undergone rapid expansion. Following conventional radiology, computed tomography (CT) was introduced to forensic sciences in 1977 by Wullenweber, with the aim to describe radiographic patterns of gunshot injuries to the head. In 1990, Ros introduced pre-autopsy postmortem magnetic resonance (MRI) imaging. So, besides conventional radiology, also cross-sectional imaging has been introduced in forensic radiologist's armamentarium. The development of such discipline has been so tumultuous, and its ramification have gained such importance, that as a result, today postmortem whole-body imaging prior to autopsy is a standard practice in many institutes across the world.

5.3 Conventional Radiology

Conventional radiology (CR) is the oldest technique of forensic imaging and examination with X-ray is the most established imaging assessment tool. CR is very rapid and cost-efficient, easy to perform but offers limited results. The permanent nature of X-ray plates makes them available for reevaluation and reinterpretation as additional evidence regarding the case investigated. Although there have been many technological advancements in imaging, CR has remained widely used in forensic pathology for decades. Actually, notwithstanding, the conventional X-ray has almost been eclipsed by CT and MRI in modern imaging.

CR still remains the most common modality used in the forensic setting and the gold standard method for many forensic challenges.

X-rays are commonly used for visualization and localization of foreign bodies, and for body identification and identities confirmation (Fig. 5.1).

5.3.1 Foreign Bodies

Conventional radiology is useful in localizing radiopaque foreign bodies, i.e., medical implants or swallowed and aspirated objects. CR, trough abdominal radiography, often helps identify drugs smuggled by body packing (i.e., condom, balloon, rubber, or latex packet) filled with illicit drugs inserted into the body, usually via the rectum. Foreign bodies in the vagina, rectum, bladder, or other tissues can also indicate sexual abuse, autoeroticism, or psychosis.

Conventional radiology is also a useful tool for gunshot wounds, because it can localize bullets, expose their number, and delineate if bullets of different caliber are present. CR is useful also in determining whether metallic fragments of a bullet's jacket are present within the body for a ballistic identification.

5.3.2 Deceased and Human Remains Identification

In forensic anthropology and odontology, positive identification of unknown human remains is obtained by comparison of antemortem and postmortem radiographs. In particular, personal identification of human remains is achieved when specific features detected on the cadaver match data recorded during the life, such as signs of medical intervention, normal anatomical variation, and healed trauma. Otherwise, dental identification is the most useful and powerful tool. Most often, these identification techniques CR-based are applied in out-of-ordinary casework, as well as in mass disaster situations.

A comprehensive overview of the fields of application, advantages, and disadvantages of conventional radiology is reported in Table 5.1.

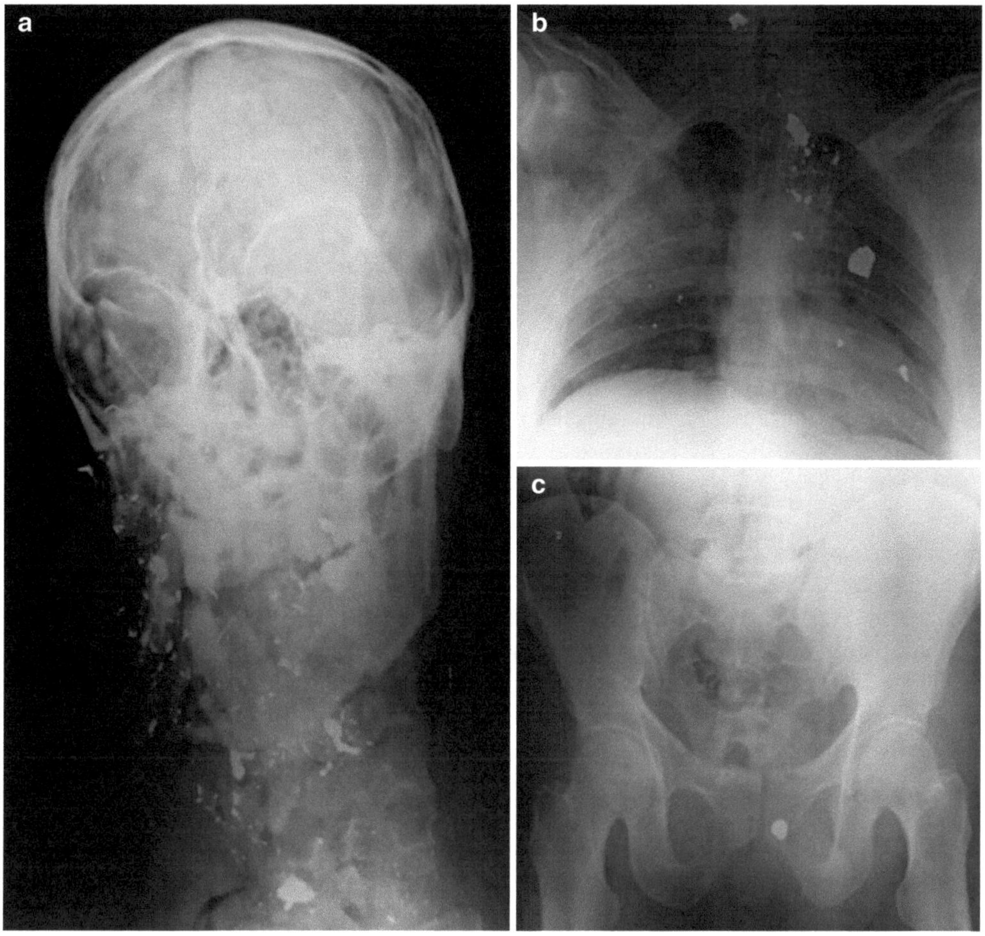

Fig. 5.1 Localization metallic foreign bodies with conventional X-Rays on craniocervical region (**a**), thorax (**b**), and hip region (**c**)

Table 5.1 Applications, advantages, and disadvantages of conventional radiology

Conventional radiology		
Fields of application	Advantages	Disadvantages
Visualization and localization of foreign bodies (i.e., medical implants, swallowed and aspirated objects, body packing, bullets) Body identification and identities confirmation for deceased and human remains	Rapidity Cost-efficiency Easiness to perform Availability for reevaluation and reinterpretation in the time	Radiation No 3D reconstructions Limited visualization of soft tissue Quality dependent on acquisition

5.4 Virtopsy

Due to the rapid development of radiological techniques, cross-sectional imaging methods have been introduced in forensic sciences besides conventional radiology. In general, the different techniques can be divided into basic methods (CT and MRI) and complementary methods (imaging-guided biopsies and postmortem angiography).

Pre-autopsy CT and MRI gained a central role in forensic case assessment over the last decade. Both CT and MRI, in fact, are primarily used to document injury or pathological findings.

These approaches can noninvasively amply contribute to support forensic medicine both for diagnostic reasons and documentation of findings. One of the further potential advantages, in fact, is the possibility to store the imaging data and to facilitate second opinions.

5.4.1 Computed Tomography

Computed tomography is the most frequent imaging tool in forensic pathology besides X-ray. At the present time, postmortem imaging is for the most part accomplished by postmortem CT (PMCT), which has become the most widespread technique in forensic imaging.

PMCT is an excellent complement to autopsy because it's a really rapid technique, easy to use, and compatible with metallic fragments. The costs and availability of CT scanners and personnel are the most important limitation in using cross-sectional imaging in addition to autopsy. In the best-case scenario the Forensic Medicine Departments should have their own CT scanners, in order to screen bodies prior to autopsy; as an alternative to an on-site scanner, forensic facilities may choose to collaborate with local radiology practices or hospitals in order to obtain CT studies on specific cases.

Furthermore, PMCT is advantageous because it is noninvasive and can substitute conventional autopsy in some particular cases, i.e., for communities where autopsy isn't widely accepted for religious or social reasons, like Buddhists, Muslims, or Orthodox Jews.

PMCT is also useful for demonstration at judges, police officers, and other subjects operating in the field of legal medicine. In fact, clear, accessible and understandable presentation of the findings is essential, and clean-bloodless images obtained by CT, also with 3D post-processing reconstruction, are better tolerated than a photography.

High resolution, rapid execution, and easy handling, besides possibility to detect any foreign material (i.e., projectiles, prosthesis and surgical material), make PMCT an excellent screening tool before the conventional autopsy. These characteristics also renders PMCT, besides CR, applicable to the investigation of victims of mass catastrophes, since it allows a rapid inspection of lesions and detection of specific elements, such as medical implants, that may aid the identification of the victim. Additionally, by investigating the virtual skeleton, it is possible to estimate age and gender. PMCT is the most suitable and permits rapid detection even in putrefied, carbonized, or otherwise highly damaged bodies, sustaining the pathologist in his activity.

Another important information given by PMCT concerns the infection surveillance, such as pulmonary tuberculosis confirmed by CT scan before autopsy.

The main weakness of the method is the low capacity for organ visualization and thus a limited sensitivity for the detection of organ findings. PMCT, moreover, can depict calcifications of the coronary arteries, but as no blood flow is evident, so that possible stenoses or occlusions cannot be assessed. PMCT, in fact, is suitable for examining cases of traumatic death, but is only of relatively small help in investigating cases of natural death.

Definitively, PMCT allows the study of body parts or areas that are not routinely dissected during a standard autopsy, such as the viscerocranium, shoulder girdle, extremities, outer pelvis, craniocervical junction, larynx, and soft tissue of the back. Moreover, PMCT allows an easy view of presence of gas and fluid accumulations, such as blood, and is especially useful in examining the skeletal system, for the presence of fractures (even very small ones) in poorly accessible skeletal parts.

In view of the above, indications of PMCT are especially focused on cases of unnatural deaths: traumatic events such as bone fractures and nonaccidental injury in children; gunshot injuries (Figs. 5.2 and 5.3); hanging (Fig. 5.4), strangulation, and drowning cases (Fig. 5.5); and putrefied (Fig. 5.6), carbonized, and badly damaged bodies.

5.4.1.1 Bone Fractures

PMCT is the method of choice for investigating cases of traumatic death, providing a great deal of

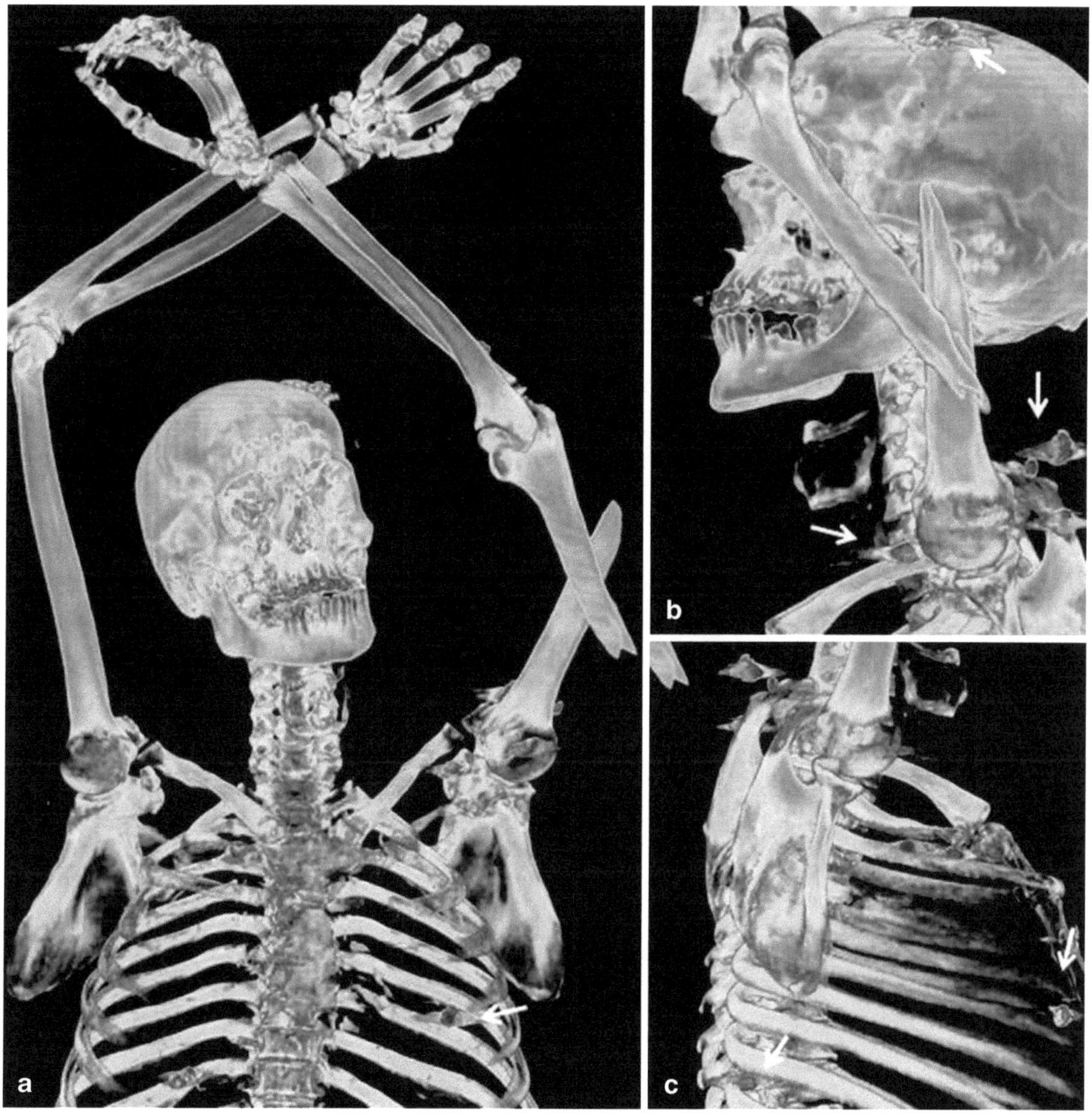

Fig. 5.2 Specific VR reconstructions are helpful in recognizing foreign bodies that have metallic densities. In this case we can point out in a different color (violet) multiple bullets from a gunshot (white arrow) and a denture with 3D reconstruction in anterior view (**a**) and lateral view on both side (**b, c**)

information concerning the biomechanical origins of fractures, thereby contributing to the forensic reconstruction of a case. PMCT allows high resolution 3D multiplanar scans of bodies and offers excellent contrast resolution, particularly for bone structure. Although soft tissues can also be seen and assessed with CT, the main strength of this technique lies in the detection and depiction of fractures, because the sensitivity for osseous findings is higher than in conventional autopsy.

The location and type of fracture, considered with reference to the age and expected level of activity of the individual, may be highly suggestive of whether the injury is accidental or inflicted. The configuration and direction of fractures in the skull may locate the impact point and direction of impact, indicate the sequence of

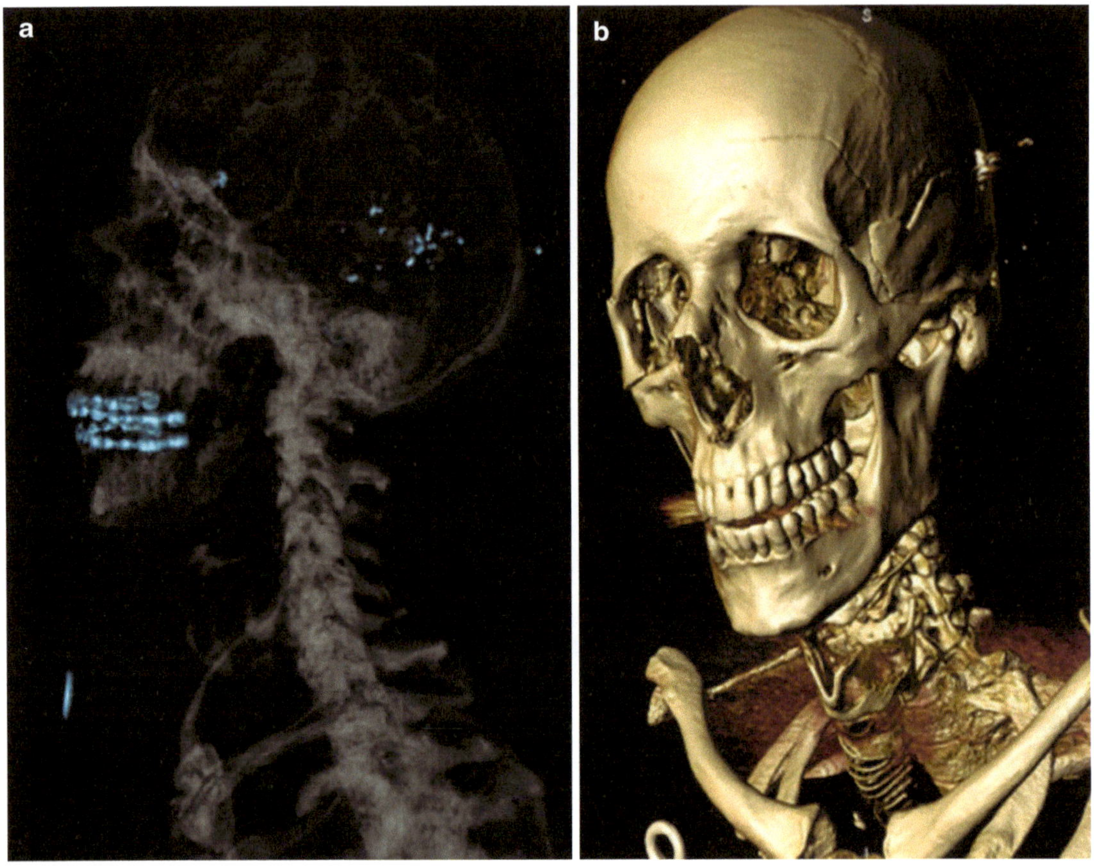

Fig. 5.3 3D reconstruction shows metallic fragments of bullets from a gunshot injury inside (**a**) and outside the cranial bones (**b**)

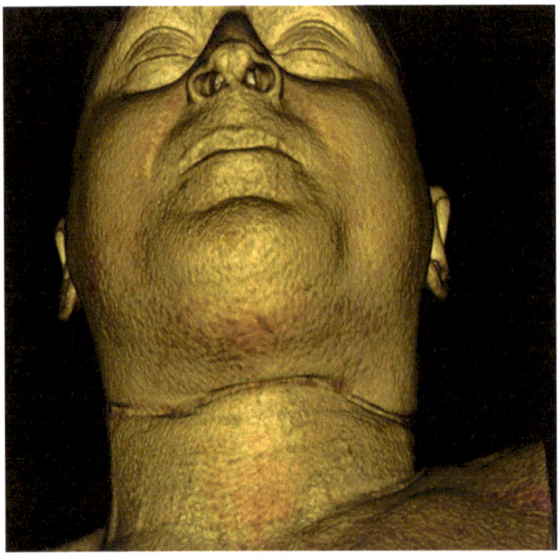

Fig. 5.4 3D reconstruction of a hanging man

repetitive blows and, sometimes, the shape of the wounding object or weapon.

5.4.1.2 Child Abuse

Identification of old or multiple fractures trough PMCT, particularly in cases of suspected nonaccidental injury (NAI) in pediatric population, has also a great relevance. Characteristic nonaccidental injuries include multiple posterior rib fractures, long bone metaphyseal fractures, vertebral body compression fractures, small bowel hematomas, and shearing-type brain injuries.

5.4.1.3 Gunshot Wounds

PMCT can be used in investigating gunshot victims. It is a useful tool for gunshot wounds because it reveals the beveling of bones from a

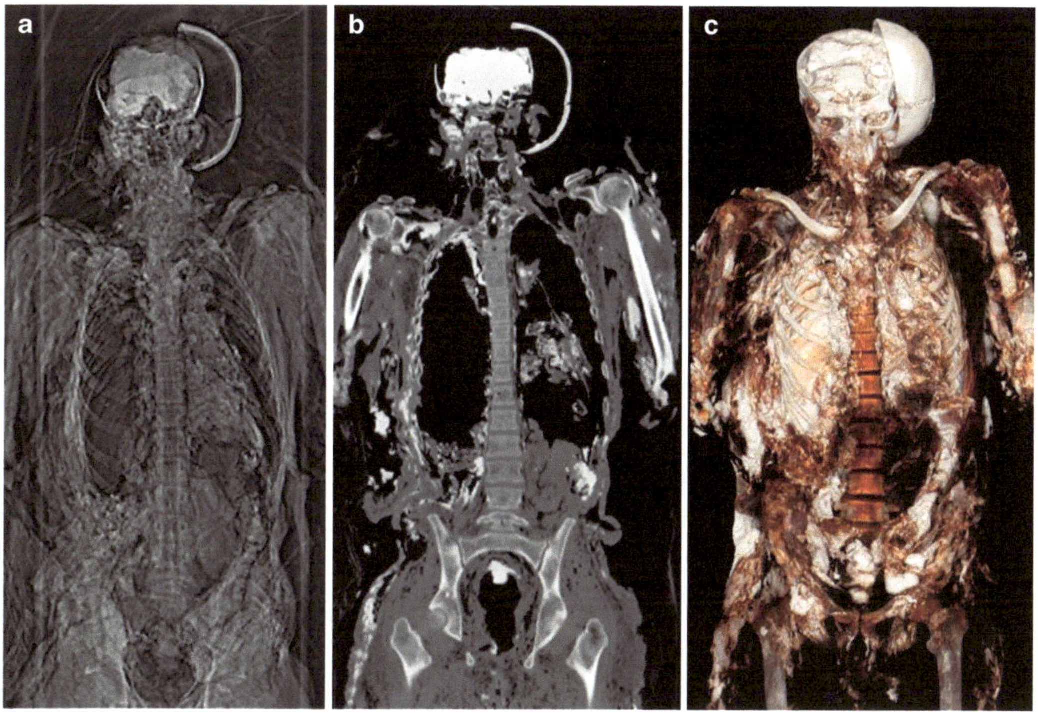

Fig. 5.5 Postmortem CT of a drowned and saponified man. The scanogram or scout (**a**) precede CT scan. Post-processing can be very useful to integrate traditional autopsy; after image acquisition it's possible to obtain multiplanar reconstruction, like this coronal view (**b**) and achieve Volume Rendering (**c**)

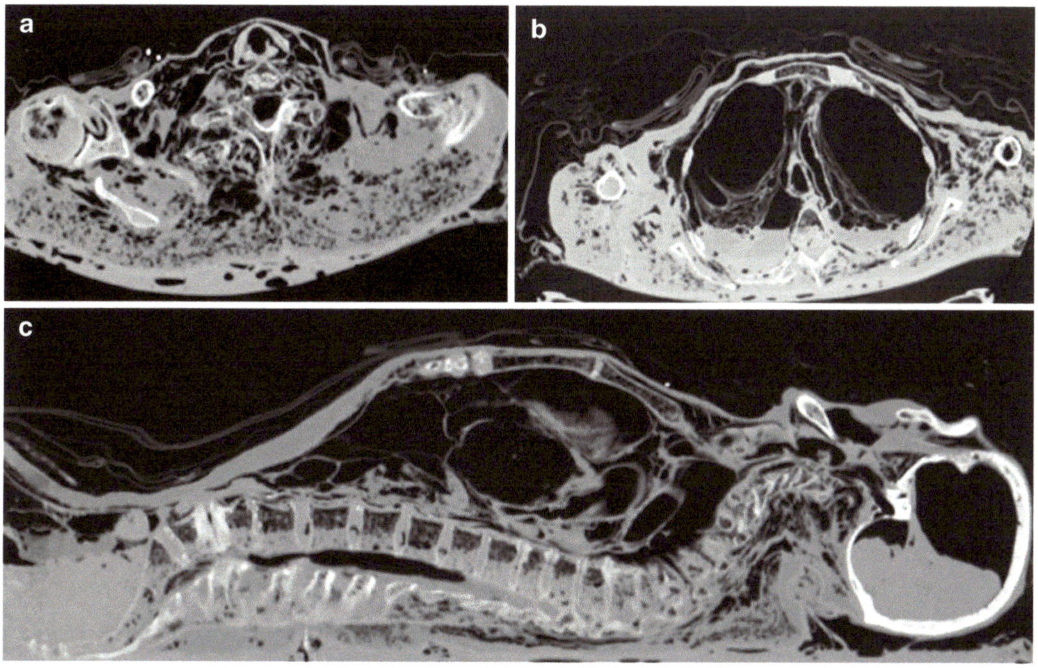

Fig. 5.6 Postmortem CT of an exhumed body in axial view (**a**, **b**) and sagittal (**c**). Imaging demonstrates natural decomposition processes of organs and bones after years and sometimes represents the unique way to assess a body when it takes so long from the time of death

bullet's impact, the existence and the number of entrance and exit wounds, the detection of bullets and bullet fragments, the bullet tracks, associated injuries, and, finally, the cause of death. PMCT can localize bullets and expose their number, delineate if bullets of different caliber are present, and reveal angle and direction of fire. Gunshot tracks through the cerebrum, neck, and visceral abdomen can also be demonstrated. In fact, although CT is less sensitive to soft tissue than MRI, it is possible to acquire images demonstrating bullet tracks through soft tissue structures.

5.4.1.4 Violent Mechanic Asphyxias

PMCT is useful for the recognition of typical hanging and strangulation findings. In strangulation and hanging cases, hemorrhage into the skin, subcutaneous and intramuscular tissues can be found, sternocleidomastoid and platysma muscle are frequently affected, glottic edema and perilaryngeal bleeding are often associated, and laryngohyoid fracture or vessel disruption are detectability better at PMCT than classic autopsy.

In drowning victims, fluid or froth in the airways from central aspiration into trachea or main bronchi, with emphysema aquosum and low standing diaphragm, can usually be observed. Furthermore, aspiration and swallowing of water or high-density materials (sand, mud, or silt) can lead to pulmonary edema, fill the paranasal sinuses, and distend stomach and duodenum.

5.4.1.5 Putrefied Bodies

When the body to be examined is badly decomposed, for instance, in exhumed cadavers, it is highly recommended to conduct a full CT study that might help visualize otherwise hidden injuries and pathological findings. The most well-known and commonly observed feature of decomposition on PMCT are the presences of gases in all anatomic spaces and loss of density in soft tissues. In advanced putrefaction, the texture can be completely dissolved, leading to a liquefaction of entire organs.

A comprehensive overview of the fields of application, advantages, and disadvantages of PMCT is reported in Table 5.2.

Table 5.2 Applications, advantages, and disadvantages of PMCT

PMCT		
Fields of application	Advantages	Disadvantages
Bone fractures Child abuse Gunshot injuries Violent mechanic asphyxia (hanging, strangulation, and drowning) Putrefied, carbonized, and badly damaged bodies	Rapidity Cost-efficiency Easiness to perform Availability for reevaluation and reinterpretation in the time Availability for 3D reconstructions Visualization of bone and gas	Radiation Limited visualization of soft tissue Data storage

5.4.2 Magnetic Resonance

In order to visualize the soft tissue, especially organs, MRI can be used. Although this technique has the potential to overcome the limitations of PCMT, it is only rarely used in forensic imaging as it is a complex technology requiring specific training, expensive, and with some complication in execution due to body size, artifact, and protocols.

The high soft-tissue resolution makes MRI a perfect tool for detecting natural causes of death and for examining traumatic soft-tissue injuries, with high sensitivity and accuracy. PMMR offers excellent anatomical detail and is especially useful to visualize pathologies of the brain, heart, subcutaneous fat tissue, and abdominal organs. PMMR is useful to assess the abdominal organs and to detect traumatic abdominal injuries of liver, spleen, pancreas, and kidneys. MRI is very useful to investigate neurological injuries, for the study of brain and spine; even if fractures can be better visualized with CT, the cord itself is not well detectable so MRI is the best way to study it.

For these reasons, MRI is recommended for the assessment of traumatic soft-tissue injuries such as impact injuries after a traffic accident, in cases of blunt force, stab wounds, medical errors, and age estimation.

T2-weighted MRI images are of paramount importance in postmortem imaging: its ability to highlight fluid accumulations makes PMMR an ideal diagnostic tool for a wide range of pathologies, including subcutaneous hematoma, bone contusion, organ laceration, internal hemorrhage and fluid collections, ischemic injury of the heart, brain edema, pericardial or pleural effusion and pulmonary edema.

Current limitations are disease states (i.e., bowel dilatation as obstruction, pneumonia, renal dysplasias and disseminated sepsis), which often have no imaging correlate, and bone alterations.

MRI has sufficient diagnostic accuracy to be used in conjunction with conventional postmortem methods, even if the precise contribution that PMMR makes to a forensic autopsy is on a case-by-case basis.

Definitively, MRI is of special significance for the diagnosis of natural death, especially related to diseases of the cardiovascular or central nervous system, and for investigations concerning neonatal and perinatal deaths (Fig. 5.7).

5.4.2.1 Sudden Cardiac Death

In cases of sudden cardiac death, the method of choice is PMMRI, which shows the myocardium and eventual lesions within it, eventually associated to MPMCTA, which permits a detailed investigation of stenosis or other lesions of coronary arteries.

Cardiovascular imaging is a core area of PMMR imaging and growing evidence indicates that PMMR is able to detect ischemic injury (acute, subacute, and chronic infarction) at an earlier stage than traditional autopsy and routine histology. In this way, cardio-PMMR could be a promising and changeling tool in forensic investigations for sudden cardiac death, besides immunohistochemical staining.

5.4.2.2 Sudden Unexpected Infant Death

MRI is suggested also in fetal (perinatal and neonatal) imaging in postmortem examinations, since congenital issues and cardiac anomalies can be seen (reported sensitivity 69% and specificity 95%), so that postmortem MRI (PMMRI) compared to conventional postmortem techniques can provide additional information regarding cause of death. In particular, PMMR is increasingly used to investigate particular deaths in childhood, such as sudden unexpected death in infancy (SUDI). The largest prospective trial of PMMR versus standard traditional autopsy reported >90% concordance in fetuses and stillbirths, and 75% concordance in children. PMMR is particularly good for congenital anatomical abnormalities (intracranial hemorrhage, brain malformations, renal anomalies, congenital heart disease, and skeletal dysplasias) and internal hemorrhage (intracranial injury, visceral or mesenteric injury associated with blunt or penetrating trauma to the body, soft tissue injuries associated with rib fractures and soft tissue limb injury). As last, PMMR imaging is considered useful to distinguish live birth from stillbirth by assessment of lung aeration.

A comprehensive overview of the fields of application, advantages, and disadvantages of PMMR is reported in Table 5.3.

5.5 Ancillary Techniques

5.5.1 Imaging-Guided Biopsies

In order to increase the sensibility of the above-described techniques, "complements" can be added. By performing imaging-guided biopsies or liquid aspiration, different matrices such as organ tissues or body fluids can be obtained in a minimally invasive way. This approach permits a combination of postmortem imaging with histological, toxicological, or microbiological investigations.

In particular, by performing a PMCT, the localization of a liquid or a gas can be detected and the biopsy performed.

5.5.2 Angiography

One of the most promising methods in forensic radiology is postmortem angiography (PMA).

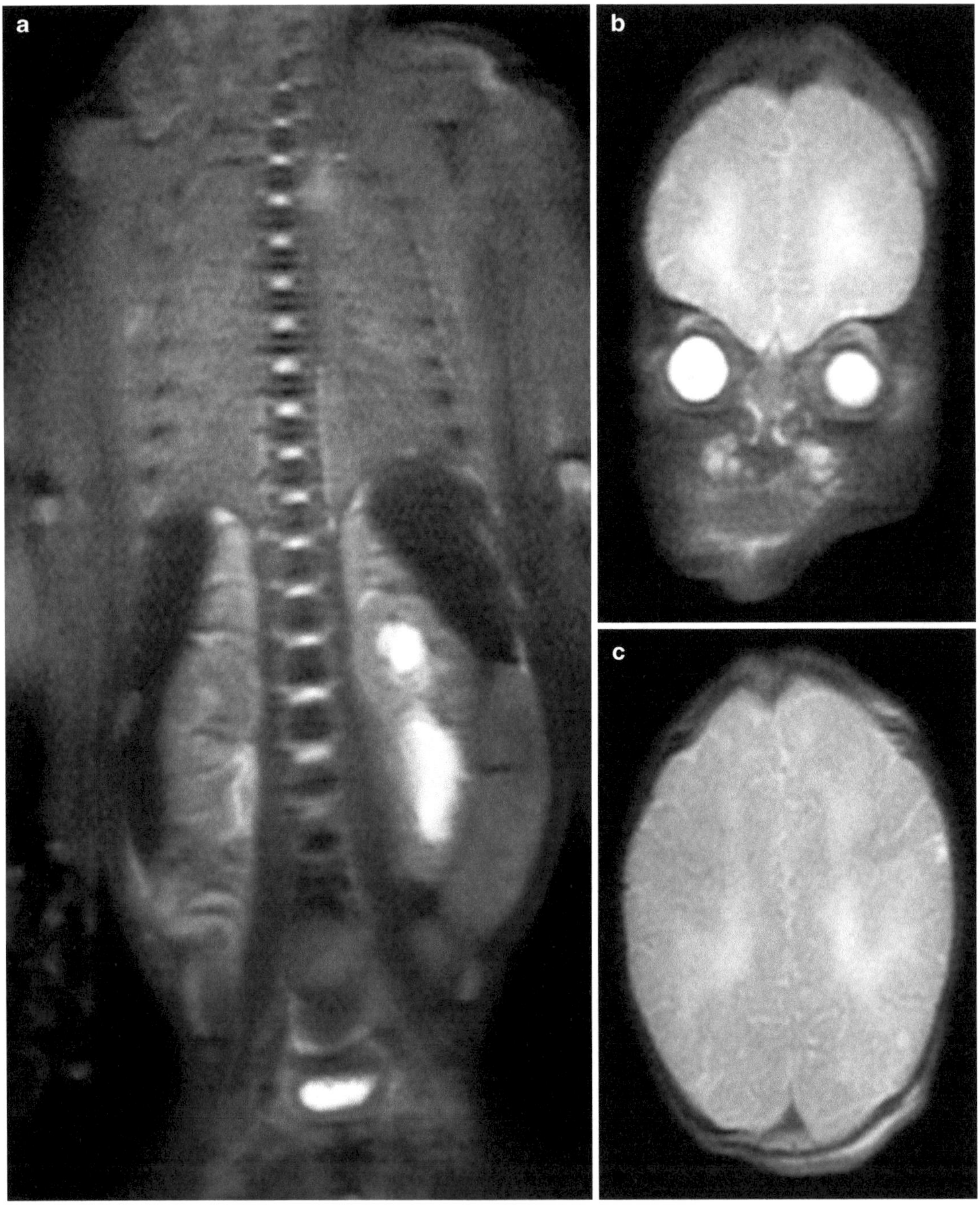

Fig. 5.7 Fetal MRI T2-weighted images show hydronephrosis (**a**) and encephalopathy of hypoxic-ischemic genesis on coronal (**b**) and axial (**c**) view

Postmortem angiography represents a validated method to document injuries of the vascular system, by injecting a contrast agent into the vascular system. Furthermore, injection of the contrast agent leads to an increase of contrast in the soft tissue, allowing the detection of organ findings.

Despite the advantages provided by contrast enhanced PMCT and PMMR, the additional cost

Table 5.3 Applications, advantages, and disadvantages of PMMR

PMMR		
Fields of application	Advantages	Disadvantages
Sudden cardiac death Sudden unexpected infant death	Availability for reevaluation and reinterpretation in the time No radiation Visualization of soft tissues	Time of execution High costs Data storage Difficulty in handle

and effort of angiography, as well as the apprehension that contrast media might negatively affect a subsequent autopsy, are possible factors that prevent this method from being used more frequently.

5.5.2.1 MPMCTA

Multi-phase PMCT angiography (MPMCTA) procedures allow for precise vascular and parenchymal localization of pathologies, extremely useful in forensic diagnoses, by administering additional intravascular contrast media using a roller-pump or modified heart–lung machine.

This method consists in the performance of a native CT scan in order to document the body prior to any manipulation. Subsequently, a contrast medium is injected by using a perfusion device. Consecutive CT acquisitions are made after the filling of the arterial system (arterial phase) and the venous system (venous phase) and during an ongoing perfusion of the body (dynamic phase). By performing this standardized technique of PMA, the sensitivity of PMCT can be increased.

This technique allows an excellent direct visualization, localization, and characterization of vascular (venous, arterial, or both) and solid organ lesion. In particular, MPMCTA has been shown to have advantages in cases of sudden cardiac death (allowing investigation of coronary arteries), stab and gunshot trauma, suspected medical error, fatal hemorrhage (finding sources of bleeding). Referring to fatal hemorrhage, contrast extravasations can be easily identified at multiple sites usually poorly accessible: disc space due to vertebral fracture, intraperitoneal space due to multiple hepatic and splenic fractures, and peri-cerebral space due to multiple skull bone fractures. It can also be suited to analysis of coronary arteries, as an important tool for investigating the causes of natural cardiac death (Fig. 5.8).

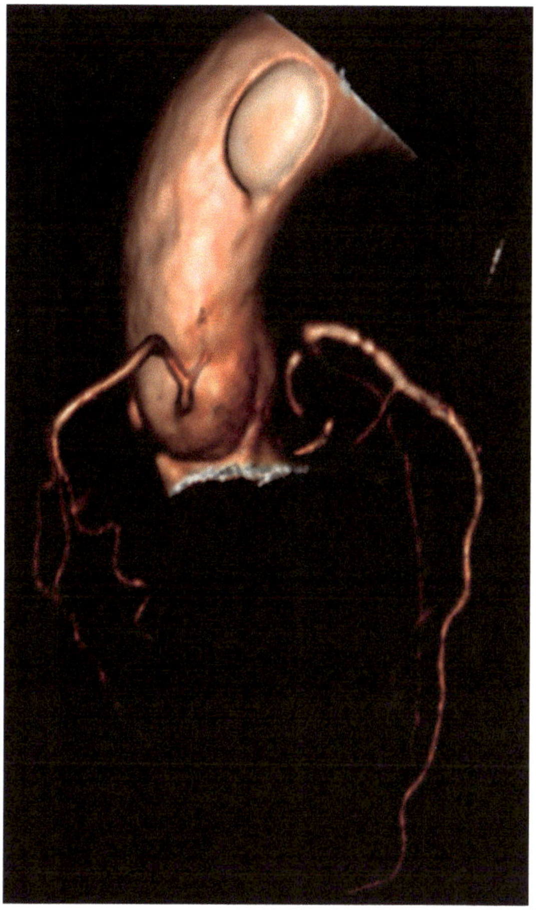

Fig. 5.8 MPMCTA demonstrate a stenosis on the anterior descending coronary artery

A comprehensive overview of the fields of application, advantages, and disadvantages of MPMCTA is reported in Table 5.4.

5.5.2.2 PMMRA

As an adjunct, a combination of the soft tissue detail provided by MRI and the information afforded by angiography is useful in investigating vascular pathology and solid organ laceration.

Basic evaluation of the coronary arteries and the assessment of coronary artery disease in

Table 5.4 Applications, advantages, and disadvantages of MPMCTA

MPMCTA		
Fields of application	Advantages	Disadvantages
Sudden cardiac death (coronary artery disease) Stab and gunshot trauma Suspected medical error Fatal hemorrhage	No invasive 3D reconstructions available Visualization of soft tissues	Relative time of execution Medium costs Data storage Difficulty in handle

PMMR non-contrast T2 weighted imaging is difficult, while PMMRA fat-saturated T1-weighted offer good possibilities. PEG-diluted contrast medium, hyperintense in T1-weighted images and hypointense in T2-weighted images, provides, in fact, visualization of vascular pathologies.

Overall, all vascular pathology identified at PMMRA can be also seen at PMCTA, so that its diffusion and utilization remains again limited.

5.6 Postmortem Imaging Applications

In summary, the indication for postmortem imaging strongly depends on the applied technique.

In different studies, evaluating the relative accuracy of PMCT and PMMR in the diagnosis of cause of death, PMMR has shown significant advantages in evaluating the central nervous system and the musculoskeletal system, in detecting abnormalities within the myocardium and lesions in the solid organs in the abdomen, due to its excellent soft tissue discrimination. On the other hand, PMCT has resulted more sensitive in the detection of abnormalities in the lungs and in the abdomen (i.e., pneumothorax and pneumoperitoneum) and in the detection of calcification (i.e., coronary artery calcification).

PMCT has important practical advantages, being more widely available, less expensive, and rapid than PMMR. PMMR limitations are, in fact, speed of acquisition and availability in most hospitals.

In this way, as each technique has its own advantages and limitations, knowledge is essential to enable the choice of correct method for solving a forensic case.

As a major advantage, common to all these techniques and missing in forensic autopsy, there is the possibility of 3D reconstruction for the corpse to be re-investigated years later, without loss of imaging detail. 3D reconstructions are also extremely useful when demonstrating medical technicalities to a court of law as they are more easily interpreted. Additional advantages of postmortem imaging are its noninvasive nature, the uninfluence of radiation dosing, the reasonably brief time of execution, and the ability to detect alterations that may not be apparent on traditional autopsies.

Nevertheless, current limitations are represented by the possibility to miss certain relatively minor but critical findings, the possibility of common major error in missed diagnoses (i.e., coronary heart disease and pneumonia), the lack of ability to demonstrate causes of death due to certain medical conditions (i.e., metabolic disorders), and the possibility to find certain imaging artifacts.

Direct comparison of autopsy findings and imaging findings is not easy. Each technique has its advantages and disadvantages, and sensitivity and specificity of imaging versus autopsy depend on the modality used and the case itself.

Comparing the results of postmortem imaging with subsequent autopsies, rates of major discrepancies between cause of death identified by radiology and autopsy of 32% for PMCT, 43% for PMMR, and 30% for PMCT + PMMRI have been reported.

Vice versa, different studies have demonstrated that PMCT or PMMRI in conjunction with conventional postmortem examinations can augment the value of postmortem examinations, providing more information than either examination alone.

For these reasons postmortem imaging is a double-edged knife, with clear superiority in specific diagnostic areas but also with certain shortcomings compared with autopsy. As a result, the gold standard for postmortem forensic assessment is still the forensic autopsy, and growing amount of evidence supports the use of postmortem imaging as complementary to traditional autopsy. In this way, these advanced techniques could be utilized as helpful adjunct to the conventional method.

Although the postmortem imaging cannot be regarded as a substitute for autopsy, it has meanwhile been proven to be a useful tool to determine the cause of death, to augment autopsy, and to improve the legal certainty in complex cases. For these reasons, postmortem imaging is becoming increasingly accepted in the field of forensic pathology. As a consequence, the increasing need of imaging techniques in forensic medicine will open new and interesting fields of activity for radiologists.

It remains that forensic pathologists have to choose the most accurate method for each case and to consider the advantages and disadvantages of each modality. Pathologists must also establish an equilibrium between exam quality and need for complementary analyses. On the other hand, radiologists should play an important role in this future assessment of forensic cases, in the frame of increasing interdisciplinar forensic-radiologic collaborations.

Further Reading

Appleby J, Rutty GN, Hainsworth SV, Woosnam-Savage RC, Morgan B, Brough A, Earp RW, Robinson C, King TE, Morris M, Buckley R (2015) Perimortem trauma in King Richard III: a skeletal analysis. Lancet 385(9964):253–259

Arthurs OJ, Hutchinson JC, Sebire NJ (2017) Current issues in postmortem imaging of perinatal and forensic childhood deaths. Forensic Sci Med Pathol 13(1):58–66

Bolliger SA, Thali MJ (2015) Imaging and virtual autopsy: looking back and forward. Philos Trans R Soc Lond Ser B Biol Sci 370(1674):20140253

Bonney HE (2015) Richard III: skeletal evidence of perimortem. Lancet 385(9964):210

Brogdon BG (2000) Scope of forensic radiology. Crit Rev Diagn Imaging 41(1):43–67

Busardò FP, Frati P, Guglielmi G, Grilli G, Pinto A, Rotondo A, Panebianco V, Fineschi V (2015) Postmortem-computed tomography and postmortem-computed tomography-angiography: a focused update. Radiol Med 120(9):810–823

Chevallier C, Doenz F, Vaucher P, Palmiere C, Dominguez A, Binaghi S, Mangin P, Grabherr S (2013) Postmortem computed tomography angiography vs. conventional autopsy: advantages and inconveniences of each method. Int J Legal Med 127(5):981–989

De Marco E, Vacchiano G, Frati P, La Russa R, Santurro A, Scopetti M, Guglielmi G, Fineschi V (2018) Evolution of post-mortem coronary imaging: from selective coronary arteriography to post-mortem CT-angiography and beyond. Radiol Med 123(5):351–358

Dirnhofer R, Jackowski C, Vock P, Potter K, Thali MJ (2006) VIRTOPSY: minimally invasive, imaging-guided virtual autopsy. Radiographics 26(5):1305–1333

Elifritz JM, Nolte KB, Hatch GM, Adolphi NL, Gerrard C (2014) Radiology, forensic imaging and the 'virtual autopsy'. In: Pathobiology of human disease: a dynamic encyclopedia of disease mechanisms. Elsevier, Amsterdam, pp 3448–3458

Fais P, Giraudo C, Viero A, Miotto D, Bortolotti F, Tagliaro F, Montisci M, Cecchetto G (2016) Micro computed tomography features of laryngeal fractures in a case of fatal manual strangulation. Leg Med (Tokyo) 18:85–89

Flach PM, Gascho D, Schweitzer W, Ruder TD, Berger N, Ross SG, Thali MJ, Ampanozi G (2014a) Imaging in forensic radiology: an illustrated guide for postmortem computed tomography technique and protocols. Forensic Sci Med Pathol 10(4):583–606

Flach PM, Thali MJ, Germerott T (2014b) Times have changed! Forensic radiology—a new challenge for radiology and forensic pathology. AJR Am J Roentgenol 202(4):W325–W334

Fukutake K, Ishiwatari T, Takahashi H, Tsuchiya K, Okubo Y, Shinozaki M, Tochigi N, Wakayama M, Nemoto T, Shibuya K, Wada A (2015) Investigation of ossification in the posterior longitudinal ligament using micro-focus X-ray CT scanning and histological examination. Diagn Pathol 10:205

Grabherr S, Baumann P, Minoiu C, Fahrni S, Mangin P (2016) Post-mortem imaging in forensic investigations: current utility, limitations, and ongoing developments. Res Rep Forensic Med Sci 6:25–37

Grabherr S, Doenz F, Steger B, Dirnhofer R, Dominguez A, Sollberger B, Gygax E, Rizzo E, Chevallier C, Meuli R, Mangin P (2011) Multi-phase post-mortem CT angiography: development of a standardized protocol. Int J Legal Med 125(6):791–802

Grabherr S, Grimm J, Baumann P, Mangin P (2015) Application of contrast media in post-mortem imaging (CT and MRI). Radiol Med 120(9):824–834

Grabherr S, Grimm J, Dominguez A, Vanhaebost J, Mangin P (2014) Advances in post-mortem CT-angiography. Br J Radiol 87(1036):20130488

Grabherr S, Gygax E, Sollberger B, Ross S, Oesterhelweg L, Bolliger S, Christe A, Djonov V, Thali MJ, Dirnhofer R (2008) Two-step postmortem angiography with a modified heart-lung machine: preliminary results. AJR Am J Roentgenol 190(2):345–351

Guidi B, Aquaro GD, Gesi M, Emdin M, Di Paolo M (2018) Postmortem cardiac magnetic resonance in sudden cardiac death. Heart Fail Rev 23(5):651–665

Hughes N, Baker M (1997) The use of radiography in forensic medicine. Radiography 3(4):311–320

Hutchinson JC, Arthurs OJ, Ashworth MT, Ramsey AT, Mifsud W, Lombardi CM, Sebire NJ (2016) Clinical utility of postmortem microcomputed tomography of the fetal heart: diagnostic imaging vs macroscopic dissection. Ultrasound Obstet Gynecol 47(1):58–64

Kahana T, Hiss J (2005) Forensic radiology. In: Forensic pathology reviews, vol 3. Humana Press, Totowa, NJ, pp 443–460

Kettner M, Potente S, Schulz B, Knauff P, Schmidt PH, Ramsthaler F (2014) Analysis of laryngeal fractures in decomposed bodies using microfocus computed tomography (mfCT). Forensic Sci Med Pathol 10(4):607–612

Kudlas M, Odle T (2010) The state of forensic radiography. Radiol Technol 81(5):484–490

La Russa R, Catalano C, Di Sanzo M, Scopetti M, Gatto V, Santurro A, Viola RV, Panebianco V, Frati P, Fineschi V (2019) Postmortem computed tomography angiography (PMCTA) and traditional autopsy in cases of sudden cardiac death due to coronary artery disease: a systematic review and meta-analysis. Radiol Med 124(2):109–117

Lundström C, Persson A, Ross S, Ljung P, Lindholm S, Gyllensvärd F, Ynnerman A (2012) State-of-the-art of visualization in post-mortem imaging. APMIS 120(4):316–326

Mokrane FZ, Savall F, Dercle L, Crubezy E, Telmon N, Rousseau H, Dedouit F (2017) A preliminary comparative study between classical and interventional radiological approaches for multi-phase post-mortem CT angiography. Forensic Sci Int 271:23–32

O'Donnell C, Woodford N (2008) Post-mortem radiology—a new sub-speciality? Clin Radiol 63(11):1189–1194

Pomara C, Bello S, Grilli G, Guglielmi G, Turillazzi E (2015) Multi-phase postmortem CT angiography (MPMCTA): a new axillary approach suitable in fatal thromboembolism. Radiol Med 120(7):670–673

Pomara C, Fineschi V, Scalzo G, Guglielmi G (2009) Virtopsy versus digital autopsy: virtual autopsy. Radiol Med 114(8):1367–1382

Reynolds A (2010) Forensic radiography: an overview. Radiol Technol 81(4):361–379

Roberts IS, Benamore RE, Benbow EW, Lee SH, Harris JN, Jackson A, Mallett S, Patankar T, Peebles C, Roobottom C, Traill ZC (2012) Post-mortem imaging as an alternative to autopsy in the diagnosis of adult deaths: a validation study. Lancet 379(9811):136–142

Ross S, Ebner L, Flach P, Brodhage R, Bolliger SA, Christe A, Thali MJ (2012a) Postmortem whole-body MRI in traumatic causes of death. AJR Am J Roentgenol 199(6):1186–1192

Ross SG, Bolliger SA, Ampanozi G, Oesterhelweg L, Thali MJ, Flach PM (2014) Postmortem CT angiography: capabilities and limitations in traumatic and natural causes of death. Radiographics 34(3):830–846

Ross SG, Thali MJ, Bolliger S, Germerott T, Ruder TD, Flach PM (2012b) Sudden death after chest pain: feasibility of virtual autopsy with postmortem CT angiography and biopsy. Radiology 264(1):250–259

Ruder TD, Flach PM, Thali MJ (2013) Virtual autopsy. Forensic Sci Med Pathol 9(3):435–436

Ruder TD, Hatch GM, Ebert LC, Flach PM, Ross S, Ampanozi G, Thali MJ (2012) Whole body postmortem magnetic resonance angiography. J Forensic Sci 57(3):778–782

Ruder TD, Thali MJ, Hatch GM (2014) Essentials of forensic post-mortem MR imaging in adults. Br J Radiol 87:20130567

Sieswerda-Hoogendoorn T, van Rijn RR (2010) Current techniques in postmortem imaging with specific attention to paediatric applications. Pediatr Radiol 40(2):141–152

Swift B, Rutty GN (2006) Recent advances in postmortem forensic radiology. Computed tomography and magnetic resonance imaging applications. In: Forensic pathology reviews, vol 4. Humana Press, Totowa, NJ, pp 355–404

Thali MJ, Yen K, Schweitzer W, Vock P, Boesch C, Ozdoba C, Schroth G, Ith M, Sonnenschein M, Doernhoefer T, Scheurer E, Plattner T, Dirnhofer R (2003) Virtopsy, a new imaging horizon in forensic pathology: virtual autopsy by post-mortem multislice computed tomography (MSCT) and magnetic resonance imaging (MRI)—a feasibility study. J Forensic Sci 48(2):386–403

Turillazzi E, Frati P, Pascale N, Pomara C, Grilli G, Viola RV, Fineschi V (2016) Multi-phase post-mortem CT-angiography: a pathologic correlation study on cardiovascular sudden death. J Geriatr Cardiol 13(10):855–865

Underwood J (2012) Post-mortem imaging and autopsy: rivals or allies? Lancet 379(9811):100–102

Vullo A, Panebianco V, Cannavale G, Aromatario M, Cipolloni L, Frati P, Santurro A, Vullo F, Catalano C, Fineschi V (2016) Post-mortem magnetic resonance foetal imaging: a study of morphological correlation with conventional autopsy and histopathological findings. Radiol Med 121(11):847–856

Wichmann D, Heinemann A, Weinberg C, Vogel H, Hoepker WW, Grabherr S, Pueschel K, Kluge S (2014) Virtual autopsy with multiphase postmortem computed tomographic angiography versus traditional medical autopsy to investigate unexpected deaths of hospitalized patients: a cohort study. Ann Intern Med 160(8):534–541

6 Radiology in Archaeology: Fundamentals and Perspective—Examination of the Living

Marta Licata and Antonio Pinto

Radiology is an important investigative tool for archaeologists, anthropologists and museum conservators. Radiological analyses on archaeological material, artefact or biological remains, allow us to retrieve a great deal of information from the finds. The first application of X-rays were addressed to the mummies and skeletonised remains and later applied to man-made cultural artefacts [1]. In the field of archaeological heritage, different types of items are radiologically inspected, depending on the information we would like to obtain from them. In regard to anthropologists and paleopathologists, the imaging used on human remains allows analysis of the biological features of skeletons or burial sites, whereas the application on relics allows archaeologists to acquire knowledge such as the manufacturing techniques and the materials used [2]. Due to their precious and unique nature, the integrity of objects recovered in archaeological excavations, being artefacts or ecofacts, need to be safeguarded. For this reason, radiological techniques are perfectly indicated to investigate archaeological items without damaging them. They are hence inserted among the Non-Destructive Examination (NDE) techniques. Another benefit guaranteed by diagnostic imaging is the accessibility of the data as a whole, including any hidden structure not visible from the outside [3–5]. Moreover, this approach allows the analysis of the structure and composition of the archaeological finds and consequently plan the restoration works accordingly [6]. These are few of the reasons why archaeologists regularly use radiology.

This chapter reviews the application of radiology in archaeological investigations since its first application to the present day.

6.1 The History of "Archaeoradiology"

Immediately after the discovery of X-rays by Wilhelm Roentgen in 1895, this new technique was used to investigate an Egyptian mummy [7]. The following year 14 archaeological finds, including a mummy of an Egyptian child, were radiologically investigated by the German scientist Walter Koenig. The radiograph showed of a mummified child's knee, which represented the first radiological image of a mummy. Since that moment, mummies were X-rayed in order to investigate their interior and to reveal hidden artefacts, embalming techniques and pathological signs. In the same year, Van Heurck analyzed

M. Licata (✉)
Department of Biotechnology and Life Sciences, Centre of Research in Osteoarchaeology and Paleopathology, University of Insubria, Varese, Italy
e-mail: marta.licata@uninsubria.it

A. Pinto
Department of Radiology, C.T.O., Hospital, Azienda Ospedaliera dei Colli, Naples, Italy

G. Lo Re et al. (eds.), *Radiology in Forensic Medicine*,
https://doi.org/10.1007/978-3-319-96737-0_6

an ibis mummy in Belgium. Around the same time, Thurstan Holland and Sir Flinders Petrie X-rayed, respectively, a mummified bird and Egyptian mummies [8, 9]. The results of these investigations were diffused through scientific publication in 1898. From this moment, numerous related studies followed. After Roentgen's first experiment, others by Elliot Smith and Howard Carter in 1904 were completed. X-rays have been largely used since the early 1920s because they represented a non-invasive and very useful investigative tool, especially for paleopathological studies. In 1931 [10], Ray L. Moodie published the results of X-ray examinations on several Egyptian and Peruvian mummies, from collections of the Field Museum in Chicago. In his book, *Roentgenologic Studies of Egyptian and Peruvian Mummies*, we find detailed reports on pathological and anthropological interpretations of human remains and we can read the first considerations on the developments of Roentgenologic studies in paleopathology [10]. Before 1954, year of the first publication of Moss's guide on the use of X-rays, the technique was seldom used [1, 11, 12]. It was only after the 1960s that radiography gained great importance in archaeological studies, and museum conservators, archaeologists and paleopathologists adopted the X-ray analysis as the gold standard. In the 1960s the British radiologist, Louis Harold Gray, accomplished the first comprehensive X-ray study of paleopathology on Egyptian mummies. A third of the 133 mummies investigated presented osteoarthritis of the spine [13]. In 1967, the important project of radiological investigation of all the royal mummies housed at the Cairo Museum, enrichens this field of research [14, 15]. With the archaeological and medical focus, the radiological application on ancient mummies became one of the main tools used in historical studies, especially in Egyptology.

In 1987, Derek Notman, a radiologist at Park Nicollet Medical Center of Minneapolis, gave birth in his article to the term "Paleoradiology", even though the etymological meaning is "ancient radiology", when referring to the radiological study of ancient human remains [16]. The radiologist, together with other researchers of the University of Alberta (Canada), examined two frozen mummies from the Franklin expedition (1845–1848), those of men who perished in the Canadian arctic [17] and highlighted the differences between the first autopsy and the following radiological exams conducted on the mummies.

The following developments of radiology with the invention of the Computed Tomography scanner had a great influence on archaeoradiological studies. CT scans entered into the clinical practice in 1970 [18] and allowed us to obtain 3D images of the body with high-resolution detail. Physical anthropologists availed themselves of newly developed biomedical image processing and Computer Tomography (CT), in order to study archaeological human remains [19, 20]. CT has allowed us to obtain more detailed information from the analysed material through virtual reconstructions of the entire body, providing a significant overall view and meticulous high-resolution detail [21]. The first CT scan of mummies was performed in 1977; in this report, Lewin and Harwood Nash examined the internal structure of mummified tissue proving that some ancient human diseases can be discovered in preserved soft tissues rather than from skeletal ones [22]. The Computer Tomography investigative method was subsequently extended to the field of cultural heritage. Different kind of artefacts could be examined in order to explain the nature of the archaeological finds. Such investigations help to have a better view on the living habits of ancient cultures. In some ways, CT investigation is better than the physical inspection of the artefacts as it offers information about the internal structure. In particular, they allow us to obtain 3D reconstruction of the archaeological finds, usually recovered fragmented from the excavations. In this regard, CT scanners have a distinctive edge over plain X-ray.

6.2 Radiological Investigation on Archaeological Artefacts

Archaeologists frequently ask radiologists to analyse artefacts in order to obtain information about the objects. The application of imaging techniques on archaeological finds allows us to obtain information on ancient technological skills and utilised material; this permits planning of an appropriate maintenance or restoration of the finds. Radiological examinations on archaeological material also allow the recognition of falsifications.

Currently many radiological applications can be useful to cultural heritage: CT, X-ray radiography and infrared reflectography in addition to UV photography [23]. Moreover, to not being invasive, these techniques offer another advantage: they can be mobile. We know that it is difficult to organise and especially to authorise the movement of archaeological finds belonging to a museum collection, both for insurance costs and for the fragility of the findings. These methodologies represent a great chance to examine the archaeological finds in situ.

In addition, we are aware of the fact that museum collection heritage is destined to disappear because of deterioration. Outside monuments can be target of degradation by atmospheric agents, such as pollution or acid rain, for instance, but the finds housed in museums suffer degradation too [24]. Radiological investigations can slow down or even hinder this phenomenon, producing permanent images, making an immortal copy of the studied item.

Today, radiological methodologies are applied to different kind of archaeological artefacts: metalworks (coins, vessels, statues, weapons…), pottery (vessels, written tables, statuettes…), glass and other finds from archaeological sites.

6.2.1 Radiology and Ancient Metallography

Metalworks are frequently recovered in archaeological excavations, especially in the necropolis contexts. The stylistic interpretation of these artefacts is often very important to date the chronological phases of the site. The radiological analyses enable the retrieval of the artefacts' shape, and the investigation of the stylistic traces, which are often obscured by the soil matrix in which the artefacts are trapped or by the deterioration of the objects. In fact, ancient metalworks are subjected to the interaction with the environment, and the factors that most influence the deterioration of archaeological finds are the composition, depth, humidity of the soil and amount of glass in it. The in-depth analysis of metalworks through radiology images also allows the recovery of the information regarding the type of metalwork, wrought with the hammer and worked on the lathe. Vessels, coins, weapons, etc. are ancient metalworks that archaeology delivers frequently to museums and that are proof of the past populations' knowledge and living habits.

In this regard, the *Guidelines of the X-radiography of archaeological metalwork*, published by the English Heritage in 2006, recommends a series of measures in proceeding with radiological investigations of archaeological metal artefacts. Firstly, the guide highlights the need to adopt X-ray investigations during the archaeological post excavation phase. This technique makes it possible to record the findings in the condition in which they were recovered. Besides explaining when, how and which radiological techniques can be used in order to retrieve data from the finds, the guide also shows us some of the results of radiological examinations on several metal artefacts recovered from excavations funded by the Archaeological Services University of Durham and by the Chester City Council.

From the first X-rayed investigations we want to remember the study by Corfield published in 1982. The author analysed a series of late Roman and Anglo Saxon ironworks and highlighted the complexity of the development of metallurgical techniques. From the Saxon Cemetery at Mucking in Essex, several metalworks were recovered and X-rayed. The great quality of the analysed artefacts is due to the development of carburisation techniques used to produce the items. This metal manufacture was also observed on weapons made of unmodified wrought iron, which were easily bent [25]. Indeed, a great development on the metallurgical techniques was the perfection of the so-called "pattern-welded blade". The analysis carried out on bronze finds deserves our interest. From some radiological images of bronze swords, spearheads and daggers it is possible to grasp the distribution and orientation of the void gas and allowing a better understanding of the process of casting [26]. Deborah Scorsch, in 1988, examined ancient Egyptian theriomorphic hollow bronze casts from several artefacts preserved in the United Kingdom Institute for Conservation [27]. The authors clearly showed the technique "lost wax" adopted by ancient Egyptians.

We want to point out to the readers' attention, the digital radioscopic examination of eight Chinese bronze ritual vessels dating back between the thirteenth and sixth centuries BC. The vessels were made during the classical production phase of the Shang Dynasty and are characterised by an elaborate surface decoration, a series of fantastic animal motifs. Eight vessels were analysed. The purpose of the CT analysis was to identify the hidden damages and repairs and to find out more about casting techniques. In particular, CT investigation on the *Jia*, a tripod vessel used for ritual warming of wine, brought to light several repairs, on the handle, in the legs and along the rim. These areas appear as "bright white" in the CT images. Some repairs were made in ancient times and these are diagnosable by the fact that they are no visible signs of breakage on the surface, while others repairs were carried out in more recent times [28].

Radiological investigations can offer an important contribution in the numismatic field. Coins represent one of the most important "fossil guide", which usually allows the dating of an archaeological site. For this reason, it is very important to verify the authenticity of these artefacts, since there are contemporary imitations or later copies of coins. Firstly, the authenticity of the coins are verified by stylistic interpretations, and radiological investigation can support this reading by recuperating the original surface of the coins usually obscured beneath corrosion layers [24]. Representative in this regard is the tomographic study conducted at the University of Southampton on the Selby treasure coins in ancient burials of East Riding, York. Thanks to the CT investigation, it was possible to analyze the details of the coins and to investigate the iconography and inscriptions. It was possible to identify the governors ruling at the time: Vespasiano, Adriano, Traiano and Marco Aurelio [29].

The following parameters are generally used when analysing metalwork: 3 mA, 110 kV and 60s to 300 s.

6.2.2 Radiology and the Study of Ancient Glass

Excavated glass can be analysed to highlight the extent of surface deterioration, composition of materials and shape of the artefacts. In this regard we want to recall a study conducted on ancient Roman glass fragments from the burial site discovered near the Dutch village of Bocholtz in 2003. The University of Amsterdam carried out high-resolution spiral computer tomography with multiplane reformation to obtain detailed information about the number, position, shape and glass fragments from the burial site. For these reasons, researchers decided that the only way to avoid further damage to the finds was to extract the objects in the blocks of soil in which they were trapped. The blocks with the highest concentration of glass were subjected to CT examination which then revealed the presence of 14 objects in glass. CT investigation allowed the identification of the type of glass which consisted mainly of clear and transparent green glass. The parameters used for this investigation were: 120 kV, 200 mA, 1.3 section thickness and 0.6 increments [30].

Another example of radiological analysis of glass is the exam conducted on Art Nouveau iridescent glass objects. The project was carried out by the Museum of Applied Arts in Vienna and the Research Center Seibersdorf (Austria) and the Academy of Fine Arts in collaboration with the Historical Society in New York. The study was based on a non-destructive analysis with XRF. This kind of analysis allowed the exploration of the manufacturing technology and investigation of the elements remaining in the iridescent surface layer [24].

6.2.3 Radiological Investigation Study of Clay and Ceramic

The radiological investigation of ceramics allows us to acquire a lot of information about the materials present, manufacturing techniques, etc. Generally, in X-ray images, it is possible to differentiate the opacity of the mineral grains in respect to clay particles. The latter do not obtain a spectrum, but their shape can be appreciated: the particles follow the direction of the shaping wheel that moulded them. Radiological inspections of glazed ceramics show the use of heavy metals in the pigments and permit the identification of the application of the lead glazes. The ceramic analysis also allows us to observe the contrast between the air voids and filled surfaces.

An interesting study is that of the archaeological artefacts from Ancient Near East conducted by the Institute of Radiology of the Hadassah University in Jerusalem. The researchers presented the results of the imaging studies conducted on clay and ceramic artefacts from an archaeological site in Israel. CT investigation on clay tablets of UR III (Neo-Sumerian Period) showed the lines of cuneiform writing and the imaging of the inner text. Indeed, it was determined that in some cases the scribe wrapped the inner tablet in two layers of clay. Another interesting CT investigation was conducted on an anthropomorphic figurine from the Pottery Neolithic Period Site of Shaar Hagolan because it could reveal important information about the beginning of ceramic technology. The author of this figurine carried out the work starting from a single slab of clay placed along the longitudinal axis and later he applied the other parts of the body [31].

In the same year, a group at the University of Kentucky formulated an algorithm for extracting inscription from CT scans of manuscripts made of clay [32].

6.3 Radiology and the Study of Ancient Human Remains

In the past, autopsies on mummies were frequently performed. This obviously did not appeal to archaeologists and anthropologists because these procedures strongly damaged the finds. Indeed, autopsies caused the physical destruction of the mummies in the sense that the body was unwrapped and opened. Therefore, greater attention has been addressed on the advancing non-invasive techniques for the examination of ancient human remains. As mentioned above, radiology, since its beginnings, has been made available to the study of mummies, and today radiological methods such as CT scanning-3D visualisation [33] and Magnetic Resonance Imaging (MRI) [17] represent the most important analytical tools for anthropological and paleopathological analyses of ancient human remains (Fig. 6.1a, b). Furthermore, conventional radiographs have acquired a benefit with the development of high spatial resolution and the possibility to better examine the soft tissue [34, 35]. The main advantages offered by radiological investigations are the accessibility to many anatomical areas, including hidden structures (endocranium, tooth roots, sinuses and cavities of the long bones), the opportunity to obtain useful information for morphometric analyses and to share data conveniently [3]. Perhaps the term "Bioarchaeoradiology" could summarise the radiological investigations that today are used frequently on human remains. They examine artificial or natural mummies, skeletonised bodies and fossils remains. The objectives of these studies are anthropological, when making identification analysis (ethnicity, gender, age at death, stature and anthropometric indices) [36–38], paleopathological [39–41] (Fig. 6.2), when diagnosing diseases, taphonomic, when focusing on the changes occurring post-mortem and paleoanthropological, when investigating the anatomical changes during the stages of human evolution.

6.3.1 Radiological Investigation on Artificial Mummies

Everyone knows that the history of "Paleoradiology" started with the study of the Pharaonic mummies, the ultimate artificial mummies. The first mummy examined with X-rays is Thutmose IV, 8th Pharaoh of the 18th dynasty, in 1903 by the Egyptian radiologist Khayat. The radiological image established the age at death of the subject did not exceed

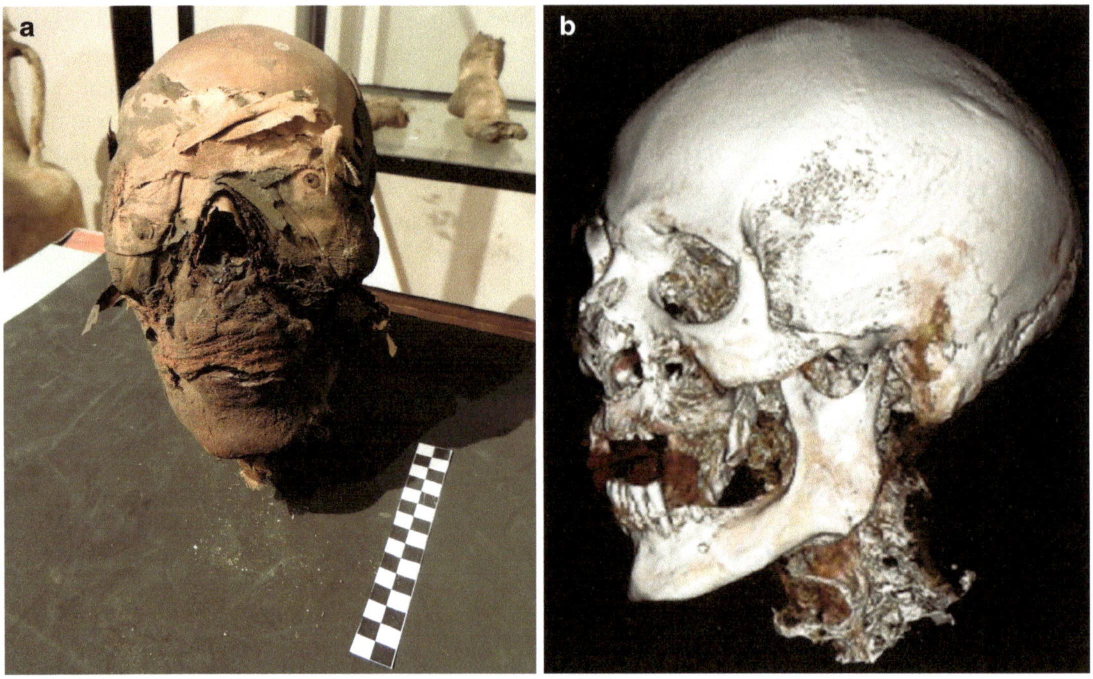

Fig. 6.1 (**a**) Embalmed head of an Egyptian mummy housed in the Civic Museum of Erba (Northern Italy); (**b**) CT of the embalmed head

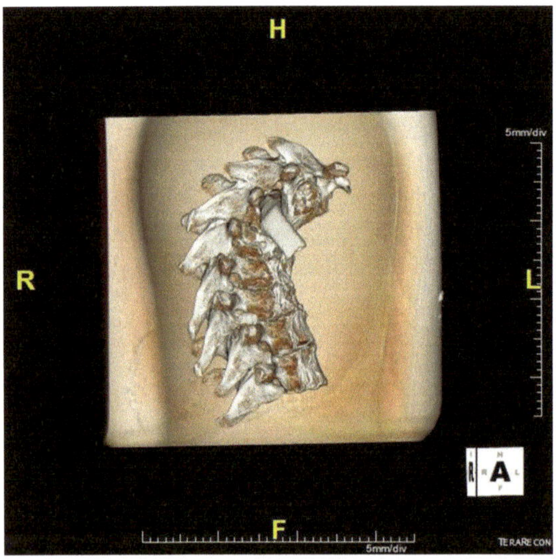

Fig. 6.2 CT of the spine affected by Pott's disease, from Azzio (Northern Italy) archaeological site

25 years. "The epiphysis of the crest of ilium was in process of being united in the front but still free behind…" [17, 42]. After 30 years, the second Pharaoh of the 18th dynasty was analysed by Dr. Douglas Derry. By using X-rays it was possible to hypothesise an age at death between 40 and 50 years. In addition to this, the author also reported that into the cranial cavity were of residues, perhaps the remains of the brain, and, in the middle of the right arm, was a small amulet [43].

In 1968, the mummy of the famous Pharaoh Tutankhamun, of the 18th dynasty, was X-rayed. From the skull radiography, through observation of the teeth, they estimated age at death between 18 and 22 years. The X-ray of the abdominal cavity revealed the presence of embalmed material but did not show any form of pathology. The skull fracture was noted and the hypothesis of a "traumatic or homicidal death" was made. Nevertheless, this theory was denied and later a post-mortem fracture was suggested [19]. The mummy of Ramses II, the third Pharaoh of the 18th dynasty, was analysed in 1976. From the first X-ray investigations conducted in 1976 it was supposed that the Pharaoh suffered of ankylosing spondylitis, but in 2004 Chhem contested this diagnosis. In fact, CT investigation of the spine and sacroiliac joints clearly revealed the diagnosis of diffuse idiopathic skeletal hyperostosis [44].

As previously mentioned, it was only from 1977 that mummies started to be investigated with CT. We would like to remember the study carried out by Notman in 1983 on four Egyptian mummies belonging to the 18th to 25th dynasty. The investigations were performed in Minnesota. Of particular importance is the mummy of Lady Tashat, of the 25th dynasty. Notman carried out the CT scan and diagnosed an infection on her knee. Radiological investigations allowed the detection of several bone lesions but is not yet clear whether these occurred before or after death [45]. Since the early 1990s, 3D CT imagining has been used to investigate possible bone fractures. The benefits of 3D imaging include the visualisation of pathological changes and, in some cases, the presence of *intra vitam* foreign objects. The study published in 1986 by Marx and D'Auria showed the results of CT scan investigation of 15 mummies from the Museum of Fine Arts in Boston. The CT images revealed soft tissue packing material, and pathological conditions such as Schmorl's nodes, arthrosis and aortic calcifications. Another example of CT investigation of an artificial mummy is the analysis of the body of the Braids Lady of Arezzo, which highlighted bone erosions and joint subluxation typical of rheumatoid arthritis [46].

The CT study of the mummies also gave better investigate interventions of embalming and therefore to understand more about the ancient funerary rituals. Egyptians were mummified because they thought that by doing this the soul could rejoin the body in the afterlife. At first, mummification was reserved for nobles, and later was diffused among the common people. Interesting, in this regard, is the study of Christian Jackowski, Stephan Bolliger, Michael J. Thali, "*Common and Unexpected Findings in Mummies from Ancient Egypt and South America as Revealed by CT*" published in 2008. The authors compared the written sources, in particular Herodotus, with the CT images of the Egyptian mummies. In particular, some skulls were examined to confirm if the removal of the brain through the nasal cavity was performed as described in the texts. CT images showed that the brain was often removed by perforating the cribriform plate. Commonly, only one nostril was designated, although this procedure was performed in a very coarse and it caused damage to some anatomical structures such as the orbital wall and ethmoid cells. Long metallic or wooden nails were passed through the nose and cribriform plate into the cranial cavity. Radiological images in some skulls showed that the brain was not removed and in others incisions were revealed at the level of the occipital bones. CT imaging performed on several mummies confirmed the removal of thoracic and abdominal organs, from making an abdominal incision on the left side of the body. Radiological investigation confirmed that the kidneys and the heart were usually left inside the body [47]. There are other mummification practices furthest from the Egyptian world that still need to be investigated. We are talking about the practice of mummification of the Buddhist monks. The process of self-mummification is a tradition known in countries such as Japan, China and Thailand, that had been practised over a thousand years ago. The elaborate and difficult process includes a special diet and drinking a poisonous tea so that the body would be too toxic to be eaten by worms. The few monks who were able to successfully complete the process were highly revered and finally exposed in the temples. An extraordinary discovery was found inside a golden statue, dating back 1000 years, through radiological examination. CT images revealed the presence of a mummified body inside it, placed in the lotus position. The images also revealed that there were no abdominal organs.

In Italy, an important paleoradiological project was carried out on the Sicilian mummies to determine information relating to the funerary treatments. Radiological investigations have made it possible to clarify that in the majority of cases the mummified bodies were not eviscerated. The bodies, after a careful preparation, were laid out in crypts and subterranean chapels [35].

6.3.2 Radiological Investigation on Natural Mummies

Many natural mummies were radiologically examined with the aim to analyse the degree of preservation, the morphological features and pathological conditions present. The most ancient natural mummy that we know of is Ötzi, found in 1991 in the Val Senales glacier in the Ötztal Alps, near Hauslabjoch on the border between Austria and Italy. This mummy belonged to a man from about 3300 BC. The reason of his death was a mystery for a long time, until radiologists intervened. At first, it was supposed that Ötzi died from exposure during a winter storm. After, it was hypothesised that Ötzi was the victim of a ritual sacrifice. Finally, in 2001, X-rays and a CT scan showed an arrowhead lodged in the shoulder, most probably the cause of death. Radiological investigation showed a lesion of an artery close-to-the-shoulder, in the dorsal wall of the left subclavian artery [48].

It is difficult to apply CT scans to other natural mummies like the bog bodies, the bodies of the swamps. The acidity of the soil of the swamps causes demineralisation of the bones. The bog bodies were recovered in Denmark and date back to between 500 BC and 500 AD. The CT study of these bodies has, in many cases, confirmed the identification, gender and age at death, and clarified the entities of some post-mortal injuries, initially interpreted as perimortem. Exemplary in this regard is the CT analysis on human remains of Grauballe, which allowed the identification of several lesions as post-mortem [33].

An interesting case is that of the 13 natural mummies of a Roccapelago Crypt in the Italian Apennines. The crypt was used as a cemetery from the sixteenth century until the Napoleonic law, where burials inside churches were prohibited (late eighteenth century). Among 281 burials, 60 showed signs of mummification; probably some little lateral windows guaranteed the constant aeration and thus maintenance of the mummification. CT scan allowed the analysis of anatomical integrity, identification features, pathological changes and occupational and nutritional markers. In particular, CT analysis diagnosed important pathological conditions on three mummies: one affected by dysplasia, one a case of a giant cell tumour and another with the presence of a large infectious oto-mastoiditis [49]. Mummification similar to those of Roccapelago is now housed in our laboratory: a skull and a child's lower limb, both mummified. The skull was recovered in the sanctuary of Sacro Monte, in a burial chamber utilised as common ossuary. It presents a facial area covered by soft tissue, while in the fronto-parieto-occipital area, the tissue is completely missing. The full exposure of the occipital bone permitted proceeding with macroscopic investigations. In particular, the morphological analysis of the skull identified some masculine dimorphic traits such as the muscle insertions on the occipital portion, and the degree of obliteration of the cranial sutures; the analysis of these traits gave an estimation of an age at death to be 40 years. The CT analyses observed some neutral feminine facial traits covered by mummified tissue: a less prominent supraorbital ridge, absence of a subversion gonial mandible, straight marginal mandibular branch and a v-shaped chin; some masculine facial traits were noted: a square-shaped upper margin of the orbit, large and vertical direction of the mastoid process, and zygomatic arch extending posteriorly beyond the external auditory meatus. The X-ray of the child's lower limb allowed us to diagnose a fracture of the fibula (Fig. 6.3) [3].

6.3.3 Radiological Investigation on Fossil Remains

Since its birth, paleoanthropology based its considerations on information acquired from the external morphological study of the samples (Fig. 6.4). These approaches obviously limit the study of human evolution. The destructive processes occurring during fossilisation make it extremely difficult to analyse the findings. The radiological analysis could help the study of Human Evolution. Among the first analysed fossils are the Neanderthal remains from Krapina. Subsequent studies were made on the remains of *Homo erectus* that were published by Weidenreich

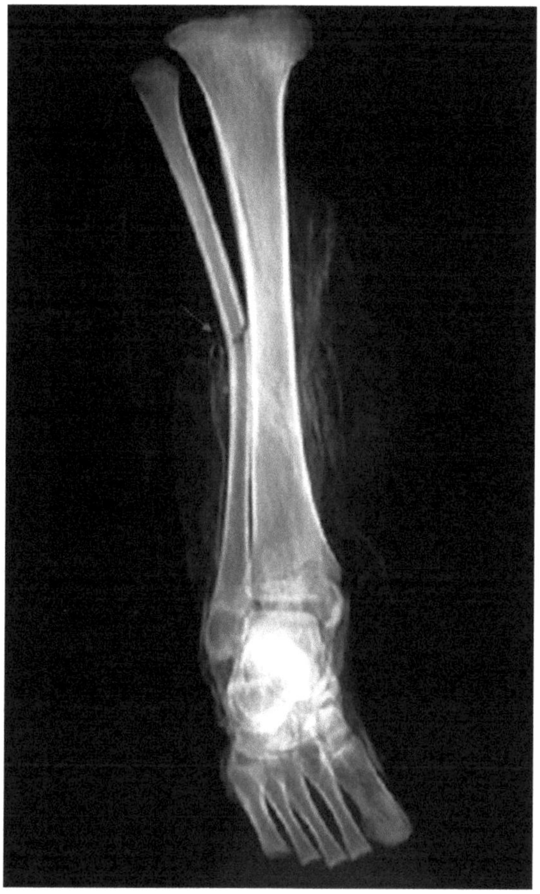

Fig. 6.3 Radiography of mummified lower limb of a child, from post-medieval ossuary, Sacro Monte Ossuary (Varese, Northern Italy)

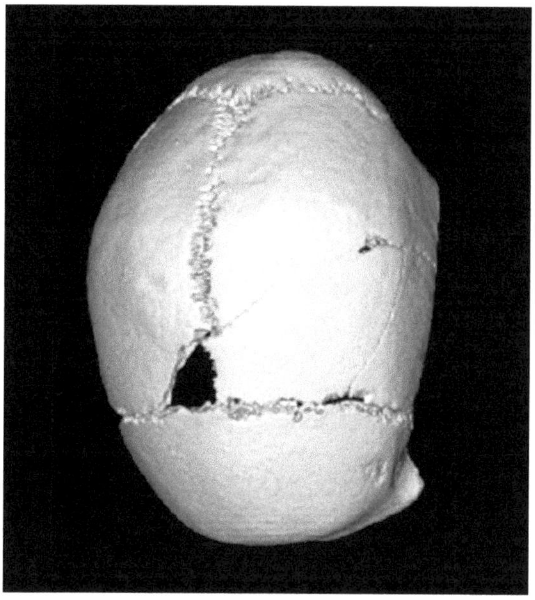

Fig. 6.4 CT of the skull of Valganna (Varese-Northern Italy)

[50]. In 1956, in the book dedicated to the centenary of the Neanderthal discovery, a radiological comparative study of three paleoanthropological skulls is showed. Thanks to the radiological contribution, it was possible to highlight the different paleoanthropological features of the finds [51]. Another interesting analysis is the study of a parietal fossil from Cova Negra, where the X-ray investigation revealed a trauma [52].

The hominid fossils are usually fragmented and trapped in a heavily calcified matrix when they come to light. Extrapolating the fossil from the calcified matrix is an operation that can definitely affect the finding. CT investigations can solve these problems by distinguishing the two materials and guiding the 3D reconstructions. The application of CT has undoubtedly facilitated the development of paleoanthropology. In 1984, CT was applied for the first time to a fossilised skull by the paleoanthropologist Conroy with radiologist Vannier. The examination was intended to identify the density of the bones of the skull. From that moment, paleoanthropologists used CT with a certain frequency [53]. An important study was carried out on the fossil skull of Neanderthals by Zollikofer in 2002 [54]. Starting from isolated fragments from the matrix, virtual reconstructions of the analysed district were made on computer through mirror imaging. Even the skull of Toumai (*Sahelanthropus tchadensis*) found in Chad in 2001 was radiologically examined to better investigate the morphological features of the fossil [55].

Tomographic investigations on fossilised endocranium reproduce the external morphology of the right cerebral hemisphere of the Taung child. They revealed important data for paleoneurological studies that indicated developmental elements in the design of the convolutions.

In regard to important discoveries in the field of paleoneurology is the study of the skulls of *Homo Florensis*, recovered on the Indonesian Island of Flores in 2003 and dating back 18,000 years. The *LB1* skull was examined by CT and the results showed that its shape was similar to those of *Homo Erectus* but an extended zone of the left broca's area and the large temporal lobes presented features associated with the complex cognition and language of modern humans [56].

6.4 Perspective

The application of radiological methodologies in archaeological fields will continue to proliferate. X-ray and CT scan are versatile and valuable as non-invasive tools of investigation in the multidisciplinary study of archaeology. Today, Magnetic Resonance Imaging (MRI) is especially used to study mummified remains. Ruhli has been able to efficaciously use MRI to image Egyptian and Peruvian mummies using an ultrashort pulse sequence, analysis that was not possible on earlier generations of MR scanners [57]. Other further radiological methodologies were adopted. In 2009 terahertz (THz) imaging was performed on parts of a mummy in conjunction with CT. THz gave more information regarding the tissues compared to CT. The THz waves being absorbed by water can penetrate deep into the mummified tissue. THz will find an increasingly important role in archaeological imaging.

In general, the progression of radiological methods will certainly have a relapse in the archaeological field. Being able to analyse objects without damaging them, to produce 3D images of the exhibits are all benefits necessary for archaeologists. Moreover, finds' digital data could be deposited in a Virtual Museum and the artefacts can be preserved in digital form, being available in the future [8].

Access to this equipment, however, continues to be a problem. CT scanners are still expensive when applied to a field other than the clinical one, in archaeology for instance, but from literature we noticed the growing collaboration between archaeology and radiology. This continuous approach could be formalised in the term "Archaeoradiology", with all other subspecialties such as "Bioarchaeoradiology" and "Paleoradiology". The birth of this scientific discipline could delineate a new professional profile of research. Only with such communication between radiologists and archaeologists an acceptable degree of accuracy in a field can be reached.

References

1. Corfield M (1973) Radiography in archaeology. University of London, Institute of Archaeology, London
2. Casali F (2006) X-ray digital radiography and computed tomography for cultural heritage. Archeometriai Műhely 1:24–28
3. Licata M, Borgo M, Armocida G, Nicosia L, Ferioli E (2015) New paleoradiological investigations of ancient human remains from North West Lombardy archaeological excavations. Skel Radiol 45:323–331
4. Licata M, Tosi A, Larentis O, Rossetti C, Iorio S, Pinto A (2019) Radiology of mummies. Semin Ultrasound CT MR 40(1):5–11
5. Licata M, Tosi A, Ciliberti R, Badino P, Pinto A (2019) Role of radiology in the assessment of skeletons from archeological sites. Semin Ultrasound CT MR 40(1):12–17
6. Cosmacini P, Piacentini P (2008) Notes on the history of the radiological study of Egyptian mummies: from X-rays to new imaging techniques. Radiol Med 133(5):615–626
7. Koenig W (1896) 14 Photographien mit RöngtenStrahlen. Johann Ambrosius Barth Verlag, Leipzig
8. Hughes S (2011) CT scanning in archaeology. In: Saba L (ed) Computer tomography-special applications. In Tech, Rijeka, pp 57–70
9. Petrie WMF (1898) Deshahesh 1897: fifteenth memoir of the Egyptian exploration fund. Egypt Exploration Fund, London
10. Moodie RL (1931) Roentgenologic studies of Egyptian and Peruvian mummies. Field Museum of Chicago, Chicago
11. Moss AA (1954a) The application of Zmys, gamma rays, ultra-violet and lnfra-red rays to the study of antiquities handbook for curators. The Museums Association) Part B Museum Technique Section, London
12. Moss AA (1954) The application of x-rays, gamma rays, ultra-violet and infra-red rays to the study of antiquities. Handbook for museum techniques. Section 4. The Museum Association, London
13. Dawson WR, Gary PHK (1968) Catalogue of Egyptian antiquities in the British museum: mummies and human remains 1. BMP, London

14. Harris JE, Weeks KR (1973) X-raying the pharaohs. Schribner & Sons, Chicago
15. Harris JE, Wente EF (1980) An X-ray atlas of the royal mummies. Chicago University Press, Chicago
16. Notman DNH, Anderson L, Beattie OB, Amy R (1987) Arctic paleoradiology: portable radiographic examination of two frozen sailors from the Franklin expedition (1845–1848). AJR 149:347–350
17. Chhem RK, Brothwell DR (2008) Paleoradiology: history and new developments paleoradiology imaging mummies and fossils. Springer, New York, pp 1–14
18. Beckmann EC (2006) CT scanning the early days. Br J Radiol 9:5–8
19. Boyer RS, Rodin EA, Grey TC, Connolly RC (2003) The skull and cervical spine radiographs of Tutankhamen: a critical appraisal. Am J Neuroradiol 24:1142–1147
20. Schulze D, Heiland M, Thurmann H, Adam G (2004) Radiation exposure during midfacial imaging using 4-and 16-slice computer tomography, cone bean computed tomography systems and conventional radiography. Dentomaxillofac Radiol 33:83–86
21. Cesarani F, Martina MC, Grilletto R, Boano R, Roveri AM, Capussotto V, Giuliano A, Celia M, Gandini G (2004) Facial reconstruction of a wrapped Egyptian mummy using MDCT. AJR Am J Roentgenol 183(3):755–758
22. Aufderheide AC (2003) The scientific study of mummies. Cambridge University Press, Cambridge
23. Hocquet FP, Calvo del Castillo H, Cervera Xicotencatl A, Bourgeois C, Oger C, Marchal A, Clar M, Rakkaa S, Micha E, Strivay D (2011) Elemental 2D imaging of paintings with a mobile EDXRF system. Anal Bioanal Chem 399(9):3109–3116
24. Schreiner M, Frühmann B, Jembrih-Simbürger D, Linke R (2004) X-rays in art and archaeology: an overview. Adv X-ray Anal 19(1):3–11
25. Corfield M (1982) Radiography of archaeological ironwork. In: Clarke RW, Blackshaw SM (eds) Conservation of iron. Trustees of the National Maritime Museum, London, pp 8–12
26. Rockley JC (1964) An introduction to industrial radiology. Butterworths, London
27. Scorsch D (1988) Technical examinations of ancient Egyptian theriomorphic hollow cast bronzes, some case studies conservation of ancient Egyptian materials. United Kingdom Institute for Conservation, London
28. Sturges D, McQueeney K, Avril E, Bonadies S (1991) Digital radioscopic examination of ancient bronze castings. In: Thompson DO, Chimenti DE (eds) Quantitative nondestructive evaluation. Plenum Press, New York, pp 1775–1781
29. University of Southampton: HTTP. www.sciencedaily.com/releases/2012/07/120710093520. Accessed 10 Jul 2012
30. Jansen RJ, Poulus M, Kotttman J, De Groot T, Huisman DJ, Stoker J (2006) CT: a new non-destructive method for visualizing and characterizing ancient Roman glass fragments in situ in blocks of soil. Radiographics 26(6):1837–1844
31. Applbaum N, Applbaum YH (2005) The use of medical computed tomography (CT) imaging in the study of ceramic and clay archaeological artifacts from the ancient near east. In: Uda M, Demortier G, Nakai I (eds) X-rays for archaeology. Springer, New York, pp 231–245
32. Lin Y, Seales WB (2005) Opaque document imaging: building images of inaccessible texts. Proceedings of the Tenth IEEE International Conference on Computer Vision (ICCV'05), p 662–669
33. Lynnerup N (2007) Mummies. Yrbk Phys Anthropol 50:162–190
34. Katalin TB, Veronika S, Attila K, Aufderheide AC (2000) Progress in soft tissue paleopathology. J Am Med Assoc 284(20):2571–2573
35. Piombino-Mascali D, Jankauskas R, Zink AR, Todesco MS, Aufderheide AC, Panzer S (2015) Paleoradiology of the Savoca Mummies, Sicily, Italy (18th–19th centuries AD). Anat Rec 298:988–1000. https://doi.org/10.1002/ar.23132
36. Carneiro C, Curate F, Borralho P, Cunha E (2013) Radiographic fetal osteometry: approach on age estimation for the Portuguese population. Forensic Sci Int 231:397
37. Dedouit F, Savall F, Mokrane FZ, Rousseau H, Crubézy E, Rougé D, Telmon N (2014) Virtual anthropology and forensic identification using multidetector CT. Br J Radiol 87:20130468
38. Kranioti EF, Vorniotakis N, Galiatsou C, Işcan MY, Michalodimitrakis M (2009) Sex identification and software development using digital femoral head radiographs. Forensic Sci Int 1189(1–3):113.e1–113.e7
39. Capasso L, Licata M, Pinto A, Fernianos F, Azizi T, Manzoli L, Centrella D, D'anastasio R (2017) A giant urinary bladder stone in the mummy of Lebanese Maronite Patriarch Joseph Tyan (1760–1820) and its environmental and nutritional implications. Radiography 23(1):67–72
40. Licata M, Armocida G, Broggini M, Borgo M (2017) To investigate the degenerative alterations of the spine in paleopathology. Acta Reumatol Port 42(1):94–95
41. Tonina E, Licata M, Pangrazzi C, Maspero U, Romano L, Larentis O (2018) A case of Concha Bullosa and potentially related evidences. Concha bullosa discovered in the bones of a medieval skeleton from Brentonico, Northeast Italy: a case report. Med Histor 2(2):94–98
42. Smith E (1912) The royal mummies. Duckworth Egyptology, London
43. Derry DE (1933) An X-ray examination of the mummy of King Amenophis I. Trans ASAE 34:47–48
44. Chhem RK, Schmit P, Fauré C (2004) Did Ramesses II really have ankylosing spondylitis? A reappraisal. Can Assoc Radiol J 55(4):211–217
45. Notman DNH (1986) Ancient scannings: computed tomography of Egyptian mummies. In: David AR (ed) Science in Egyptology. Manchester University Press, Manchester, pp 251–320

46. Ciranni R, Garbini F, Neri E, Melai L, Giusti L, Fornaciari G (2002) "The Braid s Lady" of Arezzo: a case of rheumatoid arthritis in a 16th century mummy. Clin Exp Rheumatol 20:745–752
47. Jackowski C, Bolliger S, Thali MJ (2008) Common and unexpected findings in mummies from ancient Egypt and South America as revealed by CT. Radiographics 28(5):1477–1492. https://doi.org/10.1148/rg.285075112
48. Murphy WA, zur Nedden D, Gostner P, Knapp R, Recheis W, Seidler H (2003) The iceman: discovery and imaging. Radiology 226(3):614–629
49. Petrella E, Piciucchi S, Feletti F, Barone D, Piraccini A, Minghetti C, Gruppioni G, Poletti V, Bertocco M, Traversari M (2016) CT scan of thirteen natural mummies dating back to the XVI–XVIII centuries: an emerging tool to investigate living conditions and diseases in history. PLoS One 11(6):e0154349
50. Weidenreich F (1935) The Sinanthropus population of Choukoutien (locality 1) with a preliminary report on new discoveries. Bull Geol Soc China 14:427–461
51. Singer R, Archangelsky SA (1958) A pietrified basidiomycete from Patagonia. Am J Bot 45:194–195
52. Lumley-Woodyear MA (1973) Anténéandertaliens et néandertaliens du Bassin méditerraneéen occidental européen: Cova Negra, Le Lazaret, Bañolas, Grotte du Prince, Carigüela, Hortus, Agut, Macassargues, LA Masque, Rigabe, La Crouzade, Les Peyrards, Bau de l'Aubesier. Université de Provence, Marseille
53. Conroy GC, Vannier MW (1984) Noninvasive three-dimensional computer imaging of matrix-filled fossil skulls by high-resolution computed tomography. Science 226:456–458
54. Zollikofer CP, Ponce de León MS, Lieberman DE, Guy F, Pilbeam D, Likius A, Mackaye HT, Vignaud P, Brunet M (2005) Virtual cranial reconstruction of Sahelanthropus tchadensis. Nature 434(7):755–759
55. Zollikofer CP, Ponce de Leon MS (2005) Virtual reconstruction: a primer in computer-assisted paleontology and biomedicine. John Wiley & Sons, New York
56. Jatmiko A, Falk D, Hildebolt C, Smith K, Morwood MJ, Sutikna T, Brown P, Jatmiko A, Saptomo EW, Brunsden B, Prior F (2005) The brain of LB1, Homo floresiensis. Science 308(5719):242–245
57. Rühli FJ, von Waldburg H, Nielles-Vallespin S, Böni T, Speier P (2007) Clinical magnetic resonance imaging of ancient dry human mummies without rehydration. JAMA 298(22):2618–2620

Interpretation of Diagnostic Imaging for Medicolegal Issues

7

Federica Vernuccio, Giuseppe Lo Re, Stefania Zerbo, Federico Midiri, Dario Picone, Sergio Salerno, Elvira Ventura, and Antonina Argo

7.1 Introduction

Forensic radiology is a relative recently emergent part of forensic medicine characterized by the application of radiological methods in criminal investigations, including the forensic M.E's radiological reports in civil or penal matters for judicial technical advice.

In the last 20 years there has been an increasing interest in the literature in forensic topics [1, 2]: publications in the last 5 years have doubled compared to the previous 5 years, as shown in Fig. 7.1. Among the different topics concerning forensic medicine, the main increase has been registered in forensic radiology topics, as shown in Fig. 7.2.

The different imaging modalities - i.e. X-rays, Computed Tomography (CT), Magnetic Resonance Imaging (MRI), and ultrasonography can be used depending on the individual case.

As Computed Tomography and Magnetic Resonance scanners are being integrated into forensic facilities, the pros and cons of forensic imaging investigations are still being explored, due to their enormous potential contribution in forensic medicine.

The application areas of forensic radiology are mainly represented by studies on living person to demonstrate bone age, search for foreign bodies, assess gunshot wounds, and forensic traumatology diagnostic examinations, which includes road accidents and acts of violence or abuse, and by investigations on dead corpses, including identification (age, sex, race) and evaluation of the cause, way and manner of death.

To date, the application of cross-sectional diagnostic imaging techniques to forensic medicine is more and more emerging as a new approach in disasters and mass-casualty situations [3–5]. The use of CT in many mass-casualty operations proved the utility of this technique not just in the identification of human cadavers, clothing and personal objects preserving evidences in an undisturbed state, but also in the "safety screening" prior to forensic assessment of the remains preventing dangers to the workers who handle the remains [3–5].

F. Vernuccio (✉)
Dipartimento di Biomedicina, Neuroscienze e Diagnostica avanzata, University of Palermo, Palermo, Italy

Department of Sciences for the Promotion of Health and Maternal and Child Care "G. D'Alessandro", University of Palermo, Palermo, Italy

G. Lo Re · F. Midiri · D. Picone
Dipartimento di Biomedicina, Neuroscienze e Diagnostica avanzata, University of Palermo, Palermo, Italy

S. Zerbo · E. Ventura · A. Argo
Department of Sciences for the Promotion of Health and Maternal and Child Care "G. D'Alessandro", University of Palermo, Palermo, Italy
e-mail: stefania.zerbo@unipa.it; Elvira.ventura@unipa.it; antonina.argo@unipa.it

S. Salerno
University of Palermo, Palermo, Italy
e-mail: sergio.salerno@unipa.it

G. Lo Re et al. (eds.), *Radiology in Forensic Medicine*,
https://doi.org/10.1007/978-3-319-96737-0_7

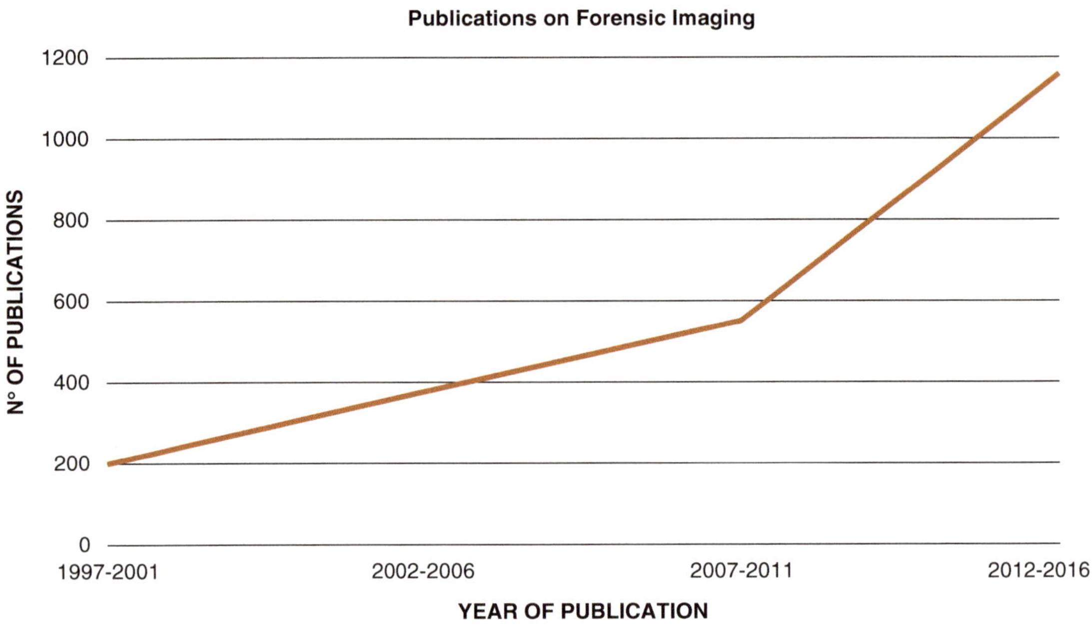

Fig. 7.1 Trends of the publications on forensic topics during the last 20 years, considering year-ranges of 5 years

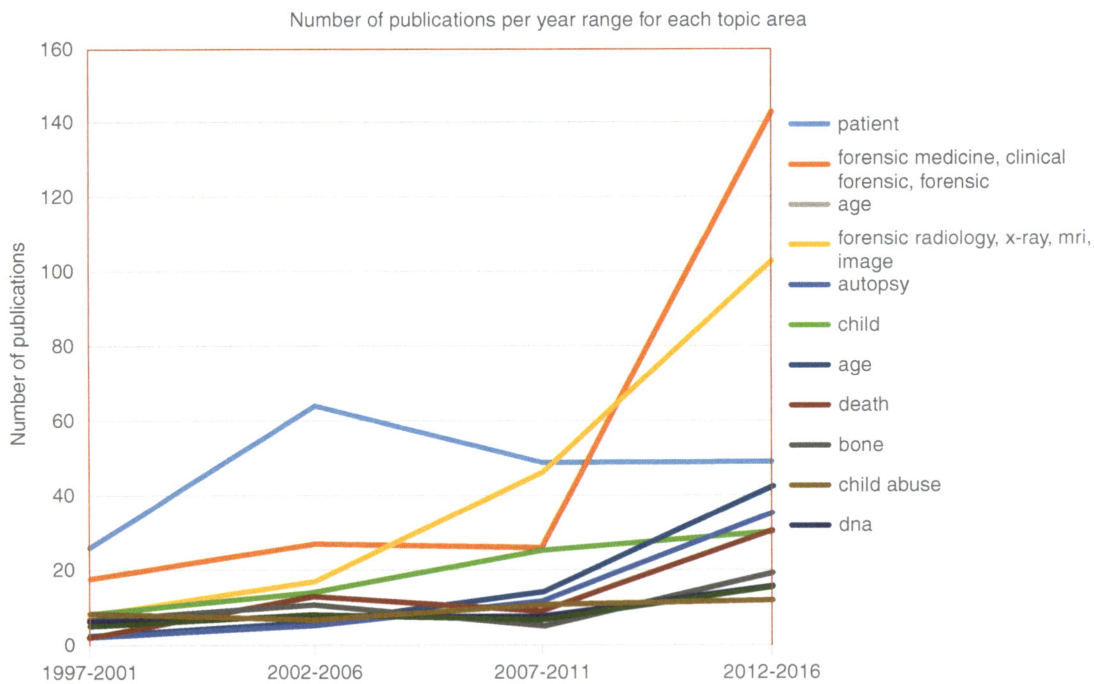

Fig. 7.2 Trends of the publications on the specific topic concerning forensic medicine during the last 20 years, considering year-ranges of 5 years

The value of diagnostic imaging techniques, from the old to the new ones depends upon timely and effective communication of the results. Interpretation of specimen images poses a number of particular challenges for the forensic radiologist that are not typical for a clinical radiologist. For this reason, the figure of a forensic radiologist as a sub specialist should be advised for medicolegal issues and interdisciplinary skills and knowledge would improve the economy and effectiveness of investigative efforts expanding scientific horizons and avoiding reinvention of well-proved tools.

The central function of forensic radiologist is to provide an imaging report that best fits the scope of the legal matter. Thus, the knowledge of the legal matter involved for each imaging acquisition, the information needed by the other forensic scientists, and the knowledge of which added value can be provided by the imaging technique compared to other forensic tests is mandatory for providing a report that will be of great value in the medicolegal study.

In accordance with these prerequisites, forensic radiologist is required to collect appropriate imaging objective foundations in which he will display and determinate the needed findings and will document what we will report eventual using multiplanar reconstructions to better elucidate the findings. However, the forensic radiologist is requested not just to collect data but also to give a qualified expert opinion as a subjective interpretation of the findings, always basing its evaluation on existing up-to-date literature and on knowledge of the legal context behind the images he evaluates. Finally, it is fundamental that a forensic radiological reconstruction of a legally relevant event must be accompanied by accurate and precise geometric ordering and written expression in the radiological report that is understandable to laypeople that will be involved in judging the legal matter. Interdisciplinary and multidisciplinary approach is mandatory to fulfill serve justice, in the view of old and emerging issues of forensic radiology. In order to gain this methodological accuracy, many American, European and Italian radiological societies are more and more publishing guidelines for imaging acquisition and reporting, with the purpose of make radiologist use the same language, provide clinicians all the information they need, but also to help the radiologist to have a national or international guideline to follow when reporting different radiological examinations. However, there are still some growing areas of radiology, as postmortem imaging, for which guidelines are still not available. Thanks to our experience on postmortem imaging, in particular the one related to mass disaster, our team of radiologists and coroners created a radiological template for postmortem imaging in mass disaster. Interdisciplinary and multidisciplinary approach is mandatory to fulfill serve justice, in the view of old and emerging issues of forensic radiology.

7.2 Legal Issue-Based Radiological Acquisition, Interpretation, and Report: From Conventional Radiology to Cross-Sectional Imaging

When approaching to forensic medical examiner radiological imaging documentation and report in civil or penal matters, it is mandatory to know which is the best imaging technique and approach to provide as much as possible information the judicial radiological technical advice is expected to furnish.

Conventional radiology has been widely used in the forensic field since the discovery of X-rays by William Roentgen in 1895. In 1896 Angerer proposed in Germany the use of the assessment of the development of the bones of the wrist to measure bone age. Levinsohn understood that X-rays could provide more accurate measures of skeletal method developed in 1883 by Bertillon and that included the evaluation of anthropometric measures. Radiography of the hand and left wrist is acquired in the anteroposterior view for age estimation and is most commonly assessed by using the method of Tanner Whitehouse [6, 7] or that of Greulich Pyle [8].

Concerning trauma, violence, and abuses [9–11], conventional radiography in emergency departments plays a role as a method of first level in the assessment of skeletal trauma findings as it allows the diagnosis of the presence and the type of fracture, the evaluation of the dislocation and/or angulation of the bone ends pre- and posttreatment, the identification of any dislocations or subluxations, identification of some complications due to the fracture, and to determine if the fracture occurred on structurally abnormal bone (pathological fracture).

The head, neck, and face are the body parts most commonly injured as more easily accessible for the abuses. The most commonly affected areas are the nose, likely secondary to its prominence; the left side of the face is the one most often injured perhaps because 90% of the population is right-handed. Another possible site affected by trauma in cases of domestic violence is the jaw and in particular the angle and the mandibular condyles. Another type of physical domestic violence is strangulation. Chest X-ray can shows, what result of strangulation, the presence of pulmonary edema, aspiration pneumonia and adult respiratory distress syndrome, findings already reported in the literature as characteristic lesions by strangulation. In the case of laryngeal fracture, it is possible to highlight the presence at radiography of subcutaneous emphysema in the soft tissues of the neck, sometimes associated to tracheal deviation due to edema or hematoma.

Another medicolegal issue that may require radiologists' advice is the search of foreign objects within human body: this may be due to different scenarios as voluntary injection of drug ovules, bullets in gunshot injuries, or surgical sponges accidentally left inside a patient. In these cases conventional radiography may highlight the presence of radiopaque objects but CT provides a better definition. Moreover, imaging may demonstrate the path of the bullet as a cloud of minute metallic fragments detached from the projectile, a phenomenon called "lead snowstorm" (Fig. 7.3).

Diagnostic imaging is also used for mass disasters, defined by the criticality of casualties and resources (personnel and equipment) involved in the disaster [3–5]. The term disaster is usually referred to unexpected and sudden events of various kinds (large accidents and natural disasters). The role of radiologist in this case vary from personal identification of cadavers, identification of bone and internal organ damages to security measures for involved working personnel. Conventional radiography was and is widely used in mass disaster because of its wider availability, albeit CT and MRI are also more and more used when available and needed.

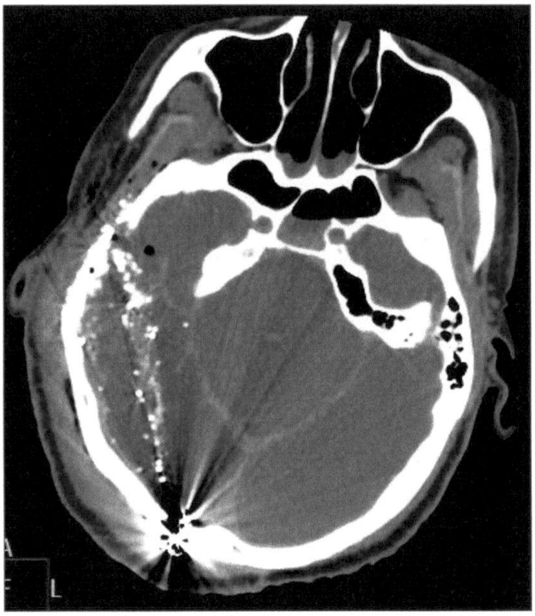

Fig. 7.3 CT scan shows a bullet in the occipital bone and the fragments along the path of the bullet in a 45-year-old photograph who was accidentally gunshotted during a wedding

Conventional radiographies provide a bi-dimensional view of a three-dimensional object: this basic knowledge is particularly important to be kept in mind when forensic scientists dispose just of skull bones of infants for evaluation of cranial sutures for age estimation or when the discontiguous arrangement of injured bones can make identification of a fracture difficult, thus limiting the eventual role of the judicial radiological technical advice. Moreover, in case of important traumatic injuries or of foreign objects in the body, the presence of damages to internal organs should be considered.

An important matter during mass disaster is cadaver identification. This procedure takes into account the comparison of antemortem and postmortem diagnostic images, mainly radiographies, age estimation obtained through dental and skeletal imaging, sex determination through the measurement of craniometrical and pelvic parameters and the evaluation of internal/external organs on CT (Fig. 7.4), and finally also the detection of personal belongings (Fig. 7.5).

Ultrasound, especially the so-called "fast ultrasound" (Focused Assessment with Sonography for Trauma), helps to identify lesions that require urgent surgery without creating the risk of a non-therapeutic laparotomy approach.

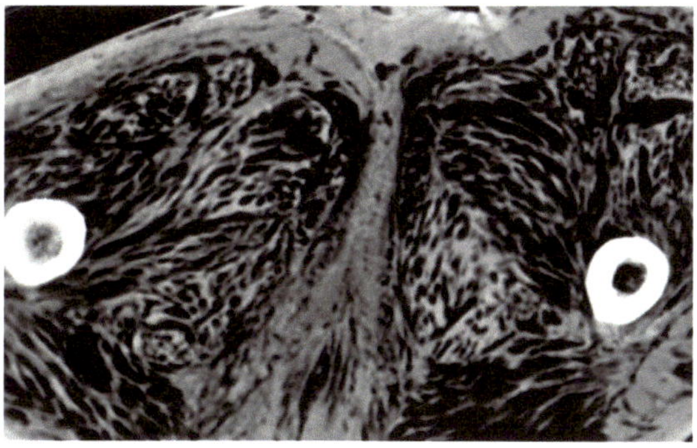

Fig. 7.4 Axial CT scan shows the residual cavernous corpses in a male victim recovered from water some months after a shipwreck

However, internal organ damages as brain hemorrhage and some damages to thoracic and abdominal organs cannot be adequately displayed at ultrasound and conventional radiography and their identification could turn to be useful in the determination of the entity of the damage to the individual and death diagnosis. In these cases, cross-sectional imaging through CT, and in few specific cases MRI, is particularly suited. Another growing field for cross-sectional imaging is the so-called "Virtopsy" [12], in which CT, and less frequently MRI, is used to study a dead corpse as a complement to conventional autopsy. CT is performed by scanning of the entire cadaver with millimetric slice and submillimetric reconstruction. The regions of particular interest, as complex fractures or teeth, can be subsequently reconstructed with sub-millimetric thickness, starting from the raw data of the examination. Workstations allow to obtain sagittal, coronal, oblique, and three-dimensional reconstructions that can then be sent to a departmental PACS.

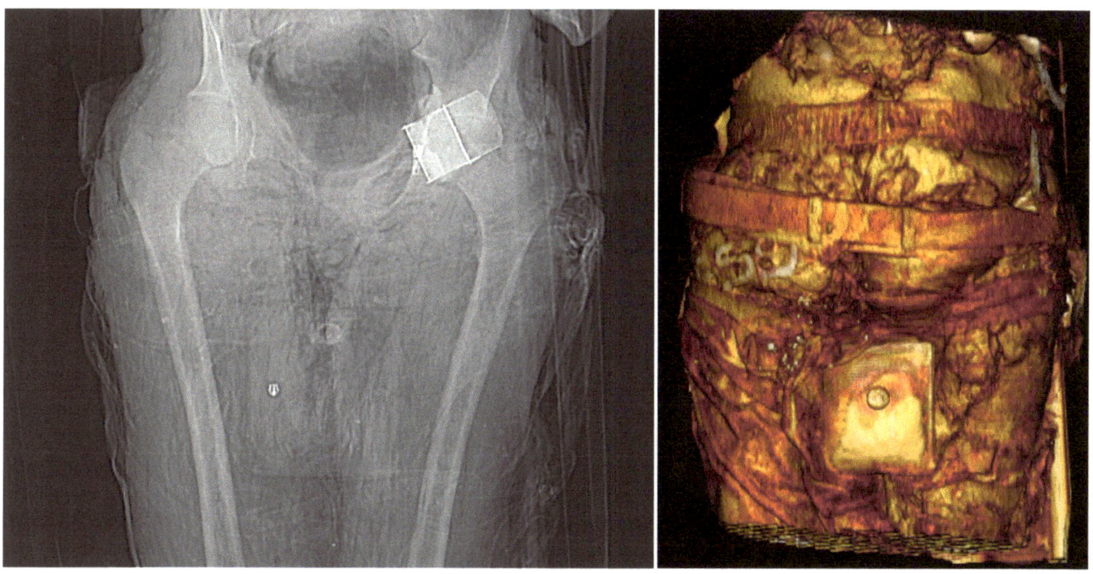

Fig. 7.5 Shows the presence of a wallet in a male victim recovered from water some months after a shipwreck; on the right, on conventional X-ray the wallet is located between the femurs but it is hardly detectable, while on the left through the Volume Rendering CT reconstruction it is possible to easily detect not just the wallet but also the "written" part "50" in the trousers of the victim

7.3 Malpractice in Radiology: A Growing Medicolegal Issue

A final consideration that cannot be avoided in this chapter regards legal issues encountered in diagnostic imaging, and in particular what is widely known as medical malpractice [13, 14].

Our society is actually changed as consumer rights are considered as a priority; thus, whenever the consumer demands anything, his demands must be promptly fulfilled. When this misconception is applied in medicine, the patient will think that physicians are responsible for every atypical or undesirable outcome resulting from the practice of medicine.

Spoken and written media often pursue journalistic and sensationalist profits submitting physicians to prejudgment on their medical practice long before proper technical and detailed investigation on the facts is carried out [15]. This leads to moral and material damages to both physicians and patients, increasing defensive and costly medical practice [16] without any benefit for the patient and maybe causing some negative effects on public health [17]. This is particularly true in diagnostic imaging: inappropriate prescriptions of CT and MRI have been demonstrated and lead to not justified ionizing radiation exposure and to increased health care costs [18].

Moreover, health, certainty of correct diagnosis, therapy, and resolution of any disease cannot be bought anywhere and the idea that all, including health, can be reduced to money is sickening. Thus, patients are not consumers, doctors are not vendors, and hospital are not supermarkets.

On the other hand, in opposition to the Hippocratic Oath that enjoins physicians to maintain their deportment and privileges while keeping patient's interests foremost, a "patient-centered medicine" is actually required to physicians: medical attention has to be focused on the individual patient's needs and concerns [19].

For this reason, more and more national and international guidelines have been published throughout the last two decades by many radiological societies. There is a guideline for any step of medical practice in diagnostic imaging: appropriateness criteria for prescription, definite protocols of exam acquisition, rules on ionizing radiation exposure and communication, rules on informed consent for diagnostic procedures that involve ionizing radiation, radiological templates for adequate reporting, and prescribed and well-defined imaging-based follow-up. Guidelines have been created to sum-up literature, to apply as much as possible the evidence-based medicine and to make all physicians speak a common language [20].

Worldwide law reform has been made to reduce the practice of so-called defensive medicine [21].

In Italy, according to the sentence n. 40708/2015 of the Penal High Court, only in case of existence of guidelines in conformity with medical practice it is possible to use them as a parameter for judging medical responsibility. The Law n. 8/2017 has just come into force in Italy, which highlights significance of guidelines and good clinical practices in relation to judgment of health care professional liability, in favor rei [22].

A guideline is still considered a sort of recommendation which equally brings benefit for the physician and the patient, when it is not as mandatory protocol to apply; it is not a law and it must be this way considering that each patient is a different and unique universe.

However, we agree with criticism of Authors who emphasize "to assure that the guidelines are at the service of the person, we must ask on what kind of evidence are they based and whether they will be beneficial to the individual patient" [23].

It is a common sense among all physicians who experience everyday practice that clinical practice guidelines cannot be assumed as an objective code of action and, according to the Italian High Penal Court, the respect of the guidelines by the physicians does not exempt from being considered as "guilty" if the clinical context imposes a deviation from them. Medicolegal responsibility in clinical practice is such a complex issue and the study of this topic goes beyond the intent of this chapter.

Concerning radiologic claims that have led to medical malpractice lawsuits most frequently have been due to "failure to diagnose" [24, 25]. Around 4% of radiological reports contain errors, but most of them are of minor degree or do not cause injury to patients [26]. The most common generic errors subject to an initial malpractice suit–failure of diagnosis concern breast cancer and injuries of all non-vertebral bones [24].

The presence of error is a necessary but not a sole requisite for the determination of negligence [27]. Firstly, the main concern is if the error was relevant for patient's treatment and prognosis and secondly if the radiologist was really negligent, that means, according to the Wisconsin appellate court, if the physician used the degree of skill and care that a reasonable physician, or an average physician would in the same or similar circumstances [28]. The question of whether a missed radiologic diagnosis can be defined as malpractice has confounded radiologists, patients, attorneys, judges, jurors, and the general public for years, and it is not likely to be easily and uniquely resolved in the foreseeable future [27].

References

1. Baglivo M, Winklhofer S, Hatch GM, Ampanozi G, Thali MJ, Ruder TD (2013) The rise of forensic and post-mortem radiology—analysis of the literature between the year 2000 and 2011. J Forensic Radiol Imaging 1:3–9
2. De Bakker HM, Soerdjbalie-Maikoe V, Kubat B, Maes A, de Bakker BS (2016) Forensic imaging in legal medicine in the Netherlands: retrospective analysis of over 1700 cases in 15 years' experience. J Forensic Radiol Imaging 6:1–7
3. Young VS, Eggesbø HB, Gaarder C, Næss PA, Enden T (2017) Radiology response in the emergency department during a mass casualty incident: a retrospective study of the two terrorist attacks on 22 July 2011 in Norway. Eur Radiol 27:2828–2834
4. Bolster F, Linnau K, Mitchell S, Roberge E, Nguyen Q, Robinson J, Lehnert B, Gross J (2017) Emergency radiology and mass casualty incidents-report of a mass casualty incident at a level 1 trauma center. Emerg Radiol 24:47–53
5. Brunner J, Rocha TC, Chudgar AA, Goralnick E, Havens JM, Raja AS, Sodickson A (2014) The Boston Marathon bombing: after-action review of the Brigham and Women's Hospital emergency radiology response. Radiology 273:78–87
6. Tanner JM, Healy M, Goldstein H et al (2001) Assessment of skeletal maturity and prediction of adult height (TW3 method), 3rd edn. WB Saunders, Harcourt Publishers Ltd, London
7. Tanner JM, Whitehouse RH, Cameron N et al (1983) Assessment of skeletal maturity and prediction of adult height (TW2 method), 2nd edn. Academic Press, London
8. Greulich WW, Pyle SI (1959) Radiographic atlas of skeletal development of the hand and wrist, 2nd edn. Stanford University Press, Stanford, CA
9. Bhole S, Bhole A, Harmath C (2014) The black and white truth about domestic violence. Emerg Radiol 21:407–412
10. Giurani F, Hasan M (2000) Abuse in elderly people: the granny battering revisited. Arch Gerontol Geriatr 31:215–220
11. Kemp AM, Butler A, Morris S, Mann M, Kemp KW, Rolfe K, Sibert JR, Maguire S (2006) Which radiological investigations should be performed to identify fractures in suspected child abuse? Clin Radiol 61:723–736
12. Thali MJ, Jackowski C, Oesterhelweg L, Ross SG, Dirnhofer R (2007) VIRTOPSY—the Swiss virtual autopsy approach. Legal Med 9:100–104
13. Jena AB, Seabury S, Lakdawalla D, Chandra A (2011) Malpractice risk according to physician specialty. N Engl J Med 365:629–636
14. Filograna L, Tartaglione T, Filograna E, Cittadini F, Oliva A, Pascali VL (2010) Computed tomography (CT) virtual autopsy and classical autopsy discrepancies: radiologist's error or a demonstration of post-mortem multi-detector computed tomography (MDCT) limitation? Forensic Sci Int 195:e13–e17
15. Prestes LCL Jr, Tourinho EK, Rangel M (2012) Medico-legal analysis of lawsuits in medical imaging. Radiol Bras 45:98–100
16. Chen J, Majercik S, Bledsoe J, Connor K, Morris B, Gardner S, Scully C, Wilson E, Dickerson J, White T, Dillon D (2015) The prevalence and impact of defensive medicine in the radiographic workup of the trauma patient: a pilot study. Am J Surg 210:462–467
17. Squillaci E, Bolacchi F, Scaggiante J, Ricci F, Pugliese L, Bergamini A, Garaci F, Floris R (2016) Inappropriateness of diagnostic imaging examinations in the inpatient setting: a case study research. Radiol Med 122:221–227
18. American College of Radiology/American Roentgen Ray Society (2010) Significant amount of inappropriate CT and MRI referrals from primary care physicians, study finds. ScienceDaily. www.sciencedaily.com/releases/2010/03/100301091308.htm
19. Bardes CL (2012) Defining "patient-centered medicine". N Engl J Med 366:782–783
20. Grilli R, Magrini N, Penna A, Mura G, Liberati A (2000) Quality of practice guidelines developed by specialty societies. The need for a critical appraisal. Lancet 355:103
21. Waxman DA, Greenberg MD, Ridgely MS, Kellermann AL, Heaton P (2014) The effect of mal-

practice reform on emergency department care. N Engl J Med 371:1518–1525
22. Ferrara SD, Baccino E, Bajanowski T et al (2013) Malpractice and medical liability. European guidelines on methods of ascertainment and criteria of evaluation. Int J Legal Med 127:545–557
23. Balducci L (2014) Practice guidelines that may kill. J Med Pers 12:96–98
24. Whang JS, Baker SR, Patel R, Luk L, Castro A (2013) The causes of medical malpractice suits against radiologists in the United States. Radiology 266(2):548–554
25. Baker SR, Shah S, Ghosh S, Castro A (2015) Radiology medical malpractice suits in gastrointestinal radiology: prevalence, causes, and outcomes. Emerg Radiol 22:141–145. https://doi.org/10.1007/s10140-014-1268-3
26. Borgstede JP, Lewis RS, Bhargavan M, Sunshine JH (2004) RADPEER quality assurance program: a multifacility study of interpretive disagreement rates. J Am Coll Radiol 1:59–65
27. Berlin L (2007) Radiologic errors and malpractice: a blurry distinction. AJR Am J Roentgenol 189(3):517–522
28. Department of Regulation and Licensing v. State of Wisconsin Medical Examining Board, 572 NW2d 508 (Wis App1997)

Forensic Radiology and Identification

8

Danilo De Angelis, Carmelo Messina, Luca Sconfienza, Francesco Sardanelli, Cristina Cattaneo, and Daniele Gibelli

8.1 Personal Identification of the Dead

When personal identification is requested, several disciplines can be applied, such as odontology, genetics and dactyloscopy. However, when no dactyloscopic or genetic profiles can be retrieved, forensic radiology is one of the most successful manners of reaching a positive identification.

Forensic radiology is crucial in the identification protocol of cadavers, thanks to the wide diffusion of radiological examinations within the population which may function as ante-mortem material and the possibility to perform radiological analysis on the same anatomical area of the body. Conventional radiology was historically one of the first radiographic techniques applied by experts [1], but with time more advanced radiographic techniques, such as computed tomography, have recently been used [2].

Radiological images represent a valuable source of information for this type of identification, as not only the presence or absence of some features but also their topographical and morphological comparisons may lead the judgment towards identification. In the same spirit of identification approaches in forensic genetics, frequency of a specific feature may be analysed in a population to obtain a numerical indication about the empiric probability that two individuals share the same characteristic. In literature, several articles have, for example, analysed the diffusion of specific odontological features in a population or the presence of peculiarities of frontal sinuses [3, 4].

In addition to this merely statistical information which expresses the probability that two persons may share the same number of septa within the frontal sinuses or a filling in the same tooth, the comparison between radiological images allows to verify the true topographical and morphological concordance of the same features.

Personal identification means assigning human remains to a specific identity based on individualising characteristics that can be recognised both in ante-mortem and in post-mortem data [5–7]. These characteristics have to be permanent or subject to minimal morphological changes in the time lapse between the ante-mortem and post-mortem radiographic comparison and individual in shape and size. From an aetiological point of view, they may belong to three main categories:

- Therapeutical features: they include joint and dental prostheses, dental works, as well as

D. De Angelis (✉) · C. Messina · L. Sconfienza
F. Sardanelli · C. Cattaneo · D. Gibelli
Dipartimento di Scienze Biomediche per la Salute, Università Degli Studi di Milano, Milan, Italy
e-mail: danilo.deangelis@unimi.it; carmelo.messina@unimi.it; luca.sconfienza@unimi.it; francesco.sardanelli@unimi.it; cristina.cattaneo@unimi.it; daniele.gibelli@unimi.it

G. Lo Re et al. (eds.), *Radiology in Forensic Medicine*,
https://doi.org/10.1007/978-3-319-96737-0_8

other structures usually inserted in soft tissues (i.e. artificial lens and mammary prostheses).

- Pathological features: they include bone calluses, caries, osteomas, etc.
- Anatomical features: as they are not frequently taken into consideration in daily practice by clinicians, they could be less detectable by unexperienced forensic practitioners. They include the natural shape and morphology of different skeletal and dental structures, as well as anatomical variants.

8.1.1 Radiology in Forensic Odontology

Odontological identification is one of the most used and reliable manners of identification, widely accepted by all scientific communities. The use of radiographs in dental identifications is massive as, in most of the cases, the final judgment relies on the comparison between a missing person's radiographic images from a dental clinic and radiographs performed on an unknown corpse.

In odontological identification, besides the possibility of quantifying the probability that another individual shares the same distribution of dental features in a specific population [8], the forensic odontologist uses ante-mortem radiographs to detect peculiar and unique features to be looked for on an unknown cadaver. As previously mentioned, morphological uniqueness can be found in anatomic, pathologic and therapeutic features; the forensic operator should therefore have a deep knowledge of dentistry to correctly focus the attention on paramount features and to be ready to explain in an official report or in a court of law the reasons of his/her choices.

The classical ante-mortem radiographic dental material is represented by "intra oral" exams (periapical, bitewings, occlusal radiographs) and "extra oral" exams as orthopantomograms (Fig. 8.1). Nowadays, as most advanced extra oral techniques such as computed tomography and cone-beam computed tomography are often used in dentistry, ante-mortem peculiarities are frequently looked for on this material (Fig. 8.1). Moreover, data from computed tomography give the forensic operator the possibility to detect the presence of even minimal abnormalities and to compare also volumes and three-dimensional surfaces. To better compare ante-mortem with post-mortem shapes, the adopted post-mortem radiographic technique should take into consideration the projection of the ante-mortem image: the best solution to produce post-mortem dental radiographs is to use the same technique and technology that was used to produce the radiograph of the missing person. Unfortunately, this is not always possible, for example, it is not common and easy to perform an orthopantomogram on a dead body, but periapical post-mortem radiographs can easily simulate the correct projection and can be used to produce comparable images (Fig. 8.2).

Dental identification data could also come from radiographs not performed for dental purposes. For example, a frontal or lateral view of the head of a subject may show some potentially useful dental features (Fig. 8.3).

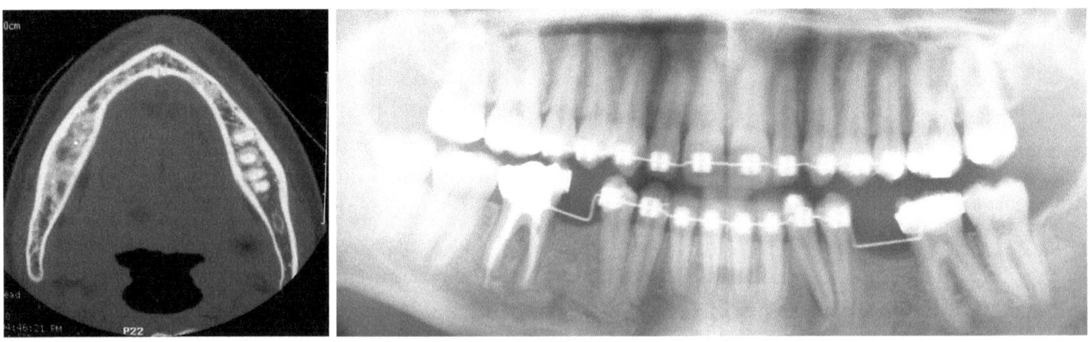

Fig. 8.1 CT and OPG as ante-mortem material of a missing subject

Especially in cases of mass disasters, the availability of a portable X-ray machine and a digital intraoral sensor can improve the efficiency of dental identification; anyway, self-developing intraoral films are a user-friendly alternative to digital sensors. We show some examples of radiographic dental identification in which anatomic, pathologic and therapeutic features are taken into consideration.

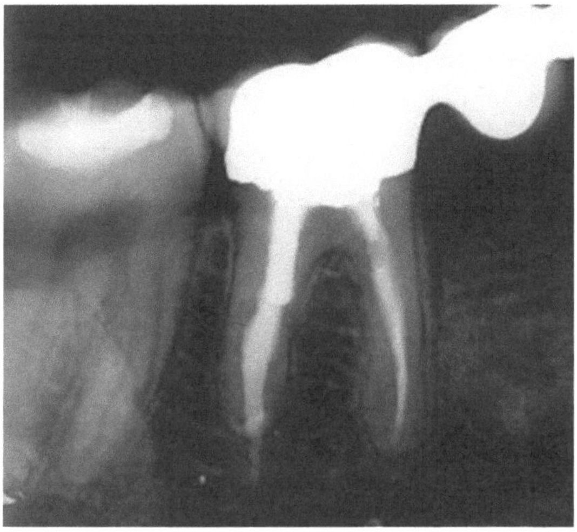

Fig. 8.2 Post-mortem periapical radiograph to be compared with ante-mortem images in Fig. 8.1: even if two different techniques are used (OPG and periapical) the post-mortem radiograph shows the first right lower molar with the same projection of the ante-mortem one

Orthopantomograms and periapical radiographs clearly show, for instance, the peculiar relationships between an impacted wisdom tooth and the surrounding mineralised structures (Fig. 8.4) or the unique morphology of the apical third of a second inferior premolar root and the shape of a molar pulp chamber (Fig. 8.5).

Caries and periodontosis create unique shapes easily detectable using X-rays; if the time interval between the ante-mortem and the post-mortem images is short, these characteristics are very useful from an identification point of view (Fig. 8.6).

Root canal therapies, endodontic posts, crowns, bridges and filling are all handcrafted and their morphology is unique by definition; all these features are very well detectable through radiology and used in odontological identifications (Fig. 8.7).

8.1.2 The Skeleton in Identification

Apart from the teeth, everything else in the skeleton and body can be used for identification.

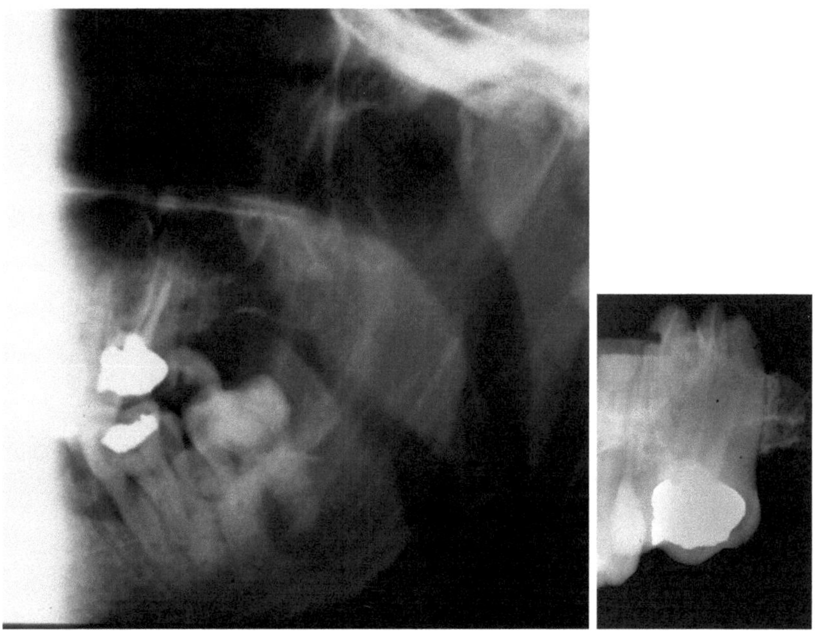

Fig. 8.3 On the left, lateral radiograph of the head of a missing person that shows interesting and peculiar therapeutic features of an upper molar; on the right the post-mortem periapical radiograph taken with the right orientation for a positive identification

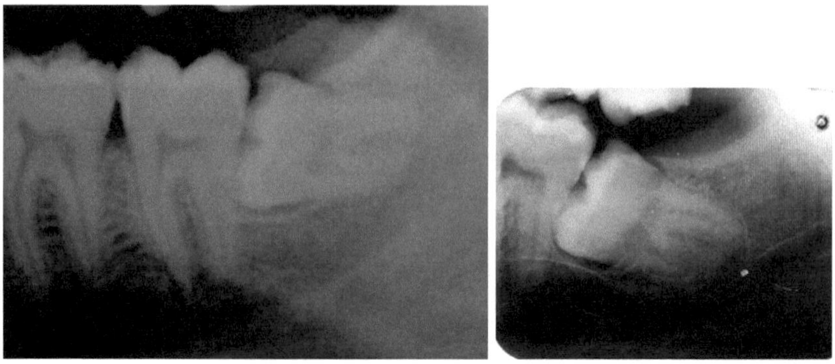

Fig. 8.4 On the left, an ante-mortem portion of an OPG showing a wisdom tooth; on the right the post-mortem periapical radiograph performed for identification purposes

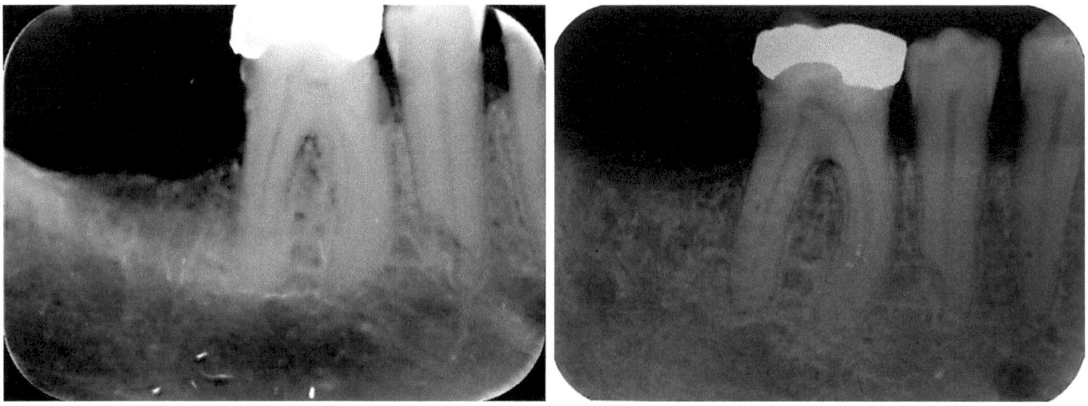

Fig. 8.5 On the left a periapical radiograph of a missing person; on the right the periapical radiograph of an unknown corpse showing the same morphological peculiarities of the molar pulp chamber and of the second premolar apex

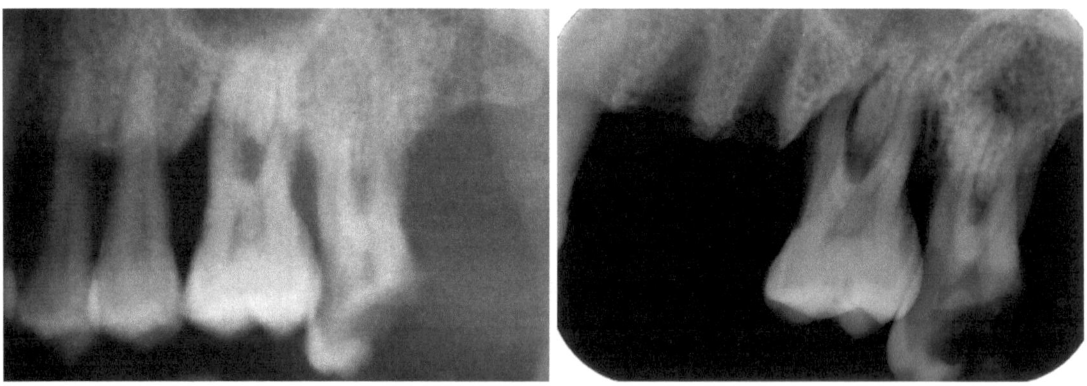

Fig. 8.6 On left the ante-mortem radiograph of a missing person with a severe bone resorption and a cavity on the second molar; on the right a post-mortem image of an unknown body showing the same bone resorption pattern and the same cavity morphology. As the time gap between ante- and post-mortem material is very short these pathologic features are usable for an identification case

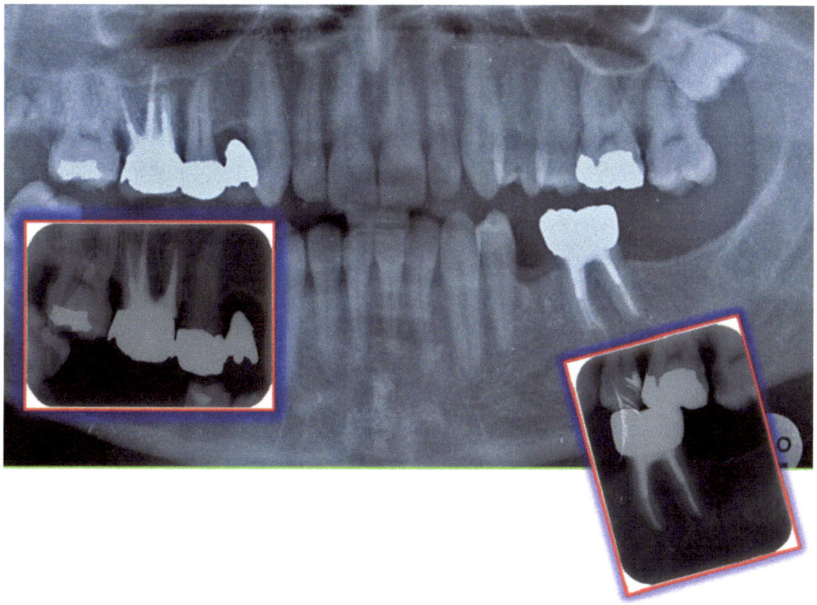

Fig. 8.7 Ante-mortem OPG showing root canal therapies, endodontic posts, a crown, a bridge and fillings; the superimposed periapical post-mortem radiographs show the correspondent morphology of all the handcrafted dental works

In forensic radiology, research for identification has been performed on several body areas through different procedures of imaging.

8.1.2.1 Head

In the head, there are several structures which can be used for identification, the frontal sinuses being the most standardised. In particular, frontal sinuses have been widely analysed, both for the variability of shape and size and individuality of sinus profile. In fact, even homozygotic twins have different frontal sinuses [9]. Different authors focused on the application of advanced techniques, applied to the frontal sinuses, aiming at reaching an objective and quantitative method of analysis that could replace the simple visual comparison with encouraging results [10].

Several authors attempted at assessing the anatomical uniqueness of frontal sinuses through different approaches: an example is provided by Yoshino et al. who in 1987 proposed a classification of frontal sinuses according to size, shape, asymmetry, outline of the superior border, presence of accessory septa, possible presence of supraorbital cells and invasion of orbital areas. The total number of possible combinations was above 20,000 [4].

Calculation of inter-observer error between several operators in correctly matching radiographic images of frontal sinuses belonging to the same individual was performed: some experiments of this type show percentages of repeatability close to 100% [11, 12].

Conventional radiography is one of the most frequently observed ante-mortem materials in case of frontal sinus comparison, and therefore several methods of identification have been developed specifically on this type of procedure (Figs. 8.8 and 8.9).

The most important source of error in using X-ray examination concerns the radiographic quality: Brogdon considered also the position of the cadaver in the PM X-ray as a relevant source of error [13].

Recent clinical approaches concern the use of computer tomography, which is expected to gain more and more importance in the forensic scenario, with its increased use as a diagnostic tool. The main approach concerns the improvement of existing methods of identification previously based on conventional radiography. For example, Tatlisumak and co-workers [14] defined for frontal sinuses a simple and useful method for identification using computed tomography scans.

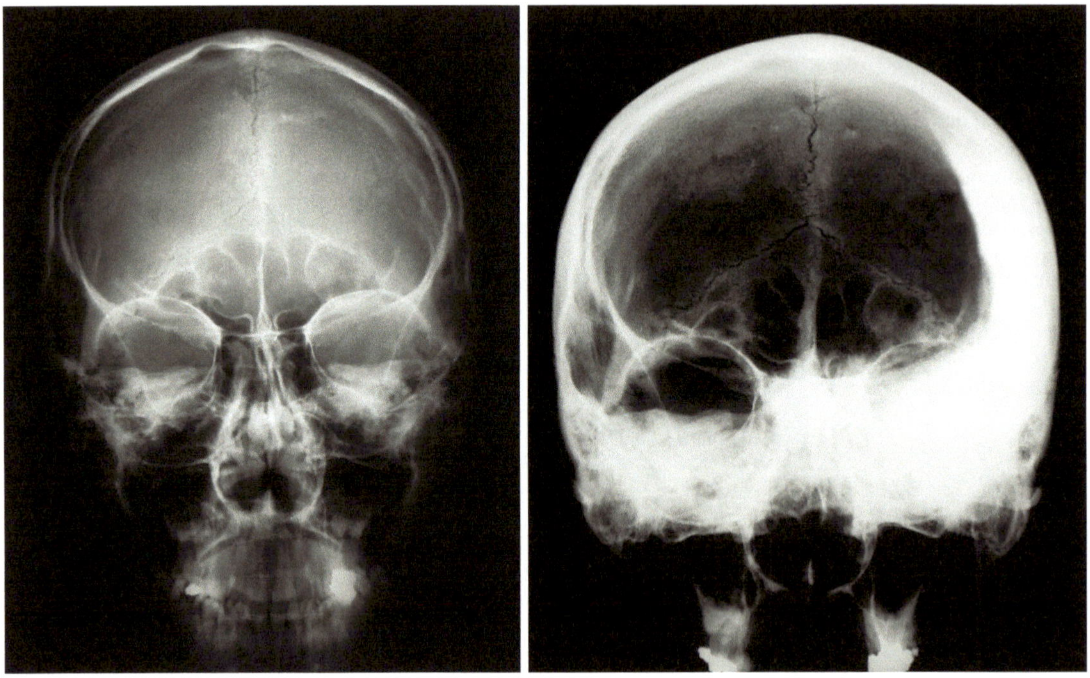

Fig. 8.8 Comparison of frontal sinuses from AM material (on the left) and PM material (on the right)

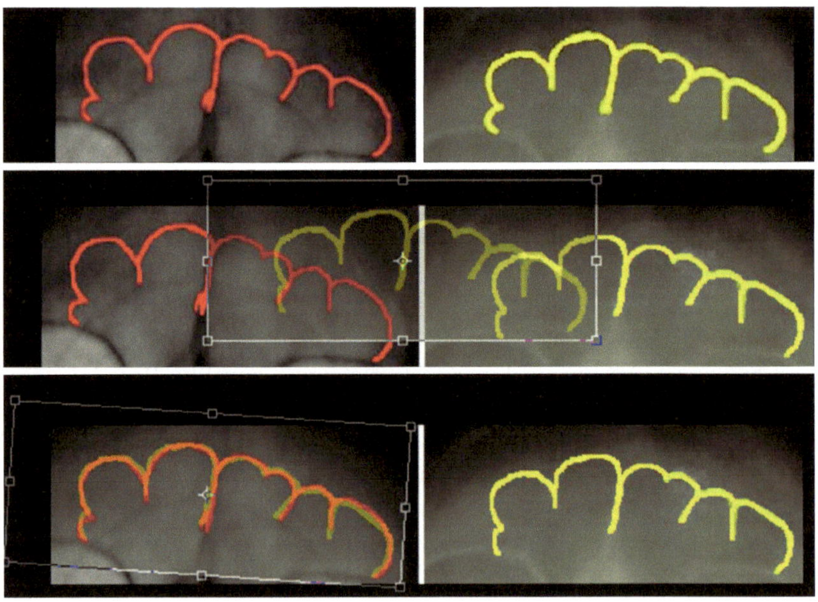

Fig. 8.9 Personal identification through frontal sinuses: on the left, the AM material, on the right the PM material

They studied both morphological and metrical features, concluding that the morphological descriptions (presence or absence of the sinuses, presence, absence or incompleteness of intra-sinus septum, etc.) were found significantly different in the study population. Concerning the quantitative measurement, they found that the anteroposterior lengths of the sinuses only were significant in that series. Adding this measurement to the morphological approach, the success

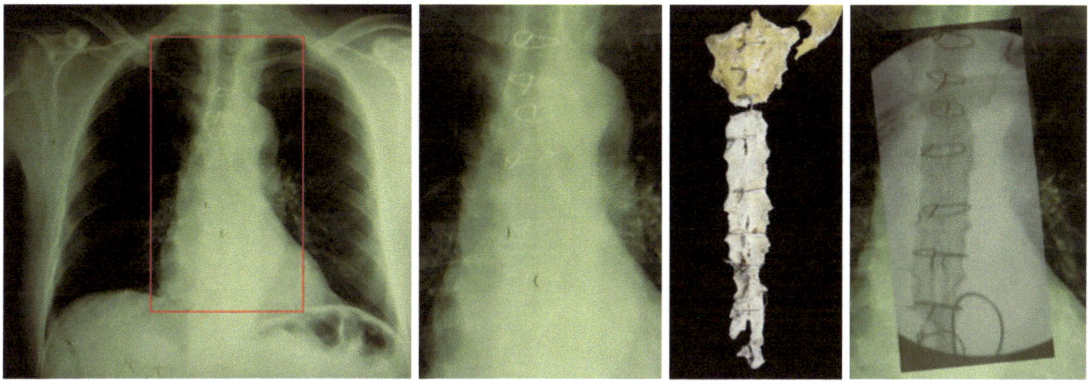

Fig. 8.10 Personal identification through the metallic sutures of previous thoracotomy; on the left, details of AM material; in the middle, skeletonised sternum; on the right, superimposition between PM X-ray of the sternum and AM material

rate significantly increased. Tatlisumak and colleagues stressed the need of a common approach for comparison of frontal sinus, as observed for the analysis of fingerprints [14].

However the most important advancement provided by computed tomography scan concerns the chance of volume segmentation and reconstruction of 3D volume of anatomical structures. A pilot study has been performed by Beaini et al. in 2015, who segmented volumes of frontal sinuses from 20 cone-beam computed tomography scans and verified the reproducibility of a correct match of 3D models belonging to the same individual, based on the mean point-to-point distance between the two surfaces. In 100% of cases, the two operators correctly identified the frontal sinuses as belonging to the same individual [15].

However, the other paranasal sinuses can be used for personal identification, as they develop randomly with a high variability. The assessment of maxillary and sphenoid sinuses may be valid as well, although their use is less standardised than the frontal sinuses.

8.1.2.2 Trunk

Another area often analysed for personal identification is the thorax, which proved to be very useful in several forensic cases because of the remarkable number of features offered and the high availability of thoracic X-rays as antemortem material [16].

Kuehn et al., for example, measured the reliability of visual comparison, in pointing out the useful features in the identification process and in evaluating the possible sources of error [17]. According to the examiners, the most useful elements come from the anatomical features of vertebrae, ribs and clavicle (Figs. 8.10 and 8.11).

Valenzuela reported a case of identification conducted throughout the comparison of lumbar X-rays, underlying the unique shape of osteophytes, transverse and spinous processes, and trabecular pattern of the vertebral body [18].

Another promising field of research concerns validation studies, where quantification of the error is reached by the mismatch rate given by operators in assigning ante-mortem with post-mortem radiographs: a recent example is provided by Stephan et al. who validated the comparison of chest X-rays [19], although similar experiments were applied also to other bone districts [20, 21]. In all these cases operators provide a manual identification through the observation of bone profiles and the quantification is given by the percentage of correct match.

8.1.2.3 Limbs

Identification from a single bone is based on the observation of single morphological characteristics, keeping in mind that the individuality increases with the number of pathological, deformative and therapeutical characteristics. As for the other districts cited above, the morphological analysis of the

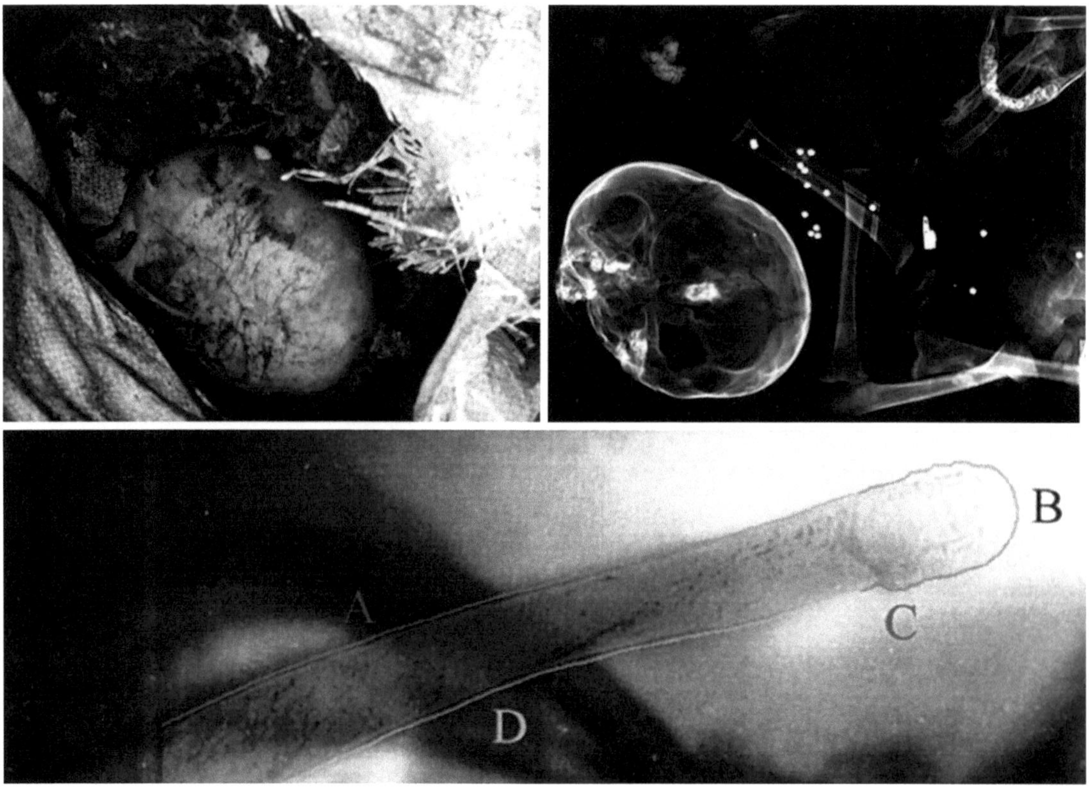

Fig. 8.11 Personal identification performed through X-ray superimposition of the clavicle; the letters indicate the individualising anatomical features

bones may lead to personal identification: an example is given by Dean et al., who simulated a comparison between fictitious ante-mortem and post-mortem material using pre- and postsurgical radiographs of the ankle [22]. In 2005, Koot and colleagues published an article concerning the visual comparison of hand radiographs, reporting that the observers with the lowest experience are less skilful than those with a greater experience. The accuracy of the method is exclusively based on expert experience, but the study proposes a numerical evaluation of their skills.

One of the most recent fields of application consists in the quantification of shapes and bone silhouettes through morphological evaluation such as Fourier analysis: an example concerns clavicle bones [23]. With time, engineering models of shape assessment have acquired more and more popularity in forensic anthropology, and seem promising in order to reach the final quantification of skeletal identification.

Concerning bone trabecular pattern, both quantitative and qualitative approaches are found in the literature [20]. Kahana and colleagues proposed a quantification method based on a software that could numerically describe the optical density of trabeculae through the creation of densitographs (Kahana et al., 1994).

Limb prostheses are useful for personal identification as well, as they allow a morphological comparison and often report a code on the metallic parts which may be useful for reconstructing the identity suspect (Figs. 8.12, 8.13, and 8.14).

8.1.2.4 The Issue of Quantification

Although personal identification is widely applied to forensic cases, the forensic experts have not yet defined a common method to express the results. Fischman, for example, states that one to four concordant features without discrepancies are usually considered to claim an identity [6]. On the other side, Brogdon states that a minimum number

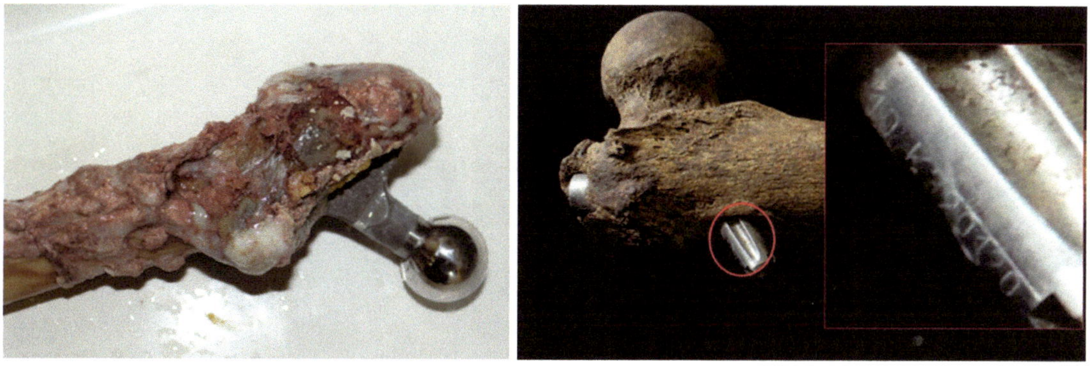

Fig. 8.12 Example of femoral prosthesis; detail of code on the metallic device

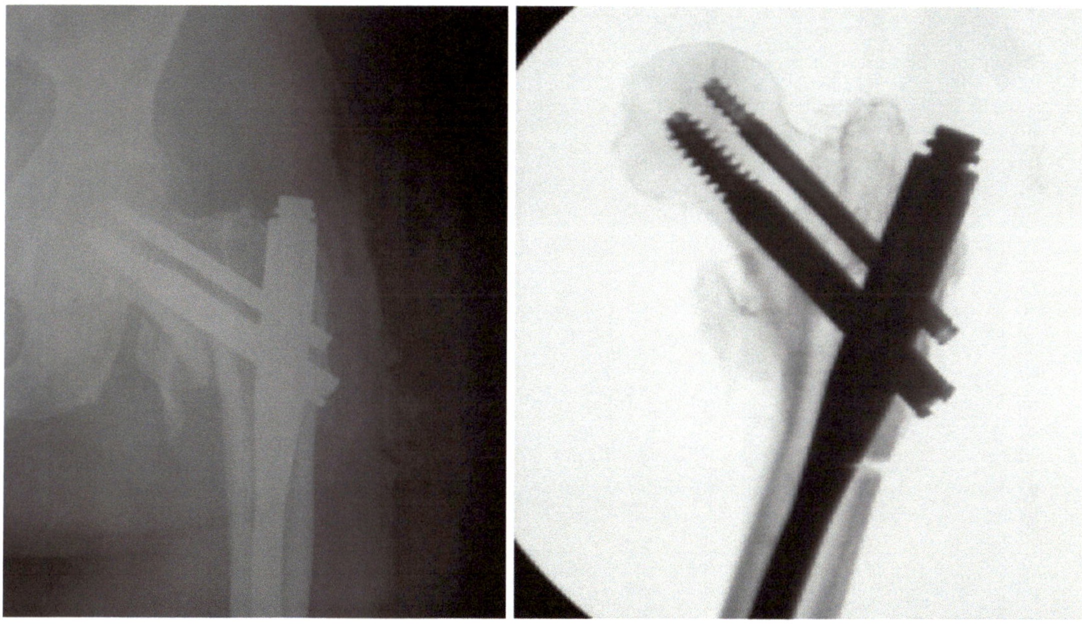

Fig. 8.13 Personal identification performed through metallic device: on the left, AM material, on the right PM material

should not be pursued since a series of common and non-specific features is sometimes enough to claim an identity. Finally, Kuehn and colleagues [17] claim that several concordant traits in at least two different body parts are needed. In general, the identification process is quite easy and straightforward when dealing with bone prosthesis, bone calluses, osteoarthritis and other exceptional traits; indeed, Mann and Brogdon state that one feature is enough when it is unique and unmistakable [24], but the verification of identity is more difficult when no particular feature is involved. Moreover, a research carried out on the frequencies of morphological characteristics of the skeleton, such as fractures, pathological conditions and surgical hardware, suggested that some features previously supposed to be sufficiently unique may be quite common [25].

Some experts claim that quantifying and standardising the features useful for personal identification is not requested and that the expert "qualitative" opinion is valid and sufficient [26].

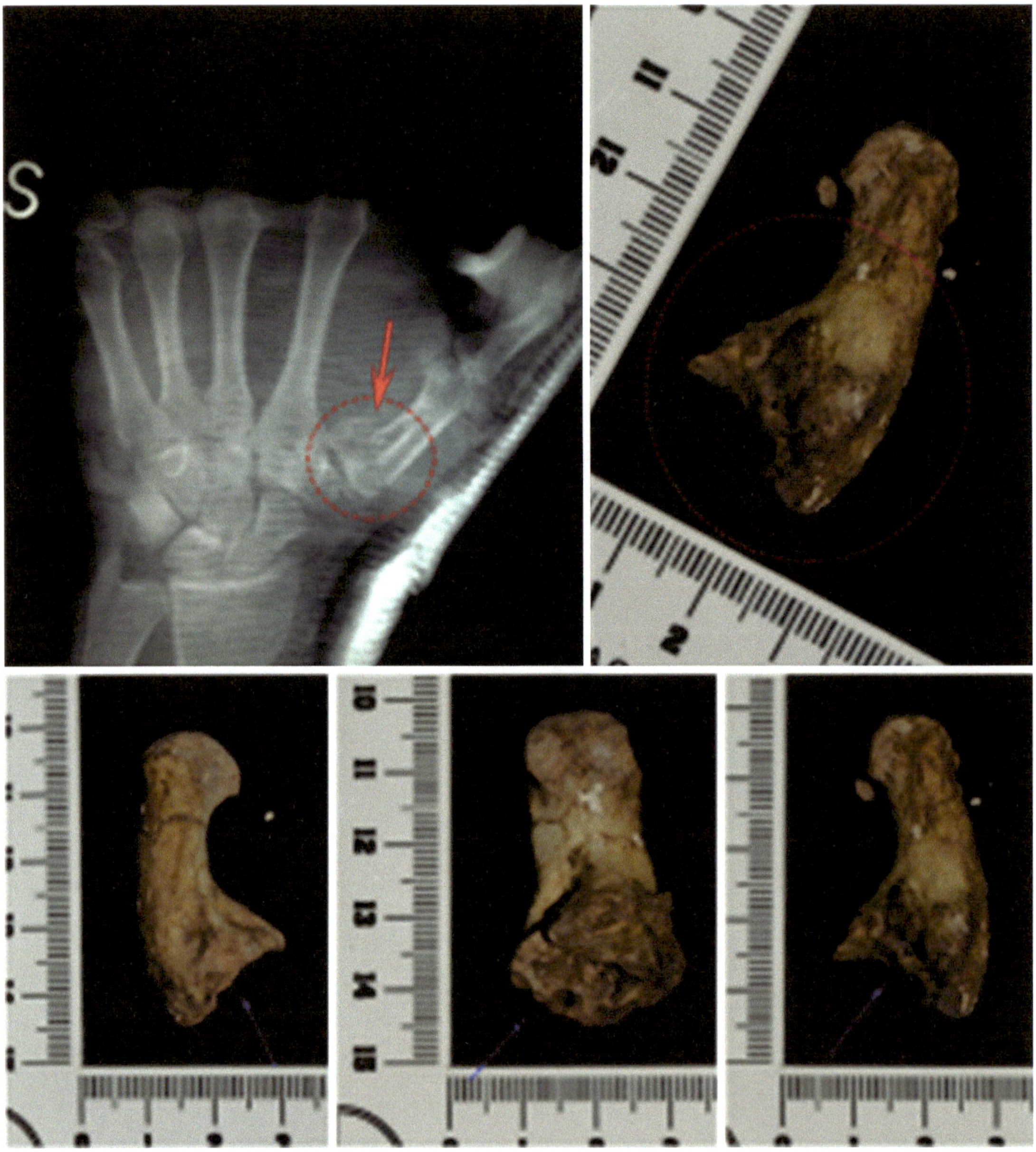

Fig. 8.14 Even the details of an old fracture and spiculae from callus formation can be useful for identification. To the left, an ante-mortem X-ray of the left hand showing a fracture on the first metatarsal; to the right the post-mortem image of a skeletonised first left metacarpal showing a similar detail

Anthropology and pathology in fact naturally deal with morphological and anatomical features, deriving both from genetics and environment, which represent a unique sample of markers useful to distinguish an individual from the other. Although radiological methods can be considered as the most natural and immediate to provide identification, in the forensic practice they suffer the limit of quantification, as data concerning shape and position are difficult to describe through numbers, and therefore cannot provide a percentage of correct (or incorrect identification). This is the most relevant point of weakness of morphological methods in comparison with DNA, which on the other side can give a probability based on allelic frequencies. Nevertheless, such methods are becoming acknowledged more and more as valid identifiers even by Interpol (http://www.interpol.int/INTERPOL-expertise/Forensics/DVI-Pages/DVI-guide).

For this reason, research in forensic anthropology has attempted to provide surrogates for a quantification concerning anthropological comparisons. An example is represented by validation studies, where quantification is reached by the assessment of disagreement among operators in assigning ante-mortem with post-mortem materials: this however does not correctly express the actual error of the method. On the other hand, as mentioned in the previous paragraphs, quantification of frequency of traits as well as strength of morphological matches is currently being assessed in literature with some success [27].

One point of discussion at this point could concern the real need for quantification in personal identification: we all know that Daubert guidelines request that the application of a method has to be linked to an error; on the other hand, Kumho has overcome this limit, recognising the existence of fields where the quantification cannot be performed [28]. This debate however is still open.

In conclusion, X-ray technology has given a great contribution to forensic sciences; the first historical application of X-rays in fact were for forensic purposes [13]. The importance of X-ray examination in forensic practise is proven also by the increasing development in the field of virtopsy with CT scanning and more recently MRI [29]. The use of radiology in personal identification brings on several advantages; above all, X-ray examination is the most common diagnostic test in clinical practice, and therefore is usually one of the most frequent ante-mortem source of information, when there is a suspicion of identity. In addition, the same radiograph with the same characteristic of an ante-mortem X-ray examination can be performed on the unidentified corpse, and this means a more reliable comparison between ante-mortem and post-mortem data.

8.2 Identification of the Living: Age Estimation

Another major application of radiology in identification concerns the estimation age in the living. Such requests usually concern the verification of a person being under 18 years of age (or under the age representing adulthood which may change depending on the country) mainly for two reasons: assessing imputability (in other words if the author of a crime is old enough to be tried and judged), or checking the age of unaccompanied minors to verify if they are indeed minors, in which case municipalities will take them in charge until they reach adulthood (this is the general orientation at least in Europe). Occasionally, this kind of assessment can be requested for adopted children whose age needs to be redefined because of the uncertainties or lack of birth certificates; in such cases all age ranges may be involved.

Exceptionally it can be requested for assessing age on adult individuals, mainly for old age pension or other civil purposes [30]. In addition, the same procedure may be performed in cases of adults affected by amnesia for personal identification [31]. This is often the most critical field of application, as very few scientifically based methods of age estimation exist for adults. The development of novel age estimation techniques is crucial in cases of age estimation involving adults.

In all such cases, but particularly in verifying imputability or the age of an asylum seeker, the importance of the application of a precise and accurate method is crucial, considering the obvious consequences arising from the incorrect diagnosis of adulthood in a minor or vice versa; for all these reasons the approach must be holistic, in other words comprise a full medical assessment, full radiological assessment, calibration of methods on the relevant ancestry and expression of the result with an error range. Age estimation may be affected by many variables, including pathology, nutrition and, especially, ancestry. The importance of population variability in this scenario is highlighted by the development of specific sections of population data within the most important scientific forensic journals, aimed at collecting information on the efficiency of age estimation methods in different ethnic groups. Today, each method needs to be tested on different population groups to verify possible variations and provide a correction factor. Estimated age and real age can differ according to ancestry. Every process of age estimation must therefore involve a thorough assessment of the health status as some diseases may slow down or accelerate growth and of ancestry. In this last case in particular results must be based on a comparison with available population data which should be adequately discussed within the expertise.

Guidelines and scientific societies dealing with age estimation procedures exist, whose aim is to work in favour of homogeneous modalities of intervention and reporting. In Europe, the most important associations are the Forensic Anthropology Society of Europe (FASE), a dedicated section of the International Academy of Legal Medicine (IALM), and the German Arbeitsgemeinschaft fur Forensische Altersdiagnostik—Study Group on Forensic Age diagnostics (AGFAD). The last one organises a proficiency test every year.

These associations have released guidelines which are superimposable for what concerns the operative modalities of the procedures for age estimation [32, 33]. In all cases, three basilar operations are required to perform a reliable age estimation:

- Clinical examination, completed by the assessment of maturation degree of sexual characteristics.
- Left hand and wrist X-ray (right hand and wrist if the subject is left-handed) and a panoramic dental X-ray.
- Radiological examination of the sternal end of the clavicle (only if doubts persist, [34]).

Hence, all cases where judgment is based only on sexual characteristics or on a single type of X-ray examination have to be considered as partial and incomplete.

One has always to keep on mind that age estimation is in all the cases a medical procedure before being a forensic act, and therefore it requires the collection of complete clinical history and a correct clinical examination. The following information should be recorded:

- Familiar medical history (information on parents, relatives, possible familiar pathologies, etc.).
- Pathological medical history (pathologies suffered during infancy, previous diseases focusing on infections and malnutrition, surgery, accidents, bone fractures, dental cares).
- Pathological information (current diseases, present health conditions).
- Physiological data (nutrition, type of alimentation, drugs and possible abuse, etc.).

Clinical history should be taken preliminarily, as it allows to correctly interpret possible alterations of the skeletal and dental development highlighted by X-ray examinations. Information on malnutrition or a prolonged infection, a parasitosis, may make suspicions arise on possible growth delay. In addition, some pathologies such as hormone-related conditions may speed up growth processes.

In all cases, registration of these possible variables is not sufficient to draw a correction of age estimation. For example, if a child has been undernourished for a long time, probably the skeleton suffered a growth delay, which may bring to possible age underestimation, but its entity cannot be verified. However, the same data may explain possible aberrations highlighted by X-ray exams [35].

The following points should be considered when writing the report of age estimation procedures.

First, the discussion must focus on the results provided by different methods of age estimation, followed by the selection of methods more reliably applicable to the present case, for example, for a wider approval by the scientific community or a stricter adherence to the ancestry group to which the subject belongs. The expert witness in fact should provide a single result, justified by the discussion of all data collected from different age estimation procedures. Reports where only one method is applied without any further discussion should be avoided.

Second, provide results in the most readable form for the judge, possibly in numeric form and with statistical information. Data about the statistical probability of having reached the legal threshold according to general population data may help in justifying a decision but, obviously, does not represent the actual probability that a single individual reached a specific age. In all cases a discussion concerning the limits of age estimation should be given.

Third, verify and discuss possible bias (pathologies, environmental conditions, ancestry characteristics) which may have influenced the results, and explain possible discordances arising from the application of different methods. In all cases, the final result has to be individualised according to the singular biological characteristics of each patient.

Age estimation of the living is ruled by different international laws and regulations, stating the principles of respect and the guarantee of juridical rights of the single individual. Hereby we provide a list of main juridical references concerning this topic:

- Guidelines on policies and procedures in dealing with unaccompanied children seeking asylum (Office of the United Nations—High Commissioner for Refugees, Geneva), February 1997.
- General comment n° 6 (2005), Committee on the Rights of the Child (CRC), UN, Treatment of unaccompanied and separated children outside their Country of origin.

Before we proceed to provide details on the radiological input, it is convenient to mention briefly health hazards of radiological assessment, since most of the standard procedures involve X-rays.

One issue that has frequently arisen concerning the ageing of minors is the potential biological hazard. While in the clinical context a balance between advantages and risks coming from a specific radiological procedures needs to be ascertained (the so-called *justification* process) under the radiologist's responsibility, in the forensic scenario no direct diagnostic or therapeutic advantage exists. Therefore, only diagnostic procedures which minimise biological hazard can be accepted.

In fact, the European Council Directive 2013/59/EURATOM of December 5th, 2013, defined the following principles: "the so-called "medico-legal" exposures introduced in Directive 97/43/Euratom have now been clearly identified as the deliberate exposure of individuals for other than medical purposes, or "non-medical imaging exposures". Such practices need to be placed under appropriate regulatory control and should be justified in a similar way as for medical exposures. However, a different approach is needed on the one hand for procedures using medical radiological equipment and on the other hand for procedures not using such equipment. In general, the annual dose limits and corresponding constraints for public exposure should apply".

For example, ultrasound evaluation is always allowed, as ultrasound in clinical practice is not considered invasive. Conversely, a computed tomography scan administers a non-negligible amount of ionising radiation. Even the most recent equipment strongly reduced the radiation dose per examination. A responsible use of X-ray (including both radiography and computed tomography) in the forensic practice requires a critical selection of methods applicable to specific age intervals. Available data suggests considering not only the application of imaging techniques at low X-ray exposure, but also the general age to which the subject belongs. In this context, hand-wrist and dental panoramic X-ray examinations provide an acceptable risk according to the scientific community [32]. The choice of the radiological examination clearly depends upon the local judicial authority.

A possible solution may come from the use of radiation-free approaches, including not only above-mentioned ultrasound methods but also magnetic resonance imaging. Some studies have already been reported with interesting results for the application of such methods to age estimation, for example, for the assessment of the degree of fusion of the clavicular sternal end [36] and of hand and wrist bones. In the latter case, the assessment is performed using ultrasound with a high concordance with traditional radiological methods of analysis according to the Greulich and Pyle Atlas [37]. The use of these technologies for forensic purposes still requires adequate standardisation and operators' training. In the future they may provide more precise and accurate information.

8.2.1 Radiology in Skeletal Age Estimation

Given that all bones during their development may provide information on age, modern literature has narrowed the field of age estimation on the skeleton down to the hand and wrist. The main advantages are represented by the high number of bones (29, including also the distal epiphysis of radius and ulna) and their age of growth, which covers the entire lifespan from birth to 18–19 years. In addition, hand and wrist X-rays do not involve highly radiosensitive anatomical structures and are considered a substantially safe analysis.

Several procedures have been developed focusing on hand and wrist. The most famous ones are represented by the Greulich and Pyle atlas [38], the Tanner-Whitehouse method (TW3 being the third, most recent version) [39] and the FELS [40] as well as the Maturos 4.0 software. They are characterised by different procedures of assessment of skeletal growth of hand and wrist bones through scoring criteria, although the Greulich and Pyle atlas still represents the most common method applied to the forensic practice and the main method used by the authors of most articles published nowadays.

The Greulich and Pyle atlas is based on a series of hand and wrist X-ray examination performed on a child population and published in 1959 (Fig. 8.15).

This method is based on a mere comparison of X-ray examinations with the standard descriptions provided by the atlas, divided according to sex; each stage has a description which may help in the correct assessment. In addition, each standard has specific error ranges based on the original populations used for the study.

The method represents a unique atlas, as its reproduction is not admitted according to the present ethical standards. As a consequence, it

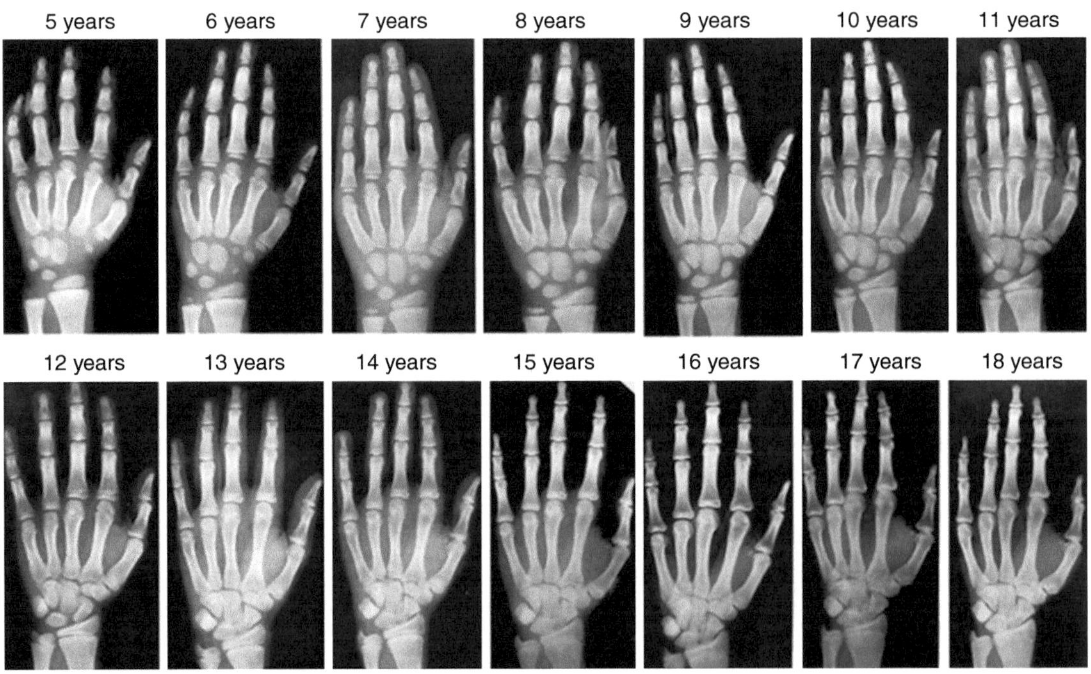

Fig. 8.15 Example of hand and wrist development at different ages according to Greulich and Pyle (male stadiation)

represents one of the most commonly used procedures for age estimation, with a high population dataset: among Europe, it has been already tested on Portuguese [41], Spanish [42], French [43], Italian [44–46], German [47], Scottish [48], Dutch [49], Danish [50], Central European [51] and Turkish ones [52–54]. In Africa it was applied to Sudanese [55] and Morocco [56]; in Asia to Indian [57–59], Pakistani [60–62], Sri Lankan [63], Lebanese [64], Chinese [65], Iran [66] and Korean groups [67, 68]. Finally it has been applied to US populations of different ancestry [69] and Australian group [70].

Although the Greulich and Pyle atlas is easy to use and widely recognised as the reference standard, it has some disadvantages. For example, it seems not to perform as well on some ethnic groups, including black populations [69]. In addition, thanks to its easy applicability, the Greulich and Pyle atlas is often used for age estimation by unskilled personnel, who may give erroneous interpretations, for example, ignoring the provided error range or applying the method inappropriately to different ethnic groups. From a practical point of view, although the atlas is easy to use, it requires awareness towards the general limits of age estimation and internationally adopted procedures.

On the other hand, the Tanner-Whitehouse method (at its third edition, TW3) assesses skeletal growth of hand and wrist based on a scoring system, divided according to bones and their developmental degree. It is more difficult to apply than the Greulich and Pyle atlas, as it requires classifying and collecting scores from different bones and gives a general age estimation according to the final sum [39]. As a consequence, it is also less applied to forensic practice, and finds less population data.

In addition, automatic systems exist, such as the FELS method, basically relying on the same procedure of the Tanner-Whitehouse method, with a scoring system based on different morphological and metric characteristics of each bone. It requires a longer time than other methods and also experience in correctly assessing subtle characteristics of each bone. As a consequence, it has been applied in a limited number of articles and seems to be an out-dated method.

Other districts may be involved in age estimation, according to the local legal age threshold: for example, fusion of iliac crest has been widely analysed in literature, but may be important in assessing 14-year subjects [71], whereas it is practically useless in cases of subjects close to 18 years. In addition, population data are very limited.

On the other hand, fusion of the sternal end of clavicle is important in countries where legal age threshold is more advanced, for example, at 21 years ([34], Figs. 8.16 and 8.17). In this case, chest X-rays represents the reference standard,

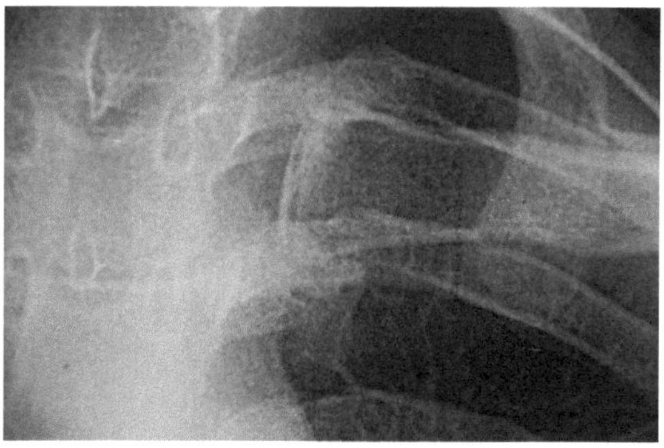

Fig. 8.17 Chest X-ray (sternal end of the clavicle, male, 17 years)

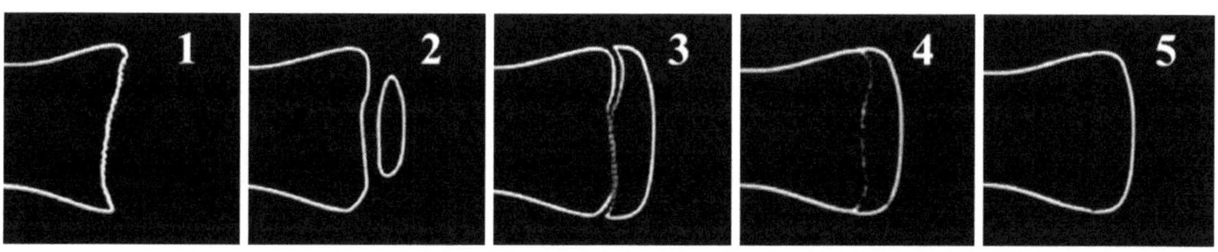

Fig. 8.16 Fusion stages of the sternal end of clavicle [34]

but the method has been standardised also for computed tomography, magnetic resonance imaging and ultrasound. However, population data are still limited also for this approach.

8.2.2 Radiology in Dental Age Estimation

Teeth have always been used as an age indicator probably starting from Ancient Romans who observed tooth eruption to evaluate the readiness for the military service; in more recent times, due to the "British Factory Act" (1833), Sanders published in 1837 "The Teeth as a test of Age, with Reference to Factory Children" [72]. In that paper, he explained the importance of tooth development when assessing the age of a juvenile for employment.

Dental age estimation techniques have been established as the most accurate indicators of chronological age in sub-adults. Many endocrine and maturational diseases affect dental development at a quarter of the rate of the skeleton [73]. Furthermore, in 2007 Meindl et al. in their paper stated that dental development underlies "strong regulation mechanisms which seem difficult to alter, even under pathological conditions" [74].

Teeth are indeed one of the most reliable biological indicators to perform age estimation in sub-adult subjects, but they are useful even in adult cases. Moreover, they are not used only in age estimation of the living, but they are routinely used when reconstructing a biological profile of an unknown corpse to give an age to human remains. Dental methods are therefore used in cases of foeticide, infanticide, biological profile reconstruction and even in palaeodemography studies.

As previously mentioned in this chapter, the practical application of forensic dental age estimation in the living comprises cases of lack of official documents, asylum seekers, criminals and victims of human trafficking, child pornography, adoptive children from countries without reliable birth registry, age categories in sports, child labour, eligibility for state-founded pensions.

Dental methods are mainly based on atlases (frequently developed using radiographic material) that depict and describe the developmental stages of the entire dentition or of every single tooth, or are based on measurements of biological variables correlated to the chronological age, such as the area of a tooth pulp chamber visible in a radiograph.

In the forensic research scenario, dental age estimation methods are constantly published and updated but, for actual cases, only the most validated ones thorough population data tests should be taken into consideration.

Tooth mineralisation begins in the foetus in its intrauterine growth. The stage of primary teeth development, highly related to the week of pregnancy, can be investigated via a radiograph of a dead foetus. The radiographic image can then be compared to atlases (Figs. 8.18 and 8.19, Ubelaker 1989; AlQahtani 2010) or is interpreted using published tables regarding foetal dental development [75].

Following the same approach, Ubelaker atlas (Fig. 8.20) or AlQahtani atlas (Fig. 8.21) can be used to estimate the age of a subject whose teeth are not completely developed just comparing the

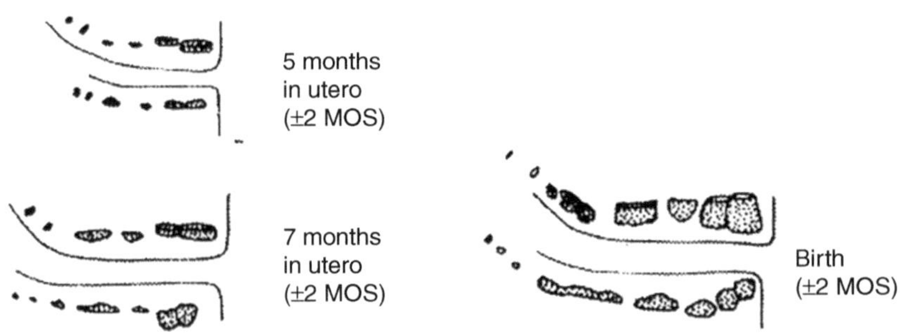

Fig. 8.18 Ubelaker schemes of foetal dental development

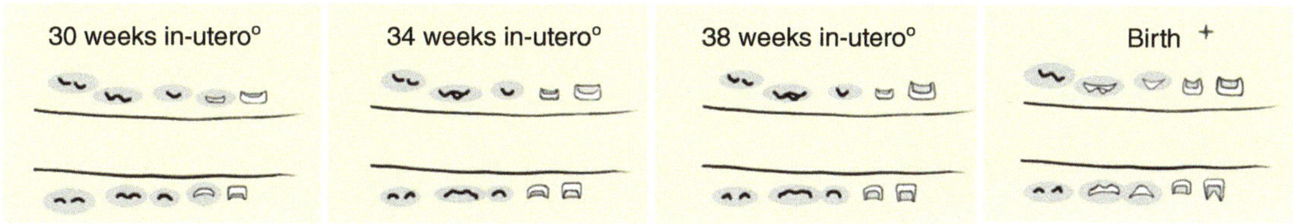

Fig. 8.19 AlQahtani schemes of foetal dental development; the first three schemes represent the midpoint of 1 month; the last one represents the midpoint of 2 weeks

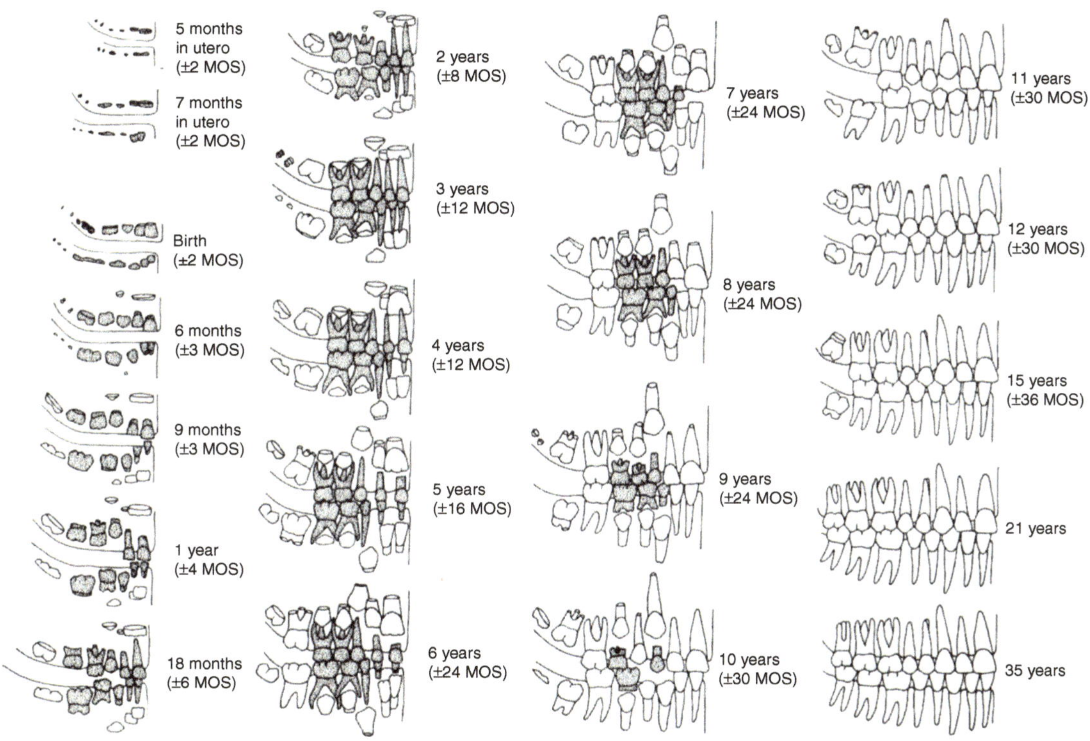

Fig. 8.20 Ubelaker atlas. Dark teeth are primary ones

radiographic image of the dentition with the published drawings (Fig. 8.22).

Radiological methods are useful as well to evaluate the degree of primary teeth root resorption [76] or the development of primary and permanent teeth using the Moorrees classification of 14 stages [76]. The development stage of one or more teeth is associated to one of the 14 stages, and then, using the published tables, is possible to associate the development stage to a chronological age interval (Fig. 8.23).

After these first publications by Moorrees, a lot of authors applied the same teeth development schemes to different populations to study the chronological age interval in which each stage is reached [77].

A radiographic dental method widely adopted and tested on several populations is the Demirijian method, published in 1973. It takes into consideration the radiographic image of the first seven permanent teeth. Each tooth is associated to a schematic representation of dental development

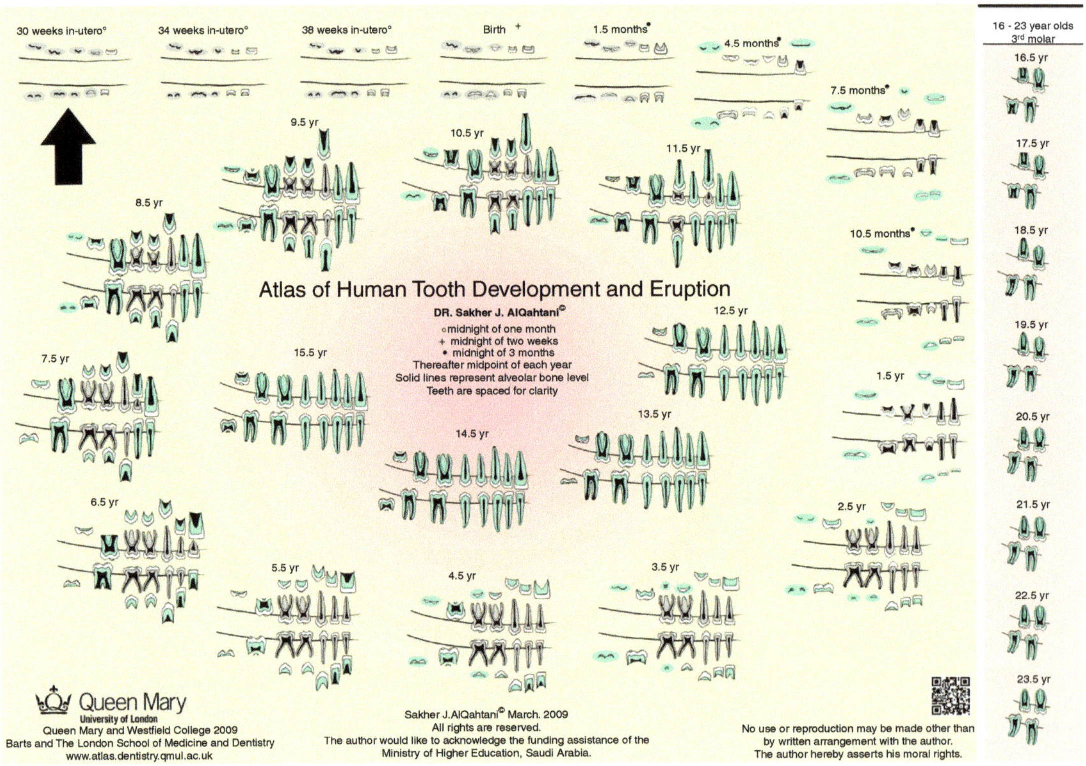

Fig. 8.21 AlQahtani Atlas

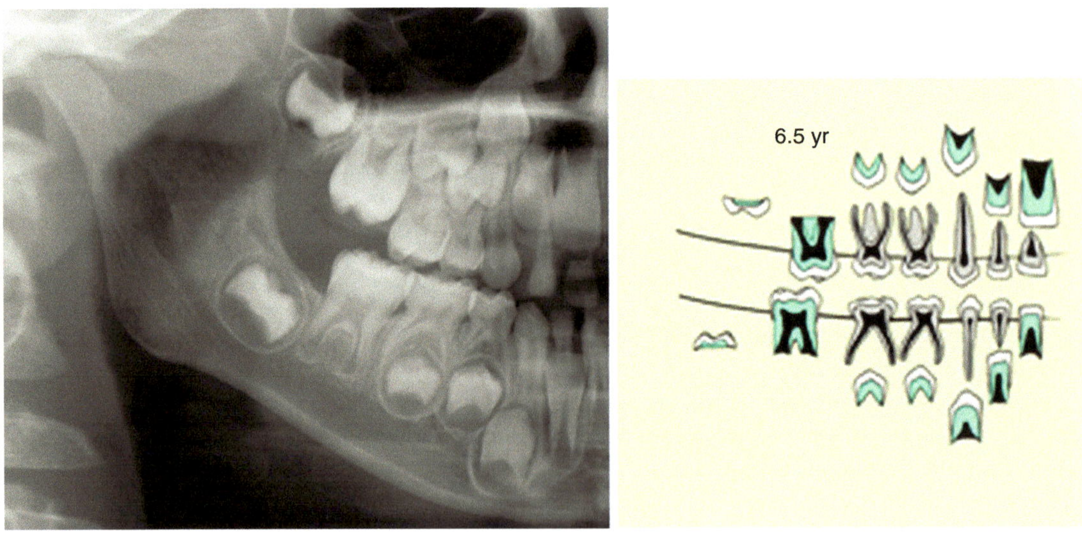

Fig. 8.22 The radiographic image of a developing dentition is associated to one of the schemes in the atlas

Description of Moorrees' stages (1963)
used to identify tooth developmental stages of single rooted teeth

ci: initial cusp formation	Ri: initial root formation with diverge edges
Cco: Coalescence of cusps	R 1/4: root length less than crown length
Coc: Cusp outline complete	R 1/2: root length equals crown length
Cr 1/2: crown half completed with dentine formation	R 3/4: three quarters of root length developed with diverge ends
Cr 3/4: crown three quarters completed	Rc: root length completed with parallel ends
Crc: crown completed with defined pulp roof	A 1/2: apex closed (root ends converge) with wide PDL
	Ac: apex closed with normal PDL width

Description of Moorrees' stages (1963)
used to identify tooth developmental stages of multirooted teeth

Ci: initial cusp formation	
Cco: Coalescence of cusps	R 1/4: root length less than crown length with visible bifurcatio area
Coc: Cusp outline complete	R 1/2: root length equals crown length
Cr 1/2: crown half completed with dentine formation	R 3/4: three quarters of root length developed with diverge ends
Cr 3/4: crown three quarters completed	Rc: root length completed with parallel ends
Crc: crown completed with defined pulp roof	A 1/2: apex closed (root ends converge) with wide PDL
Ri: initial root formation with diverge edges	Ac: apex closed with normal PDL width

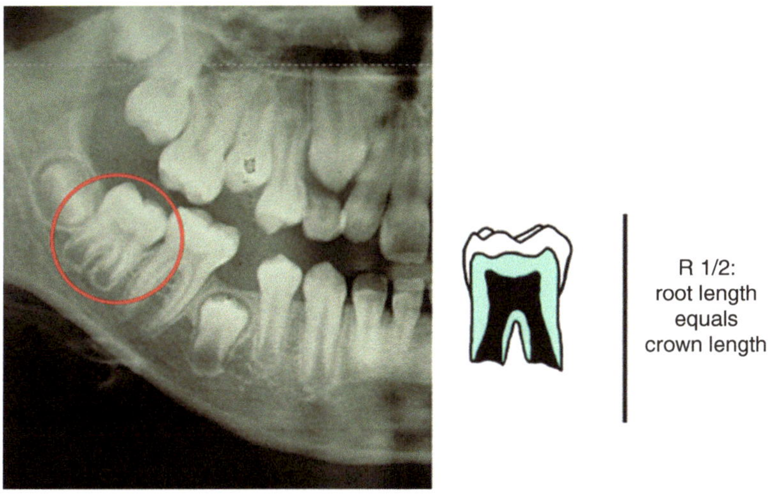

Fig. 8.23 Moorrees stages and an example of association between the development degree of a second permanent lower molar and the Moorrees stage "R1/2"

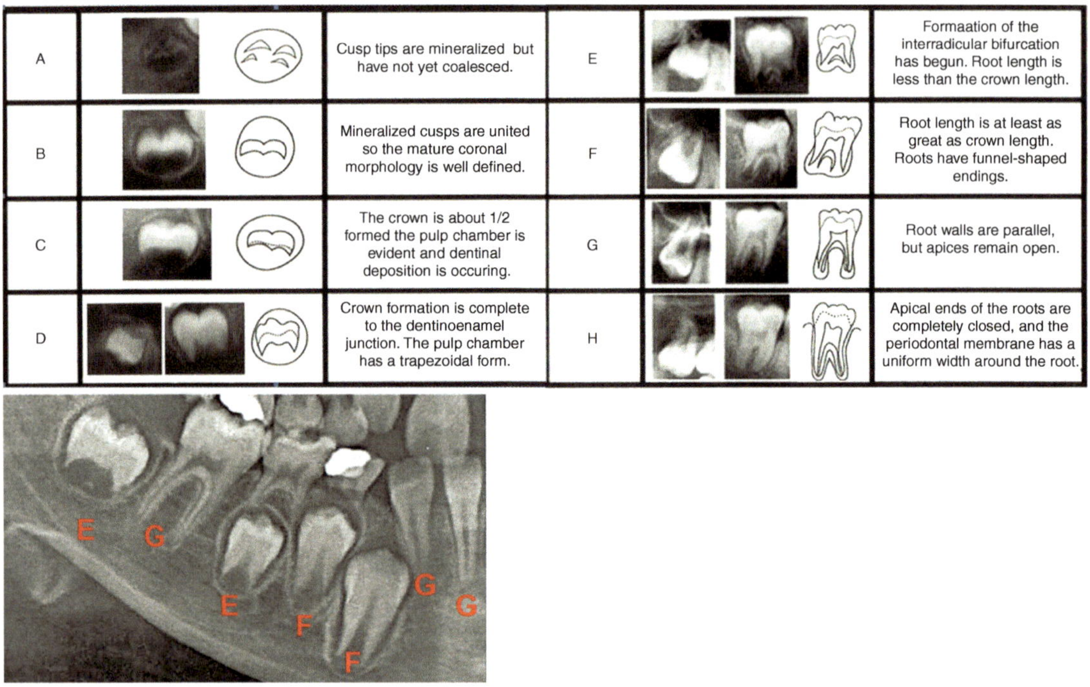

Fig. 8.24 Demirijian stages and an example of permanent developing teeth classification (the third molar, not visible in this radiographs, is never taken into consideration by the Demirijian method)

(eight stages) and a score is assigned to each tooth stage (Fig. 8.24). The scores sum is then associated to an age interval.

The Demirijian development stages have been also used by various authors (Mincer 1993; Kasper 2009; Solari 2002; Blankenship 2007; Olze 2003) to study wisdom tooth development chronology.

Radiographic sub-adult dental age estimation procedures also comprise methods based on some measurements of biological variables as the degree of tooth apex closure [78].

Finally, radiology is also used in adult age estimation cases as one of the most useful biological parameters, the pulp chamber contraction due to the continuous dentine deposition, is easily assessable through common radiographs or computed tomography (Kvaal 1994; Cameriere 2007; [31]).

In conclusion, in forensic age estimation what is performed is a quantitative or qualitative evaluation of a biological feature; this means that what is evaluated is the biological age. Scientific studies aim to correlate biological age with the chronological age as closely as possible, but biological age will never be perfectly superimposable to chronological age. Research and population data are mandatory to narrow down as much as possible this chronological age interval ("the error range").

As previously described, age estimation represents a complex procedure because of its specific characteristics and different fields of application. In fact, it requires an estimation through the quantification and classification of specific variables. Therefore, the final result should be a number, with an adequate error range and the age interval should always be discussed.

From this point of view, age estimation reports need to be objective and easily readable by the judge or other "customers"; in addition, the chance of giving a known error range is well in line with the Daubert criteria for the ascertainment of scientific evidence in expert witnessing [79–82].

References

1. Kahana T, Hiss J (1997) Identification of human remains: forensic radiology. J Clin Forensic Med 4:7–15
2. Blau S, Robertson S, Johnstone M (2008) Disaster victim identification: new applications for post-mortem computed tomography. J Forensic Sci 53:956–961
3. Adams BJ (2003) Establishing personal identification based on specific patterns of missing, filled, and unrestored teeth. Forensic Sci 48(3):487–496
4. Yoshino M, Miyasaka S, Sato H, Seta S (1987) Classification system of frontal sinus patterns by radiography. Its application to identification of unknown skeletal remains. Forensic Sci Int 34(4):289–299
5. De Angelis D, Cattaneo C, Grandi M (2007) Dental superimposition: a pilot study for standardising the method. Int J Legal Med 121(6):501–506
6. Fischman SL (1985) The use of medical and dental radiographs in identification. Int Dent J 35:301–306
7. Kahana T, Hiss J, Smith P (1998) Quantitative assessment of trabecular bone pattern identification. J Forensic Sci 43:1144–1147
8. Modesti LDM, Vieira GM, Galvão MF, de Amorim RFB (2014) Human identification by oral prosthesis analysis with probability rates higher than DNA analysis. J Forensic Sci 59:825–829
9. Pfaefli M, Vock P, Dirnhofer R, Braun M, Bolliger SA, Thali MJ (2007) Post-mortem radiological CT identification based on classical ante-mortem X-ray examinations. Forensic Sci Int 171:111–117
10. Christensen AM (2005) Testing the reliability of frontal sinuses in positive identification. J Forensic Sci 50:18–22
11. Kullman L, Eklund B, Grundin R (1990) Value of the frontal sinus in identification of unknown persons. J Forensic Odontostomatol 8:3–10
12. Patil N, Karjodkar FR, Sontakke S, Sansare K, Salvi R (2012) Uniqueness of radiographic patterns of the frontal sinus for personal identification. Imaging Sci Dent 42:213–217
13. Brogdon BG (1998) Forensic radiology. CRC Press, New York
14. Tatlisumak E, Ovali GY, Aslan A, Asirdizer M, Zeyfeoglu Y, Tarhan S (2007) Identification of unknown bodies by using CT images of frontal sinus. Forensic Sci Int 166:42–48
15. Beaini TL, Duailibi-Neto EF, Chilvarquer I, Melani RF (2015) Human identification through frontal sinus 3D superimposition: pilot study with cone beam computer tomography. J Forensic Legal Med 36:63–69
16. Brogdon BG (1998) The scope of forensic radiology. Clin Lab Med 18:203–240
17. Kuehn CM, Taylor KM, Mann FA, Wilson AJ, Harruff RC (2002) Validation of chest X-ray comparisons for unknown decedent identification. J Forensic Sci 47:725–729
18. Valenzuela A (1997) Radiographic comparison of the lumbar spine for positive identification of human remains: a case report. Am J Forensic Med Pathol 18:215–217
19. Stephan CN, Winburn AP, Christensen AF, Tyrrell AJ (2011) Skeletal identification by radiographic comparison: blind tests of a morphoscopic method using ante mortem chest radiographs. J Forensic Sci:320–332
20. Koot MG, Sauer NJ, Fenton TW (2005) Radiographic human identification using bones of the hand: a validation study. J Forensic Sci 50(2):263–268
21. Mundorff AZ, Vidoli G, Melinek J (2006) Anthropological and radiographic comparison of vertebrae for identification of decomposed human remains. J Forensic Sci 51:1002–1004
22. Dean DE, Tatarek NE, Rich J et al (2005) Human identification from the ankle with pre- and postsurgical radiographs. J Clin Forensic Med 12:5–9
23. Stephan CN, Amidan B, Rease H, Guyomarc'h P, Pulsipher T, Byrd JE (2014) Morphometric comparison of clavicle outlines from 3D bone scans and 2D chest radiographs: a shortlisting tool to assist radiographic identification of human skeletons. J Forensic Sci 59:306–313
24. Mann RW (1998) Use of bone trabeculae to establish positive identification. Forensic Sci Int 98:91–99
25. Cattaneo C (2007) Forensic anthropology: developments of a classical discipline in the new millennium. Forensic Sci Int 165:185–193
26. Rogers TL, Allard TT (2004) Expert testimony and positive identification of human remains through cranial suture patterns. J Forensic Sci 49:203–207
27. Ross AH, Lanfear AK, Maxwell AB (2016) Establishing standards for side by side radiographic comparisons. Am J Forensic Med Pathol 37:86–94
28. Grivas CR, Komar DA (2008) Kumho, Daubert, and the nature of scientific inquiry: implications for forensic anthropology. J Forensic Sci 53(4):771–776
29. Dirnhofer R, Jackowski C, Vock P, Potter K, Thali MJ (2006) VIRTOPSY: minimally invasive, imaging-guided virtual autopsy. Radiographics 26(5):1305–1333
30. Cattaneo C, De Angelis D, Ruspa M, Gibelli D, Cameriere R, Grandi M (2008) How old am I? Age estimation in living adults: a case report. J Forensic Odontostomatol 26(2):39–43
31. De Angelis D, Gibelli D, Fabbri P, Cattaneo C (2015) Dental age estimation helps create a new identity. Am J Forensic Med Pathol 36(3):219–220
32. Cunha E, Baccino E, Martrille L, Ramsthaler F, Prieto J, Schuliar Y, Lynnerup N, Cattaneo C (2009) The problem of aging human remains and living individuals: a review. Forensic Sci Int 193(1–3):1–13
33. Schmeling A, Grundmann C, Fuhrmann A, Kaatsch HJ, Knell B, Ramsthaler F, Reisinger W, Reipert T, Ritz-Timme S, Rosing FW, Rotzscher K, Geserick G (2008) Criteria for age estimation in living individuals. Int J Legal Med 122(6):457–460
34. Schmeling A, Shulz R, Reisinger W, Mulher M, Wernecke KG, Geserick G (2004) Studies on the time frame for ossification of the medial clavicular epiphy-

seal cartilage in conventional radiography. Int J Legal Med 118:5–8
35. Gibelli D, De Angelis D, Cattaneo C (2015) Radiological pitfalls of age estimation in adopted children: a case report. Minerva Pediatr 67(2):203–208
36. Schulz R, Zwiesigk P, Schiborr M, Schmidt S, Schmeling A (2008) Ultrasound studies on the time course of clavicular ossification. Int J Legal Med 122(2):163–167
37. Bilgili Y, Hizel S, Kara SA, Sanli C, Erdal HH, Altinok D (2003) Accuracy of skeletal age assessment in children from birth to 6 years of age with the ultrasonographic version of the Greulich-Pyle atlas. J Ultrasound Med 22(7):683–690
38. Greulich WW, Pyle SI (1959) Radiographic atlas of skeletal development of the hand and wrist. Stanford University Press, Stanford
39. Tanner JM, Whitehouse RH (1984) Growth and development reference charts. Castlemead Publications, Hertford
40. Roche AF, Chumlea WC, Thissen D (1988) Assessing the skeletal maturity of the hand wrist: Fels method. Charles C Thomas, New York
41. Santos C, Ferreira M, Alves FC, Cunha E (2011) Comparative study of Greulich and Pyle Atlas and Maturos 4.0 program for age estimation in a Portuguese sample. Forensic Sci Int 212(1–3):276.e1–276.e7
42. Alcina M, Lucea A, Salicrú M, Turbón D (2018) Reliability of the Greulich and Pyle method for chronological age estimation and age majority prediction in a Spanish sample. Int J Legal Med 132:1139–1149
43. Zabet D, Rérolle C, Pucheux J, Telmon N, Saint-Martin P (2015) Can the Greulich and Pyle method be used on French contemporary individuals? Int J Legal Med 129(1):171–177
44. De Donno A, Santoro V, Lubelli S, Marrone M, Lozito P, Introna F (2013) Age assessment using the Greulich and Pyle method on a heterogeneous sample of 300 Italian healthy and pathologic subjects. Forensic Sci Int 229(1–3):157.e1–157.e6
45. Santoro V, Roca R, De Donno A, Fiandaca C, Pinto G, Tafuri S, Introna F (2012) Applicability of Greulich and Pyle and Demirijan aging methods to a sample of Italian population. Forensic Sci Int 221(1–3):153.e1–153.e5
46. Tisè M, Mazzarini L, Fabrizzi G, Ferrante L, Giorgetti R, Tagliabracci A (2011) Applicability of Greulich and Pyle method for age assessment in forensic practice on an Italian sample. Int J Legal Med 125(3):411–416
47. Schmidt S, Koch B, Schulz R, Reisinger W, Schmeling A (2008) Studies in use of the Greulich-Pyle skeletal age method to assess criminal liability. Leg Med (Tokyo) 10(4):190–195
48. Hackman L, Black S (2013) The reliability of the Greulich and Pyle atlas when applied to a modern Scottish population. J Forensic Sci 58(1):114–119
49. van Rijn RR, Lequin MH, Thodberg HH (2009) Automatic determination of Greulich and Pyle bone age in healthy Dutch children. Pediatr Radiol 39(6):591–597
50. Lynnerup N, Belard E, Buch-Olsen K, Sejrsen B, Damgaard-Pedersen K (2008) Intra- and interobserver error of the Greulich-Pyle method as used on a Danish forensic sample. Forensic Sci Int 179(2–3):242.e1–242.e6
51. Groell R, Lindbichler F, Riepl T, Gherra L, Roposch A, Fotter R (1999) The reliability of bone age determination in central European children using the Greulich and Pyle method. Br J Radiol 72(857):461–464
52. Cantekin K, Celikoglu M, Miloglu O, Dane A, Erdem A (2012) Bone age assessment: the applicability of the Greulich-Pyle method in eastern Turkish children. J Forensic Sci 57(3):679–682
53. Gungor OE, Celikoglu M, Kale B, Gungor AY, Sari Z (2015) The reliability of the Greulich and Pyle atlas when applied to a Southern Turkish population. Eur J Dent 9(2):251–254
54. Koc A, Karaoglanoglu M, Erdogan M, Kosecik M, Cesur Y (2001) Assessment of bone ages: is the Greulich-Pyle method sufficient for Turkish boys? Pediatr Int 43(6):662–665
55. Elamin F, Abdelazeem N, Elamin A, Saif D, Liversidge HM (2017) Skeletal maturity of the hand in an East African group from Sudan. Am J Phys Anthropol 163(4):816–823
56. Garamendi PM, Landa MI, Ballesteros J, Solano MA (2005) Reliability of the methods applied to assess age minority in living subjects around 18 years old. A survey on a Moroccan origin population. Forensic Sci Int 154(1):3–12
57. Keny SM, Sonawane DV, Pawar E, Saraogi AA, Singh V, Khan F, Bande PP, Chandanwale A (2018) Comparison of two radiological methods in the determination of skeletal maturity in the Indian pediatric population. J Pediatr Orthop B 27:362–365
58. Mohammed RB, Rao DS, Goud AS, Sailaja S, Thetay AA, Gopalakrishnan M (2015) Is Greulich and Pyle standards of skeletal maturation applicable for age estimation in South Indian Andhra children? J Pharm Bioallied Sci 7(3):218–225
59. Patel PS, Chaudhary AR, Dudhia BB, Bhatia PV, Soni NC, Jani YV (2015) Accuracy of two dental and one skeletal age estimation methods in 6-16 year old Gujarati children. J Forensic Dent Sci 7(1):18–27
60. Awais M, Nadeem N, Husen Y, Rehman A, Beg M, Khattak YJ (2014) Comparison between Greulich-Pyle and Girdany-Golden methods for estimating skeletal age of children in Pakistan. J Coll Physicians Surg Pak 24(12):889–893
61. Manzoor Mughal A, Hassan N, Ahmed A (2014) The applicability of the Greulich & Pyle Atlas for bone age assessment in primary school-going children of Karachi, Pakistan. Pak J Med Sci 30(2):409–411
62. Rikhasor RM, Qureshi AM, Rathi SL, Channa NA (1999) Skeletal maturity in Pakistani children. J Anat 195(Pt 2):305–308
63. Gunawardena SA, Liyanage UA, Weeratna JB, Mendis NDNA, Perera HJM, Jayasekara RW, Fernando R (2017) Forensic age estimation in anti-piracy tri-

als in Seychelles: experiences and challenges faced. Forensic Sci Int 270:278.e1–278.e7
64. Saadé A, Baron P, Noujeim Z, Azar D (2017) Dental and skeletal age estimations in Lebanese children: a retrospective cross-sectional study. J Int Soc Prev Community Dent 7(3):90–97
65. Lin FQ, Zhang J, Zhu Z, Wu YM (2015) Comparative study of Gilsanz-Ratib digital atlas and Greulich-Pyle atlas for bone age estimation in a Chinese sample. Ann Hum Biol 42(6):523–527
66. Moradi M, Sirous M, Morovatti P (2012) The reliability of skeletal age determination in an Iranian sample using Greulich and Pyle method. Forensic Sci Int 223(1–3):372.e1–372.e4
67. Kim JR, Lee YS, Yu J (2015) Assessment of bone age in prepubertal healthy Korean children: comparison among the Korean standard bone age chart, Greulich-Pyle method, and Tanner-Whitehouse method. Korean J Radiol 16(1):201–205
68. Oh Y, Lee R, Kim HS (2012) Evaluation of skeletal maturity score for Korean children and the standard for comparison of bone age and chronological age in normal children. J Pediatr Endocrinol Metab 25(3–4):279–284
69. Ontell FK, Ivanovic M, Ablin DS, Barlow TW (1996) Bone age in children of diverse ethnicity. AJR Am J Roentgenol 167(6):1395–1398
70. Paxton ML, Lamont AC, Stillwell AP (2013) The reliability of the Greulich-Pyle method in bone age determination among Australian children. J Med Imaging Radiat Oncol 57(1):21–24
71. Kotwicki T (2008) Improved accuracy in Risser sign grading with lateral spinal radiography. Eur Spine J 17(12):1676–1685
72. Saunders E (1837) The teeth a test of age, considered with reference to the factory children. Addressed to the members of both Houses of Parliament. H. Renshaw, London
73. DH Ubelaker (1999) cited in Senn DR, Weems RA (2013) Manual of forensic odontology CRC Press: Boca Raton
74. Meinl A, Tangl S, Huber C, Maurer B, Watzek G (2007) The chronology of third molar mineralization in the Austrian population—a contribution to forensic age assessment. Forensic Sci Int 169(2–3):161–167
75. Lunt RC, Law DB (1974) A review of the chronology of eruption of deciduous teeth. J Am Dent Assoc 89:872–879
76. Moorrees CFA, Fanning EA, Hunt EE (1963) Formation and resorption of three deciduous teeth in children. Am J Phys Anthrop 21(2):205–213
77. Liversidge HM, Marsden PH (2010) Estimating age and the likelihood of having attained 18 years of age using mandibular third molars. Br Dent J 209(8):E13
78. Cameriere R, Ferrante L, De Angelis D, Scarpino F, Galli F (2008) The comparison between measurement of open apices of third molars and Demirjian stages to test chronological age of over 18 year olds in living subjects. Int J Legal Med 122(6):493–497
79. Daubert v. Merrell Dow Pharmaceuticals (1993) Supreme Court of the United States. 113 S.Ct. 2786
80. Cattaneo C, Grandi M (2004) Antropologia e Odontologia Forense, Guida alla studio dei resti umani. Testo atlante. Monduzzi Editore, Bologna
81. Cattaneo C, Tidball Binz M, Penados L, Prieto J, Finegan O, Grandi M (2015) The forgotten tragedy of unidentified in the Mediterranean. Forensic Sci Int 250:e1–e2
82. Rich J, Tatarek NE, Powers RH, Brogdon BG, Lewis BJ, Dean DE (2002) Using pre- and post-surgical foot and ankle radiographs for identification. J Forensic Sci 47:1319–1322

The Essential of Bone Histology for Forensic Applications

9

Giovanni Francesco Spatola, Maria Laura Uzzo, Antonietta Lanzarone, Donatella Piscionieri, Daniele Daricello, and Stefania Zerbo

Bone is a specialized connective tissue where the extracellular matrix calcified imprisons the same cells that produced it. Although the bone is one of the most hard body constituents, it has substantial dynamic capacity and able to renew itself and to change the form in relation to the forces and pressures acting on it. For example, the pressure exerted on the bone leading to its resorption, while the traction stimulates the production of new tissue. At the specialized cartilage-covered ends, it permits articulation or movement. Bone is a vascular connective tissue consisting of cells and calcified extracellular materials, known as the matrix. The elements that make up the bone matrix can be distinguished in organic and inorganic: 90% of the organic matrix is approximately composed of type I collagen fibers, but there are also type V, III, XI, and XIII, and only 10% by an amorphous component rich in proteoglycans, adhesive glycoproteins and vitamin protein K as well as osteocalcin that favors the organization of the calcium crystals. The relationship between the two components depends on age and physiological or pathological conditions. The arrangement of the collagen fibers is essential in order to optimize the bone response to stress. The inorganic component of the matrix is composed, of 80% calcium crystals in the form of hydroxyapatite crystals, of 10% calcium carbonate and other salts. During life, the composition of the mineral component and its relationship with the organic varies as a function of physiological and pathological states.

Bone may be sponge-like or dense. Sponge-like bone, like that present inside the epiphyses (heads) of long bones, is always surrounded by compact bone. Sponge-like bone has large, open spaces surrounded by thin, anastomosing plates of bone. The large spaces are marrow spaces, and the plates of bones are trabeculae composed of several layers or lamellae. Compact bone is much denser than sponge-like bone. Its spaces are much reduced in size, and its lamellar organization is much more precise and thicker. Compact bone is always covered and lined by soft connective tissues, the endosteum lining the marrow cavity and the periosteum that covers the bone itself. In endosteum and also in the periosteum are present osteoprogenitor cells from which subsequently are differentiated osteoblasts thanks to the action of certain growth factors, including the transforming growth factor beta (TGFβ).

G. F. Spatola (✉) · M. L. Uzzo
Department of Biomedicine, Neurosciences and Advanced Diagnostics (BiND), Unit of Histology and Embryology, University of Palermo, Palermo, Italy
e-mail: giovannifrancesco.spatola@unipa.it; marialaura.uzzo@unipa.it

A. Lanzarone · D. Piscionieri · D. Daricello · S. Zerbo
Department for Health Promotion, Maternal and Child Care, University of Palermo, Palermo, Italy
e-mail: stefania.zerbo@unipa.it

G. Lo Re et al. (eds.), *Radiology in Forensic Medicine*,
https://doi.org/10.1007/978-3-319-96737-0_9

The periosteum covering the outer surface of compact bone is composed of two layers, one external and one internal where are present, in addition to the osteoprogenitor cells, osteoblasts and osteoclasts. In particular, the inner layer plays osteogenic function and consists of some collagen fibers and mostly osteoprogenitor cells and their progeny, the osteoblasts. The periosteum is affixed to bone via Sharpey's fibers, collagenous bundles trapped in the calcified bone matrix during ossification.

9.1 Cells of Bone

Bone possesses four types of cells: osteoprogenitor cells, osteoblasts, osteocytes, and osteoclasts.

- *Osteoprogenitor cells* give rise to osteoblasts under the influence of transforming growth factor-β and bone morphogenic protein.
- *Osteoblasts* elaborate bone matrix, become surrounded by the matrix they synthesized, and calcify the matrix via matrix vesicles that they release. When osteoblasts are quiescent, they lose much of their protein synthetic machinery and resemble osteoprogenitor cells. Osteoblasts function not only in the control of bone matrix mineralization but also in the formation, recruitment, and maintenance of osteoclasts as well as for the initiation of bone resorption. Osteoblasts participate in the mineralization process releasing vesicles in the external environment that contain alkaline phosphatase (matrix vesicle). The alkaline phosphatase is an important enzyme in the initial phase of precipitation of calcium phosphate salts. Osteoblasts have within them, in the cytoplasm, the typical kit of organelles of all cells delegated to an active protein synthesis: plentiful RER and a highly developed Golgi complex, mitochondria and vesicles, all that gives to the cell a strong affinity for basic dyes. Osteoblasts are directly involved in calcium homeostasis mechanisms, and in particular present on their membrane receptors for parathyroid hormone that causes them to produce a factor of the macrophage colony stimulation (M-CSF) which induces CFU-M (forming units monocyte macrophage colony) to differentiate into osteoclast precursors.
- *Osteocytes* (Fig. 9.1) are osteoblasts trapped in the matrix that they have synthesized. They occupy lacunae, lenticular-shaped spaces, and possess long osteocytic processes that are housed in tiny canals or tunnels known as canaliculi. Osteocytes are responsible for the maintenance of bone. Their cytoplasmic processes contact and form gap junctions with processes of other osteocytes within canaliculi; thus, these cells sustain a communication network.
- *Osteoclasts* (Fig. 9.2), large, multinucleated cells derived from monocyte-macrophage precursors are responsible for the resorption of bone. As they remove bone, they appear to

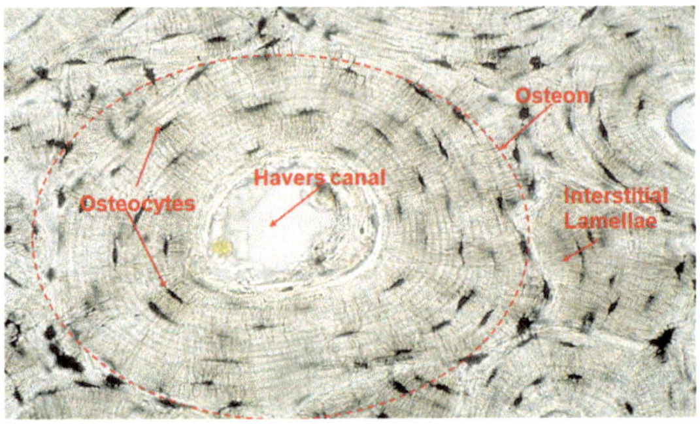

Fig. 9.1 Haversian system: osteons, evidence of osteocytes and interstitial lamellae, human bone—abrasion method, brightfield microscopy 20×

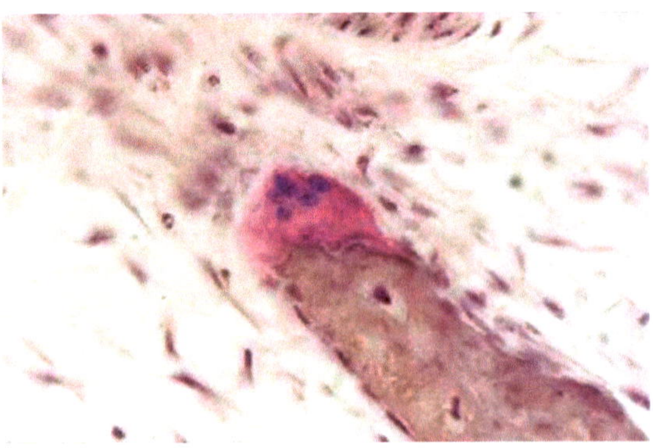

Fig. 9.2 Osteoclast: evidence of multiple nuclei and presence of Howship's lacuna, human bone—EE Brightfield microscopy 63×

occupy a shallow cavity, Howship's lacuna (subosteoclastic compartment). Osteoclasts have various regions:

- The basal zone, housing nuclei and organelles of the cell.
- The ruffled border, composed of finger-like processes that are suspended in the subosteoclastic compartment where the resorption of bone is actively proceeding.

The ruffled border possesses many proton pumps that deliver hydrogen ions from the osteoclast into the subosteoclastic compartment. Additionally, aquapores and chloride channels permit the delivery of water and chloride ions, respectively, forming a concentrated solution of HCl in the subosteoclastic compartment, thus decalcifying bone. Enzymes are delivered via vesicles into the subosteoclastic compartment to degrade the organic components of bone. The by-products of degradation are endocytosed by endocytic vesicles and are used by the osteoclast or are exocytosed into the extracellular space where they enter the vascular system for distribution to the rest of the body—the vesicular zone, housing numerous vesicles that ferry material out of the cell and into the cell from the subosteoclastic compartment, and the clear zone, where the osteoclast forms a seal with the bone, isolating the subosteoclastic compartment from the external milieu. The osteoclast cell membrane also possesses calcitonin receptors; when calcitonin is bound to the receptors, these cells become inhibited; they stop bone resorption, leave the bone surface, and dissociate into individual cells or disintegrate and are eliminated by macrophages. Cooperation between osteoclasts and osteoblasts is responsible not only for the formation, remodeling, and repair of bone but also for the long-term maintenance of calcium and phosphate homeostasis of the body.

9.2 Concentric or Haversian System

In the long bones the compact bone tissue is organized in Haversian system, where a variable number of cylindrical lamellae (8–15) are placed concentrically the one with the other. This structure takes the name of osteon (Fig. 9.1) and presents its major axis parallel to the major axis of the bone. At the center of the osteon, always along the major axis, runs a channel where vessels and nerves (Haversian canal) are, while peripherally forms a jagged line (cementing line) more mineralized and more reflective, which interposes from neighboring osteons. The bone vascularity is provided through the presence of vessels in the Haversian canal; these channels are connected among them through oblique channels with respect to the major axis of the bone and often anastomosed between them, the Volkmann canals. They cross the cementing lines and open in correspondence of the periosteum and of the endosteum. The blood supply comes from the vessels that flow in these two systems. There is a remarkable communication between the osteocytes through the system of canaliculi osteocytic gaps and the osteonic channels and this allows an effective contribution to the metabolic osteocytes arranged in all regions of the bone tissue. Most osteons have a cylindric aspect and appears circular in cross section, although some may appear distorted or incomplete; this aspect is linked to bone remodeling processes. The osteons, in fact, are continually reshaped, whereby the existing lamellae undergo a degradation and are replaced by newly formed lamellae. The inner lamella of the osteon is always the most recent available. The degradation of osteon, without a complete reconstruction, can be responsible for its aspect distorted and incomplete. A fundamental fact, with important implications in the forensic study, is that in elderly patients remodeling slows and shape of osteons becomes more regular. The collagen fibers in the lamellae shall run in parallel. The oblique and parallel arrangement of the collagen fibers in a cylindric lamella makes the helical course with respect to the axis of osteon. The fibers in adjacent lamellae intersect forming varying angles. The lamellar organization and arrangement of the collagen fibers are responsible for the resistance to traction, bending and pressure to the bone (Figs. 9.3 and 9.4).

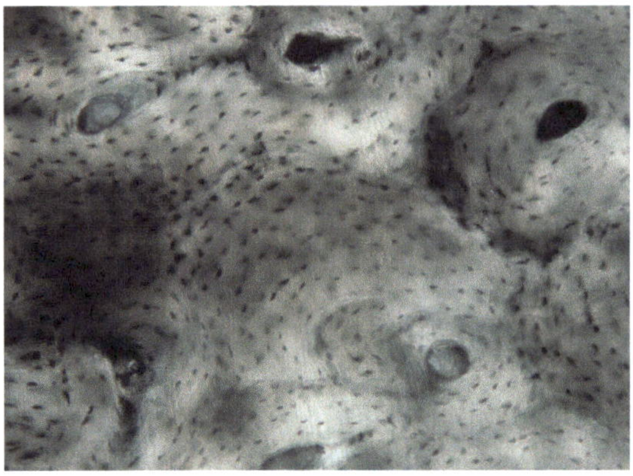

Fig. 9.3 Haversian system—human bone, abrasion method, brightfield microscopy 20×

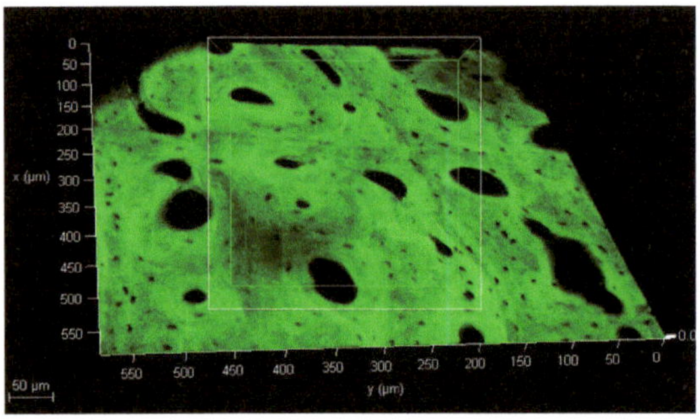

Fig. 9.4 Haversian system—pig bone, osteons, and interstitial lamellae in confocal microscopy 20×

9.3 Interstitial Lamellae System

The space between the adjacent osteon surfaces is bridged by interstitial lamellae system. It is tendentially parallel lamellae bounded by cementing lines. Within each interstice among osteons the orientation of the lamellae can be variable. The interstitial system represents the residue of concentric lamellae of degraded osteons and is therefore the result of bone remodeling. Being older interstitial lamellae of the osteons, their level of mineralization is higher (Fig. 9.1).

9.4 Systems of Internal and External Circumferential Lamellae

Outside and inside the compact bone layer formed by concentric and interstitial systems, the lamellae are arranged concentrically with respect to the major axis of the diaphysis of a long bone or along the surface of a bone plate. So two outer circumferential lamellae systems (subperiosteal) and internal (subendosteal) form. Those often subperiosteal are crossed by Sharpey's fibers.

9.5 Bone Remodeling

Adult bone is continuously being remodeled to compensate for changes in the forces being placed on it. As the remodeling of compact bone occurs, haversian canal systems have to be modified by osteoclastic resorption followed by osteoblastic bone formation. Since this progression takes place completely within the substance of compact bone, it is frequently called internal remodeling. The haversian canal system is being remodeled by what is known as a bone remodeling unit, which has two components: *resorption cavity (cutting cone) and lamellar formation (closing zone).*

- A resorption cavity is formed as osteoclasts enter the haversian canal and begin resorbing bone. Osteoclastic activity is followed by an invasion by capillaries, osteoprogenitor cells, and osteoblasts.
- Once the osteoclastic activity ceases, the osteoprogenitor cells divide, forming osteoblasts, which manufacture lamellae of bone until a new haversian canal system is completed.

The remodeling processes continue throughout the individual's life, slowing in intensity and with considerable differences depending on the considered bone segment. In the third decade of life a complex and intricate system of interstitial lamellae will form because of the incomplete degradation of preexisting osteons, while the outer and inner circumferential lamellae tend to persist only in limited areas. In old age the shape of osteons is more regular than in the young and the regressive processes prevail over those plastic, so it is established as a senile osteoporosis (after the 60th year of age) which leads to an increase in the lumen of osteonic channels and you can appreciate of the cavities which are formed by erosion with few lamellae of new deposition. These data are essential in the forensic practice, as they allow, albeit with some difficulties related to the histological methods, with a good approximation to obtain from bone segments (shaft of long bones in particular the femur or radio) data that help us to determine the chronological age of the subject. There are various methods to obtain this estimate but all take into account in particular of the presence of complete osteon (identifiable thanks to their cementing line) and interstitial lamellae which are a sign of bone remodeling. Greater is the number of interstitial lamellae and more younger the age of the subject.

Further Readings

Abbott S, Trinkaus E, Burr DB (1996) Dynamic bone remodeling in later Pleistocene fossil hominids. Am J Phys Anthropol 99(4):585–601

Abou-Arab M, Thomsen JL, Frohlich B, Lynnerup N (1995) Technical note: histological staining of secondary osteons. Am J Phys Anthropol 98(3):391–394

Baccino E, Ubelaker DH, Hayek LA, Zerilli A (1999) Evaluation of seven methods of estimating age at death from mature human skeletal remains. J Forensic Sci 44(5):931–936

Báca V, Kachlík D, Horák Z, Stingl J (2007) The course of osteons in the compact bone of the human proximal femur with clinical and biomechanical significance. Surg Radiol Anat 29(3):201–207

Boela LW, Boldsenb JL, Melsena F (2007) Double lamellae in trabecular osteons: towards a new method for age estimation by bone microscopy. Homo 58:269–277

Britz HM, Thomas CD, Clement JG, Cooper DM (2009) The relation of femoral osteon geometry to age, sex, height and weight. Bone 45(1):77–83. https://doi.org/10.1016/j.bone.2009.03.654

Cho H, Stout SD, Madsen RW, Streeter MA (2002) Population-specific histological age-estimating method: a model for known African-American and European-American skeletal remains. J Forensic Sci 47(1):12–18

Clement JG (2005) The Melbourne Femur Collection: the gift of tissue underpins important medical and forensic research. VIFM Rev 3:7–11

Dillon S, Cunningham C, Felts P (2016) Quantification of osteon morphology using geometric histomorphometrics. J Forensic Sci 61(2):402–408. https://doi.org/10.1111/1556-4029.12966

Ericksen MF (1991) Histologic estimation of age at death using the anterior cortex of the femur. Am J Phys Anthropol 84(2):171–179

Ericksen MF (1979) Aging changes in the medullary cavity of the proximal femur in American Blacks and Whites. Am J Phys Anthropol 51(4):563–569

Ferretti A, Cardini A, Crampton JS, Serpagli E, Sheets HD, Štorch P (2013) Rings without a lord? Enigmatic fossils from the lower Palaeozoic of Bohemia and the Carnic Alps. Lethaia 46(2):211–222

Franklin D (2010) Forensic age estimation in human skeletal remains: current concepts and future directions. Leg Med (Tokyo) 12(1):1–7. https://doi.org/10.1016/j.legalmed.2009.09.001

Frost HM (1987) Secondary osteon population densities: an algorithm for determining mean bone tissue age. Yearbook Phys Anthropol 30:221–238

Frost HM (1987) Secondary osteon population densities: an algorithm for. Estimating the missing osteons. Yearbook Phys Anthropol 30:239–254

Goldman HM, Bromage TG, Thomas CD, Clement JG (2003) Preferred collagen fiber orientation in the human mid-shaft femur. Anat Rec A Discov Mol Cell Evol Biol 272(1):434–445

Gundersen HJ, Bendtsen TF, Korbo L, Marcussen N, Møller A, Nielsen K, Nyengaard JR, Pakkenberg B, Sørensen FB, Vesterby A et al (1988) Some new, simple and efficient stereological methods and their use in pathological research and diagnosis. APMIS 96(5):379–394

Hillier ML, Bell LS (2007) Differentiating human bone from animal bone: a review of histological methods. J Forensic Sci 52(2):249–263

Katzenberg MA, Saunders SR, Robling AG, Stout SD (2008) Histomorphometry of human cortical bone: applications to age estimation. In: Biological anthropology of the human skeleton, 2nd edn. Wiley, New York

Kerley ER (1965) The microscopic determination of age in human bone. Am J Phys Anthropol 23:149–163

Keough N, L'Abbé EN, Steyn M (2009) The evaluation of age-related histomorphometric variables in a cadaver sample of lower socioeconomic status: implications for estimating age at death. Forensic Sci Int 191(1–3):114.e1–114.e6. https://doi.org/10.1016/j.forsciint.2009.07.012

Kerley ER, Ubelaker DH (1978) Revisions in the microscopic method of estimating age at death in human cortical bone. Am J Phys Anthropol 49(4):545–546

Konigsberg LW, Frankenberg SR (1992) Estimation of age structure in anthropological demography. Am J Phys Anthropol 89(2):235–256

Kragstrup J, Melsen F, Mosekilde L (1983–1984) Thickness of bone formed at remodeling sites in normal human iliac trabecular bone: variations with age and sex. Metab Bone Dis Relat Res 5(1):17–21

Laitman JT, Albertine KH (2015) The anatomical record by the numbers: seeing anatomy through the lens of mathematics and geometry. Anat Rec (Hoboken) 298(1):1–2. https://doi.org/10.1002/ar.23077

Lovejoy CO, Meindl RS, Pryzbeck TR, Mensforth RP (1985) Chronological metamorphosis of the auricular surface of the ilium: a new method for the determination of adult skeletal age at death. Am J Phys Anthropol 68(1):15–28

Lynnerup N, Thomsen JL, Frohlich B (1998) Intra- and inter-observer variation in histological criteria used in age at death determination based on femoral cortical bone. Forensic Sci Int 91(3):219–230

Lynnerup N, Frohlich B, Thomsen JL (2006) Assessment of age at death by microscopy: unbiased quantification of secondary osteons in femoral cross sections. Forensic Sci Int 159(Suppl 1):S100–S103

Maat GJR, Van Den Bos RPM, Aarents MJ (2001) Manual preparation of ground sections for the microscopy of natural bone tissue: update and modification of Frost's 'rapid manual method. J Osteoarcheol 11:366–374

Maat GJR, Aarents MJ, Nagelkerke NJD (2005) Age prediction from bone replacement: remodeling of circumferential lamellar bone tissue in the anterior cortex of the femoral shaft of the present Dutch population. Barge's Anthropologica, Leiden University Medical Center, Leiden

Maat GJ, Maes A, Aarents MJ, Nagelkerke NJ (2006) Histological age prediction from the femur in a contemporary Dutch sample. The decrease of nonremodeled bone in the anterior cortex. J Forensic Sci 51(2):230–237

Martrille L, Irinopoulou T, Bruneval P, Baccino E, Fornes P (2009) Age at death estimation in adults by computer-assisted histomorphometry of decalcified femur cortex. J Forensic Sci 54(6):1231–1237. https://doi.org/10.1111/j.1556-4029.2009.01178.x

Meissner C, Ritz-Timme S (2010) Molecular pathology and age estimation. Forensic Sci Int 203(1–3):34–43. https://doi.org/10.1016/j.forsciint.2010.07.010

Parfitt AM, Drezner MK, Glorieux FH, Kanis JA, Malluche H, Meunier PJ, Ott SM, Recker RR (1987) Bone histomorphometry: standardization of nomenclature, symbols, and units. Report of the ASBMR Histomorphometry Nomenclature Committee. J Bone Miner Res 2(6):595–610

Pfeiffer S, Lazenby R, Chiang J (1995) Brief communication: cortical remodeling data are affected by sampling location. Am J Phys Anthropol 96(1):89–92

Pratte DG, Pfeiffer S (1999) Histological age estimation of a cadaveral sample of diverse origins. Can Soc Forensic Sci J 32(4):155–167

Stout SD, Paine RR (1992) Histological age estimation using rib and clavicle. Am J Phys Anthropol 87:11–15

Stout SD, Gehlert SJ (1980) The relative accuracy and reliability of histological aging methods. Forensic Sci Int 15(3):181–190

Stout SD, Stanley SC (1991) Percent osteonal bone versus osteon counts: the variable of choice for estimating age at death. Am J Phys Anthropol 86(4):515–519

Stout SD, Saunders SR, Katzenberg MA (1992) Methods of determining age at death using bone microstructures. In: Skeletal biology of past peoples: research methods. Wiley-Liss, Inc, New York, pp 21–35

Thomas CDL, Stein MS, Feik SA, Wark JD, Clement JG (2000) Determination of age at death using combined morphology and histology of the femur. J Anat 196(Pt 3):463–471

Thomas CDL, Cooper DML, Clement JG, Peele AG, Hannah K (2007) Intra-osteon distribution of osteocyte lacunae in human cortical bone assessed by synchrotron radiation micro-CT. Australas Phys Eng Sci Med 30(4):433

Watanabe Y, Konishi M, Shimada M, Ohara H, Iwamoto S (1998) Estimation of age from the femur of Japanese cadavers. Forensic Sci Int 98(1–2):55–65

Yoshino M, Imaizumi K, Miyasaka S, Seta S (1994) Histological estimation of age at death using microradiographs of humeral compact bone. Forensic Sci Int 64(2–3):191–198

Lethal Traumatic Injuries due to Traffic Accidents

10

S. Zerbo, A. Di Piazza, S. Procaccianti, E. Ventura Spagnolo, and G. Lo Re

Although in recent years there has been progress towards improving road safety legislation and in making vehicles safer, the report highlights that the action to combat this global challenge has been insufficient [1].

Lethal injuries occur in all forms of transportation but statistically road traffic accidents account for the vast majority in the world.

Most common cause of death in car accidents is head injuries followed by chest and abdomino-pelvic injuries [2]. A. Ndiaye report that the most frequently injuries responsible for death affected the thorax (62% of casualties), the head (49%), the abdomen (10%), and the spine (9%) [3].

There is some evidence on effectiveness of digital autopsy in determining the cause of death due to blunt trauma following traffic accidents [4].

Postmortem cross-sectional imaging, including computed tomography (CT) and magnetic resonance imaging (MR), has been an established adjunct to forensic pathology for approximately a decade [5].

Although imaging in postmortem investigation is performed since radiography (X-rays) itself exists, recently the use of heavy imaging techniques has been improved to assist or supplant conventional autopsy in postmortem investigation [5].

PMCT technique is increasingly implemented into forensic medicine thanks to the possibility to re-assess data through the use of multiplanar and volume rendering reconstructions.

While there are few who doubt the ability of PMCT to detect fractures, foreign bodies, and major hemorrhagic injuries, there have been many false dawns in this field.

On the other hand, a growing filed is represented by postmortem MRI (PMMR) which has a high sensitivity and specificity especially in the evaluation of soft tissue, nervous and cardiovascular systems. A major limiting factor of PMMR is the high cost of the technique, which is not widely available. Furthermore another limitation is the long examination time for a whole-body study, which is required to completely evaluate the deceased.

For this specific reason, PMMR evaluation, when requested and possible to apply, must be focused on specific anatomic region of interest.

An important tool of PMMR is the evaluation of certain areas, such as the subcutaneous fat of the extremities, the spine and the back of the torso improving examination before autopsy.

S. Zerbo (✉) · S. Procaccianti · E. Ventura Spagnolo
Department for Health Promotion, Maternal and Child Care, University of Palermo, Palermo, Italy
e-mail: stefania.zerbo@unipa.it; salvatore.procaccianti@unipa.it; elvira.venturaspagnolo@unipa.it

A. Di Piazza · G. Lo Re
Policlinic Hospital, University of Palermo, Palermo, Italy

G. Lo Re et al. (eds.), *Radiology in Forensic Medicine*,
https://doi.org/10.1007/978-3-319-96737-0_10

However, it has been reported in literature that whole-body MRI for postmortem imaging compared with classic autopsy in cases of a traumatic cause of death showed overall good performance of this technique in the visualization of major life-threatening pathologic conditions [6].

It is important to underline also that some findings, easily recognized at PMCT and PMMR, can be missed during autopsy if not depicted before the beginning of the conventional procedure such as pneumothorax, pneumomediastinum, and gas bubble in the vessels.

10.1 Head Injuries

Head injuries commonly occur as consequence of direct impact to the head; rapid acceleration/deceleration of the head with or without a head impact. The probability of lethal injuries depends on the impact velocity and on the size and type of vehicle involved in a crash.

The most common head lethal injuries include:

- Skull fractures.
- Vertebral dislocations and fractures.
- Epidural, subdural, subarachnoid hemorrhages.
- Brain and spinal cord contusions, lacerations and hemorrhages.
- Intraventricular hemorrhage.
- Diffuse brain injury (swelling, axonal injury, hypoxic-ischemic injury, vascular injury).

The fracture skull bones are distinguished into linear fracture, depressed fracture, comminuted fracture, and ring fracture. The various pattern of injuries are caused by direct contact from objects and/or energy transfer to sites remote from the impact site.

Basilar skull fractures are defined as linear fractures in the skull base, and are often associated with facial fractures that extend to the skull base. The sphenoid sinus, foramen magnum, temporal bone, and sphenoid wings are the most common areas of these fractures.

The most common site of skull base fracture is the anterior vault followed by the middle and the posterior region. Basilar fractures tend to run along the length of the petrous ridges passing through the sella turcica ("hinge fractures"). Less common are ring fractures and multiple fracture lines of the base of the skull.

The clivus is the strongest bone of the skull base and provides mechanical support for the cranial vault and protection for the brainstem and adjacent major vascular structures. Despite its deep location it is very susceptible to related fractures and a high mortality or at least a poor outcome for survivors related to concomitant injuries of the brainstem, lower cranial nerves, and vertebro-basilar artery.

In general, clivus fractures are hardly detected on conventional radiography, contrariwise to cross-sectional imaging such as CT, and is usually a detectable autoptical finding (Figs. 10.1 and 10.2).

As reported by Corradino et al. [7] the clival fractures are classified according their CT

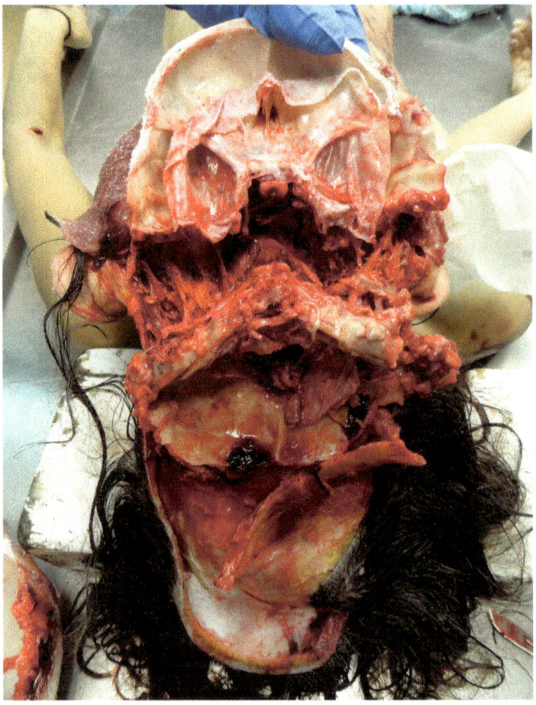

Fig. 10.1 A hinge fracture of the base of the skull. The fracture line runs from side to side across the floor of the middle cranial fossa, passing through the pituitary fossa in the midline. The victim was a young who died following front impact crash while sitting in the front passenger seat

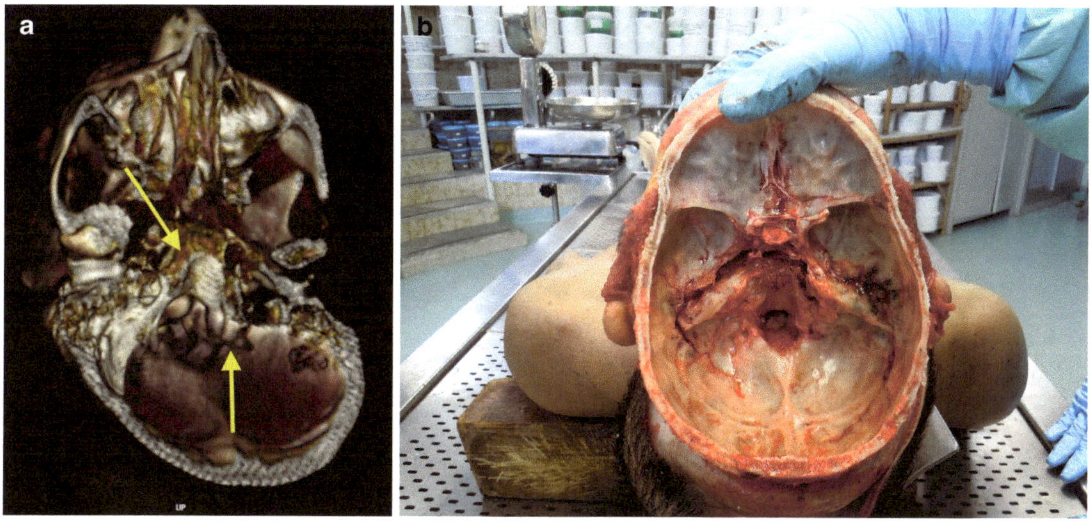

Fig. 10.2 (**a**) Para-axial volume rendering reconstruction image shows two fractures of the base of the skull with their direction and length (yellow arrows). The victim was a young man who died after a smash-up while he was stopping on his motorcycle. (**b**) The same traumatic fracture of the skull base at autopsy

imaging as longitudinal, transverse, and oblique. Longitudinal types are usually caused by frontal or axial impact and are associated with the highest mortality (67–80%), related to the concomitant injuries of the brainstem, lower cranial nerves, and vertebro-basilar artery. As reported in forensic literature, the oblique or transverse clival fractures usually occur after a severe axial blow and have been often implicated in damage of the carotid arteries [8].

Traumatic intracranial hemorrhages occur in the following sites:

- Epidural space
- Subdural space
- Subarachnoid space.
- Intracerebral hemorrhages

The **epidural hemorrhage** is generally due to avulsion and rupture of the diploic veins or stretching and tearing of a sinus wall. It may be the result of transection of the middle meningeal artery by a skull fracture that passes through the middle meningeal groove. Extradural hematomas is usually in the temporal or parietal regions, where an impact to the temporal bone causes a fracture of the squamous temporal bone. These hemorrhages may occur over any portion of the hemispheres or in the posterior fossa and are much slower.

The **acute subdural hematomas** is caused by a tear of the bridging veins between the cortical surface and the dural sinuses or small artery on the cortical surface. Acute subdural hematomas is usually associated with head trauma severe enough to cause skull fracture and cerebral contusion or laceration. Acute subdural hematoma (ASDH) is generally associated to diffuse axonal injury (DAI) produced acceleration/deceleration forces. The mortality is extremely high and the residual dysfunction of survivors is severe.

The **subarachnoid hemorrhage** may be focal or diffuse as sequel of head blunt trauma or it is secondary to a rupture of vertebral artery or dissection of vertebra-basilar artery due to blunt cervical trauma particularly by rapid deceleration of the high-speed motor vehicle crashes.

Rarely a closed head injury is complicated by a rupture of vertebral artery or vertebral artery aneurysm [9].

Generally, a vascular injury after a blunt cervical trauma results either from shearing forces secondary to rotational injuries or from direct trauma to the vessel wall from bony prominences. Distraction/extension, distraction/flexion, and lateral flexion injuries have been implicated as

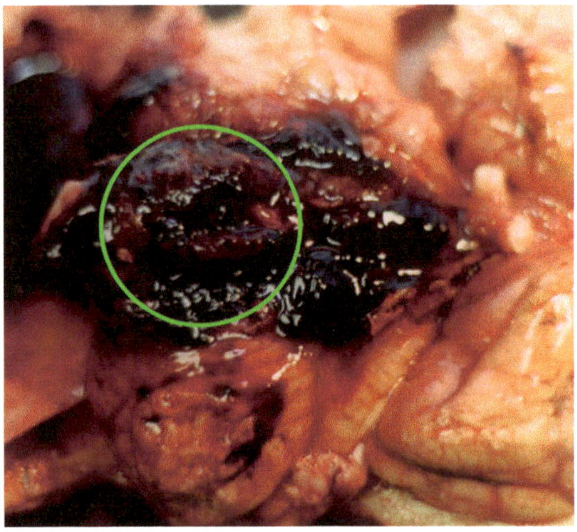

Fig. 10.3 A rupture of fusiform aneurysm of right vertebral artery observed in a 13-year-old female due to blunt cervical trauma following a traffic accident

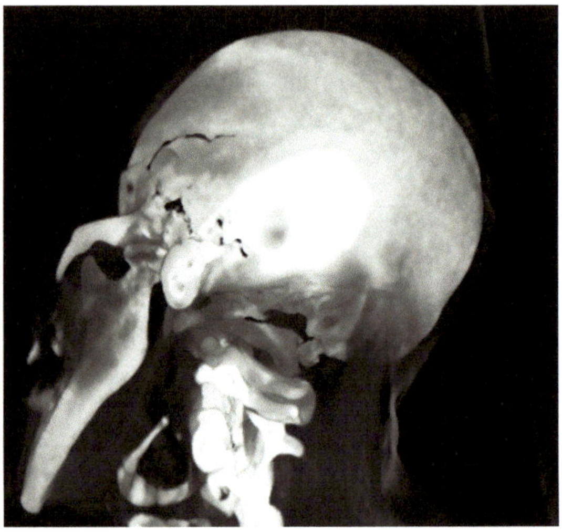

Fig. 10.4 MIP 3D volume rendering reconstruction shows a wide fractures of the plank head from the medial third of the occipital bone suture to parietal bone and subluxations of the atlo-occipital articulation

major mechanisms of injury in vertebral artery. Moreover, either distraction/extension or distraction/flexion injuries could easily be elicited by the rapid deceleration of the high-speed motor vehicle crash (Fig. 10.3).

Intracerebral hemorrhages are, also, common in severe head injuries. Some are primary, occurring at the time of impact or soon afterwards; others are secondary and caused by changes in intracranial pressure or bleeding into infarcts caused by vascular damage.

At PMCT intracranial hemorrhages are not different if compared with alive and are well detectable as intraparenchymal, epidural, subdural, or subarachnoid hemorrhage [10] (Figs. 10.4 and 10.5).

Fractures of the calvarium, the skull base, and the facial bones can be rapidly detected at PMCT before tissue dissection [11].

Despite PMCT has a low performance value in detecting soft tissue injuries and parenchymal injuries, PMCT findings such as traumatic decerebration, external brain herniation, crush fracture of skulls, massive intraventricular hemorrhage, and cerebral venous gas emboli due to secondary open skull-fractures are sufficient to underline the cause of death [11–13].

Another important tool of traumatic lesions detected at PMCT is intraocular hemorrhage: in the most of cases it is due to orbital and skull base fractures which sometimes can be not evidentiated by performing conventional autopsy [14].

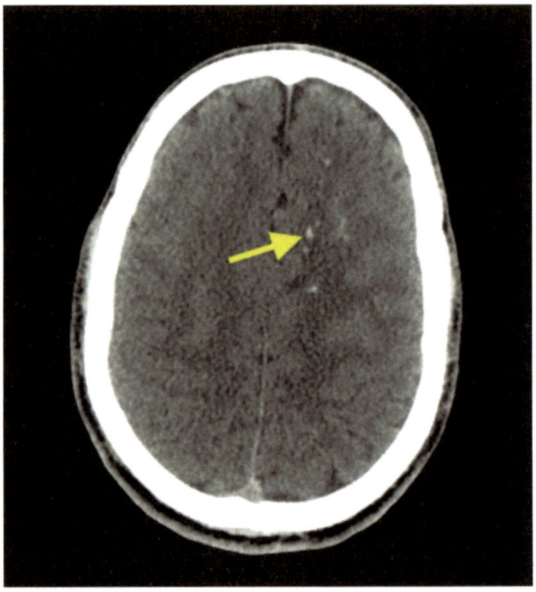

Fig. 10.5 Unenhanced CT of the head after motorcycle accident highlights the presence of subarachnoid hemorrhage and microhemorrhages in the corona radiata

The role of PMCT in cases of cerebral venous gas emboli is important because it could be missed during conventional autopsy although modified autopsy techniques to detect air are employed.

Moreover signs which make high suspicion of cerebral venous gas emboli include gas in the cerebral venous sinuses, right heart, supracardiac neck veins, and pulmonary artery [11].

Embolism has to be suspected when there are the absence of subcutaneous emphysema, absence of air in the left side of the heart, and air only in the hepatic veins without portal venous gas [15]. Specificity, sensitivity, and accuracy in the detection of subarachnoid hematoma, subdural hematoma, and epidural hematoma are really high at PMMR, as reported by Ross et al. [6]. In the same study, in cases of intraparenchymal hemorrhage of brain tissue, PMMR had a sensitivity of 80%, with good concordance with that of autopsy [6].

Moreover PMMR is sufficient for the evaluation of findings identified as coup or contrecoup lesions by the autopsy [16].

As reported in literature, the coup lesion occurs in the same site of the primarily impacted area, with the contrecoup lesion occurring on the opposite site. About this, when possible, it is important both for the pathologist and the radiologist to know how was the trauma to calculate the impact vector, important for the forensic reconstruction of the head trauma [16].

During PMCT of the head after trauma it is important to be aware about some unspecific postmortem signs which may not be related to the trauma itself. In particular, loss of cortico-medullary differentiation, brain swelling, hyperdensity of sagittal sinus and cerebral veins, and the presence of gas bubbles are not necessarily related to the trauma.

The loss of cortico-medullary differentiations is due to postmortem hypoxia which leads to edema reducing the border between the cortex and medulla of the brain. However, to increase the specificity of postmortem imaging investigation, we have to underline that performing PMMR, the cortico-medullary differentiation remains after weeks and can help to identify brain structure in other type of traumatic death.

Brain swelling is also related to hypoxic edema formation and results in the increasing size of the brain with reduction of the volume of the sulci, cisterns, and ventricles, often associated with intracranial hernias [17].

Thanks to the sedimentation effect of the static flow of the blood after death, hyperdensity of the vessels is a common finding. Blood clots are always located on the backside of the body, if the deceased lies on the back, and at imaging revealed a brighter imaging of the posterior sagittal sinus compared with other sinus. Also cerebral veins may appear brighter but it has to be not confused with subarachnoid hemorrhage.

Moreover the presence of gas bubbles has to be correlated to bacterial putrefaction that begins after a short time after death. The same pattern is seen in the whole body. The most important feature to underline in this case is the diffuse distribution of putrefaction gasses, which is not common in cases of embolism or trauma [18].

Postmortem fractures of the body can occur due to accidentally sloppy during transfer to and from the CT couch. Communication with the forensic pathologist regarding the initial external inspection or later inspection during autopsy is relevant to avoid mistaking postmortem fractures for antemortem findings. On the other hand, indirect signs of antemortem fractures, such as hematoma on PMCT or bone bruises on PMMR, might be present. Nevertheless, bone marrow edema can also occur as a result of heat-related bone changes due to thermal impact with potential pitfalls findings [19].

10.2 PMMR vs. PMCT vs. Autopsy

Radiological techniques and conventional autopsy are equivalent for the diagnosis of skull fractures. Facial bone fractures are better identified at PMCT than autopsy. In the evaluation of brain tissue injuries, PMMR is found to be sufficient for the evaluation of typical blunt head trauma injuries [6, 20].

Hemorrhages are well identified with a good diagnostic agreement both by autopsy and radiological techniques, although subdural hematomas and subarachnoid hemorrhages are visualized slightly better with autopsy than PMCT and

PMMR. However intraventricular hemorrhages are well detected at PMCT, due to the complexity of findings of the injured brain tissue after meninges are opened at autopsy [11].

Smaller hemorrhages are often missed with both PMCT and PMMR, although the role of these injuries is important in forensic medicine.

Extra-axial hemorrhages are better investigated with higher specificity through PMMR than PMCT [20, 21].

10.2.1 Brainstem Injuries

Traumatic lesions of brainstem most commonly occur on pontomedullary junction. The most common mechanisms of pontomedullary lacerations include impact to the chin, with or without a skull base fracture, lateral and posterior head impacts with subsequent hinge fractures, frontoposterior hyperextension of the head [22].

In all the cases with pontomedullary laceration posterior neck dissection should be performed during the autopsy, since upper spine injuries are often associated with this type of injury (Fig. 10.6).

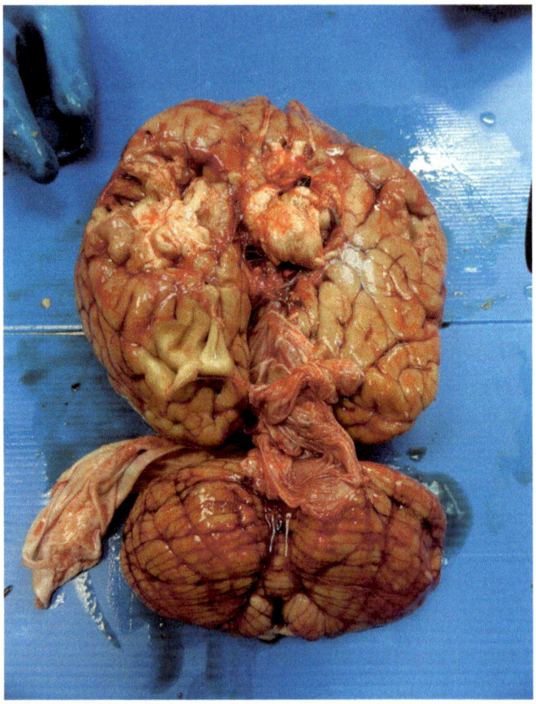

Fig. 10.6 Longitudinal brainstem laceration associated with complex basilar skull fractures observed in a young woman due to blunt head trauma following a traffic accident

10.2.2 Spine Injuries

The cervical spine is susceptible to injuries during hyperextension or hyperflexion of the neck. The introduction of PMCT has significantly improved diagnostic accuracy of cervical spine examination [23] (Fig. 10.7).

One injury that is frequently overlooked at autopsy is the atlanto-occipital dislocation not easily detected at conventional autopsy. Other fractures can occur anywhere in the cervical spine, often at about C5–C6 level. Seatbelt restraint cannot prevent cervical spine damage, though a rigid head restraint can reduce injuries resulting from hyperextension. The thoracic spine is less often damaged, but in unrestrained drivers the same "whiplash" effect can fracture or dislocate the upper dorsal spine, often around T5–6–7 level.

PMCT has a strong limit in the detection of cervical cord injury and discoligamentous injury which can be seen only on PMMR, although it can be suspected if spine fractures are present [12].

Spinal cord injuries without radiographic abnormalities (SCIWORA) are well-known entity, first described in 1982 by Pang and Wilberg. This entity includes normal findings on radiographs, but detectable on MRI studies only if spinal cord has been visualized.

However, most traumatic changes can be easily detected and characterized at PMCT, although SCIWORA are a potential pitfall in PMCT. Spinal cord injuries (SCIs) characterized by bone fractures at PMCT can be easily detected at PMCT.

Ossification of the posterior longitudinal ligament, spinal stenosis due to cervical spondylosis, ossification of the ligamentum flavum, diffuse idiopathic skeletal hyperostosis, fused vertebral bodies, and ankylosing spondylitis are often detected at PMCT and can be considered

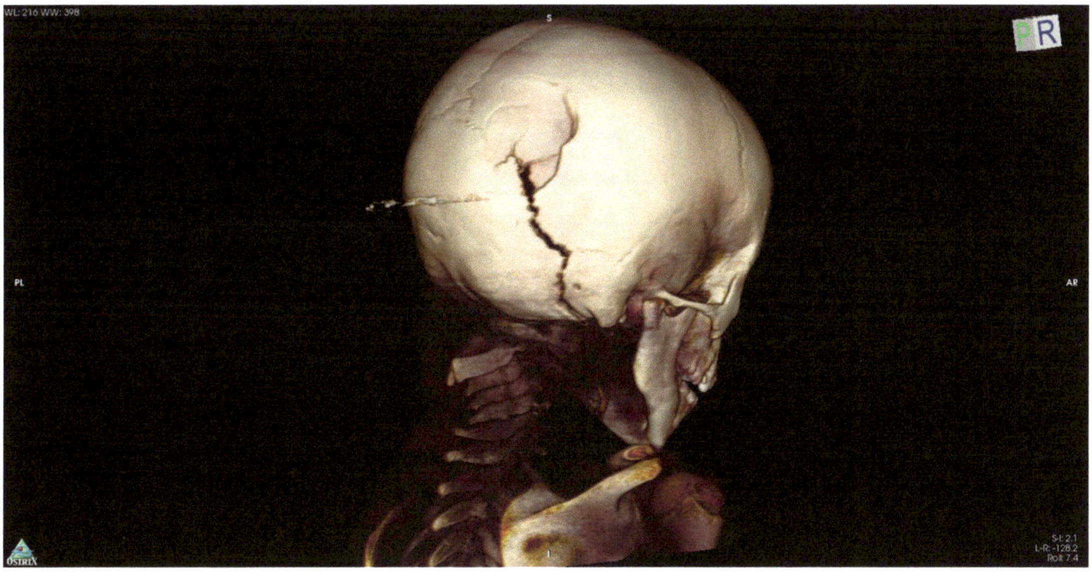

Fig. 10.7 Atlanto-axial joint dislocation associated with fracture of odontoid process at CT scan image observed in a young woman due to airbag

to be associated with SCIs and also with SCIWORAs [24, 25].

Spinal cord injuries can be seen at PMCT and are identified also by the presence of hemorrhages and contusion in the spinal cord also without transection or severe deformity, some only detectable microscopically.

Fractures, on one hand, are well recognizable at PMCT. On the other hand, it is not easy to detect intervertebral disk injuries, although PMCT is useful in identifying dislocations, tears, and hemorrhage, but sometimes are very difficult to identify without subluxations. Perivertebral hemorrhage is always associated with SCIs and easily recognized at PMCT.

As reported by Makino et al., SCIs with apparent transection or severe deformity, which can lead to immediate death, are sometimes detectable at PMCT. However contusions and tiny hemorrhages were more frequent at autopsy, but could not be identified at PMCT because of artifacts from teeth and bones. On the other side, SCIWORAs typically were associated with occult disk injuries and occult perivertebral hemorrhage, but not with fractures. Because of apart mentioned reasons about disk dislocation, occult disk herniation or spontaneously reduced subluxations could cause spinal cord compression, but are not evidentiated at PMCT.

A specific pitfall about SCIs and SCIWORAs is represented by postmortem positional changes which can lead to a reduction of subluxations, also associated with reduced blood circulation caused by the death [26].

10.3 PMMR vs. PMCT vs. Autopsy

PMCT and PMMR are equivalent or superior to conventional autopsy in identifying spine fractures to conventional autopsy. PMCT can identify upper cervical spine injuries, with a good agreement with autopsy, but cranio-vertebral dislocations are better identified with autopsy [20, 27].

10.3.1 Chest and Abdomen Blunt Injury

Chest blunt injury is usually associated with injuries in other body parts. They are caused by different and combined mechanism such as a direct impact, compression, and deceleration.

A direct compression of chest causes ribs and sternal fractures. Typical fracture patterns depend on the site of compression: sternal and anterolateral rib fractures are due to anterior compression; posterior rib fractures are due to posterior compression, and a lateral compression causes costochondral disruption. Multiple ribs fractures are generally associated with hemothorax and pneumothorax, lacerations and contusion of the lungs and the heart. Mechanical heart lacerations are usually associated with injury to other structures of the chest. The causative force is typically applied to the anterior precordium. Due to its position between the sternum and the thoracic vertebrae, the heart is exposed to any sudden impact on the sternum and to compression forces applied to the chest. High energy blunt traumas (injury severity scores—ISS) can lead to different types of cardiac injury such as valve or myocardial contusions, cardiac rupture, and aortic lacerations with hemopericardium. These lesions are usually associated with a high mortality rate either by hemorrhagic or arrhythmic complications. The incidence rate of cardiac injury after blunt chest trauma in postmortem studies is reported between 14% and 20%. Cardiac lacerations are rare and usually fatal.

Heart lacerations may involve the right and left atria, the right and left ventricles, the atrial septum, the interventricular septum as well as the intrapericardial portion of the superior or inferior vena cava, the pulmonary veins, the atrioventricular valves, and their chordae tendineae. The rupture of interventricular septum with or without other cardiac injuries after blunt thoracic trauma in car accidents is rare as reported in the literature. The severity and degree of injuries depends upon the phase of the cardiac cycle at the time of injury. Late diastole or early systoles are periods of increased vulnerability because the chambers are full and the valves are closed. Autopsy studies have shown that the right ventricle is most frequently ruptured, followed by the left ventricle, right atrium, intraventricular septum, left atrium, and inter atrial septum in decreasing frequency (Figs. 10.8 and 10.9).

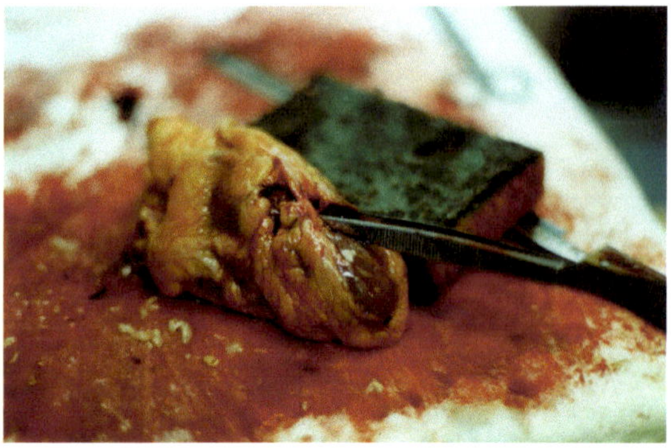

Fig. 10.8 A 40-year-old Caucasian woman died in a traffic accident. The woman wasn't seat-belted in the front passenger seat. At autopsy the anterior surface of the heart shows two transmural lacerations: the first cm 3 × 2 in size, located on the interventricular sulcus 3 cm from the atrioventricular sulcus; the second cm 3 × 2.5 cm in size located on the margo obtusus cordis

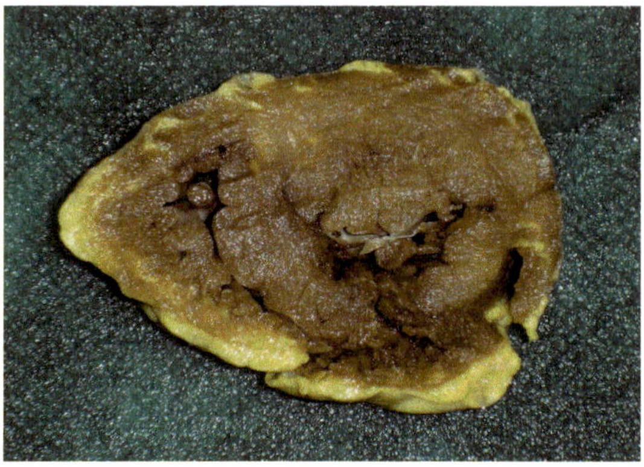

Fig. 10.9 The same case after parallel cuts made perpendicularly to the longitudinal axis, a laceration of the anterior side of the right and left ventricles and of the interventricular septum was observed

Possible mechanisms of laceration include a direct blow to the chest, compression of the heart through bidirectional forces between the sternum and the spine during early systole, with the ventricular cavity filled and the atrioventricular valves closed, deceleration or rapid rotation with fixation of the great vessels, transmission of high hydraulic venous pressure following compression of the abdomen or extremities and rupture of the myocardium by a fractured rib [28, 29].

In all these injuries, the sudden great pressure applied to the chest seems to be the key factor in determining explosive cardiac laceration, frequently involving the roof of the atria and/or apex of both ventricular. Chamber or valvular

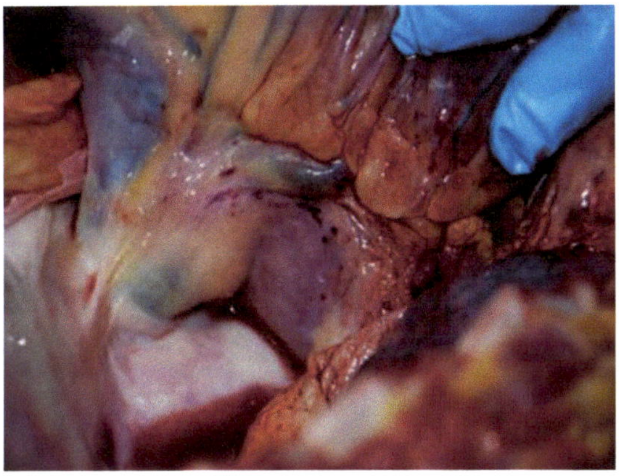

Fig. 10.10 On the posterior surface of the right atrium, punctiform ecchymosis were observed, specifically between the superior and inferior vein caval connection and the wall of the right atrium. The autopsy did not show external signs of thoracic trauma, no evident rib or sternum fractures

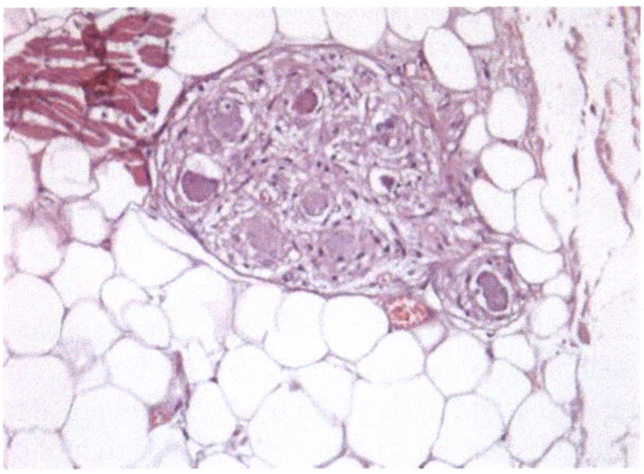

Fig. 10.11 In the atrioventricular conduction tissue, plurifocal petechial hemorrhagic infiltration of the interatrial septum involving the myelinic fibers in the contest of adipose tissue. E E 40×

rupture is more likely if impact occurs at end diastole, when the heart is maximally distended with blood. The severity of the lesion depends on the impact velocity and chest compression (Figs. 10.10 and 10.11).

- Blunt thoracic trauma can rarely cause coronary artery injury. Blunt trauma can result in occlusion of any of the coronary arteries or can lead to its rupture [30].
- Traffic accidents are, also, the most frequent causes of cardiac contusion (contusions) resulting from a direct blow to the chest. Rarely blunt cardiac contusion can result in cardiac conduction system injury leading to a fatal arrhythmia [31].

PMCT has a useful role in the detection of chest wall injuries such as hemothorax, pneumothorax, hemopericardium, pneumopericardium, pulmonary injuries, fractures of ribs and dorsal vertebras and the application of contrast medium does not much improve sensitivity of the technique in the recognition of chest wall lesions [4].

In some cases the cause of death can be also tension pneumothorax due to a chest wall trauma: in fact gas may induce pneumorachis and pneumocephalus which can be responsible of the death [32].

The presence of gas, as discussed, may be underestimated at conventional autopsy without using special techniques such as opening the body under water or using aspirometers. In these cases performing PMCT before autopsy can be useful to apply as the gold technique [11].

The presence of fracture of the ribs and thoracic spine with a flail chest and subsequent pneumothorax, pneumomediastinum, and hemothorax at PMCT may suggest exsanguination as the cause of death [17, 33].

At PMMRI hemothorax can be detected with high sensitivity and specificity, as reported in literature [6].

On PMMR images the typical pattern is characterized by sedimented corpuscular blood components at the bottom and a serous layer on top, due to the effect of gravity [6].

Moreover, in the same study conducted in 2012, it has been reported that pneumothorax was diagnosed with sensitivity of 100% and specificity and accuracy of 73%, while in ten cases was not detected at autopsy [6].

Aortic lacerations may occur in both head-on and side-impact crashes. Traumatic aortic rupture is the second most common cause of death in victims of blunt chest trauma from motor vehicle accidents [34]. Aortic rupture in blunt trauma results most commonly from sudden high speed deceleration or less frequently from chest compression. Other mechanisms involved in blunt aortic injuries might include compression of the vessels between bony structures, such as sternum and spine. The most common site of injury is the aortic isthmus [35, 36].

Specific signs of exsanguination include "vanishing aorta" sign, "hyperdense armored heart," and "flattened heart," which also correlate with cardiac tamponade [4].

Vanishing aorta refers to the collapse of the vessel, an important feature in fatal hemorrhage, but can be also seen in all the big vessels such as pulmonary arteries and caval veins. However it can also be seen in other causes of death due to a pressure loss from a decreased cardiac ejection [17].

Traumatic aortic rupture is not always detectable at unenhanced PMCT. It can be assumed when there is a big intrathoracic hematoma adjacent to the aorta without any fat plane in between. However PMMRI better recognizes aortic tears than in unenhanced PMCT, although at PMCT angiography an eventual "active" extravasation of contrast medium can be detected.

Overall sensitivity for ruptured aorta in postmortem CT and MRI together is between 75% and 100% [37].

Sometimes the presence of hyperdensities and nondependent air foci may be suggestive of thrombus formation [4].

Pulmonary embolism, as a secondary cause of death after trauma, is impossible to detect at unenhanced PMCT [17].

Myocardial ruptures are simply recognized at PMMR [6].

However aortic tears, despite the excellent soft-tissue image contrast of PMMR, are not easily recognized and localized in cases of exsanguination because of the collapse of the vessel lumen [6].

As in PMCT, the site of the lesion has to be suspected in case of perivascular and intramural hematomas.

The appearance of hyperdense aortic wall can be related to a contraction of the aortic wall, luminal loss of pressure and decreased attenuation of the lumen due to dilution of blood after massive infusion at resuscitation or sedimentation of the blood away from aorta. The possibility of atherosclerotic disease and the presence of intracardiac bypass or other devices can be useful at non-contrast PMCT in the recognition of the aorta after rupture within mediastinal bleeding [17] (Fig. 10.12).

Diaphragmatic injuries may occur rarely with blunt chest trauma. The rupture of the left side is more common than the right side probably because the right half of diaphragm is protected by the liver. The rupture of diaphragm is often associated with a herniation of abdominal organs and is generally associated with liver, spleen, and lungs blunt injuries.

Traumatic diaphragmatic hernias, characterized by the elevation of the diaphragm and abdominal organ herniation into the thorax, can be seen at PMCT. It could be very challenging to recognize at non-contrast PMCT the right side hernias: in fact the liver having the same attenua-

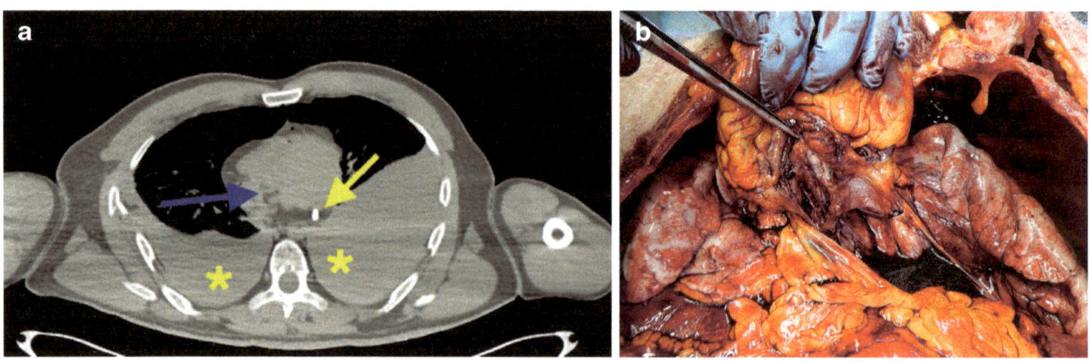

Fig. 10.12 (**a**) Unenhanced CT after a motorcycle accident shows the presence of a wide hematic pleural effusion due to the direct chest blunt trauma. It is also possible to recognize the presence of a cardiac bypass verified at autopsy (yellow arrow) and to conjecture a lesion of the posterior wall of the right atrium (blue arrow), demonstrated at autopsy. (**b**) Shows the traumatic laceration of the posterior wall of the right atrium

tion of hemothorax can make right diaphragmatic hernias missed. On the other hand, left-sided hernias are more simple to distinguish thanks to the natural contrast between the lung and the left-sided abdominal organs (stomach, bowel) [11].

10.4 Lung Lesions

However atelectasis can be easily recognized at contrast-PMCT because pulmonary tissue shows significative enhancement after administration of iodinated contrast medium [17].

The evaluation of lung parenchyma may include pulmonary contusions and lacerations. The direct damage to the parenchyma can be a cause of death through the formation of a pulmonary alveolo-venous fistula which leads to systemic arterial gas emboli. It has to be suspected in cases of open chest wall injuries and gas in the left side of the heart and systemic arteries without specific signs of putrefactive changes [38].

The evaluation of pulmonary parenchyma findings at PMCT can be difficult especially considering nonspecific signs associated with hypostasis which is not always simple to distinguish from pulmonary contusions or pulmonary hemorrhage or pulmonary edema with its different causes [38].

PMMR has an important role also in the detection of the lung parenchymal contusions and lacerations; however diagnostic value can be reduced by superimposition of postmortem alteration of lung tissue, as described for PMCT [6].

10.5 PMMR vs. PMCT vs. Autopsy

PMCT has a strong agreement with autopsy in the detection of ribs fractures [6].

Autopsy is superior in the identification of intrathoracic injuries, with the exception of pneumothorax and hemothorax. Moreover thoracic gas-related injuries can be missed with autopsy [39].

All studies state that autopsy was equal or superior to PMCT or PMMRI in identifying pulmonary injuries such as contusions and lacerations.

Several authors argue this to be the result of postmortem changes that render it difficult to distinguish between hypostasis, putrefaction, alveolar hemorrhage or even pneumonia on PMCT or PMMRI.

In concordance with other soft tissue and organ injuries, autopsy is the method that detects more cardiac and pericardial injuries.

Ross et al. investigated myocardial ruptures and found a sensitivity of 75% with PMMRI [6].

Schnider et al. conclude that PMCT sufficed in the detection of cardiac lesions [40].

Similar to fluid and gas in the pleural space, pneumomediastinum, hemomediastinum, pneumopericardium, and hemopericardium are often missed with autopsy. In contrast, PMCT detects even small amounts of fluid or gas in these injuries that are missed at autopsy [33].

Moreover, mediastinal shift remains undetected at autopsy in many cases [20, 33].

10.6 Abdomen

Blunt force applied to the anterior or lateral surface of abdomen can lead to lacerations of abdominal organs such as liver and spleen.

Unenhanced-PMCT has a low sensitivity in the detection of solid abdominal organ injury. The sensitivity for detecting liver injuries is 53%, with even lower sensitivities for splenic and renal injuries [41].

However high grade of liver and splenic injuries are recognizable and characterized as low-attenuation regions within the liver, fractured liver and spleen, focal intrahepatic parenchyma gas bubble (to distinguish from portal veins or hepatic veins gas accumulation), perihepatic or perisplenic blood and hemoperitoneum [15, 41].

Also renal injuries are difficult to depict at unenhanced PMCT if there is no evidence of perirenal fluid or fat stranding or shattered kidneys [15].

Bowel injuries have to be suspected when significant pneumoperitoneum is evident and there is not a high grade of decomposition. In fact bowel distension, intramural air, and gastromalacia

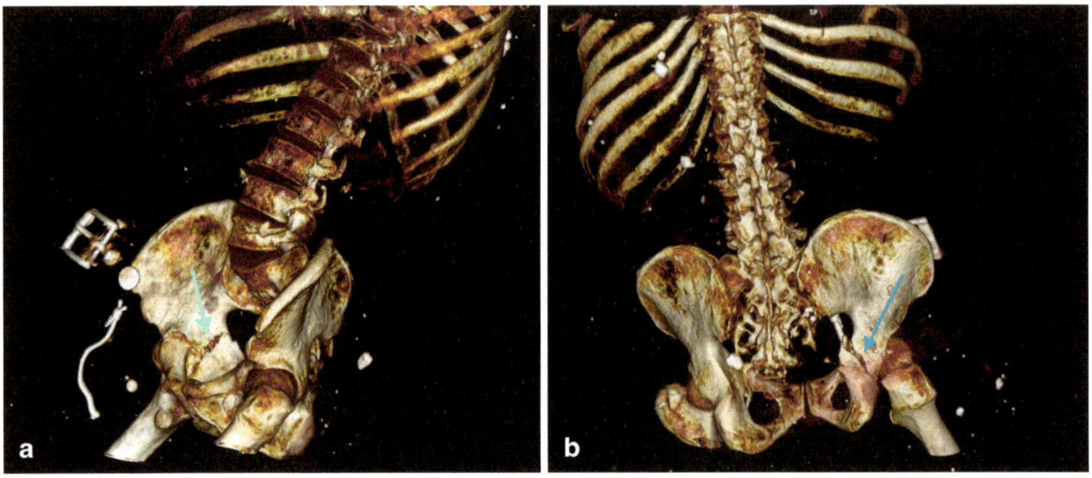

Fig. 10.13 Unenhanced CT of a young man ran over from a vehicle. The volume rendering reconstruction image highlights a length and direction of the iliac bone and of the sacro-iliac junction (**a** right; **b** left)

have to be suspected as normal postmortem changes [41].

On the other hand, the role of PMCT in the detection of lumbar spine and pelvic fracture is similar to bone's injuries in the whole body. Moreover, if pelvic fractures are associated with PMCT signs of exsanguination, these signs are high suggestive of potential cause of the death [11].

In the evaluation of abdominal organs lesions, PMMR can also be useful, especially for liver injuries. Both liver and splenic injuries have to be suspected if MRI shows fluid in the adjacent peritoneal space. For renal lesion PMMR has high specificity, while it is lower for pancreatic injuries.

In every case PMMR is very useful in the detection of peritoneal and retroperitoneal hemorrhages [6].

10.7 PMMR vs. PMCT vs. Autopsy

Autopsy remains superior to PMCT and PMMR in the detection of the injuries of organs and soft tissue of the abdomen.

PMCT and PMMR have a sensitivity of 100% in the identification of perihepatic and perisplenic fluid, although this finding does not adequately predict liver injuries [20, 41].

10.7.1 Pelvic Injuries

The bony pelvis suffers a variety of fractures and dislocations in severe trauma. The mortality is not caused by the pelvic fracture itself but is due to associated injuries such as disruption of the genitourinary and gastrointestinal system and laceration of great vessels [42].

The fracture of pubic symphysis or the posterior iliac spines and dislocation of both sacroiliac joints are due to an antero-posterior compression, as in running over by a vehicle wheel. An impact from the side may cause the superior and, rarely, the inferior pubic ramus with dislocation of the sacroiliac joint on that side [43].

The pelvic fractures are more easily detected by PMTC than conventional autopsy (Fig. 10.13).

10.8 Extremities

Post-traumatic alterations of the subcutaneous fatty tissue in fact is clearly visualized as homogeneous, well-defined accumulations of pooled liquid. Hemorrhages appeared as hypointense on T1-weighted sequences and hyperintense on T2-weighted sequences. Although a limit in the identification is the presence of extent subcutaneous fluid collection which may mask the post-traumatic findings in people who had been hospitalized and bodies that had begun to decompose [6].

Fractures of the extremities are easily recognized when 1–1.5 mm thin-section acquisition is performed, and high resolution images are reached through volume rendering and multiplanar reconstruction techniques. Moreover it is possible to define site and type of fracture and to visualize soft tissue injuries without a dissection required in autopsy to reach bones [11].

10.9 PMMR vs. PMCT vs. Autopsy

Skeletal injuries of the extremities are well detected at PMCT which also identify additional fractures missed at autopsy [11].

On the other hand, PMMR has a mixed sensitivities, from 40% for upper extremity fractures to 100% for lower extremity fractures.

However for hematomas in the extremities, PMMR revealed high sensitivity [6, 20].

References

1. WHO (2015) Global status report on road safety. World Health Organization, Geneva
2. Saukko P (2016) Knight's forensic pathology, 4th edn. CRC Press, Taylor and Francis Group, New York
3. Ndiaye A, Chambost M, Chiron M (2009) The fatal injuries of car drivers. Forensic Sci Int 184:21–27
4. Panda A, Kumar A, Gamanagatti S, Mishra B (2015) Virtopsy computed tomography in trauma: normal postmortem changes and pathologic spectrum of findings. Curr Probl Diagn Radiol 44:391–406
5. Baglivo M, Winklhofer S, Hatch GM, Ampanozi G, Thali MJ, Ruder TD (2013) The rise of forensic and post-mortem radiology—analysis of the literature between the year 2000 and 2011. J Forensic Radiol Imaging 1:3–9
6. Ross S, Ebner L, Flach P, Brodhage R, Bollinger SA, Christe A, Thali MJ (2012) Post-mortem whole-body MRI in traumatic cause of death. AJR Am J Roentgenol 199:1186–1192
7. Corradino G, Wolf AL, Mirvis S, Joslyn J (1990) Fractures of the clivus: classification and clinical features. Neurosurgery 27:592–596
8. Menkü A, Koç RK, Tucer B, Durak AC, Akdemir H (2004) Clivus fractures: clinical presentations and courses. Neurosurg Rev 27:194–198
9. Triolo V, Argo A, Zerbo S, Bono G, Bonifacio A, Pugnetti P, Procaccianti P (2009) Lethal rupture of post-traumatic aneurysm of the vertebral artery case report. J Forensic Legal Med 16:168–171
10. Añon J, Remonda L, Spreng A et al (2008) Traumatic extra-axial hemorrhage: correlation of postmortem MSCT, MRI, and forensic-pathological findings. J Magn Reson Imaging 28(4):823–836
11. Daly B, Abboud S, Ali Z et al (2013) Comparison of whole-body post mortem 3D CT and autopsy evaluation in accidental blunt force traumatic death using the abbreviated injury scale classification. Forensic Sci Int 225:20–26
12. Kasahara S, Makino Y, Hayakawa M et al (2012) Diagnosable and non-diagnosable causes of death by postmortem computed tomography: a review of 339 forensic cases. Legal Med 14:239–245
13. Jacobsen C, Lynnerup N (2010) Craniocerebral trauma—congruence between post- mortem computed tomography diagnoses and autopsy results: a 2-year retrospective study. Forensic Sci Int 194:9–14
14. Flach PM, Egli TC, Bolliger SA et al (2014) "Blind spots" in forensic autopsy: improved detection of retrobulbar hemorrhage and orbital lesions by postmortem computed tomography (PMCT). Leg Med (Tokyo) 16:274–282
15. Jackowski C, Sonnenschein M, Thali MJ et al (2007) Intrahepatic gas at postmortem computed tomography: forensic experience as a potential guide for in vivo trauma imaging. J Trauma 62:979–988
16. Besenski N (2002) Traumatic injuries: imaging of head injuries. Eur Radiol 12:1237–1252
17. Christe A, Flach P, Ross S, Spendlove D, Bolliger S, Vock P, Thali MJ (2010) Clinical radiology and postmortem imaging (Virtosy) are not the same: specific and unspecific postmortem signs. Legal Med 12:215–222
18. Patzelt D, Lignitz E, Keil W et al (1997) Diagnostic problem of air embolism in a corpse. Beitr Gerichtl Med 37:401–405
19. Flach PM, Gascho D, Schweitzer W, Ruder TD, Berger N, Ross SG, Thali MJ, Ampanozi G (2014) Imaging in forensic radiology: an illustrated guide for postmortem computed tomography technique and protocols. Forensic Sci Med Pathol 10:583–606
20. Jalalzadeh H, Giannakopoulos GF, Berger FH, Fronczek J, Van de Goot FRW, Reijnders UJ, Zuidema WP (2015) Post-mortem imaging compared with autopsy in trauma victims—a systematic review. Forensic Sci Int 257:29–48
21. Añon J, Remonda L, Spreng A, Scheurer E, Schroth G, Boesch C et al (2008) Traumatic extra-axial hemorrhage: correlation of postmortem MSCT, MRI, and forensic-pathological findings. J Magn Reson Imaging 28(4):823–836
22. Zivković V, Nikolić S, Babić D, Juković F (2010) The significance of pontomedullar laceration in car occupants following frontal collisions: a retrospective autopsy study. Forensic Sci Int 10:13

23. Burke MP (2012) Forensic pathology of fractures and mechanisms of injury: postmortem CT scanning. CRC Press - Taylor & Francis Group, Boca Raton
24. Ehara S, Shimamura T (2001) Cervical spine injury in the elderly: imaging features. Skelet Radiol 30:1–7
25. Regenbogen VS, Rogers LF, Atlas SW, Kim KS (1986) Cervical spinal cord injuries in patients with cervical spondylosis. AJR Am J Roentgenol 146:277–284
26. Mkino Y, Yokota H, Hayakawa M, Yajima D, Inokuchi G, Nakatani E, Iwase H (2014) Spinal cord injuries with normal postmortem CT findings: a Pitgall of virtual autopsy for detecting traumatic death. AJR Am J Roentgenol 203:204–244
27. Uhrenholt L, Boel LW (2010) Contributions from forensic imaging to the investigation of upper cervical fractures. J Forensic Sci 55(6):1598–1602
28. Gonin J, De la Grandmaison GL, Durigon M, Paraire F (2009) Cardiac contusion and hemopericardium in the absence of external thoracic trauma. Case report and review of the literature. Am J Forensic Med Pathol 30:373–375
29. Robinet S, Morimont P, Lambermont B, Defraigne JO (2012) Interventricular septal rupture caused by vehicular trauma. Heart Lung 41(2):200–202
30. Abu-Hmeidan JH, Arrowaili AL, Yousef RS, Alasmari S, Kassim YM, Aldakhil Allah HH, Aljenaidel AM, Alabdulqader AA, Alrashed MH, Alkhinjar MI, Al-Shammari NR (2016) Coronary artery rupture in blunt thoracic trauma: a case report and review of literature. J Cardiothorac Surg 11(1):119
31. Marshall DT, Gilbert JD, Byard RW (2008) The spectrum of findings in cases of sudden death due to blunt cardiac trauma-commotio cordis. Am J Forensic Med Pathol 29(1):1–4
32. Katz DS, Groskin SA, Wasenko JJ (1994) Pneumorachis and pneumocephalus caused by pneumothorax and multiple thoracic vertebral fractures. Clin Imaging 18:85–87
33. Aghayev E, Christe A, Sonnenschein M et al (2008) Postmortem imaging of blunt chest trauma using CT and MRI: comparison with autopsy. J Thorac Imaging 23:20–27
34. Bertrand S, Cuny S, Petit P, Trosseille X, Page Y, Guillemot H, Drazetic P (2008) Traumatic rupture of thoracic aorta in real-world motor vehicle crashes. Traffic Inj Prev 9(2):153–161
35. Harmouche M, Slimani EK, Heraudeau A, Verhoye JP (2013) Blunt traumatic aortic rupture of the proximal ascending aorta repaired by resection and direct anastomosis. Interact Cardiovasc Thorac Surg 17(4):739–740
36. Kodali S, Jamieson WR, Stephens ML, Miyagishima RT, Janusz MT, Tyers GF (1991) Traumatic rupture of the thoracic aorta. A 20-year review: 1969–1989. Circulation 84(5 Suppl):40–46
37. Aghayev E, Sonnenschein M, Jackowski C et al (2006) Postmortem radiology of fatal hemorrhage: measurements of cross-sectional areas of major blood vessels and volumes of aorta and spleen on MDCT and volumes of heart chambers on MRI. AJR Am J Roentgenol 187(1):209–215
38. Brook OR, Hirshenbaum A, Talor E et al (2012) Arterial air emboli on computed tomography (CT) autopsy. Injury 43:1556–1561
39. Leth PM, Ibsen M (2010) Abbreviated injury scale scoring in traffic fatalities: comparison of computerized tomography and autopsy. J Trauma 68(6):1413–1416
40. Schnider J, Thali MJ, Ross S, Oesterhelweg L, Spendlove D, Bolliger SA (2009) Injuries due to sharp trauma detected by post-mortem multislice computed tomography (MSCT): a feasibility study. Leg Med (Tokyo) 11(1):4–9
41. Christe A, Ross S, Oesterhelweg L, Spendlove D, Bolliger S, Vock P, Thali MJ (2009) Abdominal trauma—sensitivity and specificity of postmortem non-contrast imaging findings compared with autopsy findings. J Trauma 66:1302–1307
42. Richter M, Otte D, Gansslen A, Bartram H, Pohlemann T (2001) Injuries of the pelvic ring in road traffic accidents: a medical and technical analysis. Injury 32:123–128
43. Di Maio V, Di Maio D (2001) Forensic pathology, 2nd edn. CRC Press, Boca Raton

Violence and Abuse: Battered Child

11

Antonina Argo, Giuseppe Lo Re,
Elvira Ventura Spagnolo, Alberto Calandra,
Marija Čaplinskienė, Agata Crapanzano,
Antonio Pinto, and Sergio Salerno

Child abuse is an important social and medical problem which represents a major cause of morbidity and mortality among children. Battered Child Abuse (BCA) is a comprehensive term to indicate classical features at first described by Ambroise Tardieu (1818–1879), a French forensic pathologist, in 1860 in a series of 32 cases of cruelty to children, resulting to death in 21 cases [1].

In 1946, John Caffey (1895–1978) published his first paper where he described six infants with multiple fractures in the long bones, who additionally had chronic subdural haematoma and no history of injury [2]. He recommended that unexplained fractures of the long bones warranted investigations for subdural haematoma (SDH). In 1962, Kempe and co-workers published their study on 'The battered-child syndrome', first real recognition of child abuse as a disease and of the responsibility physicians held for its diagnosis and prevention [3–5]. Finally, Kempe et al. provided radiographic clues to whether trauma was accidental or non-accidental [6]. Worthy of noting, this article was considered one of the best paediatric research articles in the last 150 years, as Kempe et al. established that physicians have a special responsibility to children—a responsibility to help keep them safe, sometimes even from their own parents [1]. During decades scientific interest as reflected by online search of the MEDLINE database yields relevant data about the development of child maltreatment awareness by health care professionals since the article by Kempe et al. was published in 1962. In 1963, the keyword *child abuse* was added to the MEDLINE system [7]. Following keywords were first assigned to battered-child article by the National Library of Medicine (*wounds and injuries*, *child*, *child welfare*, and *infant*). Twelve articles were categorized under this keyword, in 2006 almost 600 articles were listed in MEDLINE under the keyword *child abuse* and 1989 in 2016. Not surprisingly, the marked increase in knowledge about child maltreatment has led to the development of a new paediatric subspecialty, child abuse paediatrics [8–10]. In 2009, the American Board of Pediatrics will administer the first examination for board certification in this subspecialty, legacy related. A significant result of Kempe's battered-child syndrome article has been the raising of paediatricians [11–13] who are dedicated to diagnosing, treating, and preventing child abuse

A. Argo · E. Ventura Spagnolo
Department for Health Promotion, Maternal and Child Care, University of Palermo, Palermo, Italy
e-mail: antonella.argo@unipa.it

G. Lo Re · A. Calandra · A. Crapanzano · S. Salerno
Department of Radiology, Policlinic Hospital, Palermo, Italy
e-mail: sergio.salerno@unipa.it

M. Čaplinskienė (✉)
State Forensic Medicine Service, Vilnius, Lithuania
e-mail: marija.caplinskiene@vtmt.lt

A. Pinto
Ospedale Caldarelli, Naples, Italy

G. Lo Re et al. (eds.), *Radiology in Forensic Medicine*,
https://doi.org/10.1007/978-3-319-96737-0_11

and neglect. Over the years, diagnosis of child abuse becomes more sophisticated within methods such as biomechanics [14], proteomics [15], biochemistry [16] and genetics [17] also in perspective of forensic molecular approach as epigenetic modifications [18, 19].

The 'child abuse syndrome' (also known as the 'battered baby' or 'non-accidental injury in childhood') is a clinical condition in young children who have received serious physical abuse and is a frequent cause of permanent injury or death. The syndrome should be considered in any child exhibiting evidence of fracture of any bone, subdural haematoma, failure to thrive, soft tissue swellings or skin bruising, in any child who dies suddenly, or where the degree and type of injury is at variance with the history given regarding the occurrence of the trauma [20, 21] (Fig. 11.1). After hundreds of researches and contribution of both clinical and forensic interest in decades, as emphasized (Knight's 2016) the BCA happen when an infant or child suffers repetitive physical injuries inflicted by a parent or guardian, in circumstances that exclude accident.

11.1 Fatal Physical Abuse of Children Epidemiology

Child maltreatment—the physical, sexual, mental abuse and/or neglect of children younger than 18 years—exists in every society. It is common in the WHO European Region [22] and globally, often occurring with other negative experiences (mental illness, drug or alcohol problem, prison, witnessing intimate partner, domestic violence, parental separation). While severe child maltreatment may come to [23] the attention of child protection agencies, more hidden forms that progress over many years also exist [24].

Assessments of child abuse involve the interaction of multiple disciplines, including medicine, social work, law enforcement, and the judicial system [25, 26]. This interdisciplinary approach, which is facilitated by Child Advocacy Centers or similar multidisciplinary models, can be challenging because of differing definitions of child abuse, expectations regarding information that can be determined during the medical evaluation, or interpretations of findings [22, 27].

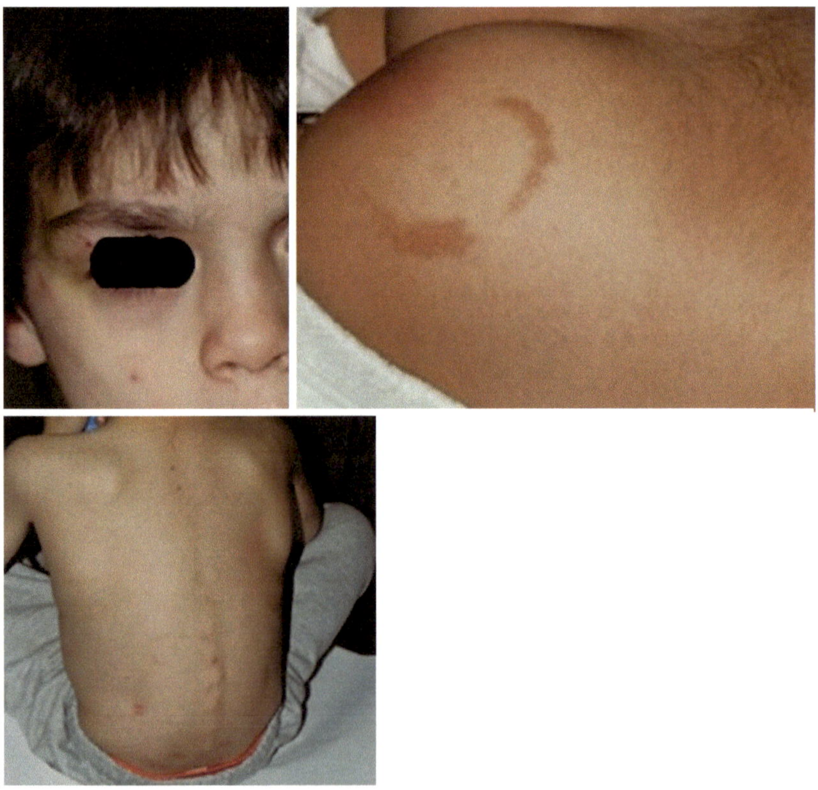

Fig. 11.1 Clinical and forensic constellation related to Battered child syndrome (authors' observation). Male patient, 6 years old at Emergency Department observation, presenting multiple skin bruises (periorbital and on the back), adult bite mark on genital area

Severe abuse can lead to homicide [28–34]. While homicide rates for children aged under 15 in the Region appear low at about 850 deaths per year, many child deaths are not investigated and the numbers may be much higher [35–37]. National statistics on child abuse in the USA show that in 2013 approximately 679,000 children were victims of maltreatment, and approximately 1520 of them died. Children in the first year of their life had the highest rate of victimization of 23.1 per 1000 children in the national population of the same age. Of the children who experienced maltreatment or abuse, 18% suffered physical abuse. Although figures vary yearly, approximately 700,000 cases of child abuse and neglect are reported annually in the United States, of which 117,772 are physical abuse, as documented by the Department of Health and Human Services in 2015 [23, 24].

Child maltreatment is considered an important public health issue in the European Region. Within data from European Report on Preventing Child Maltreatment, 2013, child maltreatment leads to the premature death of 852 children under 15 years in the European Region every year. In that document it is also properly observed that 'not all deaths from maltreatment are properly recorded and this figure is likely to be an underestimate'. Deaths are the tip of the iceberg, as it is estimated that for every death, there are between 150 and 2400 substantiated cases of physical abuse [38]. The number of children suffering from maltreatment whose plight goes unrecognized is likely to be very much higher and may only come to light through population surveys [39]. Global estimates state that prevalence ranges from 4 to 47% for moderate-to-severe physical abuse, 15 to 48% for emotional and 20% for sexual abuse in girls and 5 to 10% in boys [40], suggesting that tens of millions of children in the Region suffer different forms of maltreatment. Differences also exist within countries and child death rates are several times higher in disadvantaged populations than wealthier communities; this is also true for hospital admissions, with children from deprived neighbourhoods more likely to be admitted for assaults. Deprivation exposes children to more risk factors for abuse: these can grow over time, increasing the likelihood of violence and neglect [41].

Trauma is the most common cause of death in childhood, and inflicted head injury is the most common cause of traumatic death in infancy [40]. The physician may be asked to render a legal opinion as to whether medical findings indicate abuse [42]; many published reports on medical findings indicative of abuse are based on observational data—primarily from case series—and on clinical judgment [43]. In addition to a medical evaluation to guide treatment, findings that do not require therapy but that support an inflicted cause must also be documented [44]. The legal mandate for physicians to report suspected child abuse requires a reasonable suspicion of abuse, which is sometimes a difficult criterion to meet because of uncertainty regarding the diagnosis [45], particularly when the physician is also a paediatrician caretaker of family, possibly the physician may want to be more certain of the diagnosis [46]. Sometimes the history and/or examination findings facilitate a prompt accurate diagnosis of assault, but this is an uncommon scenario [47–50]. More commonly, the suspicion of child abuse arises after a doctor is told an uncommon story about how an injury occurred or the doctor discovers an injury frequently attributed to assault [51–53]. Suspicion can arise when the pattern of injury seems discordant with the alleged mechanism, especially after consideration of injury biomechanics. Discordance is only one of many factors [30, 54–56] that raise concern about child abuse but it is an important consideration when evaluating children's fractures [57, 58].

Once child abuse is suspected, forensic practitioners must remain open to the possibility that the history provided may be truthful, fabricated, deliberately misleading or incomplete. A careful search for other evidence of injury, such as patterned bruising [59, 60] from fingertip pressure, wounds of different ages, cigarette burns and signs of neglect must form part of the child's clinical examination [61]. Object of protection of such vulnerable persons as a minor must be an absolute imperative.

11.2 Clinical Points on Physical Abuse of Children

The diagnosis of child abuse is often not just a simple diagnosis but requires knowledge from different medical disciplines (paediatrics, neurology, ophthalmology, dermatology, surgery, forensic medicine, toxicology) to reveal a solid diagnostic basis taking into account all differential diagnoses of accidental trauma or confounding diseases [62–64] (Table 11.1). The diagnosis of child abuse may have a number of legal consequences [65]. To avoid legal consequences against the treating physicians—in cases of unreported suspected child abuse as well as in the event of reported but not proven child abuse—the diagnosis has to be confirmed and validated [66, 67].

The legal mandate for physicians to report *suspected* child abuse requires a reasonable suspicion of abuse [68], which is sometimes a difficult instance to meet because of uncertainty regarding the diagnosis, particularly when the physician has a relationship with the family, in which case the physician may want to be more certain of the diagnosis. Following key points and assessment for Suspected Physical Abuse of a Child (Table 11.1) are to be carefully considered in diagnostic approach [7]:

Table 11.1 Assessment for suspected physical abuse of a child

Step 1:	*Obtain a careful history of the alleged circumstances surrounding the injury* Were there witnesses to the event? Who was present with the child when the event occurred? Can the alleged event account for the injuries? Is the child's developmental level consistent with the proposed mechanism of injury? What was done when the event occurred or the child became symptomatic? Was there a delay in seeking medical attention?
Step 2:	*Perform a complete examination with the child fully unclothed* Document the overall clinical status of the child Document the presence of any bruises, burns, or other cutaneous findings Document the presence of intraoral lesions by carefully checking each frenulum for injury Document the presence of findings such as subconjunctival haemorrhages Photograph the findings or request that law enforcement obtain photographs
Step 3:	*Initiate a diagnostic workup on the basis of the findings and clinical condition of the child. The acuteness of the child's condition and the need for medical intervention may determine the order in which diagnostic studies are obtained* Perform CT or MRI of the head Perform CT of the abdomen with contrast enhancement if abdominal injuries are suspected Obtain complete blood count, assess bask (metabolic profile, perform coagulation studies, and measure hepatic and pancreatic enzymes) Perform a full skeletal survey Perform a funduscopic examination with photographs
Step 4:	*Manage any acute medical problem*
Step 5:	*Notify child protective services as mandated in the state. Notification of law enforcement is also mandated in some jurisdictions*
Step 6:	*Hospitalize the child if needed*
Step 7:	*Have hospital personnel or a child protective services social worker perform an extensive social evaluation*
Step 8:	*Consider an additional forensic workup if indicated or requested or refer the case to a paediatrician, team, or centre that specializes in child abuse cases. Additional tests that might be performed include:* A radionuclide scan to look for occult or acute fractures A repeat skeletal survey in 2 weeks Evaluation for blood dyscrasia Evaluation for osteogenesis imperfecta Evaluation of other medical problems as suggested by the differential diagnosis of the findings

List of the recommended steps that should be taken to assess cases of suspected child abuse

- Physically abused children, particularly infants, may present with non-specific symptoms and signs, such as vomiting or apnoea; the possibility of abusive head trauma requires consideration in such cases.
- Physical findings, such as bruising of the face, neck, or torso, or intraoral lesions, such as torn frenula, in infants who are not yet ambulatory should arouse suspicion of inflicted trauma.
- The evaluation of infants and young children for suspected inflicted trauma should include a complete physical examination of the child, with particular attention to the skin, oral cavity [69], and abdomen; imaging of the brain; an examination for retinal haemorrhages; a skeletal survey; and measurement of hepatic and pancreatic enzymes [70–72].
- Physicians are mandated to report to child protective services cases in which they have a reasonable suspicion of child abuse [73].

Detecting fragile bones is a part of clinical assessment, difficult to determine, particularly in children. Neither X-ray images nor bone densitometry scans provide a clinically useful measure of bone strength [57]. Bones have two main structural components: mineral and protein. Abnormality of bone mineralization in children is called osteomalacia or rickets, most commonly related to vitamin D deficiency but there are multiple congenital and acquired causes of rickets. Abnormality of the protein component of bones can also be due to a large number of congenital or acquired conditions and present either as part of a generalized bone disorder effecting multiple bones or joints or incidentally as a localized deformity [74]. The bones of children with reduced bone strength can fracture as a result of lesser forces than children with normal bones (Table 11.2).

Blood tests that should be performed to evaluate bone metabolism include blood levels of calcium, phosphate, alkaline phosphatase, urea, electrolytes, creatinine and vitamin D [75, 76]. There is an ongoing debate regarding the association between vitamin D levels [77], bone mineral density and bone strength at different ages [78] and the AAP have recently recommended that breast-fed infants receive vitamin D [79].

Table 11.2 Conditions that may affect bone strength in children

Abnormalities of mineralization
• Vitamin D deficiency
• Renal disease
• Hypoparathyroidism
• Vitamin D resistant rickets
• Resorption due to disuse
• Osteopaenia of prematurity
• Hypophosphatasia
Abnormalities of protein formation
• Osteogenesis imperfecta
• Congenital bone dysplasias
• Scurvy
• Osteopetrosis
• Menkes disease tumours
• Neuroblastoma
• Leukaemia
• Langerhans cell histiocytosis
Infections
• Osteomyelitis
• Syphilis
Drugs
• Methotrexate
• Vitamin A toxicity
• Prostaglandin E
Aetiology not known
• Infantile cortical hyperostosis

Second-line blood tests include parathyroid hormone levels and urine metabolic screening. Tests for metabolic disease, osteogenesis imperfecta, copper deficiency, syphilis and scurvy might be considered when there are suggestive clinical or radiological features [80]. Additional tests for rare disorders should be considered when additional information related to family history (such as family members with a history of abnormal bones) and the child's particular circumstances (such as abnormal diet, clinical findings and concurrent illness) warrant further consideration.

Bone densitometry tests are not recommended as a useful tool in the routine forensic investigation of bone injury in childhood because these tests have controversial reference ranges in children. In addition, the tests have such low sensitivity and specificity for reduced bone strength that they are of limited use in forensic evaluation of injury.

In circumstances when the diagnosis of osteogenesis imperfecta or other rare metabolic conditions are being considered, advice from an expert in metabolic and genetic conditions should be obtained [81, 82]. The diagnosis of osteogenesis imperfecta is usually a clinical one. Specific tests of collagen synthesis and the genes that code for type 1 collagen (COL1A1 and COL1A2) might be recommended when the diagnosis of osteogenesis imperfecta is being seriously considered [83]. In literature report of a case of OI type I misdiagnosed as child abuse in which treatment was successful despite a tardive diagnosis are still present [84, 85].

11.2.1 Child Fatalities Related to Physical Abuse and Head Trauma

Deaths due to child abuse can occur as a consequence of intracranial or extra cranial injuries [86]. Overall, head injuries are the leading cause of death in abused young children [87], and extensive research has been published describing the epidemiology, patterns and mechanisms of injury associated with paediatric abusive head trauma [88–95]. Uncertainties continue to surround determinations of abusive head trauma [96, 97]; the dispute about the aetiology of these injuries relies both with the advances of forensic knowledge about this matter (way and manner) [98–100] and duty against the law.

The names applied to the syndromes of Inflicted Head Injury in infancy reflect the evolving and sometimes controversial [101] understanding of the actions necessary to cause the types of injuries seen [11, 102–105], such as shaking an infant held by the arms or trunk or forcefully striking an infant's head against a surface [40, 106, 107]. A special focus concerns the triads of Subdural Haematoma, Retinal haemorrhage, brain injury patterns and Shaking syndrome [99, 108–114], with a more recent caveat of the possibility that uncommon [115], or silent 'pathological' [112, 116–126] causes determining retinal haemorrhages.

During inflicted head injury, a distinct type of trauma occurs causing more global brain injury with hypoxic-ischaemic brain injury (HII) and more severe retinal haemorrhages [127–130]. HII is not a necessary factor for severe retinal haemorrhage to develop from inflicted trauma [131].

Understanding of paediatric abusive head trauma has evolved over the last five decades. In 1962 issue of Kemp identified intracranial haemorrhage in young children as a hallmark sign in many cases. In 1971, Guthkelch suggest shaking as a form of abusive injury, reporting on 23 children (22 < 18 months of age) presenting with various combinations of subdural haemorrhage, fractures, parenchymal brain injury, and retinal haemorrhages [113]. Shortly thereafter, Caffey coined the term Whiplash-Shaken infant syndrome [1]. Both Authors noted a frequent absence of external signs of trauma and suggested the role of torn bridging vessels in the brain as the cause of the intracranial haemorrhage [3, 103, 104]. Using autopsy evidence and a dummy model, Duhaime and colleagues in 1987 suggested that blunt impact trauma may be a prerequisite to generate sufficient deceleration forces for the characteristic injuries to occur [132]; however, consistency across perpetrator confessions suggests that shaking alone is sufficient to cause such injuries, and actual injury threshold levels for infant brains have yet to be established [133]. There are currently multiple hypothesized factors in the pathogenesis of brain pathology and retinal haemorrhage in abusive head trauma [134–136], including deceleration and sheering injury, hypoxic-ischaemic injury (from decreased perfusion or apnoea), blunt impact, neck flexion-extension, and raised intracranial or venous pressures [137]. However, the relative importance of these factors cannot be determined precisely based on the published data [138–140].

The availability of diffusion-weighted magnetic resonance imaging (DW-MRI) and non-invasive vascular imaging techniques now make it possible to evaluate the role of hypoxic-ischaemic injury (HII) in traumatic paediatric head injuries [141, 142]. DW-MRI enables identification of acute cellular injury and cytotoxic oedema, which in the context of head trauma may result from hypoxic-ischaemic injury, direct traumatic injury, or both. Brain tissue damage causes shifting of water molecules from extracellular to intracellular compartments, which can be identified as reduced diffusion of water on DW-MRI, in comparison to undamaged areas. Such changes can be identified early, hours or days before changes in the appearance of tissue on T2-weighted sequences. DW-MRI (versus T1 or T2) is particularly helpful in infants, whose brains have a high water content and immature myelination. Biousse and colleagues reported a high incidence of possible HII in a cohort of infants with presumed abusive head trauma. In 2007, Ichord and colleagues demonstrated a relationship between HII and inflicted trauma using DW-MRI in a cohort of children with both accidental and inflicted head injuries [143].

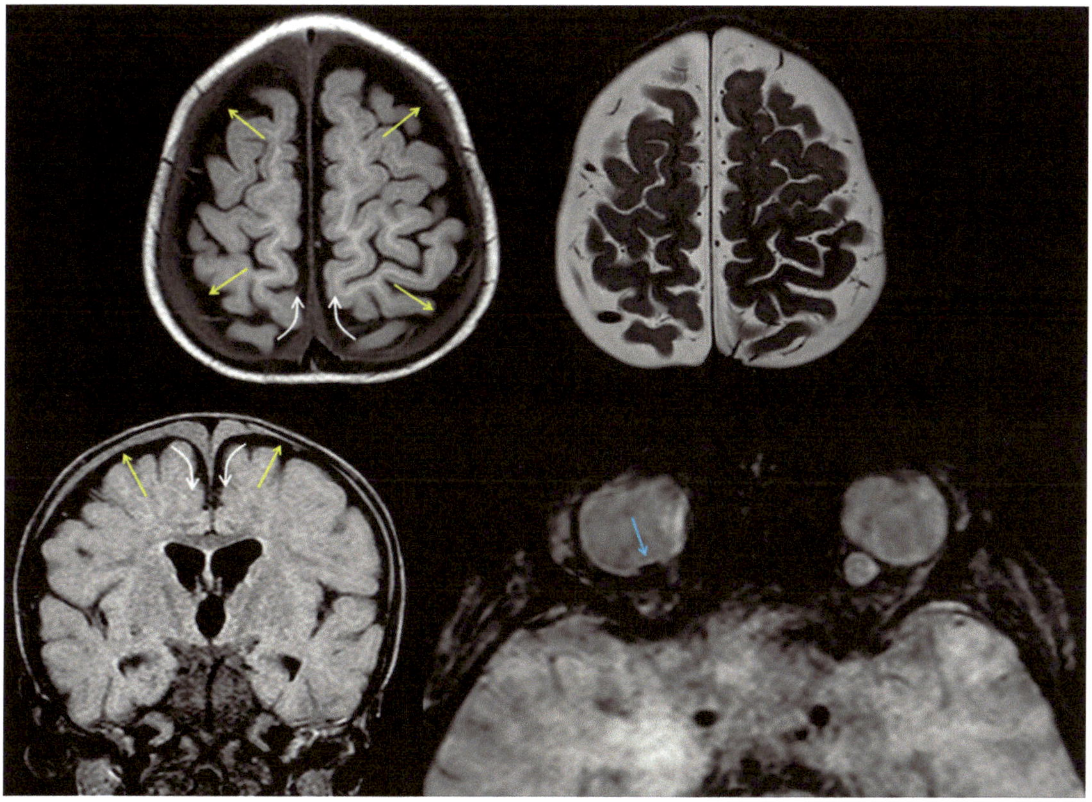

(**a**) Axial T1, (**b**) axial T2 and (**c**) coronal flair MR images of a 12-month boy affected by bilateral subdural chronic haematoma (arrows) with involvement of the interhemispheric fissure (curved arrows). (**d**) SWI MR image demonstrating retinal haemorrhage (arrow). Courtesy of Dr. Andrea Rossi Giannina Gaslini Children's Hospital, Genoa

It has been clearly established that both the presence and increasing severity of retinal haemorrhages are highly associated with abusive versus accidental injury in children presenting with traumatic intracranial haemorrhage [144–146]; however, the mechanisms underlying retinal haemorrhages are still not clearly established, and there is limited information in the literature addressing HII as it relates to ocular findings in the setting of paediatric head trauma [147, 148].

Although the available evidence suggests that it is the sudden deceleration associated with the forceful striking of the head against a surface that is responsible for most, if not all, severe, inflicted brain injuries [149, 150]. Because the histories given when infants with such injuries present for medical attention are often vague or unreliable, the events must be inferred from knowledge of the causative forces in witnessed cases of accidental trauma and experimental models of injury [151].

Studies of the biomechanics of brain injury have established that forces applied to the head that result in a rotation of the brain about its centre of gravity cause diffuse brain injuries. A differential diagnosis that includes non-accidental as well as accidental causes of skull fractures in child deaths is always required in forensic practice [94, 149, 152, 153]. Accidental deaths due to severe trauma (i.e. motor vehicle collisions, vehicles striking pedestrian, skull fractures from heavy falling objects) usually result in extensive multiple injuries together with skull fractures and intracranial findings. In accidental cases such as these, the investigative history usually corroborates the manner of death, since it corresponds with the injuries found, and excludes child abuse [154–156]. Conversely, a fall from a short height (either unwitnessed or witnessed by a single caretaker) can result in skull fractures in children with a very similar pattern to the ones found in inflicted trauma. Confounding this diagnostic dilemma, the majority of head injuries in child abuse and accidental head trauma are often both explained by parents as accidental [157–159]. According to the literature, accidental skull fractures will rarely lead to serious or life-threatening intracranial injury. Further, skull fractures due to accidental falls are rarely seen in concert with simultaneous fractures in other skeleton segments (i.e. ribs or extremities) [160, 161]. The investigative history is a fundamental part of the diagnostic process, as an accidental skull fracture can nearly always be routinely absent [157, 159, 162].

Diastases of cranial sutures are more common than skull fractures and could be either a direct consequence of trauma or due to raised intracranial pressure from any cause, because suture diastases occurred both in cases with signs of impact to the head as well as no signs of impact [163–165]. Their frequency is significantly higher in infants than in toddlers, because of the progressive fusion of the sutures during growth. Extradural haemorrhages (EDH) is rarely seen in paediatric cases due to the tight adherence of the dura mater to the skull and because of the elasticity of the young skull and not always associated with skull fractures. EDH does not occur in subjects with no signs of an impact. EDHs are typically associated with accidental trauma but have been also described in abused children. EDH may occur with relatively minor trauma to the parietal or temporal skull if the vulnerable middle meningeal artery is torn, so it is frequently observed in accidental trauma (Fig. 11.2).

Intra-dural haemorrhages are caused by physical or physiologic damage to the dural capillary plexus that, according to some researchers, can lead to SDH [166]. SDH are observed both in the subjects with and in those without visible evidence of impact injury. Infants are more affected

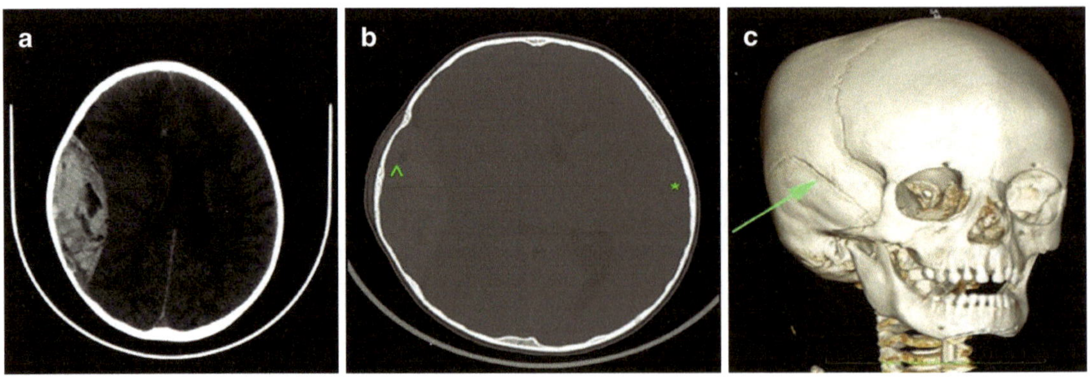

Fig. 11.2 Accidental head trauma in a 3-year-old boy. Fall from a short height (witnessed by caretakers and children) (Authors' observation). (**a**) Axial non-contrast CT scan shows a huge epidural right-side epidural haemorrhage, with inhomogeneous density of haematoma, due to different timing of haemorrhage; (**b**) axial CT scan slab-VR 3D reconstruction shows deformity of parietal and frontal bone along the squamosal (^) suture, compared to left side (*); (**c**) 3D VR image clearly shows the fracture along the squamosal suture

by subdural haematoma than toddlers and older children, because the brain of infants has more space than the brain of older children to move around in the skull upon impact. It has been reported in the literature that subdural haemorrhages in cases of abusive paediatric head trauma are rarely massive [137, 167]. This seems to confirm that SDH is not typically a lesion producing increased intracranial pressure, but rather a marker of brain movement within the cranial cavity, which may be associated with some shearing brain injury (e.g. diffuse axonal injury). In fact, because the dura is firmly attached to the skull and the arachnoid to the cerebral cortex, most brain motion occurs across the potential subdural space. The thin-walled bridging veins are thus easily vulnerable to tearing. Therefore, in every paediatric autopsy it is extremely important for the pathologist to remove the brain personally or directly observe its removal when performed by a technician. Otherwise, a thin layer of blood from subdural bleeding could easily be missed as it will tend to slide quickly off the surface of the brain as the calvarium is removed. Subdural haemorrhages caused by accidental trauma are typically produced by severe force such as a motor vehicle accident, ejection from a motor vehicle, or a fall from a significant height. Accidental SDHs usually occur at the site of impact, are limited to the cerebral convexities, and are often isolated and associated with an overlying fracture.

11.2.2 Pathology Findings at Autopsy

Closed head injury in early infancy (5 months of age and younger) produces focal lesions, parenchymal laceration—also known as contusional tears—and diffuse astrocytic reaction [168–170].

The presence of skull fractures, diffuse axonal injury, and subdural haemorrhage suggest that abused children are subject to several forms of injury, direct trauma to the skull causing fractures; brain acceleration over a short arc producing subdural haematoma; and slower acceleration in shaking where axons are damaged [171]. This inertial effect may also produce acute subdural haemorrhage as the subdural veins are sensitive to shearing forces. Diffuse axonal injury was not usually seen in the brain stem. In the diffuse axonal injury described in adults axonal discontinuities are typically seen in the dorsolateral quadrant of the brain stem [172]. In all cases in which contusional tears had occurred, diffuse axonal injury was evident [141, 173]. Thus, the presence of a contusional tear was focal evidence of more diffuse damage. The experimental studies of axonal damage to subhuman primates, using angular acceleration, suggest that there is a slower component of the acceleration which produces the diffuse axonal injury, but it is impossible to identify the varieties of trauma used in the cases [174, 175] (Fig. 11.3).

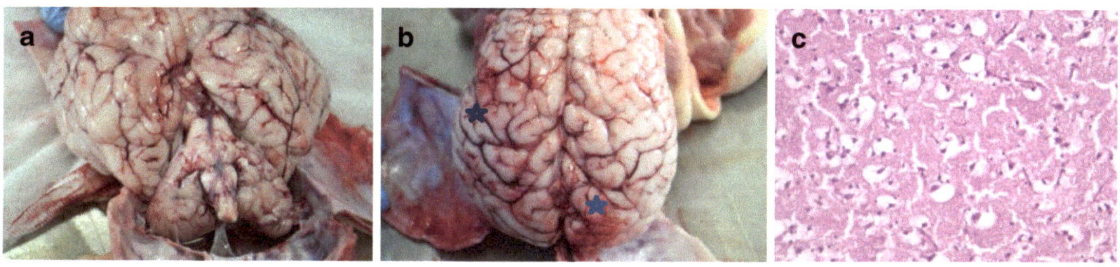

Fig. 11.3 A 3-month-old infant with accidental head trauma, with clinical and circumstantial suggesting infant shaking syndrome; the child showed coma and apnoea at presentation to first aid of health professional and died after few minutes; at autopsy gross examination showed a thin layer of subarachnoidal haemorrhage (∗) on cerebral convexities and left side (**a**) and dramatic brain swelling (**b**), with histology evidence of hypoxic ischaemic brain damage (**c**, H&E, 25×)

11.2.3 Child Abuse Imaging Protocol and Forensic

When bone trauma is suspected, the critical investigations are radiological and a classic aphorisms in the study of child abuse was stated by the forensic pathologists, Cameron, Johnson and Camps ('The skin and bones tell a story which the child is either too young or too frightened to tell'). The essence of forensic evaluation of bone trauma in children is being able to determine *whether* bone trauma has occurred, *when* bone trauma might have occurred and being able to determine the *likely mechanism* of the injury [56, 176, 177].

Forensic evaluation of bone injury in children requires a preliminary understanding of bone metabolism and growth, an understanding of injury biomechanics causing fractures and an appreciation of the power and limitations of radiological investigation to accurately detect the presence and estimate the time of bone injury.

The forensic opinion about the likely cause(s) of injury can then be compared to the offered explanation and their mutual compatibility analysed. To establish whether bone trauma has occurred, it is also essential to have an understanding of the normal structure of different bones and how they deform with application of different forces [178]. Infants and very young children have significantly different bone structure, metabolism, bone strength and reaction to mechanical trauma than older children, adolescents and adults [179]. In addition, there are a number of metabolic processes and congenital abnormalities that can affect the strength of children's bones and therefore their bones' susceptibility to injury when mechanical forces are encountered [180, 181]. Children's bones are softer, contain more cartilage than adults' bones, the growth plates are relatively fragile and the structure of the bone matrix alters with maturity.

Bone trauma in children can be difficult to detect with both clinical and radiological examination findings sometimes problematic to analyse. Errors in interpretation of findings can lead to incorrect forensic conclusions and subsequent erroneous action on the part of the state to protect vulnerable children. A misdiagnosis of child abuse can be as harmful as a missed diagnosis of child abuse. Studies attempted to compare magnetic resonance imaging (MRI) using limited sequence protocols to CT (computerized tomography) for evaluating paediatric head trauma. Although studies have some differences in sequences and population demographics, both conclude that the CT and MRI are comparable in terms of detecting acute intracranial haemorrhages. In fact, one institution claims to use MRI as the initial imaging exam in paediatric head trauma except 'if the wait for MRI is unacceptably long for appropriate patient care' [182], and moreover doesn't use ionizing radiation [183].

As it was said, if MRI could fulfil three conditions—be cheap, be available everywhere, with no or minimal wait time, and offer complete scans in very short times—every Emergency Room would have one and would use it almost exclusively for evaluating paediatric head trauma [184]. A full sequence MRI is more sensitive and specific than CT for everything in the head except for some bone lesions. Add to that the capability for diffusion imaging and diffusion tensor imaging for discovering new information and making diagnoses of brain lesions, not detectable on conventional MRI, and the user can appreciate why MRI may eventually become ubiquitous. Using MRI costs more and is more expensive to operate. It has physical limitations to access since the magnet is always on and is waiting to suck in the unwary. Also, the vast and ever growing array of possible MRI sequences causes longer and longer exam times. MRI imaging, furthermore, needs completely immobilization of patients and this condition is difficult to have in children, sometimes making necessary to anaesthetize young patients.

Some authors observe they are aware of and very sensitive to radiation exposure in children, particularly those who will need repeated studies using ionizing radiation. However, with the exception of the lens of the eye, the brain is pretty radiation insensitive, but is always necessary to consider the risk-benefit ratio of using CT imaging instead of MR one. If there is an acutely injured child it makes no sense to not perform a CT if that is what the situation demands. A properly performed head CT is highly unlikely to add much, if any, morbidity to a child's life, especially one with a critical head injury.

As with other areas of medicine, the diagnostic process builds upon the history provided and the clinical examination findings. The process of forensic evaluation of injury follows a standard pathway; this is no different for evaluation of suspected bone trauma than for any other injury that might have an inflicted cause.

Financial, political, jurisdictional and geographical considerations result in varying recommendations and practices throughout the world.

Recommendations from local health authorities, colleges and special societies guide good practice [185–187]. If access to facilities for specialist investigation is limited, alternative means of investigation need to be considered, as the following: it is also questionable the possibility to perform all investigations close to the child's home, to minimize the child's exposure to ionizing radiation and to investigate using recommended 'gold standard' tools. The long-term risks of ionizing radiation which may have a latent period of decades must be balanced against the short-term risk of further physical harm to the child. Obtaining consent for these imaging procedures should not be overlooked, but will sometimes come from a temporary Court-nominated child carer, instead of child's parents. Sometimes it is in a child's best interests for him/her and to assure physical protection to travel to a specialist centre or third level hospital, for investigation using techniques and facilities optimized for paediatric imaging. Decision-making must carefully consider the local national guidelines for health assessment of child protection. For children aged less than 2 years, consensus exists regarding the need for a high-quality radiographic skeletal survey as an essential part of the investigation of suspected non-accidental injury. Even if the injury appears to be localized to one body region, the whole skeleton is surveyed because these children are (usually) unable to give a reliable history, are vulnerable to injury because of their immature and relatively weak skeleton and their small size and the injuries may not be evident from clinical examination of the child. The recommended facilities, equipment, technique and protocols needed to obtain this high-quality skeletal survey vary slightly between countries and professional colleges, however, with each region recommending a standard protocol. The American College of radiology (ACR-SPR, Practice Parameter for the Performance and Interpretation of Skeletal Surveys in Children) recommends high-quality digital X-rays, with lowest possible radiation dose, and concurrent monitoring of the images by a radiologist (in case additional views are required in order to further define perceived abnormality) [12, 13]. A common error in acquisition of skeletal survey images by practitioners unfamiliar with accepted protocols is the failure to obtain coned views of the metaphyses and growth plates of the long bones (especially at the wrist, knees and ankles) and inadequate imaging of the ribs due to poor aeration of the lungs, patient movement, suboptimal exposure factors/image capture or poorly centred X-ray beam. A nuclear medicine scan is recommended as an additional 'first-line' investigation because the combination of nuclear medicine scan and radiographic skeletal survey increases the overall detection rate of non-accidental injury in children [180, 188–192], but really Authors think that the radiation exposition of nuclear medicine scan could be too high to be routinary accepted in clinical practice. Other imaging modalities can also be used to provide additional information when clinically indicated. Ultrasound examination of bone, for example, for ribs fractures, can help radiology in detecting fractures not clearly detectable in X-ray imaging [193–195].

In children aged more than 2 years the detection rate of occult bone injury is significantly lower and suspected bone injuries are best investigated using an X-ray of the suspected site of injury. For some children aged 2–3 years in whom occult bone injury is strongly suspected, radiological investigation with skeletal survey may be considered, leaving bone scan in doubt cases. The likelihood of detecting occult bone injury in a child aged more than 5 years is small because they are able to provide a better history and their bones require a greater force to cause injury. Consequently, for older children, radiographic skeletal surveys should be reserved for emergency or in other exceptional circumstances when the clinical suspicion is unusually high. Blood tests to evaluate bone metabolism should also be performed as a routine procedure when non-accidental bone trauma is suspected in children of all ages. The authors suggest tests such as serum calcium, phosphate, alkaline phosphatase, urea and electrolytes and serum vitamin D [196, 197]. Sometimes additional tests need to be considered. When an individual clinician lacks adequate knowledge and skill to collate this information and form a forensic opinion, it is imperative that he/she seek advice from a suitably experienced forensically trained colleague. Nuclear medicine bone scan demonstrates bone trauma by identifying the metabolic changes that occur within bone tissues as a consequence of trauma. Sometimes, the bone metabolic changes demonstrated may not be associated with a visible change in appearance on an X-ray examination.

An understanding of the physical principles of these imaging techniques is required to facilitate the identification of injuries that are not apparent on clinical examination. The changes that are demonstrated must be differentiated from normal variants and pathologies that mimic bone trauma. Some mimics of bone pathology require investigation with other laboratory tests.

The differences in the electron density of different body tissues and the properties of the different detector systems allow five different densities to be identified on conventional X-ray images or radiographs of humans. Bony trauma is most commonly identified when a gap, defect, break or alignment-abnormality is demonstrated in a bone or there are radiological signs of a healing bone injury present. Factors that influence whether bone injury will be demonstrated include the separation of the bony margins of the fracture, orientation of the fracture to the X-ray beam, position of the fracture in the body relative to other structures (is it obscured by overlying bones) and both the stage and extent of bony healing. Technical factors that can influence how well the bones are demonstrated include the resolution of the imaging system used, how well the child is immobilized, whether the images are coned to a region, the number of projections making up the examination and whether exposure factors appropriate for the size of the child are used. Coned views and different projections can be very important to identify subtle injuries of growth plates and ribs.

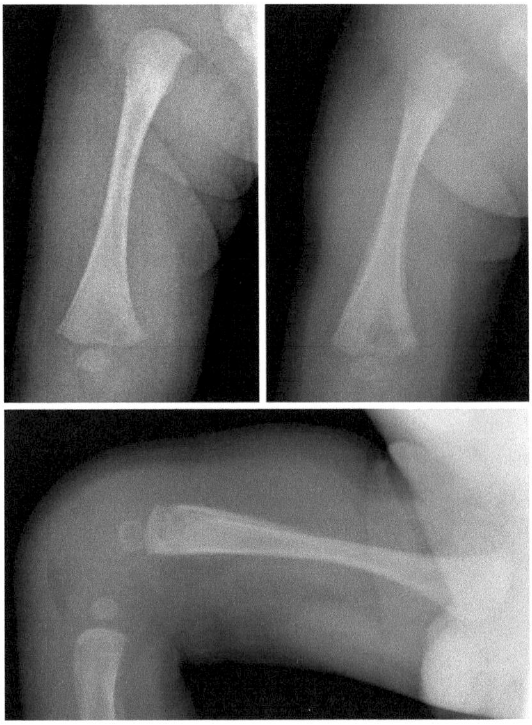

Femoral radiogram (AP view) demonstrating metaphyseal distal femoral fracture in a 6-month boy. Diffuse periosteal reaction of the distal femur after 15 days (AP and lateral views). Courtesy of Dr. Claudo Granata Giannina Gaslini Children's Hospital, Genoa

Plain radiographs are two-dimensional (2D) representations of 3D structures and this causes superimposition of body tissues and organs. This, together with the limited ability of plain radiographs to distinguish between different body tissues, can make identification of some structures difficult. However, when looking at bones in the extremities, this is less of a problem as there are fewer superimposed structures, and radiological orthogonal projections of bones help in fractures detection. Plain X-rays have the ability to produce images with very high spatial resolution (down to 100 μm or less). Despite this very high resolution, some bone fractures are not visible on plain

X-rays due to the orientation of the X-ray beam to the fracture and/or the small distance of separation of the fracture fragments. Computed tomography (CT) imaging produces images by using a collimated X-ray beam that is directed through the patient in multiple projections. The data collected from the multiple different projections allows mathematical computation of the attenuation of X-rays in individual points of the patient. A single slice used to take less than 1 min to acquire and a longer time to process. Current multidetector CT scans have a resolution of about 0.3 × 0.3 × 0.3 mm, can simultaneously acquire up to 320 slices in less than 0.5 s and are able to process all the data required to generate/construct the images in a few seconds. The improved temporal resolution reduces movement artefact and the improved spatial resolution in all imaging planes has resulted in an increased use of CT scans to identify complex fractures in multiple planes or oblique to the incident X-ray beam, with very good contrast resolution. CT scans can therefore demonstrate fractures that are not visible on conventional radiographs. Computed tomography utilizes ionizing radiation and involves a higher, more significant dose than plain radiographs. Where plain radiographs are able to differentiate five densities, CT has a much greater contrast resolution and can differentiate between tissues such as blood, white matter, grey matter and cerebrospinal fluid (CSF) in a CT scan image of the brain. The contrast between tissues of different structures can be manipulated by adjusting the image window width and level; this gives rise to terms such as 'bone window' settings. CT imaging allows superimposed structures to be individually identified and provides detail of bone anatomy which is very useful in the assessment of bones with a complex shape and around joints. CT very clearly shows focal areas of bone lysis/destruction, areas of bone sclerosis and periosteal new bone formation. CT is able to provide some information about soft tissues, particularly when there is localized soft tissue calcification or in case of subcutaneous emphysema, not easy to depict at X-ray when is of little amount. Ultrasound examinations and MRI studies usually provide superior images of soft tissues that are more likely to identify soft tissue pathology, especially in case of detection and in dating of haematomas. Forces causing bones fracture in infant is a part of diagnostic process. Planar micro-fractures at the metaphyseal-epiphyseal region in the immature primary spongiosum layer of immature long bones are believed to be caused by planar shearing forces. These injuries are referred to as classic metaphyseal lesions [198], but they are frequently referred to as 'bucket-handle' or 'corner' fractures [199]. Shearing forces occur during rapid acceleration and deceleration when an infant is shaken and when traction, compression or rotation forces are applied to cartilaginous epiphyses. While the X-ray appearance may differ depending on the projection of the X-ray beam, these radiological findings actually represent a single pathological process. Diaphyseal (shaft of long bone) fractures are more commonly seen in abused children than classic metaphyseal lesions. Diaphyseal fractures are commonly caused by accidental childhood trauma such as might be experienced during an accidental fall or sporting injury. In contrast to classic metaphyseal lesions, the site and type of diaphyseal fracture rarely contributes to differentiation of accidental from inflicted trauma. In some circumstances, for example, when the presence of a spiral fracture indicates that a torsional force has been applied, a discrepancy between the caregiver's offered explanation and the observed pattern of injury might suggest that the caregiver is not being truthful. Additional questions would need to be asked about the alleged mechanism of injury. Transverse fractures of the diaphysis can be caused by the application of force perpendicular to the shaft of the long bone (such as a direct blow) but can also be caused by bending forces transmitted along the shaft of the bone (Fig. 11.4). The periosteum is relatively poorly attached to the diaphysis of children's bones. Torsional and twisting forces can strip the periosteum from the cortex of diaphyseal bone, resulting in subperiosteal haemorrhage and resultant subperiosteal callus. When child abuse is diagnosed on the basis of skeletal injury, skull fracture is a common cause of presentation [164] (Fig. 11.5). Simple linear skull fractures occur as a result of both inflicted and accidental trauma

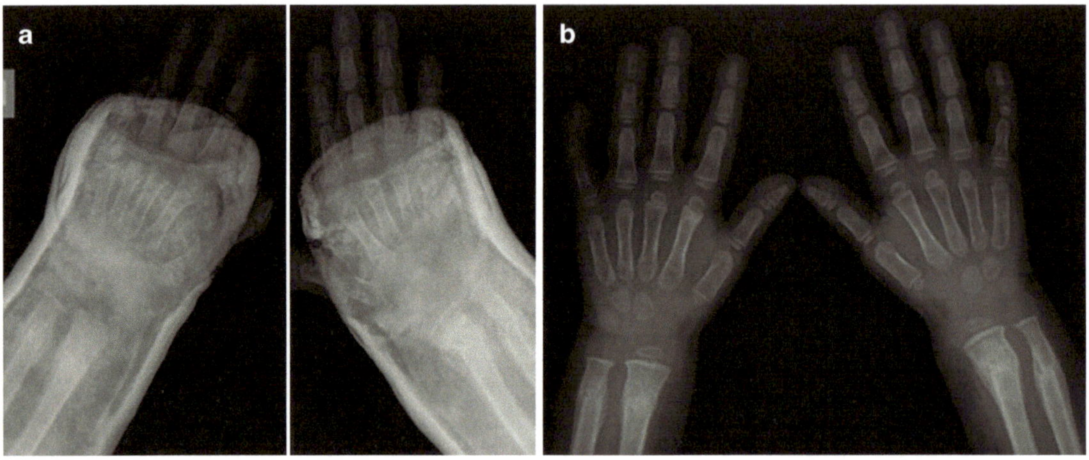

Fig. 11.4 Non-accidental fractures in a 4-year-old female (Authors' observation). (**a**) Bilateral fractures of distal radius and ulna with metaphyseal dorsal angulation and dislocation. (**b**) Nevertheless, the altered cortical bone profile, thanks to the physiological bone remodelling, may undergo to a complete resolution

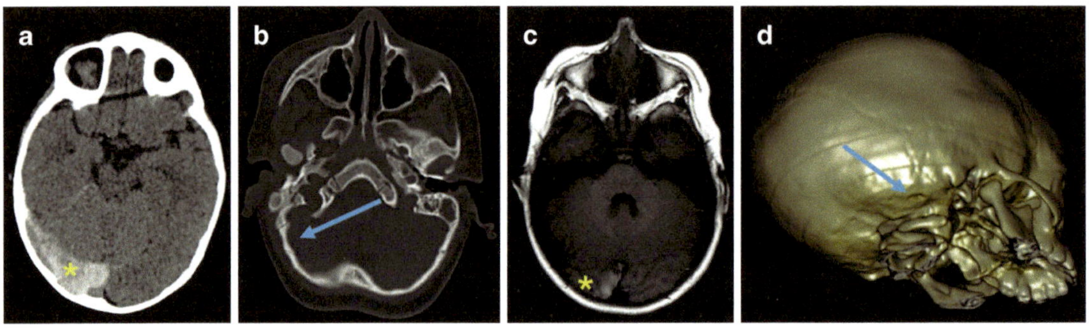

Fig. 11.5 Non-accidental brain injuries in a 2-year-old female (battered by her mother). (**a**) Brain CT scan shows right parasagittal and occipital epidural haemorrhage (∗) with ipsilateral tentorial and posterior falcine involvement; (**b**) small ipsilateral cortical lesion of the occipital/peri-mastoid skull (arrow) is present as well; (**c**) subarachnoid haemorrhage is still detected in brain MR, performed 3 month after with little haematic residuals (∗) along the occipital bone; (**d**) 3D VR reconstruction CT image shows an inflexible fracture of occipital bone (arrow)

[200–206] (Fig. 11.6). Non-parietal fractures, multiple and complex fractures, widely separated and depressed fractures and fractures associated with significant intracranial injury should all raise concern about possible inflicted injury. A single impact can result in a skull fracture that crosses a suture line. Rarely, a single impact may transmit forces such that two skull bones fracture some distance from the impact site. When bones on either side of the skull are fractured, multiple impacts and crush injury should be considered. Ping-pong fractures where there is deformity without a gap in the bone due to the pliability of the immature skull and depressed skull fractures can occur as a result of blunt impact with a contoured object in circumstances of accidental and inflicted trauma.

These fractures show transversal appearances, which are uncommon in accidental traumatic fractures in children.

Indeed, they usually show greenstick appearance, with eccentric far cortex comminution. Alternatively, but less commonly, they may show spiral appearance, caused by the involvement, during traumatic events, of diaphyseal long axis, thus resulting in oblique and longitudinal fracture rime. In this patient instead complete transverse fracture rimes are present and they can be caused

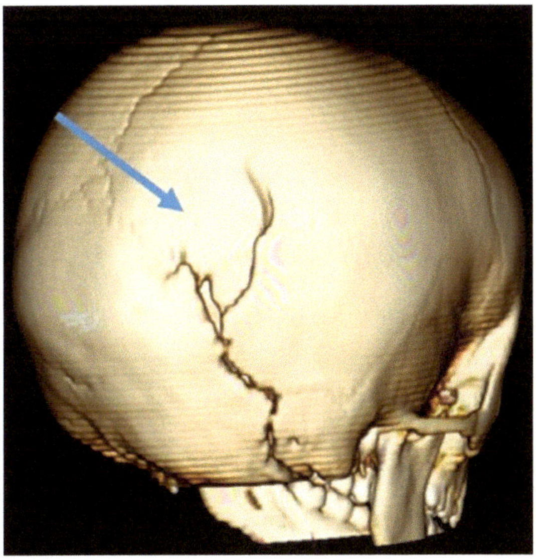

Fig. 11.6 18-month-old female. D: 3D VR reconstruction CT image shows a huge fracture of occipital bone (arrow)

by direct injury, probably painful, on the distal diaphyseal bones. Moreover, the bilateral fractures localized at the same bone portion may suggest a non-accidental injury, while they usually show different localization in the same bone, especially in cases of accidental distortion-caused fractures. Patient was treated by orthopaedic casts placement, but without surgical fractures reduction, which has lead, in 30 days, to abundant callus formation and bones deformities.

11.3 Conclusion

There are no particular bone injuries that are pathognomonic of child abuse [202–204, 207]. Although there are not bone injuries diagnostic of child abuse [208], however, some patterns of bone injury are seen much more frequently in assaulted children than in children who sustain accidental bone trauma. Classic metaphyseal lesions in children aged less than 2 years are seen far more commonly in abused children than in children experiencing trauma as a result of accidents [209].

Posterior rib fractures, fractures of the scapula, ends of clavicles, sternum and vertebral spinous processes suggest, but do not prove, injury caused by assault. Multiple bilateral symmetrical fractures, fractures judged to be of different ages, fractures of the hands and feet, vertebral body fractures, complex skull fractures and associated non-skeletal injury should raise suspicions of possible assault. Authors have referred to the 'specificity' of recognized patterns of bone injury to facilitate a diagnosis of child abuse [198, 210], but caution is imperative. Fractures seen predominantly in children known to have been abused have been categorized as 'specific' for child abuse whereas fractures occurring in both assaulted and accidentally injured children have been categorized as 'non-specific'. The most common types of fractures seen in assaulted children are fractures that are categorized as 'non-specific', including diaphyseal fractures and linear skull fractures. When forensic practitioners form an opinion about the cause of a child's bone injury, their existing knowledge base underpins opinion formation. Unfortunately, the existing literature is replete with examples of poor research methodology, dogmatic statements based on only a small number of cases and faulty reasoning by way of circular logic and other fallacies of logic. For example, the willingness of a forensic practitioner to diagnose child abuse in a toddler with an isolated spiral femur fracture is strongly influenced by the forensic practitioner's belief that in a non-ambulant child this fracture pattern is more likely to be caused by abuse than an accident. At times, circular logic, the child's poor social circumstances [211] and the presence of coexisting injuries influence the forensic practitioner's diagnosis in relation to fracture causation [212]. Knowledge of bone healing in children take a relevant part of diagnostic contribution in a suspected abusive fracture and several authors have made important contributions to our understanding of how bones recover from trauma. The times-since-injury implies particularly those working in a forensic context, are cautioned that these times are only estimates based on limited data and the understanding has been derived from the study of bone injury in children who have died as a result of accidental trauma. Histological analysis suggests that the healing process is usually no different when the cause of injury is inflicted trauma [213]. Bone healing is understood to occur in a number of phases. Firstly, the *induction phase* extends from the time of injury to the appearance of new bone at the fracture site. An inflammatory response initiated with the associated bleeding may last a few days and reveal itself on an X-ray in the form of soft tissue swelling with displacement and obliteration of normal fat and fascial planes. The initial soft tissue swelling is referred to as the pro-callus. A fracture line that initially appears sharp will change as healing progresses. Damaged bone is first resorbed as part of the inflammatory process which may blur the fracture margins. A nuclear medicine bone scan may detect increased blood flow due to inflammation and an MRI or ultrasound scan may detect soft tissue changes that are not yet evident on an X-ray. Soft or primary callus then starts to form with the fibrocartilaginous tissues laid down to stabilize the bones at the fracture site converting to loosely woven bone. In infants, this calcification/ossification is frequently seen as periosteal new bone and can occur within approximately 7–10 days but tends to occur later in older children (10–14 days after injury). Exuberant callus formation can be a sign of fracture instability and/or repetitive injury. Next, hard callus forms when disorganized periosteal and endosteal bone (sometimes called the provisional callus) begins to convert to lamellar bone with the bony trabeculae orientated along the lines of weight bearing/compression/tension. This phase begins in infants at 14–21 days at the earliest and peaks at 21–42 days. Remodelling occurs with gradual correction of deformity and resorption of the excess callus laid down as part of the initial healing process. This phase begins after bone union and may continue for 1–2 years after the injury. Remodelling of bone following bone fracture in children can result in a bone that heals completely and appears indistinguishable on X-ray from a bone that has not been injured.

Healing generally occurs more rapidly in younger infants but the rate at which bones heal and remodelling occurs varies with a number of factors: the anatomy of the injured bone; the site and nature of fracture; the degree of angulation and displacement of bone segments; the degree of immobilization of fractured bones during healing; stresses applied across the fracture during healing; and metabolic processes that enable healing of bone injury. Subtle fractures such as classic metaphyseal lesions and rib fractures may only be identified on plain X-rays once the healing process is well established, making bone scans or repeat X-ray examination essential in the evaluation of injury. With optimal healing conditions, a fractured bone may appear normal on an X-ray or nuclear bone scan examination in as short a time as a few months. Other bones, such as the skull, may not show radiological evidence of healing; dating skull fractures is notoriously imprecise. Table 11.3 identifies factors that may influence bone healing.

Table 11.3 Bone healing repairing

Factors promote bone healing	Factors that impair bone healing
Immobilization	Poor immobilization/instability
Early treatment	Delayed treatment
Simple fracture, two segments	Complex fracture, multiple segments
Good alignment, small gap (minimal displacement)	Separation, angulation or displacement of fracture segments
Good blood supply	Precarious/inadequate blood supply
Youth, good nutrition and good health	Old age, poor nutrition, poor health, local or generalized infection

When a fracture involves the growth plates or is allowed to unite with angulation or displacement, the bone may not grow normally resulting in a permanent deformity and/or limb shortening. When children's bones have been injured by inflicted trauma, other factors that might influence the healing process are a delay in presentation for medical treatment, coexisting nutritional deficiencies (possibly associated with neglect) and subsequent/repeated trauma at the fracture site. Two 1987 case reports by Perkins and Skirvin [214] and Spencer [215] reported faster healing of femoral fractures in children with coexisting severe head injury. These studies have not been replicated and the clinical significance of this association remains uncertain.

When forensic practitioners form an opinion about the cause of a child's bone injury, their existing knowledge base underpins opinion formation. Unfortunately, the existing literature is replete with examples of poor research methodology, dogmatic statements based on only a small number of cases and faulty reasoning by way of circular logic and other fallacies of logic. For example, the willingness of a forensic practitioner to diagnose child abuse in a toddler with an isolated spiral femur fracture is strongly influenced by the forensic practitioner's belief that in a non-ambulant child this fracture pattern is more likely to be caused by abuse than an accident. At times, circular logic, the child's poor social circumstances and the presence of coexisting injuries influence the forensic practitioner's diagnosis in relation to fracture causation [212]. Knowledge of bone healing in children take a relevant part of diagnostic contribution in a suspected abusive fracture and several authors have made important contributions to our understanding of how bones recover from trauma. The times-since-injury implies particularly those working in a forensic context, are cautioned that these times are only estimates based on limited data and the understanding has been derived from the study of bone injury in children who have died as a result of accidental trauma. Histological analysis suggests that the healing process is usually no different when the cause of injury is inflicted trauma [213]. Bone healing is understood to occur in a number of phases. Firstly, the *induction phase* extends from the time of injury to the appearance of new bone at the fracture site. An inflammatory response initiated with the associated bleeding may last a few days and reveal itself on an X-ray in the form of soft tissue swelling with displacement and obliteration of normal fat and fascial planes. The initial soft tissue swelling is referred to as the pro-callus. A fracture line that initially appears sharp will change as healing progresses. Damaged bone is first resorbed as part of the inflammatory process which may blur the fracture margins. A nuclear medicine bone scan may detect increased blood flow due to inflammation and an MRI or ultrasound scan may detect soft tissue changes that are not yet evident on an X-ray. Soft or primary callus then starts to form with the fibrocartilaginous tissues laid down to stabilize the bones at the fracture site converting to loosely woven bone. In infants, this calcification/ossification is frequently seen as periosteal new bone and can occur within approximately 7–10 days but tends to occur later in older children (10–14 days after injury). Exuberant callus formation can be a sign of fracture instability and/or repetitive injury. Next, hard callus forms when disorganized periosteal and endosteal bone (sometimes called the provisional callus) begins to convert to lamellar bone with the bony trabeculae orientated along the lines of weight bearing/compression/tension. This phase begins in infants at 14–21 days at the earliest and peaks at 21–42 days. Remodelling occurs with gradual correction of deformity and resorption of the excess callus laid down as part of the initial healing process. This phase begins after bone union and may continue for 1–2 years after the injury. Remodelling of bone following bone fracture in children can result in a bone that heals completely and appears indistinguishable on X-ray from a bone that has not been injured.

A radiological estimate of the time of injury involves evaluation of the appearance of soft tissues, the fracture line, the deformity and the callus. It is therefore only possible to offer an estimate of the possible date of injury within a range. However, when there are multiple sites of trauma it is often useful to assess whether the injuries are likely to have occurred at the same or different times. Repeated trauma raises suspicions of inflicted injury. In the systematic review of Prosser et al. [216], the dating of fractures in children identified only three articles that met their inclusion criteria. Of the 189 children reported (243 fractures), only 56 children were aged less than 5 years, the age group in which most fractures caused by assault occur. Kleinman's textbook (1998) offers opinion about dating fractures based on the author's personal experience. Offiah and Hall [217] recently added significantly to the literature about fracture patterns and bone healing in abused children. However, there remain few cases on which to base firm opinions about the features of healing fractures in children of different ages, in different bones and with different fracture patterns.

In addition to the physiological factors, the radiographic technique and imaging system resolution might not be optimized. It is important that high-resolution techniques be used and that imaging is performed by radiographers familiar with techniques used to optimize the imaging of children. Radiologists who are less familiar in interpreting children's X-rays might not detect signs of bone injury that are recognized more readily by experienced paediatric radiologists. Ultrasound is very operator-dependent and requires specialist skills. Its nature is more suited to localized examination of a clinically suspicious area rather than generalized screening for evidence of injury. However, it can be used to identify soft tissue changes when there is a focus of clinical concern such as bruising or swelling when the X-ray is normal.

References

1. Tardieu A (1860) Étude médico-légale sur les sévices et mauvais traitements exercés sur des enfants. Ann Hyg Pub Med Leg 13:361–398
2. Caffey J (1946) Multiple fractures in the long bones of infants suffering from chronic subdural hematoma. Am J Roentgenol Radium Ther 56:163–173
3. Caffey J (1972) The parent-infant traumatic stress syndrome; (Caffey-Kempe syndrome), (battered babe syndrome). Am J Roentgenol Radium Therapy, Nucl Med 114:218–229
4. Cameron JM, Johnson HR, Camps FE (1966) The battered child syndrome. Med Sci Law 6(1):2–21
5. Cameron JM, Rae LJ (1975) Atlas of the battered child syndrome. Churchill Livingstone, Edinburgh, London
6. Kempe CH, Silverman FN, Steele BF, Droegemueller W, Silver HK (1962) The battered-child syndrome. JAMA 181:17–24
7. Berkowitz CD (2017) Physical abuse of children. N Engl J Med 376:1659–1666
8. Block RW, Palusci VJ (2006) Child abuse pediatrics: a new pediatric subspecialty. J Pediatr 148(6):711–712
9. Adams G, Ainsworth J, Butler L, Bonshek R, Clarke M, Doran R, Dutton G, Green M, Hodgkinson P, Leitch J, Lloyd C, Luthert P, Parsons A, Punt J, Taylor D, Tehrani N, Willshaw H, Child Abuse Working Party (2004) Update from the child abuse working party: Royal College of Ophthalmologists. Eye (Lond) 18:795–798
10. Ross AH, Juarez CA (2014) A brief history of fatal child maltreatment and neglect. Forensic Sci Med Pathol 10(3):413–422
11. Adamsbaum C, Grabar S, Mejean N, Rey-Salmon C (2010) Abusive head trauma: judicial admissions highlight violent and repetitive shaking. Pediatrics 126:546–555
12. American Academy of Pediatrics, Section on Radiology (2000) Diagnostic imaging of child abuse. Pediatrics 105:1345–1348
13. American Academy of Pediatrics, Section on Radiology (2009) Diagnostic imaging of child abuse. Pediatrics 123:1430–1435
14. Pierce MC, Bertocci G (2008) Injury biomechanics and child abuse. Annu Rev Biomed Eng 10:85–106
15. Gao WM, Chadha MS, Berger RP, Omenn GS, Allen DL, Pisano M, Adelson PD, Clark RS, Jenkins LW, Kochanek PM (2007) A gel-based proteomic comparison of human cerebrospinal fluid between inflicted and non-inflicted pediatric traumatic brain injury. J Neurotrauma 24(1):43–53
16. Berger RP, Adelson PD, Pierce MC, Dulani T, Cassidy LD, Kochanek PM (2005) Serum neuron-specific enolase, S100B, and myelin basic protein concentrations after inflicted and noninflicted traumatic brain injury in children. J Neurosurg 103(1):61–68
17. Cicchetti D, Rogosch FA, Sturge-Apple ML (2007) Interactions of child maltreatment and serotonin transporter and monoamine oxidase A polymorphisms: depressive symptomatology among adolescents from low socioeconomic status backgrounds. Dev Psychopathol 19(4):1161–1180
18. Hecker T, Radtke KM, Hermenau K, Papassotiropoulos A, Elbert T (2016) Associations among child abuse, mental health, and epigenetic modifications in the proopiomelanocortin gene (POMC): a study with children in Tanzania. Dev Psychopathol 28:1401–1412
19. Zarate YA, Clingenpeel R, Sellars EA, Tang X, Kaylor JA, Bosanko K, Linam LE, Byers PH, Genet A (2016) COL1A1 and COL1A2 sequencing results in cohort of patients undergoing evaluation for potential child abuse. Am J Med Genet A 170(7):1858–1862
20. Maguire S, Mann MK, Sibert J, Kemp A (2005) Are there patterns of bruising in childhood which are diagnostic or suggestive of abuse? A systematic review. Arch Dis Child 90:182–186
21. Maguire S, Mann MK, Sibert J, Kemp A (2005) Can you age bruises accurately in children? A systematic review. Arch Dis Child 90:187–189
22. Vock R, Schellmann B, Schaidt G (1980) Isolated injuries of intestinal tract due to body maltreatment (author's transl). Z Rechtsmed 84(2):155–159
23. Global Burden of Disease (2013). World Health Organization, Geneva. http://www.who.int/topics/global_burden_of_disease/en/. Accessed 18 Nov 2017

24. Global Status Report on Violence Prevention (2014) WHO, Global status report on violence prevention 2014, Geneva. Accessed 15 Nov 2017
25. Child Maltreatment (2012) Washington: A.f.C.a.F. U.S. Department of Health and Human Services, Administration on Children, Youth and Families, Children's Bureau, 2012
26. U.S. Department of Health & Human Services, Administration for Children and Families, Administration on Children, Youth and Families, Children's Bureau (2016) Child maltreatment 2014. http://www.acf.hhs.gov/programs/cb/research-data-technology/statistics-research/child-maltreatment. Accessed 18 Nov 2017
27. Kleinman PL, Kleinman PK, Savageau J (2004) Suspected infant abuse: radiographic skeletal survey practices in pediatric health care facilities. Radiology 233(2):477–485
28. Chadwick DL, Chin S, Salerno C, Landsverk J, Kitchen L (1991) Deaths from falls in children: how far is fatal? J Trauma 31(10):1353–1355
29. Chadwick DL, Bertocci G, Castillo E, Frasier L, Guenther E, Hansen K, Herman B, Krous HF (2008) Annual risk of death resulting from short falls among young children: less than 1 in 1 million. Pediatrics 121:1213–1224
30. Dedouit F, Mallinger B, Guilbeau-Frugier C, Rougé D, Rousseau H, Telmon N (2011) Lethal visceral traumatic injuries secondary to child abuse: a case of practical application of autopsy, radiological and microscopic studies. Forensic Sci Int 206(1–3):e62–e66
31. Graupman P, Winston KR (2006) Nonaccidental head trauma as a cause of childhood death. J Neurosurg 104(4 Suppl):245–250
32. Hall JR, Reyes HM, Horvat M, Meller JL, Stein R (1989) The mortality of childhood falls. J Trauma 29(9):1273–1275
33. Jenny C, Isaac R (2006) The relation between child death and child maltreatment. Arch Dis Child 91(3):265–269
34. Serinelli S, Arunkumar P, Filkins JA, Gitto L (2017) Deaths due to child abuse: a 6-year review of cases in the Cook County Medical Examiner's Office. J Forensic Sci 62(1):107–118
35. World Health Organization (2013) Regional Office for Europe. European report on preventing child maltreatment. Edited by Dinesh Sethi, Mark Bellis, Karen Hughes, Ruth Gilbert, Francesco Mitis, Gauden Galea. Accessed 15 Nov 2017
36. Sidebotham P, Bailey S, Belderson P, Brandon M (2011) Fatal child maltreatment in England, 2005–2009. Child Abuse Negl 35(4):299–306
37. Spies EL, Klevens J (2016) Fatal abusive head trauma among children aged <5 years—United States, 1999–2014. MMWR Morb Mortal Wkly Rep 65:505–509
38. UNIcEF Innocenti Research Centre (2003) A league table of child maltreatment deaths in rich nations. Florence. Accessed 18 Nov 2017
39. Schnitzer PG, Gulino SP, Yuan YY (2013) Advancing public health surveillance to estimate child maltreatment fatalities: review and recommendations. Child Welfare 92(2):77–98
40. Krug EG, Mercy JA, Dahlberg LL, Zwi AB (2002) World report on violence and health. Biomedica 22(2):327–336
41. Lanzarone A, Nardello R, Conti E, Zerbo S, Argo A (2017) Child abuse in a medical setting: Case illustrations of two variants of munchausen sindrome by proxy. EMBJ 12(10):47–50
42. Argo A, Averna L, Triolo V, Francomano A, Zerbo S (2012) Validity and credibility of a child's testimony of sexual abuse: A case report. EMBJ 7(21):97–100
43. Girardet R, Lahoti S, Bolton K, Kellogg N (2016) Characteristics of cases submitted to a statewide system of child abuse experts. Child Youth Serv Rev 67:198–202
44. Lane WG, Dubowitz H, Langenberg P (2009) Screening for occult abdominal trauma in children with suspected physical abuse. Pediatrics 124:1595–1602
45. Trokel M, Discala C, Terrin NC, Sege RD (2006) Patient and injury characteristics in abusive abdominal injuries. Pediatr Emerg Care 22:700–704
46. Maguire SA, Upadhyaya M, Evans A, Mann MK, Haroon MM, Tempest V, Lumb RC, Kemp AM (2013) A systematic review of abusive visceral injuries in childhood—their range and recognition. Child Abuse Negl 37(7):430–445
47. Matthieu V, de Foort-Dhellemmes S, Desurmont M, Delestret I (2010) Confessed abuse versus witnessed accidents in infants: comparison of clinical, radiological, and ophthalmological data in corroborated cases. Childs Nerv Syst 26:637–645
48. Nimityongskul P, Anderson LD (1987) The likelihood of injuries when children fall out of bed. J Pediatr Orthop 7(2):184–186
49. Reddie IC, Bhardwaj G, Dauber SL, Jacobs MB, Moran KT (2010) Bilateral retinoschisis in a 2-year-old following a three-storey fall. Eye (Lond) 24:1426–1427
50. Reiber GD (1993) Fatal falls in childhood. How far must children fall to sustain fatal head injury? Report of cases and review of the literature. Am J Forensic Med Pathol 14(3):201–207
51. Dye DW, Peretti FJ, Kokes CP (2008) Histologic evidence of repetitive blunt force abdominal trauma in four pediatric fatalities. J Forensic Sci 53(6):1430–1433
52. Erck Lambert AB, Parks SE, Camperlengo L, Cottengim C, Anderson RL, Covington TM, Shapiro-Mendoza CK (2016) Death scene investigation and autopsy practices in sudden unexpected infant deaths. J Pediatr 174:84–90
53. Gaines BA, Shultz BS, Morrison K, Ford HR (2004) Duodenal injuries in children: beware of child abuse. J Pediatr Surg 39:600–602
54. Dashti SR, Decker DD, Razzaq A, Cohen AR (1999) Current patterns of inflicted head injury in children. Pediatr Neurosurg 31:302–306

55. Dias MS, Rottmund CM, Cappos KM, Reed ME, Wang M, Stetter C, Shaffer ML, Hollenbeak CS, Paul IM, Christian CW, Berger RP, Klevens J (2017) Association of postnatal parent education program for abusive head trauma hospitalization rates. JAMA Pediatr 171:223–229
56. Duffy SO, Squires J, Fromkin JB, Berger RP (2011) Use of skeletal surveys to evaluate for physical abuse: analysis of 703 consecutive skeletal surveys. Pediatrics 127(1):e47–e52
57. Evans KT, Knight B (1981) Forensic radiology, 1st edn. Blackwell Scientific Publications, Oxford
58. Gabaeff SC (2016) Exploring the controversy in child abuse pediatrics and false accusations od abuse. Legal Med:90–97
59. Sugar NF, Taylor JA, Feldman KW (1999) Bruises in infants and toddlers: those who don't cruise rarely bruise. Arch Pediatr Adolesc Med 153:399–403
60. Williams RA (1991) Injuries in infants and small children resulting from witnessed and corroborated free falls. J Trauma 31(10):1350–1352
61. Sheets LK, Leach ME, Koszewski IJ, Lessmeier AM, Nugent M, Simpson P (2013) Sentinel injuries in infants evaluated for child physical abuse. Pediatrics 131:701–707
62. Kellogg ND, American Academy of Pediatrics Committee on Child Abuse and Neglect (2007) Evaluation of suspected child physical abuse. Pediatrics 119:1232–1241
63. Kenney IJ (2001) Doubt, difficulties and practicalities in the diagnosis of non-accidental injury—a personal view. Imaging 13:295–301
64. Pierre-Kahn V, Roche O, Dureau P, Uteza Y, Renier D, Pierre-Kahn A, Dufier JL (2003) Ophthalmologic findings in suspected child abuse victims with subdural hematomas. Ophthalmology 110:1718–1723
65. Rini MS, Colucci C, Bucci MB, Argo A (2017) Child abuse hidden in plain sight: The dentist obligations. Dental Cadmos 85(10):647–656
66. Saukko P, Knight B (2016) Fatal child abuse (Chapter 22). In: Knight's forensic pathology, 4th edn. CRC press, Taylor and Francis Group, New York, pp 475–495
67. Minns RA, Madea B, Kernbach-Wighton G (2014) Non-accidental head injury in children historical aspects of child abuse, definitions and incidence. In: Madea B (ed) Handbook of forensic medicine. Wiley Blackwell, Chichester, pp 681–701
68. Crichton KG, Cooper JN, Minneci PC, Groner JI, Thackeray JD, Deans KJ (2016) A national survey on the use of screening tools to detect physical child abuse. Pediatr Surg Int 32(8):815–818
69. Maguire S, Hunter B, Hunter L, Sibert J, Mann M, Kemp AM (2007) Diagnosing abuse: a systematic review of torn frenulum and other intra-oral injuries. Arch Dis Child 92:1113–1117
70. Levin AV, Christian CW, Committee on Child Abuse and Neglect, Section on Ophthalmology (2010) The eye examination in the evaluation of child abuse. Pediatrics 126:376–380
71. Rangarajan N, Kamalakkannan SB, Hasija V, Shams T, Jenny C, Serbanescu I, Ho J, Rusinek M, Levin AV (2009) Finite element model of ocular injury in abusive head trauma. J AAPOS 13:364–369
72. Royal College of Ophthalmology Child Abuse Working Party (1999) Child abuse and the eye. Eye (Lond) 13:3–10
73. Averna L, Argo A, Cascino FM, D'Anna T, Procaccianti P (2012) Suspected child abuse: Unusual death in western country. Suicide or homicide? EMBJ 11(6):52–54
74. Stanley P, Gwinn JL, Sutcliffe J (1976) The osseous abnormalities in Menke's syndrome. Ann Radiol 19(1):167–172
75. Lindberg DM, Shapiro RA, Blood EA, Steiner RD, Berger RP (2013) Utility of hepatic transaminases in children with concern for abuse. Pediatrics 131:268–275
76. Suzuki K, Fukushima T, Meguro K, Aoki T, Kamezaki T, Saitoh H, Enomoto T, Nose T (1999) Intracranial hemorrhage in an infant owing to vitamin K deficiency despite prophylaxis. Childs Nerv Syst 15(6–7):292–294
77. Schilling S, Wood JN, Levine MA, Langdon D, Christian CW (2011) Vitamin D status in abused and nonabused children younger than 2 years old with fractures. Pediatrics 127:835–841
78. Cranney A, Horsley T, O'Donnell S, Weiler H, Puil L, Ooi D, Atkinson S, Ward L, Moher D, Hanley D, Fang M, Yazdi F, Garritty C, Sampson M, Barrowman N, Tsertsvadze A, Mamaladze V (2007) Effectiveness and safety of vitamin D in relation to bone health. Evid Rep Technol Assess (Full Rep) 158:1–235
79. Gartner LM, Greer FR (2003) AAP clinical report on prevention of rickets and vitamin D deficiency: new guidelines for vitamin D intake. Pediatrics 111(4):908–910
80. Flaherty EG, Perez-Rossello JM, Levine MA, Hennrikus WL, American Academy of Pediatrics Committee on Child Abuse and Neglect, Section on Radiology, American Academy of Pediatrics, Section on Endocrinology, American Academy of Pediatrics, Section on Orthopaedics, American Academy of Pediatrics, Society for Pediatric Radiology (2014) Evaluating children with fractures for child physical abuse. Pediatrics 133(2):e477–e489
81. D'Eufemia P, Palombaro M, Lodato V, Zambrano A, Celli M, Persiani P, De Bari MP, Sangiorgi L (2012) Child abuse and osteogenesis imperfecta: how can they be still misdiagnosed? A case report. Clin Cases Miner Bone Metab 9(3):195–197
82. Cheung MS, Glorieux FH (2008) Osteogenesis imperfecta: update on presentation and management. Rev Endocr Metab Disord 9:153–160

83. Genetics Home Reference Osteogenesis imperfecta (2007). http://ghr.nlm.nih.gov/condition=osteogenesisimperfecta. Accessed 18 Nov 2017
84. Ojima K, Matsumoto H, Hayase T, Fukui Y (1994) An autopsy case of osteogenesis imperfecta initially suspected as child abuse. Forensic Sci Int 65(2):97–104
85. Singh Kocher M, Dichtel L (2011) Osteogenesis imperfecta misdiagnosed as child abuse. J Pediatr Orthop B 20(6):440–443
86. Maguire SA, Kemp AM, Lumb RC, Farewell DM (2011) Estimating the probability of abusive head trauma: a pooled analysis. Pediatrics 128(3):e550–e564
87. Wright JN (2017) CNS Injuries in Abusive Head Trauma. AJR 208(5):991–1001
88. Atwal GS, Rutty GN, Carter N, Green MA (1998) Bruising in non-accidental head injured children; a retrospective study of the prevalence, distribution and pathological associations in 24 cases. Forensic Sci Int 96(2–3):215–230
89. Bacopoulou F, Henderson I, Philip SG (2006) Menkes disease mimicking non-accidental trauma. Arch Dis Child 91(11):919
90. Banaschak S, Janßen K, Schulte B, Rothschild MA (2015) Rate of deaths due to child abuse and neglect in children 0–3 years of age in Germany. Int J Legal Med 129(5):1091–1096
91. Barr RG (2012) Preventing abusive head trauma resulting from a failure of normal interaction between infants and their caregivers. Proc Natl Acad Sci U S A 109(Suppl 2):17294–17301
92. Ellingson KD, Leventhal JM, Weiss HB (2008) Using hospital discharge data to track inflicted traumatic brain injury. Am J Prev Med 34(4 Suppl):S157–S162
93. Helfer RE, Slovis TL, Black M (1977) Injuries resulting when small children fall out of bed. Pediatrics 60(4):533–535
94. Hobbs CJ, Wynne JM (1996) Fractures in infancy: are the bones brittle? Curr Paediatr 6:183–188
95. Squier W, Mack J, Jansen AC (2016) Infants dying suddenly and unexpectedly share demographic features with infants who die with retinal and dural bleeding: a review of neural mechanisms. Dev Med Child Neurol 58(12):1223–1234
96. Shuman MJ, Hutchins KD (2017) Severe retinal hemorrages with retinoschisis in infant are not pathognomonic for abusive head trauma. J Forensic Sci 62(3):807–811
97. Christian CW, Block R (2009) Abusive head trauma in infants and children. Pediatrics 123:1409–1411
98. Bell E, Shouldice M, Levin AV (2011) Abusive head trauma: a perpetrator confesses. Child Abuse Negl 35:74–77
99. Bennett S, Ward M, Moreau K, Fortin G, King J, Mackay M, Plint A (2011) Head injury secondary to suspected child maltreatment: results of a prospective Canadian national surveillance program. Child Abuse Negl 35(11):930–936
100. Billmire ME, Myers PA (1985) Serious head injury in infants: accident or abuse? Pediatrics 75(2):340–342
101. Narang SK, Estrada C, Greenberg S, Lindberg D (2016) Acceptance of shaken baby syndrome and abusive head trauma as medical diagnoses. J Pediatr 177:273–278
102. American Academy of Pediatrics, Committee on Child Abuse and Neglect (2001) Shaken baby syndrome: rotational cranial injuries—technical report. Pediatrics 108:206–210
103. Caffey J (1972) On the theory and practice of shaking infants: its potential residual effects of permanent brain damage and mental retardation. Am J Dis Child 124:161–169
104. Caffey J (1974) The whiplash shaken infant syndrome: manual shaking by the extremities with whiplash induced intracranial and intraocular bleedings, linked with residual permanent brain damage and mental retardation. Pediatrics 54:396–403
105. Matshes EW, Evan RM, Pinckard JK, Joseph JT, Lew EO (2011) Shaken infants die of neck trauma not of brain trauma. Acad Forensic Pathol 1:82–91
106. Duhaime AC, Alario AJ, Lewander WJ et al (1992) Head injury in very young children: mechanisms, injury types, and ophthalmologic findings in 100 hospitalized patients younger than 2 years of age. Pediatrics 90:179–185
107. Spivack B (2001) Fatal pediatric head injuries caused by short-distance falls. Am J Forensic Med Pathol 22(3):332–336
108. Bhardwaj G, Chowdhury V, Jacobs MB, Moran KT, Martin FJ, Coroneo MT (2010) A systematic review of the diagnostic accuracy of ocular signs in pediatric abusive head trauma. Ophthalmology 117:983–92.e17
109. Biousse V, Suh DY, Newman NJ, Davis PC, Mapstone T, Lambert SR (2002) Diffusion-weighted magnetic resonance imaging in shaken baby syndrome. Am J Ophthalmol 133:249–255
110. Brogdon BG (2011) Child abuse. In: Thali M, Viner MD, Brogdon BG (eds) Brogdon's forensic radiology. CRC Press, Boca Raton, pp 255–278
111. Budenz DL, Farber MG, Mirchandani HG, Park H, Rorke LB (1994) Ocular and optic nerve hemorrhages in abused infants with intracranial injuries. Ophthalmology 101(3):559–565
112. Gabaeff SC (2011) Challenging the pathophysiologic connection between subdural hematoma, retinal hemorrhage and shaken baby syndrome. West J Emerg Med 12(2):144–158
113. Guthkelch AN (1971) Infantile subdural haematoma and its relationship to whiplash injuries. Br Med J 2:430–431
114. Kivlin JD, Simons KB, Lazoritz S, Ruttum MS (2000) Shaken baby syndrome. Ophthalmology 107:1246–1254

115. Odom A, Christ E, Kerr N, Byrd K, Cochran J, Barr F, Bugnitz M, Ring JC, Storgion S, Walling R, Stidham G, Quasney MW (1997) Prevalence of retinal hemorrhages in pediatric patients after in-hospital cardiopulmonary resuscitation: a prospective study. Pediatrics 99:E3
116. Gago L, Wegner R, Capone A, Williams GA (2003) Intraretinal hemorrhages and chronic subdural effusions: glutaric acidurics type 1 can be mistaken for shaken baby syndrome. Retina 23(5):724–726
117. Goldman M, Dagan Z, Yair M, Elbaz U, Lahat E, Yair M (2006) Severe cough and retinal hemorrhage in infants and young children. J Pediatr 148:835–836
118. Kanter RK (1986) Retinal hemorrhage after cardiopulmonary resuscitation or child abuse. J Pediatr 108:430–432
119. Kivlin JD, Currie ML, Greenbaum VJ, Simons KB, Jentzen J (2008) Retinal hemorrhages in children following fatal motor vehicle crashes: a case series. Arch Ophthalmol 126:800–804
120. Lueder GT, Turner JW, Paschall R (2006) Perimacular retinal folds simulating nonaccidental injury in an infant. Arch Ophthalmol 124:1782–1783
121. Mei-Zahav M, Uziel Y, Raz J, Ginot N, Wolach B, Fainmesser P (2002) Convulsions and retinal haemorrhage: should we look further? Arch Dis Child 86:334–335
122. Mishra P, Naithani R, Dolai T, Bhargava R, Mahapatra M, Dixit A, Seth T, Kumar R, Saxena R (2008) Intracranial hemorrhagein patients with congenital haemostatic defects. Haemophilia 14(5):952–955
123. Pham H, Enzenauer RW, Elder JE, Levin AV (2013) Retinal hemorrhage after cardiopulmonary resuscitation with chest compressions. Am J Forensic Med Pathol 34(2):122–124
124. Sandramouli S, Robinson R, Tsaloumas M, Willshaw HE (1997) Retinal haemorrhages and convulsions. Arch Dis Child 76:449–451
125. Tyagi AK, Scotcher S, Kozeis N, Willshaw HE (1998) Can convulsions alone cause retinal haemorrhages in infants? Br J Ophthalmol 82:659–660
126. Weissgold DJ, Budenz DL, Hood I, Rorke LB (1995) Ruptured vascular malformation masquerading as battered/shaken baby syndrome: a near tragic mistake. Surv Ophthalmol 39:509–512
127. Binenbaum G, Mirza-George N, Christian CW, Forbes BJ (2009) Odds of abuse associated with retinal hemorrhages in children suspected of child abuse. J AAPOS 13:268–272
128. Binenbaum G, Forbes BJ (2014) The eye in child abuse: key points on retinal hemorrhages and abusive head trauma. Pediatr Radiol 44(4 Suppl):571S–577S
129. McCabe CF, Donahue SP (2000) Prognostic indicators for vision and mortality in shaken baby syndrome. Arch Ophthalmol 118:373–377
130. Shiau T, Levin AV (2012) Retinal hemorrhages in children. The role of intracranial pressure. Arch Pediatr Adolesc Med 166(7):623–628
131. Case ME, Graham MA, Handy TC, Jentzen JM, Monteleone JA, National Association of Medical Examiners Ad Hoc Committee on Shaken Baby Syndrome (2001) Position paper on fatal abusive head injuries in infants and young children. Am J Forensic Med Pathol 22(2):112–122
132. Duhaime AC, Gennarelli TA, Thibault LE, Bruce DA, Margulies SS, Wiser R (1987) The shaken baby syndrome: a clinical, pathological, and biomechanical study. J Neurosurg 66:409–415
133. Ludwig S, Warman M (1984) Shaken baby syndrome: a review of 20 cases. Ann Emerg Med 13:104–107
134. Christian CW, Taylor AA, Hertle RW, Duhaime AC (1999) Retinal hemorrhages caused by accidental household trauma. J Pediatr 135:125–127
135. Coats B, Binenbaum G, Peiffer RL (2010) Ocular hemorrhages in neonatal porcine eyes from single, rapid rotational events. Invest Ophthalmol Vis Sci 51:4792–4797
136. Puanglumyai S, Lekawanvijit S (2017) The importance of optic nerve sheath hemorrhage as a postmortem finding in cases of fatal abusive head trauma: a 13-year study in a tertiary hospital. Forensic Sci Int 276:5–11
137. Morad Y, Kim YM, Armstrong DC, Huyer D, Mian M, Levin AV (2002) Correlation between retinal abnormalities and intracranial abnormalities in the shaken baby syndrome. Am J Ophthalmol 134:354–359
138. Curcoy AI, Trenchs V, Morales M, Serra A, Pineda M, Pou J (2009) Do retinal haemorrhages occur in infants with convulsions? Arch Dis Child 94:873–875
139. Gleckman AM, Evans RJ, Bell MD, Smith TW (2000) Optic nerve damage in shaken baby syndrome: detection by beta-amyloid precursor protein immunohistochemistry. Arch Pathol Lab Med 124:251–256
140. Greiner MV, Berger RP, Thackeray JD, Lindberg DM (2013) Dedicated retinal examination in children evaluated for physical abuse without radiographically identified traumatic brain injury. J Pediatr 163:527–531
141. Parizel PM, Ceulemans B, Laridon A, Ozsarlak O, Van Goethem JW, Jorens PG (2003) Cortical hypoxicischemic brain damage in shaken-baby (shaken impact) syndrome: value of diffusion-weighted MRI. Pediatr Radiol 33:868–871
142. Phillips MD, Zimmerman RA (1999) Diffusion imaging in pediatric hypoxic ischemia injury. Neuroimaging Clin N Am 9:41–52
143. Ichord RN, Naim M, Pollock AN, Nance ML, Margulies SS, Christian CW (2007) Hypoxic-ischemic injury complicates inflicted and accidental traumatic brain injury in young children: the role of diffusion-weighted imaging. J Neurotrauma 24:106–118
144. Binenbaum G, Rogers DL, Forbes BJ, Levin AV, Clark SA, Christian CW, Liu GT, Avery R (2013)

Patterns of retinal hemorrhage associated with increased intracranial pressure in children. Pediatrics 132(2):e430–e434
145. Binenbaum G, Christian CW, Ichord RN, Christian CW, Ichord RN, Ying GS, Simon MA, Romero K, Pollock AN, Forbes BJ (2013) Retinal hemorrhage and brain injury patterns on diffusion-weighted magnetic resonance imaging in children with head trauma. J AAPOS 17:603–608
146. Mills M (1998) Funduscopic lesions associated with mortality in shaken baby syndrome. J AAPOS 2:67–71
147. Hymel KP, Willson DF, Boos SC, Pullin DA, Homa K, Lorenz DJ, Herman BE, Graf JM, Isaac R, Armijo-Garcia V, Narang SK, Pediatric Brain Injury Research Network (PediBIRN) Investigators (2013) Derivation of a clinical prediction rule for pediatric abusive head trauma. Pediatr Crit Care Med 14:210–220
148. Levin AV (2010) Retinal hemorrhage in abusive head trauma. Pediatrics 126:961–970
149. Hobbs CJ (1984) Skull fracture and the diagnosis of abuse. Arch Dis Child 59(3):246–252
150. Hughes LA, May K, Talbot JF, Parsons MA (2006) Incidence, distribution, and duration of birth-related retinal hemorrhages: a prospective study. J AAPOS 10:102–106
151. Prange MT, Coats B, Duhaime AC, Margulies SS (2003) Anthropomorphic simulations of falls, shakes, and inflicted impacts in infants. J Neurosurg 99:143–150
152. Keats TE, Anderson MW (2006) Atlas of normal roentgen variants that may simulate disease, 8th edn. Mosby, Philadelphia
153. Prahlow JA, Rushing EJ, Bernard JJ (1998) Death due to a ruptured berry aneurysm in a 3.5-year-old child. Am J Forensic Med Pathol 19:391–394
154. Hughes-Roberts Y, Arthurs OJ, Moss H, Set PA (2012) Post-mortem skeletal surveys in suspected non-accidental injury. Clin Radiol 67(9): 868–876
155. Jenny C, Hymel KP, Ritzen A, Reinert SE, Hay TC (1999) Analysis of missed cases of abusive head trauma. JAMA 281:621–626
156. Jenny C, Committee on Child Abuse and Neglect (2006) Evaluating infants and young children with multiple fractures. Pediatrics 118(3):1299–1303
157. John SM, Jones P, Kelly P, Vincent A (2013) Fatal pediatric head injuries: a 20-year review of cases through the Auckland coroner's office. Am J Forensic Med Pathol 34(3):277–282
158. Jones M, Darwall D, Khalid G, Prabhu R, Kemp A, Arthurs OJ, Theobald P (2017) Development and validation of a physical model to investigate the biomechanics of infant head impact. Forensic Sci Int 276:111–119
159. Jones R, Flaherty EG, Binns HJ, Price LL, Slora E, Abney D, Harris DL, Christoffel KK, Sege RD (2008) Clinicians' description of factors influencing their reporting of suspected child abuse: report of the Child Abuse Reporting Experience Study Research Group. Pediatrics 122:259–266
160. Kleinman PK, Marks SC Jr, Richmond JM, Blackbourne BD (1995) Inflicted skeletal injury: a postmortem radiologic-histopathologic study in 31 infants. Am J Roentgenol 165(3):647–650
161. Kleinman PK, Nimkin K, Spevak MR, Rayder SM, Madansky DL, Shelton YA, Patterson MM (1996) Follow-up skeletal surveys in suspected child abuse. AJR Am J Roentgenol 167:893–896
162. Karibe H, Kameyama M, Hayashi T, Narisawa A, Tominaga T (2016) Acute subdural hematoma in infants with abusive head trauma: a literature review. Neurol Med Chir (Tokyo) 56(5):264–273
163. Karmazyn B, Lewis ME, Jennings SG, Hibbard RA, Hicks RA (2011) The prevalence of uncommon fractures on skeletal surveys performed to evaluate for suspected abuse in 930 children: should practice guidelines change? Am J Roentgenol 197(1):W159–W163
164. Keeling JW, Busuttil A (2005) Paediatric forensic medicine and pathology. Edward Arnold, London
165. van Rijn RR, Spevak MR (2011) Imaging of neonatal child abuse with an emphasis on abusive head trauma. Magn Reson Imaging Clin N Am 19:791–812
166. Mack J, Squier W, Eastman JT (2009) Anatomy and development of the meninges: implications for subdural collections and CSF circulation. Pediatr Radiol 39(3):200–210
167. Matschke J, Voss J, Obi N, Görndt J, Sperhake JP, Püschel K, Glatzel M (2009) Nonaccidental head injury is the most common cause of subdural bleeding in infants <1 year of age. Pediatrics 124:1587–1594
168. Vowles GH, Scholtz CL, Cameron JM (1987) Diffuse axonal injury in early infancy. J Clin Pathol 40(2):185–189
169. Geddes JF, Hackshaw AK, Vowles GH, Nickols CD, Whitwell HL (2001) Neuropathology of inflicted head injury in children. I. Patterns of brain damage. Brain 124:1290–1298
170. Geddes JF, Vowles GH, Hackshaw AK, Nickols CD, Scott IS, Whitwell HL (2001) Neuropathology of inflicted head injury in children. II. Microscopic brain injury in infants. Brain 124:1299–1306
171. Kemp AM, Stoodley N, Cobley C, Coles L, Kemp KW (2003) Apnoea and brain swelling in nonaccidental head injury. Arch Dis Child 88:472–476
172. Smith DH, Meaney DF, Shull WH (2003) Diffuse axonal injury in head trauma. J Head Trauma Rehabil 18:307–316
173. Parker JR, Parker JC Jr, Overman JC (1990) Intracranial diffuse axonal injury at autopsy. Ann Clin Lab Sci 20(3):220–224
174. Case ME (2007) Abusive head injuries in infants and young children. Leg Med (Tokyo) 9(2):83–87
175. Case ME (2014) Distinguishing accidental from inflicted head trauma at autopsy. Pediatr Radiol 44(4 Suppl):632S–640S

176. Smit A, Cain T (2011) Assessment and interpretation of bone trauma in children (Chapter 4). In: Gall J, Payne-James J (eds) Current practice in forensic medicine. John Wiley and Sons, Hoboken, NJ
177. Harwood Nash CE, Hendrick EB, Hudson AR (1971) The significance of skull fractures in children. A study of 1,187 patients. Radiology 101(1):151–156
178. Shapiro R (1972) Anomalous parietal sutures and the bipartite parietal bone. Am J Roentgenol Radium Ther Nucl Med 115:569–577
179. Schaber B, Hart AP, Armbrustmacher V, Hirsch CS (2002) Fatal pediatric head injuries caused by short distance falls. Am J Forensic Med Pathol 23(1):101–103. author reply 103–5
180. Sty JR, Starshack RJ (1983) The role of bone scintigraphy in the evaluation of the suspected abused child. Radiology 146:369–375
181. Yason D, Jane JA, White RJ, Sugar O (1968) Traumatic subdural hematoma of infancy. Long-term follow-up of 92 patients. Arch Neurol 18(4):370–377
182. Young JY, Duhaime AC, Caruso PA, Rincon SP (2016) Comparison of non-sedated brain MRI and CT for the detection of acute traumatic injury in children 6 years of age or less. Emerg Radiol 23(4):325–331
183. Mehta H, Acharya J, Mohan AL, Tobias ME, LeCompte L, Jeevan D (2016) Minimizing radiation exposure in evaluation of pediatric head trauma: use of rapid MR imaging. Am J Neuroradiol 37:11–18
184. Ryan ME, Jaju A, Ciolino JD, Alden T (2016) Rapid MRI evaluation of acute intracranial hemorrhage in pediatric head trauma. Paediatr Neuroradiol 58(8):793–799
185. American College of Radiology (2006) Practice guidelines for skeletal surveys in children. Revised 2016 (Resolution 10) www.acr.org/SecondaryMainMenuCategories/quality_safety/guidelines/pediatric/skeletal_surveys.aspx. Accessed 18 Nov 2017
186. British Society of Paediatric Radiologists (1999) Standard for skeletal surveys in suspected non-accidental injury (NAI) in children. www.bspr.org.uk/nai.htm. Accessed 18 Nov 2017
187. Government of Western Australia (2009) (Updated 2012 and 2015) Diagnostic imaging pathways—paediatric, injury (non-accidental). www.imagingpathways.health.wa.gov.au. Accessed 18 Nov 2017
188. Kemp AM, Butler A, Morris S, Mann M, Kemp KW, Rolfe K, Sibert JR, Maguire S (2006) Which radiological investigations should be performed to identify fractures in suspected child abuse? Clin Radiol 61(9):723–736
189. Mandelstam SA, Cook D, Fitzgerald M, Ditchfield MR (2003) Complementary use of radiological skeletal survey and bone scintigraphy in detection of bony injuries in suspected child abuse. Arch Dis Child 88:387–390
190. Conway JJ, Collins M, Tanz RR, Radkowski MA, Anandappa E, Hernandez R, Freeman EL (1993) The role of bone scintigraphy in detecting child abuse. Semin Nucl Med 23:321–333
191. Haase GM, Ortiz VN, Sfakianakis GN, Morse TS (1980) The value of radionuclide bone scanning in the early recognition of deliberate child abuse. J Trauma 20:973–975
192. Jaudes PK (1984) Comparison of radiography and radionuclide bone scan in the detection of child abuse. Pediatrics 73:166–168
193. Barsness KA, Cha ES, Bensard DD, Calkins CM, Partrick DA, Karrer FM, Strain JD (2003) The positive predictive value of rib fractures as an indicator of nonaccidental trauma in children. J Trauma 54(6):1107–1110
194. Bulloch B, Schubert CJ, Brophy PD, Johnson N, Reed MH, Shapiro RA (2000) Cause and clinical characteristics of rib fractures in infants. Pediatrics 105(4):E48
195. Cadzow SP, Armstrong KL (2000) Rib fractures in infants: red alert! The clinical features, investigations and child protection outcomes. J Paediatr Child Health 36:322–326
196. Morild I, Gjerdet NR, Giertsen JC (1993) Bone strength in infants. Forensic Sci Int 60(1–2):111–119
197. Perez-Rossello JM, Feldman HA, Kleinman PK, Connolly SA, Fair RA, Myers RM, Gordon CM (2012) Rachitic changes, demineralization, and fracture risk in healthy infants and toddlers with vitamin D deficiency. Radiology 262:234–241
198. Kleinman PK (1998) Diagnostic imaging of child abuse, 2nd edn. Mosby, St. Louis, MO
199. Kleinman PK (2008) Problems in the diagnosis of metaphyseal fractures. Pediatr Radiol 38(13):388–394
200. Gill JR, Andrew T, Gilliland MGF, Love J, Matshes E, Reichar RR (2014) National Association of Medical Examiners Position Paper: recommendations for the postmortem assessment of suspected head trauma in infants and young children. Acad Forensic Pathol J 4(2):206–213
201. Leventhal JM, Thomas SA, Rosenfield NS, Markowitz RI (1993) Fractures in young children. Distinguishing child abuse from unintentional injuries. Am J Dis Child 147(1):87–92
202. Piteau SJ, Ward MG, Barrowman NJ, Plint AC (2012) Clinical and radiographic characteristics associated with abusive and nonabusive head trauma: a systematic review. Pediatrics 130(2):315–323
203. Plunkett J (2001) Fatal pediatric head injuries caused by short-distance falls. Am J Forensic Med Pathol 22(1):1–12
204. Roach JP, Acker SN, Bensard DD, Sirotnak AP, Karrer FM, Partrick DA (2014) Head injury pattern in children can help differentiate accidental from non-accidental trauma. Pediatr Surg Int 30(11):1103–1106
205. Shugerman RP, Paez A, Grossman DC, Feldman KW, Grady MS (1996) Epidural hemorrhage: is it abuse? Pediatrics 97(5):664–668

206. Worlock P, Stower M, Barbor P (1986) Patterns of fractures in accidental and non-accidental injury in children: a comparative study. Br Med J (Clin Res Ed) 293(6539):100–102
207. Reece RM, Sege R (2000) Childhood head injuries: accidental or inflicted? Arch Pediatr Adolesc Med 154(1):11–15
208. Kemp AM, Dunstan E, Harrison S, Morris S, Mann M, Rolfe K, Datta S, Thomas DP, Sibert JR, Maguire S (2008) Patterns of skeletal fractures in child abuse: systematic review. BMJ 337:a1518
209. Leventhal JM, Edwards GA (2017) Flawed theories to explain child physical abuse: what are the medical-legal consequences? JAMA 318(14):1317–1318
210. Reece RM (1994) Child abuse: medical diagnosis and management. Lea & Febiger, Philadelphia
211. Levey EJ, Gelaye B, Bain P, Rondon MB, Borba CP, Henderson DC, Williams MA (2017) A systematic review of randomized controlled trials of interventions designed to decrease child abuse in high-risk families. Child Abuse Negl 65:48–57
212. Schwend RM, Werth C, Johnston A (2000) Femur shaft fractures in toddlers and young children: rarely from child abuse. J Pediatr Orthop 20(4):475–481
213. Giardino AP, Alexander R (2005) Child maltreatment: a clinical guide and reference, 3rd edn. GW Publishing Inc., St. Louis
214. Perkins R, Skirvin A (1987) Callus formation in the rate of healing of femoral fractures in patients with head injuries. J Bone Joint Surg Br 69:521–524
215. Spencer RF (1987) The effect of head injury on fracture healing. A quantitative assessment. J Bone Joint Surg Br 69B(4):525–528
216. Prosser I, Maguire S, Harrison SK, Mann M, Sibert JR, Kemp AM (2005) How old is the fracture? Radiological dating of fractures in children: a systematic review. AJR Am J Roentgenol 184:1282–1286
217. Offiah AC, Hall CM (2009) Radiological atlas of child abuse. Radcliffe Publishing, Oxford and New York

Domestic Violence 12

Magdy Kharoshah, Mohammed Gaballah, Manal Bamousa, and Kholoud Alsowayigh

12.1 Introduction

Domestic violence (DV), including intimate partner violence, is a phenomenon that has consistently taken place throughout history across the world, and continues in the present day. DV is considered to be a major public health issue, particularly as it affects a very wide demographic of people in society, cutting across age, economic and social background, race and religion. DV is not an isolated issue; rather, it is linked to a variety of social and mental health issues such as suicide, rape, murder, and self-harm.

However, the public profile of DV as an important issue has grown over recent decades; today, in numerous countries worldwide, it is a topic discussed by politicians, lawyers, and doctors among others, and there are visible attempts not only to offer support to anyone experiencing DV, but also to stop it from happening in the first place. The Duluth Minnesota Domestic Abuse Intervention Project became a paradigm globally in 1980, providing the model for further intervention in many states and countries.

In 2002, the World Health Organization (WHO) published a comprehensive report on violence and health globally, as well as publishing several studies on violence against women, which encompassed the acts and effects of DV. In addition, the WHO organized an international network for the prevention of violence, which sought to connect campaigners against DV to one another, as part of the global challenge to the practice.

Over recent decades, Canada and the United States (US)—soon after followed by Australia and a number of countries in Europe—introduced new laws regarding DV, in an outspoken attempt to transfer experiences of and conversations about DV from the private sphere to the public [1]. One example of federal law brought in by state government is the Violence Against Women Act, established in the US in 1994. The US Department of Justice declared that "between 1993 and 2008, there was a 53% drop in the number of nonfatal, violent acts committed by intimate partners," a potential result of the efforts of the Act to amplify protector for DV survivors, and to educate and rehabilitate perpetrators of DV.

M. Kharoshah (✉) · M. Bamousa
Dammam Forensic Medicine Center, Dammam, Kingdom of Saudi Arabia

M. Gaballah
Egyptian Forensic Medicine Authority, Cairo, Egypt

K. Alsowayigh
Jeddah Forensic Medicine Center, Jeddah, Kingdom of Saudi Arabia

G. Lo Re et al. (eds.), *Radiology in Forensic Medicine*, https://doi.org/10.1007/978-3-319-96737-0_12

Due to the establishment of federal laws passed in relation to DV, and the increased enforcement of these laws and public awareness that followed, so too came a focus on the importance of optimal evidence-based criminal prosecutions in a court of law. Clinical research was pursued, seeking conclusive answers in regard to the characteristics, diagnoses, evidence and documentation of DV and the signs of a perpetrator or survivor.

The following articles seek to improve this collation of knowledge, and provide a summary of issues surrounding DV, in regard to scientific research and practices attempting to combat DV [2].

12.2 Magnitude of Domestic Abuse

Estimates contend that around 35% across the world have experienced either physical and/or sexual intimate partner violence by a non-partner at some point in their lives. In addition, national studies suggest that up to 70% of women have experienced physical and/or sexual violence from an intimate partner [3]. These statistics make it clear that DV and IPV are not individual issues faced by a small percentage of the global population, but are a systemic issue that affects a vast number of women, regardless of their different demographics.

12.3 Risk Factors for DV and PVI

According to WHO [4, 5], there are many factors that can be understood as leading to DV and IPV. These factors can be categorized into groups labeled, individual, relationship, and community/societal factors.

Individual factors relate specifically to issues surrounding the perpetrator or survivor of DV. They encompass: young age; education status; as a child witnessing or being a survivor of abuse; the use of alcohol and/or drugs to a harmful extent; personality disorders and mental health issues; acceptance of violence; and a history of abusing former partners.

Relationship factors relate to issues surrounding the couple relationship. They include: dissatisfaction in a relationship (that may lead to conflict); male dominance; polyamorous relationships; and disparity in status between male and female (including, but not limited to, educational attainment).

Community and societal factors relate to issues within the wider community and society that the perpetrator, survivor, and/or relationship develop in. These factors include: gender-inequitable social norms; poverty and the stresses induced by it; women's low economic and social status; the difficulty to legally identify or challenge IPV within marriage; the continuing low status of women's civil rights (including within institutional acts such as marriage); weak community sanctions against IPV; how violence is often used as a way to resolve conflict, as part of broader forms of violence in society.

12.4 Forms of Domestic Violence

Battered women, children, and elderly persons occur in all segments of community. In this chapter we discuss IPV child abuse and elder abuse are discussed in other chapters.

12.4.1 Role of Radiology in Diagnosis and Management of Domestic Violence and IPV

Domestic violence and intimate partner violence became a significant health burden all over the world. Unfortunately, radiological documentation of this issue is not illustrated enough in forensic radiology literature.

On the other hand, health care providers play an important role in total management of domestic violence. Consequently, radiologists can interestingly provide an early detection of victims of domestic violence with comprehensive and accurate diagnosis of radiological findings in combination with clinical manifestations [6].

However, domestic violence or intimate partner violence (IPV) has many forms and aspects including physical violence, sexual violence, stalking, and psychological hostility [7].

Nevertheless, physical abuse may include tying down or restraining woman, abandoning her in a dangerous place or situation or health status [8].

In addition, domestic violence or IPV can range from a single assault to multiple repeated battering with variable frequency and severity which is often common rather than being an isolated incident [9].

12.4.2 Settings of Diagnosis and Detection of Domestic Abuse

The diagnosis of domestic abuse is a continuing and multidisciplinary process starting from early diagnosis at emergency room, passing through complete diagnosis of all types of physical and psychological trauma, until complete management of the victim following certain diagnostic and therapeutic guidelines [8, 10].

12.4.2.1 Radiological Diagnosis at Emergency Room

Many approaches can be followed for immediate and early diagnosis of victims of domestic abuse in emergency department including verbal interrogation, clinical examination, and radiological investigations. Hopefully, radiologist is able to early detection of any sort of intentional physical abuse.

Also, the radiologist is able to suspect the possible intentional physical abuse by the inconsistency in clinical history, patterns of diagnosed trauma, and timing of detected physical complications with possibility of keeping the records for legal utilization.

Usually, repeated attendance to emergency department is more common. Also, head, face, and neck injuries seem to be more common. Multiple simultaneous injuries in the same victim may also be more common [11].

Regarding to radiological techniques for diagnosis of bone trauma, one plain radiograph view is not sufficient. It is essential to get at least two views, preferably at right angle to one another. The reason is to avoid missing of fracture's dense line. It may appear as lucent line, sclerotic line, step in the cortex, or buckling of cortex (green stick). Nevertheless, joint effusions and soft tissue swelling are supportive finding to presence of fracture [12].

Invisible injuries even with two views taken at right angles may occur. So if there is clinical suspicious to bony injury with normal radiographs, then further films should be taken as follows:

- Oblique view.
- Stress films: which taken with joint under stress and this type is mainly helpful in ankle injuries.
- Flexion-extension views.
- X-ray of other side; for comparative purposes.
- Delayed films: taken 2 weeks after injury in which resorption can be seen at fracture site.

If those tiny fracture are not seen by plain film radiography, radio-nucleotide bone scanning is helpful in detecting recent type of fractures, i.e., (2–3 days of infliction) by showing an increased activity at the injured site, often lasting several months [12].

12.4.2.2 Radiological Diagnosis for Trauma, Complications, and Follow-Up

Head and neck injuries are the most common sites for injuries result from domestic violence and abuse; however, any part of the body is at risk for injury in cases of domestic violence.

So, for making such physical injuries more feasible for diagnosis and documentation, it can be classified regarding to anatomical involvement into cranial injuries, maxillofacial trauma, musculoskeletal injuries, and visceral injuries.

1. Cranial injuries

Cranial injuries and traumatic brain injury (TBI) have a high prevalence in domestic violence with increased risk of poor physical and psychological health outcomes. Anatomically, the most affected regions in the brain are the prefrontal cortex, hypothalamus, amygdala, and hippocampus. These areas are associated functionally to behaviors, personality, memorization, decision-making, and stress responses [13].

On the other hand, direct force to the head can result in a closed or open head injury.

(a) Closed head injuries:

A closed head injury results when an injurious force impacts the head and causes brain trauma while the skull is intact [14].

The problematic issue about the closed head injury is that there may be no manifested signs of traumatic brain injury and victims usually report only that they have fallen and were not beaten [15].

Reportedly, the shaken adult syndrome is one of the most recently described types of closed head injuries and had been described in forensic literature few times, one of them was associated with domestic abuse. Typically, this syndrome can be manifested by retinal hemorrhages, subdural hematoma, or cerebral edema with or without external bruises that resulted from repetitive acceleration-deceleration injury (Figs. 12.1 and 12.2) [16].

In addition to the shaken adult syndrome, other forms of closed head trauma can be seen in cases associated with domestic or intimate partner abuse. These forms include cerebral contusion which may be multiple from single attack and seen in coup and countercoup areas.

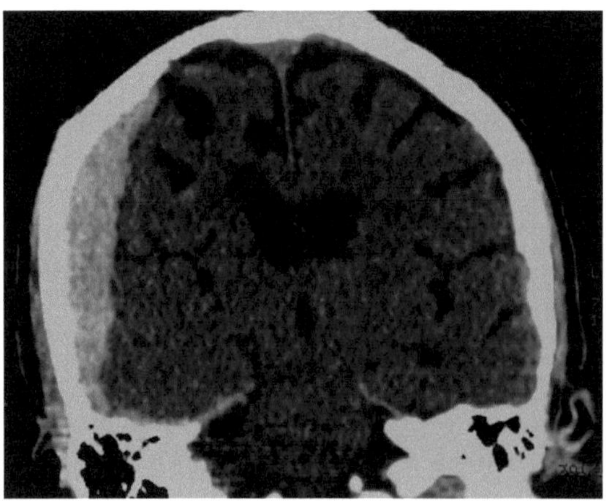

Fig. 12.1 Right parietal subdural hematoma coronal image

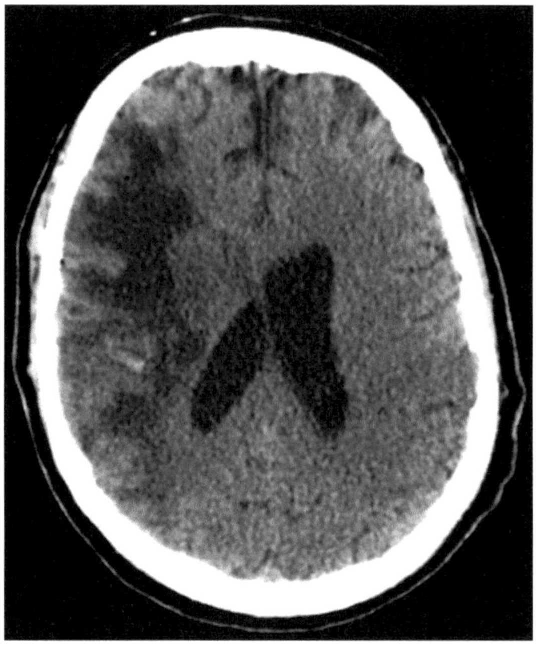

Fig. 12.2 Brain edema with axonal injury

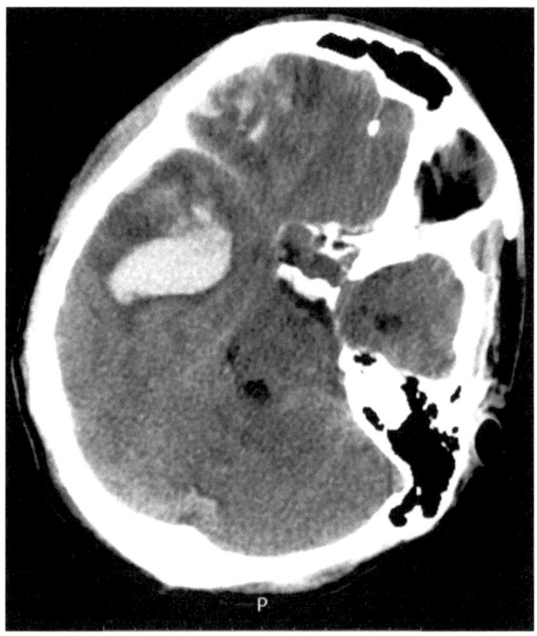

Fig. 12.3 Intracerebral hematoma in right temporal lobe

Intracerebral hematoma is mostly located at frontal or temporal lobes (Fig. 12.3).

Also, diffuse axonal injury is common with direct head trauma or violent repeated shaking to

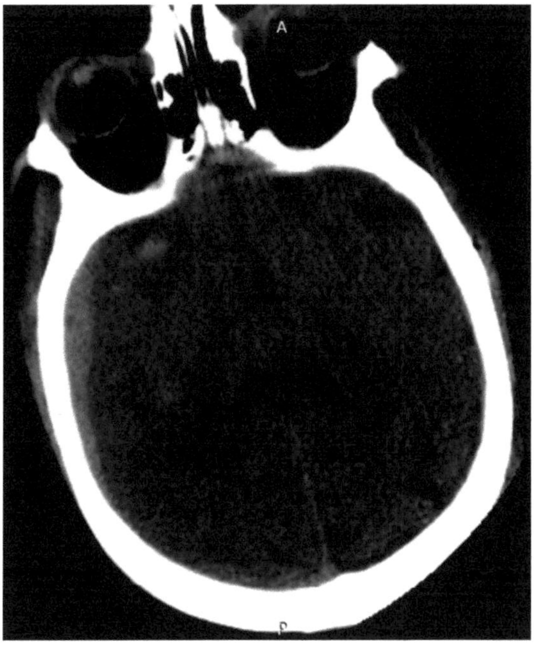

Fig. 12.4 Subdural hemorrhage with diffuse axonal injury

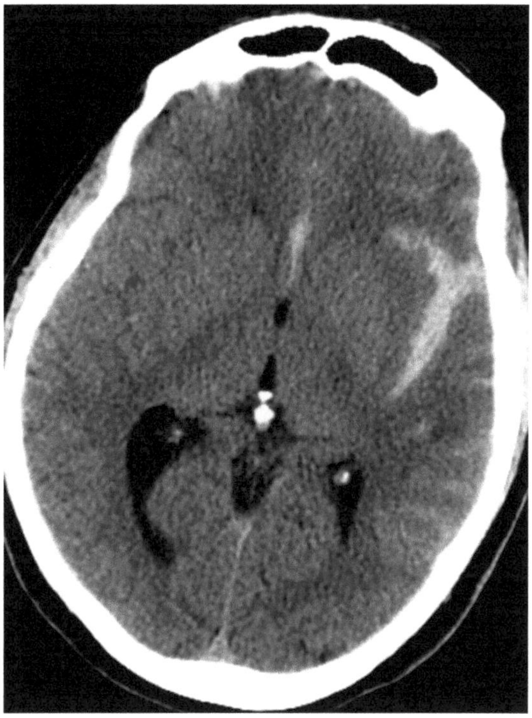

Fig. 12.5 Subarachnoid hemorrhage

the victim causes widespread tearing of axons in many areas of the brain with disruption of neuronal transmission that may produce temporary or permanent diffuse brain. It is usually more accurately diagnosed using MRI rather than CT (Fig. 12.4) [17].

Moreover, traumatic subarachnoid hemorrhage in victims of domestic abuse is usually associated with poor outcomes (Fig. 12.5).

Nevertheless, victims of domestic violence may also suffer from chronic forms of traumatic brain injury (TBI) which is an alteration in brain function caused by an external force [18].

Such chronic sequel can be manifested by chronic traumatic encephalopathy (CTE) which is a distinctive neurodegenerative disorder that occurs as a hidden complication of cumulative repetitive head impacts (RHIs), including concussion and subconcussion [19].

CTE is characterized by impaired cognitive functions (impaired attention and memory), emotional dysfunctions (irritability, depression, anxiety), and physical symptoms (fatigue and headache). On the other hand, no specific radiological criteria were established for diagnosis of CTE, hence diagnosis can be done with correlation between history of repeated head trauma, clinical signs, and existing radiological findings. The most commonly reported findings are cavum septum pellucidum which occurs when the layers of the septum pellucidum are separated and the space is occupied with CSF. Also, enlargement of the perivascular spaces, scattered tiny areas of diffuse axonal injury, spots of micro hemorrhage, and mild brain atrophy are common [20].

Generally speaking, computed tomography is less sensitive to detection of CTE changes and usually reliable only in detection of diffuse brain atrophy associated with CTE. On the other hand, MRI may be more valuable in detection of various consequences of CTE. Advanced MRI modalities used in imaging of CTE include diffusion tensor imaging (DTI), functional MRI (fMRI), and magnetic resonance spectroscopy (MRS) [21].

(b) Open head injuries:

An open head injury exists if there is skull fractures associated with brain injury. Open head

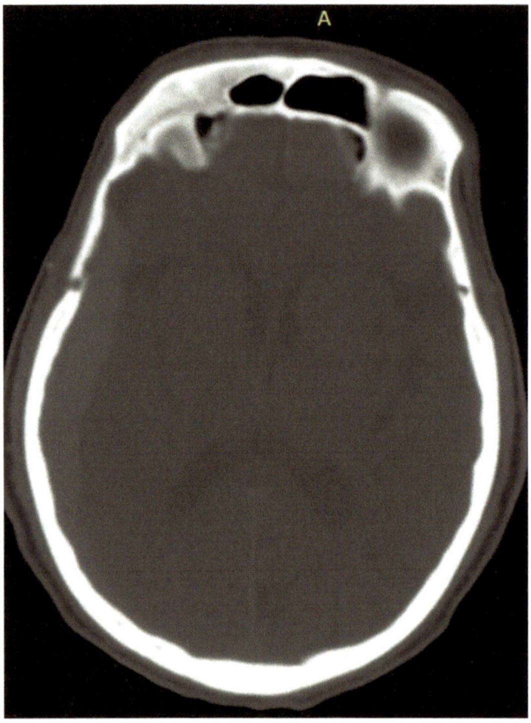

Fig. 12.6 Right parietal bone fracture

injuries may be associated with entrance of foreign bodies into the cranial cavity making extensive damage to brain tissue with increased incidence of infection (Fig. 12.6) [14].

Open head injuries include penetrating injuries due to use of firearms in intimate partner violence, which is the most lethal type of traumatic brain injury [17].

In addition, using household instrument in infliction of penetrating head trauma in domestic violence is not common although it is possible and reported [22].

2. Maxillofacial trauma

   In domestic violence and intimate partner violence, maxillofacial injuries are more common than any type of injuries and occur in about 83% of cases. It usually occurs as a result of blunt trauma and is usually associated with mandibular, nasal, and zygomatic fractures [23].

   Also, facial soft tissue injuries are more common than fractures and may be associated with epistaxis or loosening of teeth. It usually occurs as a result of punching, kicking, or smacking [24].

   Other causative instruments included hard and fragile objects like glass bottles, beverage can, and household objects [25].

   As being easily accessible, the face is mostly targeted during domestic violence assaults. Also, there is preferential distribution of types of facial trauma as the middle face (nasal fractures) is the most common site of traumas, the most prominent part of the face, and composed of fragile bones (Fig. 12.7). In addition, due to dominance of right-handed assailants, the left zygomatic region was the second most common fractured facial bone [26].

   Nevertheless, mandibular fractures can be seen in victims of domestic violence, specially fractures in the mandibular angle and condylar region (Fig. 12.8). While mandibular fractures are not fatal, but blood aspiration from hemorrhage may be life threatening in victims with disturbed level of consciousness [27].

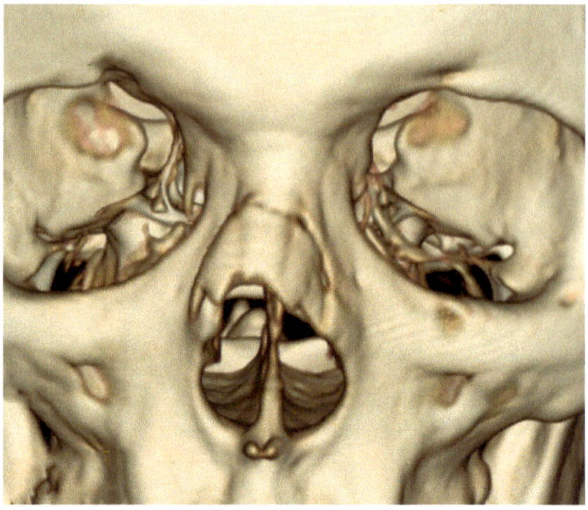

Fig. 12.7 Nasal bone fracture 3D image

On the other hand, orbital fractures from domestic violence may be missed and concealed during clinical investigations done for the victims (Fig. 12.9) [6].

In addition, ocular injuries may vary in severity from a small laceration or bruises on the eye-

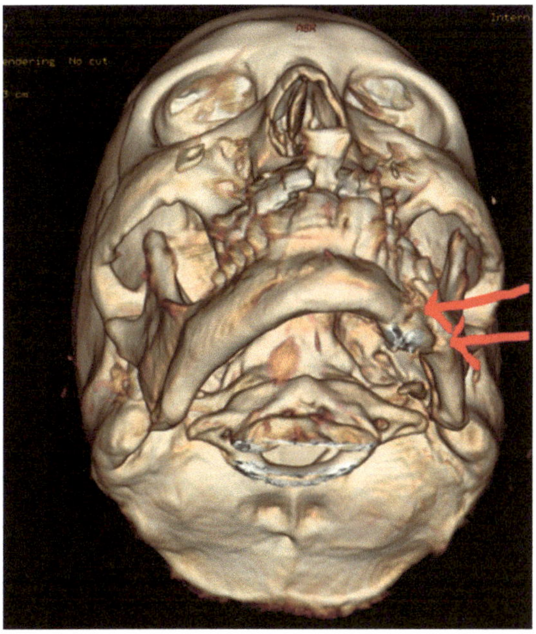

Fig. 12.8 Fracture mandible 3D image

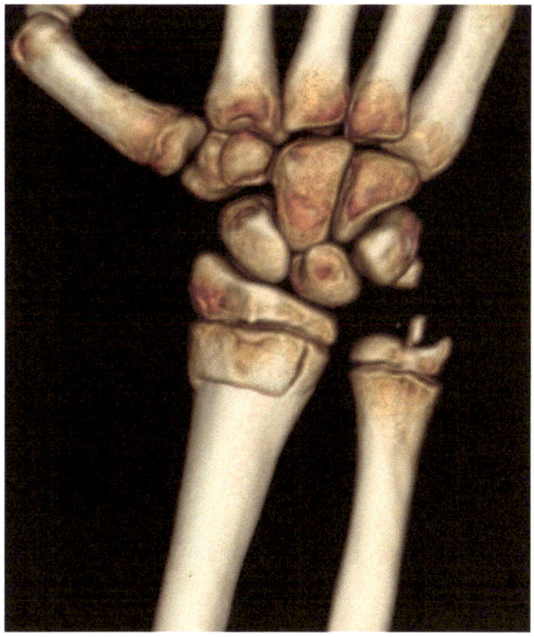

Fig. 12.10 Fracture radius 3D image

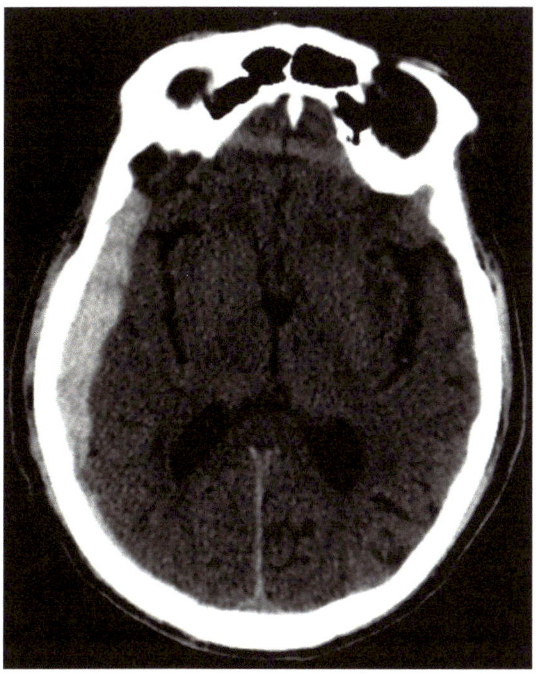

Fig. 12.9 Left orbital fracture associated with left parietal subdural hematoma

lid to an orbital fracture. Also, it may be blunt or perforating trauma [23].

3. Musculoskeletal injuries

   Following cranial and neck trauma, musculoskeletal injuries are considered in second place in occurrence during incidents related to domestic violence. Usually it may be in the form of contusions, sprains or fractures and dislocations [28].

   Regarding to upper extremity injuries, although it is difficult to distinguish between accidental and homicidal injuries, but usually injuries to upper extremities are defensive injuries when it is proximal or central (Fig. 12.10) [29].

   Intentional musculoskeletal injuries that occur in domestic violence should be suspected when it occurs in unusual sites such as upper arms and upper legs, outer side of the hand, back, shoulder, and buttocks [30].

   On the other hand, shoulder trauma is relatively rare in domestic violence and usually related to trauma with high momentum and usually suspected as being a result of domestic violence in the absence of history of extreme trauma [6].

Nevertheless, thoracic cage injuries are not commonly see

n in domestic violence victims although it is reported in some literatures [31, 32].

Thoracic trauma may be manifested by wide range of signs starting from external bruises and hematomas, rib fracture or even pneumothorax. Those signs may be first noticed by the radiologists and emergency physicians [6].

Curiously, a case report of intimate partner violence against man who was presented to emergency department with a history of right-sided falling against a table revealed afterward it was a result of assault by his female partner. Plain radiograph revealed multiple fractured ribs (old and recent) (Figs. 12.11 and 12.12) [33].

On the other hand, spinal fractures in abuse are uncommon; it requires a high-energy contact trauma such as traffic accidents. However, fracture dislocation of spine is unlikely accidental unless a bizarre shaped form of massive ambiguous trauma has occurred. It is noteworthy that any case of abuse with multiple skeletal injuries should be carefully investigated by an intensive radiological examination of spine [34].

4. Pregnancy and abdominal trauma
   Incidence of domestic violence increases with pregnancy and it is the third cause of trauma during pregnancy. Also, trauma during pregnancy is a leading cause of non-obstetric maternal mortality, as abdominal trauma has a

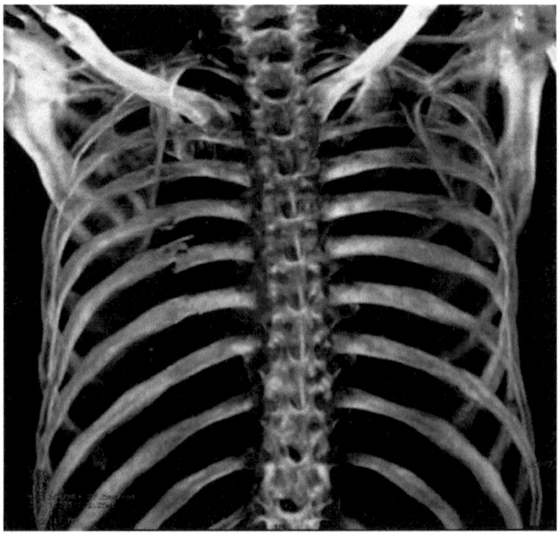

Fig. 12.11 Fracture ribs

Fig. 12.12 Multiple fracture ribs with bilateral hemothorax

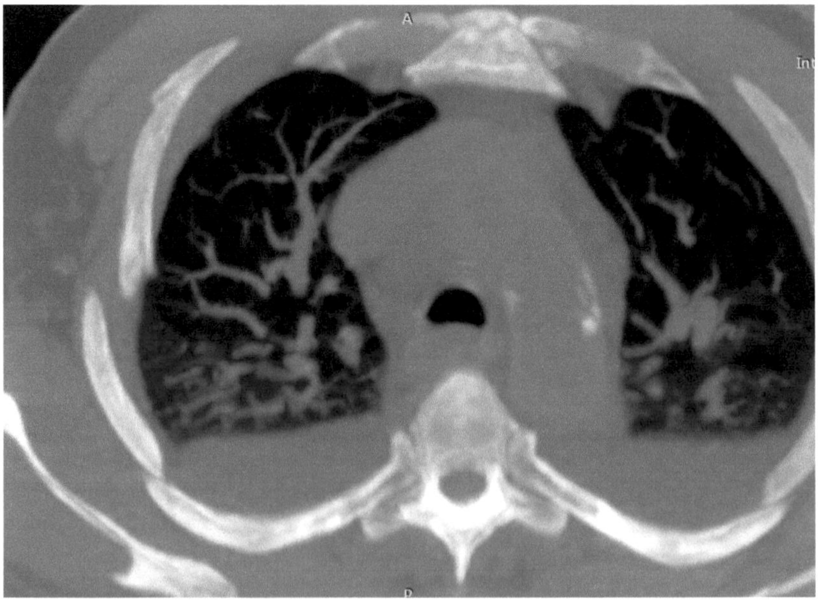

higher incidence in pregnant more than non-pregnant [35].

The pregnant victim is predisposed to all types of domestic violence trauma with increased incidence of retroperitoneal hemorrhage due to increased pelvic blood flow. Also, the liver and spleen are displaced against the ribs and the bladder is displaced out of the pelvis by the mass effect of the enlarged gravid uterus, making them more prone to injury. In addition, the kidneys and spleen become more susceptible to trauma as they enlarge during pregnancy [36].

In addition, intimate partner violence during pregnancy is highly associated with antepartum hemorrhage, and associated with high rate of fetal mortality [37].

Patterns of abdominal trauma vary according to situation and causative instrument. Mostly, domestic violence is associated with blunt trauma that usually affects spleen and liver. Fortunately, bowel is located behind the gravid uterus making it less affected by trauma. Also, domestic violence may be associated with penetrating abdominal trauma and gunshot wound injuries [38].

Initially, the basic target of the medical team is to resuscitate and stabilize the mother using standard techniques because maternal death means fetal death. Consequently, she should be placed in the 30° left lateral decubitus position to prevent systemic hypotension if she is more than 20 weeks pregnant [39].

Consequently, ultrasonography (US) should be performed periodically to evaluate fetal heart rate and gestational age, especially if the fetus with a gestational age younger than 24–26 weeks. Older fetus can be continuously monitored externally [40].

On the other hand, radiological evaluation of both maternal and fetal injuries is very beneficial regarding to many aspects. It decreases the rate of invasive unnecessary surgical intervention. Also, it helps in early detection of hidden injuries which gives the opportunity to early management and to avoid hemodynamic deterioration of both mother and fetus. Lastly, imaging helps in accurate targeting of injured site with time saving and efficient management [41].

Nevertheless, multiple imaging modalities are used for diagnosis and detection of the site of injury in pregnant woman. Ultrasonography, conventional radiography, and computed tomography are the main used modalities. Also, diagnostic imaging of abdominal trauma during pregnancy is a problematic issue as safety of both mother and fetus is a point of concern.

Ionizing radiation has a considerable risk on fetus, but the higher risk of mismanagement and misdiagnosis of trauma in injured pregnant in case of delay in use of diagnostic radiological techniques. Therefore, usage of computed tomography is preserved for highly indicated cases with guarantee of least time and frequency of exposure. In addition, informed consent must be obtained in case of use of ionizing radiation except in cases of seriously injured patients especially in emergency department [42].

Computed tomography is used for screening for trauma in pregnant woman and also ultrasonography and magnetic resonance imaging can be used for follow-up. Also, MRCP can be used for imaging of biliary and pancreatic trauma [35].

US examination is usually used initially in acute and urgent cases for assessment of gestational age and vitality. Also, US is used in assessment of maternal visceral injuries and visualization of both intraperitoneal and pericardial fluid [43].

Notably, US can't replace CT examination in visualization of injuries in solid and hollow organ injuries and revealing of such injuries and hemoperitoneum requires considerable training and skill in using US [41].

Regarding to CT scans, lowest dose should be used as possible. In case of using intravenous iodinated contrast, according to U.S. Food and Drug Administration (FDA) considered intravenous iodinated contrast one of category B drug and should be used only in cases where important information can be gained by using this modality with benefits for mother and fetus [44].

On the other hand, although magnetic resonance (MR) imaging is relatively safe for both mother and fetus, but it is not used in acute stage as it takes long time and it is used only in cases where evaluation of spinal, neurological, and soft tissue evaluation is mandatory [41].

In addition, using gadolinium as a contrast media in MRI is considered a pregnancy category C drug by the FDA, and only done in extremely rare circumstances during pregnancy [45].

12.5 Conclusion

As this work has demonstrated, DV is an important, serious, and widespread issue that needs to be addressed in not only the private sphere of society, but the public too. DV and IPV can have fatal outcomes, affecting people—particularly women—across all demographic lines. Without challenges and interventions made to DV, the acceptability of the practice in society—and thus the frequency and severity—will increase greatly. Thus, it is incredibly important that workers in areas such as health care are able to recognize the signs and symptoms of trauma resulting from DV and IPV, and provide information on the rights of survivors under government law.

References

1. Declaration on the elimination of violence against women. New York, United Nations, February 23, 1994 (Resolution No. A/RES/48/104)
2. Krug EG, Mercy JA, Dahlberg LL, Zwi AB (2002) The world report on violence and health. Lancet 360(9339):1083–1088
3. World Health Organization, Department of Reproductive Health and Research, London School of Hygiene and Tropical Medicine, South African Medical Research Council (2013) Global and regional estimates of violence against women: prevalence and health effects of intimate partner violence and non-partner sexual violence, p 2
4. Cavalin C, Garcia-Moreno C, Jansen HA, Ellsberg M, Heise L, Watts C (2010) WHO multi-country study on women's health and domestic violence against women. Initial results on prevalence, health outcomes and women's responses. World Health Organization, Geneva
5. World Health Organization (2012) Understanding and addressing violence against women: intimate partner violence. World Health Organization, Geneva
6. Bhole S, Bhole A, Harmath C (2014) The black and white truth about domestic violence. Emerg Radiol 21(4):407–412
7. Breiding MJ, Basile KC, Smith SG, Black MC, Mahendra RR (2015) Intimate partner violence surveillance: uniform definitions and recommended data elements, version 2.0. National Center for Injury Prevention and Control, Centers for Disease Control and Prevention, Atlanta, GA, p 18
8. Yawn BP, Yawn RA, Uden DL (1992) American Medical Association diagnostic and treatment guidelines on domestic violence. Arch Fam Med 1:39
9. Centers of Disease Control and Prevention (2013) Intimate partner violence: definitions. Accessed 1 Feb 2013 http://www.cdc.gov/violenceprevention/intimatepartner violence/definitions.html
10. Rudman W (2000) Coding and documentation of domestic violence. Family Violence Prevention Fund, San Francisco, pp 1–20
11. Boyle A, Robinson S, Atkinson P (2004) Domestic violence in emergency medicine patients. Emerg Med J 21(1):9
12. Armstrong P, Wastie ML (1998) Diagnostic imaging, 4th edn. Blackwell Science Ltd, Hoboken
13. Ivany AS, Schminkey D (2016) Intimate partner violence and traumatic brain injury: state of the science and next steps. Fam Commun Health 39(2):129–137
14. Senelick RC, Ryan CE (1998) Living with brain injuries: a guide for families. Healthsouth Press, Birmingham, AL
15. Grisso JA, Wishner AR, Schwarz DF, Weene BA, Holmes JH, Sutton RL (1991) A population-based study of injuries in inner-city women. Am J Epidemiol 134(1):59–68
16. Carrigan TD, Walker E, Barnes S (2000) Domestic violence: the shaken adult syndrome. J Accid Emerg Med 17(2):138–139
17. Car M (2000) Increasing awareness about possible neurological alterations in brain status secondary to intimate violence. Brain Injury Source 4(2):30–37
18. Murray CE, Lundgren K, Olson LN, Hunnicutt G (2016) Practice update what professionals who are not brain injury specialists need to know about intimate partner violence-related traumatic brain injury. Trauma Violence Abuse 17(3):298–305
19. McKee AC, Alosco ML, Huber BR (2016) Repetitive head impacts and chronic traumatic encephalopathy. Neurosurg Clin N Am 27(4):529–535

20. Shura RD, Taber KH, Brenner LA, Wortzel HS (2015) Chronic traumatic encephalopathy and traumatic brain injury: bridging pathology, function, and prognosis. Curr Phys Med Rehabil Rep 3(2):106–114
21. Mez J, Stern RA, McKee AC (2013) Chronic traumatic encephalopathy: where are we and where are we going? Curr Neurol Neurosci Rep 13(12):1–12
22. Bodwal J, Sreenivas M, Aggrawal A (2013) Intracranial penetrating injury by screw driver: a case report and review of literature. J Forensic Legal Med 20(8):972–975
23. Arosarena OA, Fritsch TA, Hsueh Y, Aynehchi B, Haug R (2009) Maxillofacial injuries and violence against women. Arch Facial Plast Surg 11(1):48–52
24. Saddki N, Suhaimi AA, Daud R (2010) Maxillofacial injuries associated with intimate partner violence in women. BMC Public Health 10(1):1
25. Beck SR, Freitag SK, Singer N (1996) Ocular injuries in battered women. Ophthalmology 103(1):148–151
26. Le BT, Dierks EJ, Ueeck BA, Homer LD, Potter BF (2001) Maxillofacial injuries associated with domestic violence. J Oral Maxillofac Surg 59(11):1277–1283
27. Matteoli M, Vinciguerra M, et al (2011) The role of radiological analysis to identify the battered women in emergency department. ECR Congress 2011. https://doi.org/10.1594/ecr2011/C-0693
28. Bhandari M, Sprague S, Dosanjh S, Petrisor B, Resendes S, Madden K, Schemitsch EH, PRAISE Investigators (2011) The prevalence of intimate partner violence across orthopedic fracture clinics in Ontario. J Bone Joint Surg Am 93(2):132–141
29. Sheridan DJ, Nash KR (2007) Acute injury patterns of intimate partner violence victims. Trauma Violence Abuse 8(3):281–289
30. Reijnders UJL, Ceelen M (2014) 7208 Victims of domestic and public violence; an exploratory study based on the reports of assaulted individuals reporting to the police. J Forensic Legal Med 24:18–23
31. Bergaminelli C, De Angelis P, Gauthier P, Salzano A, Vecchio G (1999) Thoracic drainage in trauma emergencies. Minerva Chir 54(10):697–702
32. Karangelis D, Karkos CD, Tagarakis GI, Oikonomou K, Karkos PD, Papadopoulos D, Hevas A, Tsilimingas N (2011) Thoracic injuries resulting from intimate partner violence. J Forensic Legal Med 18(3):119–120
33. Ananthakrishnan G, Alagappan D, Riyat M (2006) Rib fractures in an adult male: Unusual presentation of a victim of domestic violence. Injury Extra 37(11):428–429
34. Brogdon BG, Shwayder T, Elifritz J (2012) Child abuse and its mimics in skin and bone. CRC Press, Boca Raton
35. Sadro C, Bernstein MP, Kanal KM (2012) Imaging of trauma: Part 2, Abdominal trauma and pregnancy—a radiologist's guide to doing what is best for the mother and baby. AJR Am J Roentgenol 199(6):1207–1219
36. Pearlman MD, Tintinalli JE, Lorenz RP (1990) Blunt trauma during pregnancy. N Engl J Med 323(23):1609–1613
37. McFarlane J, Campbell JC, Sharps P, Watson K (2002) Abuse during pregnancy and femicide: urgent implications for women's health. Obstet Gynecol 100(1):27–36
38. Pearce C, Martin SR (2016) Trauma and considerations unique to pregnancy. Obstet Gynecol Clin N Am 43(4):791–808
39. Ueland K, Hansen JM (1969) Maternal cardiovascular dynamics: II. Posture and uterine contractions. Am J Obstet Gynecol 103(1):1–7
40. Sadro C, Bittle M, O'Connell K (2011) Imaging the pregnant trauma patient. Ultras Clin 6(1):97–103
41. Raptis CA, Mellnick VM, Raptis DA, Kitchin D, Fowler KJ, Lubner M, Bhalla S, Menias CO (2014) Imaging of trauma in the pregnant patient. Radiographics 34(3):748–763
42. Dauer LT, Thornton RH, Miller DL, Damilakis J, Dixon RG, Marx MV et al (2012) Radiation management for interventions using fluoroscopic or computed tomographic guidance during pregnancy: a joint guideline of the Society of Interventional Radiology and the Cardiovascular and Interventional Radiological Society of Europe with Endorsement by the Canadian Interventional Radiology Association. J Vasc Interv Radiol 23(1):19–32
43. Rose JS (2004) Ultrasound in abdominal trauma. Emerg Med Clin North Am 22(3):581–599
44. Widmark JM (2007) Imaging-related medications: a class overview. Proc (Baylor Univ Med Cent) 20(4):408–417
45. Sundgren PC, Leander P (2011) Is administration of gadolinium-based contrast media to pregnant women and small children justified? J Magn Reson Imaging 34(4):750–757

13 Imaging and Elderly Abuses

Eric Baccino and Maisy Lossois

13.1 Introduction

If forensic medicine was a business, there would be many reasons to invest in the ***elderly abuses (EA)*** as it will be the ***market of the future for forensic doctors activity***. There are several reasons to support this prevision:

- Individuals ***over 65 are the fastest growing part of western population***: 13% of the US population is over 65 and that figure is susceptible to double by 2030 [1, 2]. In France in 2016 [3], among a population of 67 millions, people over 60 were 3.3 millions. 1.3 millions of them are dependent (700,000 in nursing homes, the remaining with assistance at home) and cost 23.5 milliards euros in public expenses.
- ***Conditions favorable to crime*** are more and more present: impoverishment of young generations obliged to stay longer at parent's home with their elderly getting richer, older and thus more fragile and dependent, provides an explosive combination.
- So far EA, mentioned in medical literature only recently (1970) [4], drew much less political and public attention than the child abuse and violence against women: as a result it is ***widely underestimated and there is no real prevention, allowing EA to increase***.

As soon as western societies will be mature and aware enough to confront with this pathology, the clinical forensic medicine (CFM) community should face a very significant increase of judicial cases, as they did in the 1980 when child abuse went public and benefited from state information and media campaigns.

In this chapter after a general presentation of definitions, statistical data, and the various clinical situations which must raise the possibility of EA, we will develop the contribution of imaging for positive and differential diagnosis.

We will focus on bone trauma and on subdural hematoma, a potentially lethal condition, which, more often than now, should lead to discussing the possibility of EA (as it is systematically the case in child abuse for instance).

We will conclude with some suggestions aimed to improve the detection and management of EA.

13.2 Definitions and Clinical Features of Elderly Abuses

13.2.1 Elderly

By convention in literature (with no clear reasons) the limit to be part of elderly people is 65 years. But we do not need statistics to know

E. Baccino (✉) · M. Lossois
Forensic Medicine Unit, Montpellier University Hospital, Montpellier, France
e-mail: e-baccino@chu-montpellier.fr; m-lossois@chu-montpellier.fr

G. Lo Re et al. (eds.), *Radiology in Forensic Medicine*,
https://doi.org/10.1007/978-3-319-96737-0_13

that 66 is much younger than 89 or even 99. On the one hand, a pre senile, 77 individual, needing only 4 h weekly of domiciliary care, will become bedridden and demented after leg surgery and 5 days in hospital. On the other hand, as health professionals we all met cases of 85-year-old individuals, very fit, former sportsman and still professionally active, who recover from a leg fracture faster than a 40-year-old, obese, depressed, jobless, addict individual.

In other words, ***being an elderly person is not (only) a question of age***: it is an individual feature which has to do with vulnerability: one is "old" when vulnerable, i.e., when he lost the capacity to recover from an aggression which would be harmless and without long-term effect for the rest of the population.

We may therefore **classify an individual over 60 in one of the 3 following groups**:

Active adult: often more active than the 30–40 according to some statistics....

Retired adult: having fun and spending money

Old adult as dependent and vulnerable: who needs to be considered from a forensic point of view.

***"Elderly"* is too vague a word, from a physiological, sociological, and medical point of view (but by convention we will continue to use it...)**

13.2.2 Elderly Abuse

The United Nations (Abuse of older person 2002), the council of Europe (1992), after the JAMA classification [5], one of the oldest but still useful, provided complete definitions of elderly abuses.

For practical and operational reason it can be simplified into three types of abuses: physical, psychological, and material or financial [6], each type resulting either from a voluntary action or from neglect. It results in ***six subgroups of EA*** as illustrated in the following examples:

- Pushing an elderly to rob her bag or not providing easy access to her bedroom may both result in a fall, fracture, and eventually death.... One is voluntary violence and the other is neglect.
- Giving a high dose of sedative or not providing necessary pain killers are both physical abuse, one from action and the other from omission.
- Yelling at a former French state senator stuck to his nursing home bed, calling him "Jimmy" is psychological violence as is the fact not to talk to the person seated by you in a bar because she is old and ugly (...according to current standards).
- A grandchild receiving gift money from his granny who will not be able to change her dental prosthesis will get her into malnutrition, acquired immune deficiency, infection, and death as easily as the robbery of her bank account.

Among the huge scope ***of EA some main features*** must be underlined:

Neglect: As quite often, the victim is as weak as a baby, highly dependent from her "care taker."

Money: cognitive disorders along with valuables are, sometimes, too much a temptation for social workers and family; financial exploitation of the elderly is thus nowadays considered as a "virtual epidemic" [7].

Fragility: physical assault, lack of care, psychological distress, and loneliness can kill more effectively than in younger adults.

Sexual abuse: very rare.

Home and Nursing Homes or long-term care facilities: the profile for EA is different at home were family members (son for mother and wife for husband) are the usual abusers, whereas in nursing home the staff is the main suspect (especially in low-cost nursing homes).

13.3 Epidemiology

It is **almost impossible to get a reliable prevalence study** on EA because of the difficulty to reach the target, a population sometimes not willing to complain, as they love their abuser (child, spouse, home worker...), sometimes unable to answer (dementia, neurological disease, impossibility to get out of their living place). Moreover they are often "*protected*" from the questions by those who are involved in the abuse, the so-called "*care takers*."

As many as 10% of US older adults experience elder mistreatment each year [8, 9], and evidences suggest that victims have dramatically increased mortality and morbidity [10].

In a large (seven countries) and recent European study [11] ***prevalence of physical abuses was 1.7–4.8% in males and 1.6–6.6% in females*** (this discrepancy, probably because sexual abuse even marginal in the elderly were included in physical abuses). Financial exploitation concerned 5–8% of the elderly.

The general tendency in international studies is that 2–10% of the elderly are physically abused, and that *the oldest they are, the highest the risk of EA* [6, 7].

Data about reporting rate of EA are even more confusing: large US studies claiming that 16% of EA among a group of 400,000 cases were reported to social services in 1996, are in complete opposition with our daily practice; in a clinical forensic medicine setting where we deal yearly with 3000 living victims (child, domestic, sexual abuses etc.…) in 2015 we had only 5 victims over 65. In the mean time 100 children were examined.

Underreporting is mainly due to characteristics of the victim and her surroundings mentioned earlier in this paragraph, but our society also has a responsibility: much more money and good will is spent to prevent and fight child abuse and other domestic violence than EA. So far, politicians and media are not interested in EA, maybe because, like suicide, aging reminds us of "real death," a topic not very good for TV audience, polls, and elections…

And to be honest, who will blame professionals who have vocation to take care and protect nice "cute" babies rather than incontinent and bedridden nursing home residents?

13.4 Detection of EA

As health professionals dealing with patients, we must not be troubled by academicals classifications but rather focus on one question: "is this old person health in danger?". If the answer is yes, measures must be taken.

The easiest (but rarest) situation is when the victim reports to the police or to a nurse, a physician, with precise description of the facts. To collect these highly valuable information, the absolute necessity to interview the elderly in private, out of the presence of relative, must be underlined.

More often, the victim does not want or is not able to report and the possibility of EA must be evoked in the presence of various signs:

- Cutaneous ecchymosis, hematomas, burns, scars which are not located in area prone to accidental trauma: bruising on the back and lateral aspects of forearms and wrists was more common in EA victims than other older adults [12]. Temporal area, eyes and nose, breast, inner aspect of the arm skin are also suspicious locations for trauma. In 2013, a review of literature made it possible to define the most frequently encountered locations of injuries in elderly abuses: upper limbs (43.98%) > maxillofacial region, teeth and neck (22.88%) > skull and brain (12.28%) > lower limbs (10.61%) > trunk (10.25%) [13].
- An injury, which does not appear to match with the proposed mechanism, like a high-energy transfer fracture from an alleged slight trauma.
- Skin lesions of different colors suggesting repeated trauma (but caution is needed as color changes are not reliable dating indicators).
- Muscular skeletal pains must be considered with attention as osteopenic bones are more susceptible to fractures, which can be underdetected in patients with low mobility and difficulties to communicate.
- Dehydration, malnutrition, lack of hygiene, inappropriate clothing, bad dental care and lack of replacement of loss teeth, the recent apparition of impairment of cognitive functions, incontinence, and depression must also draw attention on EA.

It will be even more difficult when only risk factors are present, even in a highly typical situation where such as a female widow, socially isolated, over 80, with cognitive impairment and dependent living in the same place with her depressed alcoholic son, jobless and financially dependent for her pension.

It is therefore crucial that discussion with the relatives and caretakers be conducted by trained practitioners in order to get the most information possible without antagonizing them.

In a world where family doctors will soon become a "*souvenir*," the importance of social and home workers, nurses attending the patients at home, must be stressed and, consequently, the necessity of training them in the field of EA.

Despite their usual work overload, emergency room personnel should also think of EA each time such situations come to their attention. *Elder Assessment Instrument* (EAI) are available but not easy to use during the rush hours [14].

13.5 Diagnosis of EA

When possible the most effective is ***to hospitalize*** the patient in order to protect and make the necessary investigations.

The differential diagnosis, conversely to child abuse, is always complicated in EA as any symptom suggestive of abuse may also result from pathology or accident:

- Cognitive impairment may be symptoms of reactive depression to neglect, or an early stage of Alzheimer or even a chronic subdural hematoma.
- Dehydration may results from lack of liquid input or an excess of diuretic pills.
- Loss of weight from unknown cancer or starvation.
- Spontaneous fracture from myeloma can be misinterpreted for accidental or inflicted trauma.
- Brain hemorrhage can be due to hypertension or fall on the ground when taking anticoagulant treatment.
- Purpura senilis and bruises from battering.

Biological assessments (coagulation factors, nutritional indicators, hepatic and kidney metabolism…) will be necessary to make an accurate differential diagnosis.

Imaging will also be essential.

13.6 Imaging of EA

13.6.1 Particularities of Imaging in the Elderly [15]

There are mainly ***technical difficulties*** limiting the efficiency of imaging in this age group.

For the elderly maintaining, for a while, a joint in forced position, maintaining apnea, understanding or even earring the orders can be difficult, even impossible.

Thus, conventional X-ray's realization and ultrasounds will need ***a compromise between the ideal protocol and what the old person can stand***: i.e., no complementary incidences in bone investigations, chest X-rays in seated position and incomplete inspiration….

Interpretation of bone X-rays will always be limited by bone low mineralization and density making the diagnosis of small fractures and lytic lesions more difficult.

The frequent presence of calcification and previous lesions may hinder the diagnosis of trauma, tumor, and infections.

CT scans in the elderly grow at a fast pace in France (16% increase between 2004 and 2009) as they are widely used in neurology, bone trauma and spine, pulmonary parenchyma investigation. However, contrast CT scan so useful in pulmonary embolism and vascular investigation must be used with more caution in the elderly as they often present several risk factors of renal toxicity.

MRI, less accessible than CT scan, are also limited in the elderly by the time needed for acquisition and thus immobilization which must be strictly respected (not easy for some elder patients). It is also forbidden in several situations (pace maker, vascular metallic clips, vascular stents, metallic foreign bodies, severe chronic renal failure) more frequently met in the elderly than in the rest of the population.

Imaging in the elderly is never simple and thus need to have a precise evaluation of risk/benefit ratio before realization.

13.6.2 Some Imaging Findings in EA

Imaging findings pathognomonic or highly indicative for child abuse are well defined in the literature and play a critical role in child abuse detection [16, 17].On the contrary, radiology literature describing imaging indicative of elder mistreatment is very limited [10, 13, 18].

13.6.2.1 Bone Fractures

Bone is often decalcified in the elderly either from osteoporosis (Fig. 13.1) or from osteomalacia (Fig. 13.2).

This can lead to spontaneous fractures or fractures occurring after such a low-intensity trauma that the event can be missed or forgotten (Fig. 13.3).

Considering also the number of patient with vertebral body flattening detected through routine, or other motive X-rays, one must admit that some bone fractures are less painful in the elderly than in younger adults. Consequently, imaging must be considered (and done) on trauma areas

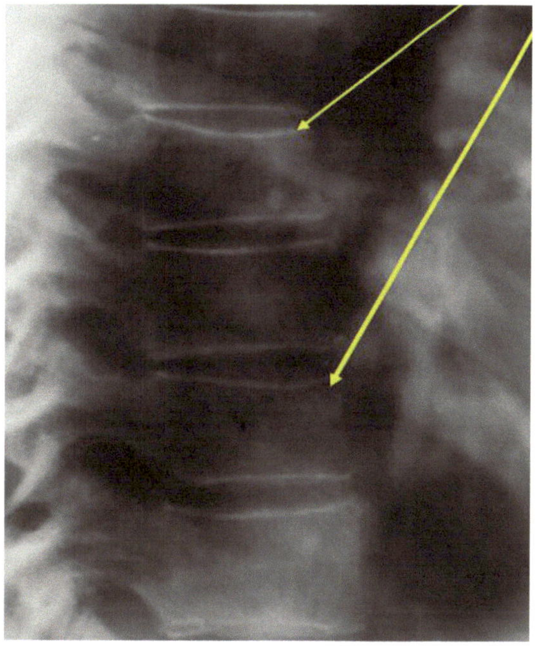

Fig. 13.1 Osteoporosis with reduction of bone density and compression fracture of a vertebral body (lateral radiography of spine)

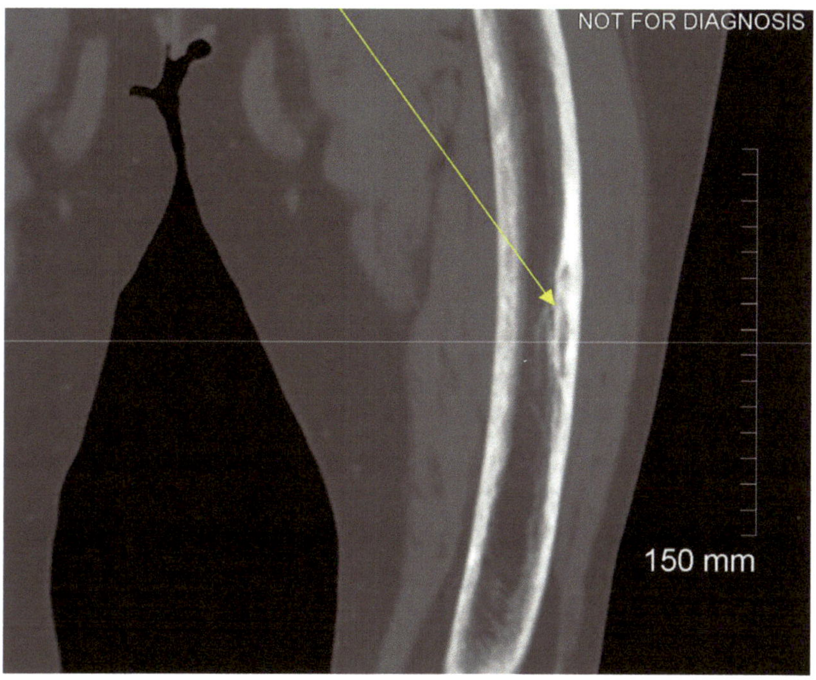

Fig. 13.2 Osteomalacia with looser transformation zone (CT scan of left lower limb in coronal section)

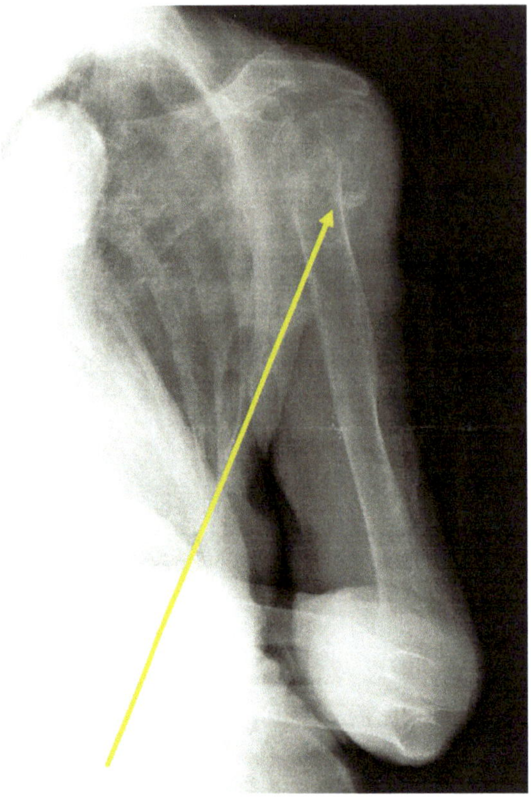

Fig. 13.3 Fracture of left humeral head (anteroposterior radiography of left arm): no history of fall

even when the victim does not complain expressively (Fig. 13.4).

Limited fractures can be underdiagnosed on bones of bad quality on X-rays. Moreover bone reconstruction is slower and dating of bone trauma from callus aspect can be misleading. Bone technetium scintigraphy can be useful in both situations providing clues for repeated trauma at various stage of healing (Figs. 13.5 and 13.6).

In order to support the hypothesis of non-accidental trauma here again (like in all types of inflicted violence's) localization is crucial.

The mechanism of fracture can be guessed from the combined analysis of the aspect of the skin (bruise or not, located in the area of bone fracture or distant) and the radiological features: classically spiroid fractures in cases of torsion or indirect trauma and transversal/horizontal in cases of direct blow, but with notable exceptions.

Inconsistencies between the reported mechanism (from accompanying person or the victim) and medical findings such as site and type of fracture must raise suspicion, in a classical forensic approach.

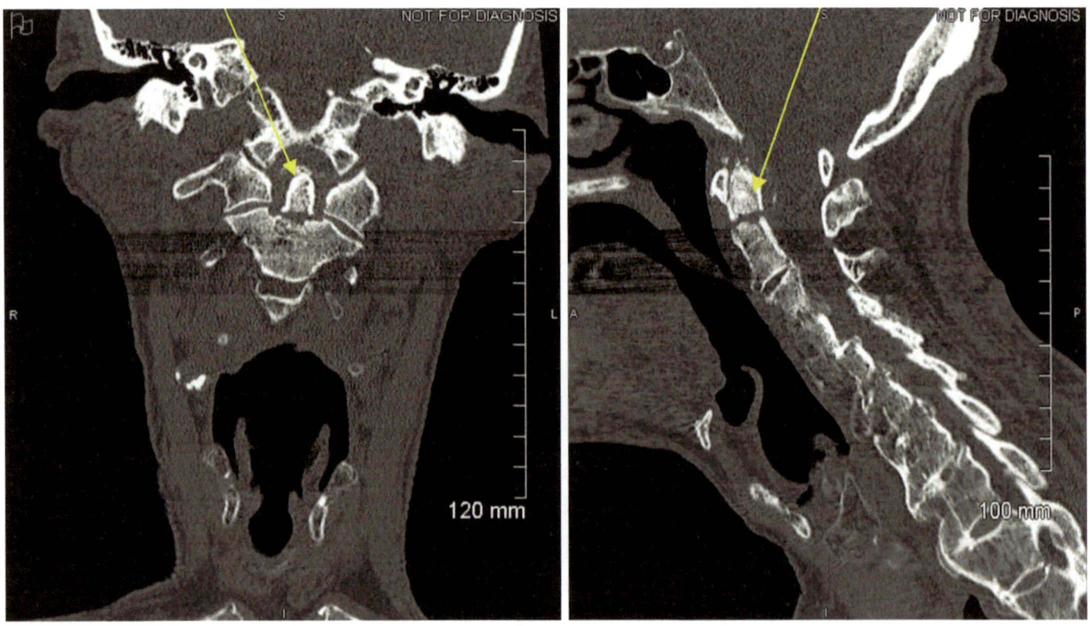

Fig. 13.4 Pseudarthrosis of odontoid process (CT scan of cervical spine in coronal and sagittal sections): not detected after a significant trauma 4 years earlier

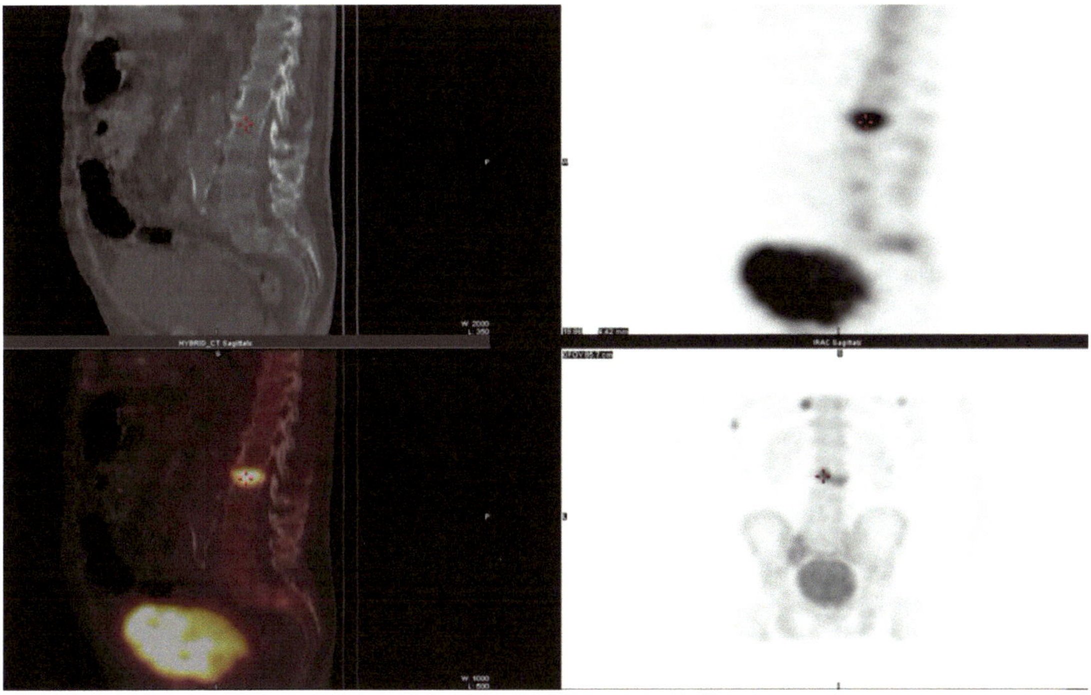

Fig. 13.5 (Scintigraphy): lesion is indicated by red spots

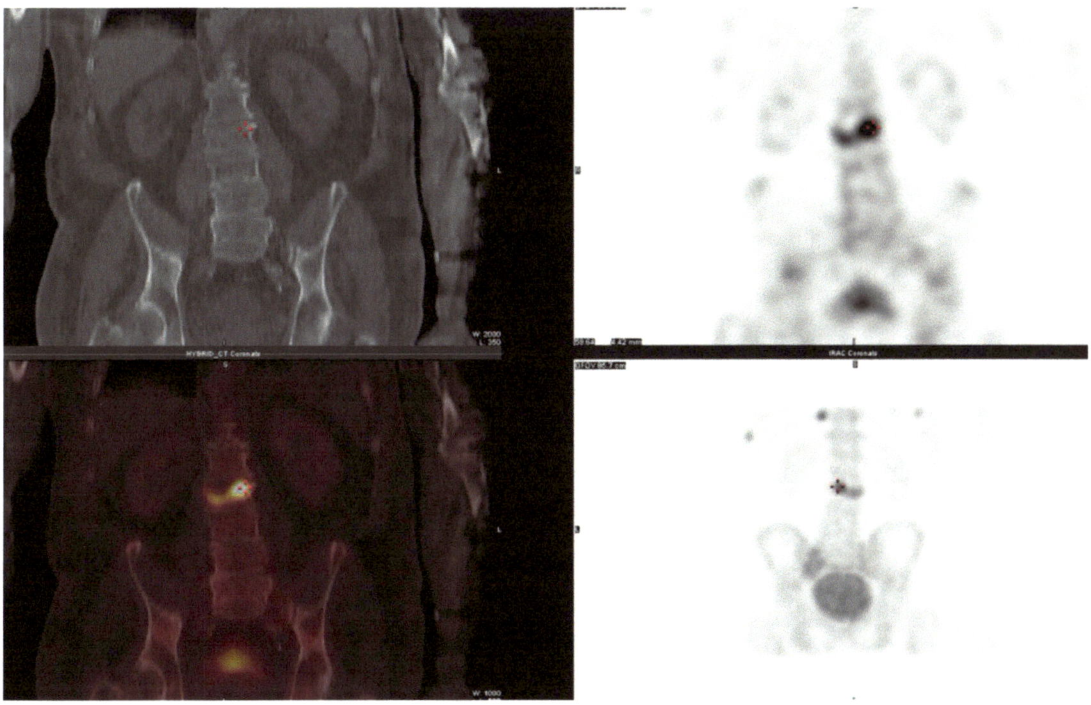

Fig. 13.6 (Scintigraphy)

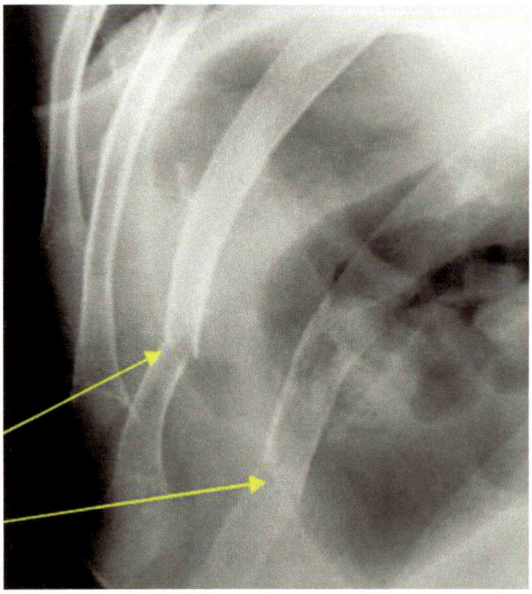

Fig. 13.7 Ribs fractures

In some cases, it can be impossible to make a clear-cut difference between accidental and not accidental fractures: are these ribs fractures (see Fig. 13.7) due to brutal handling by a nursing auxiliary or the consequence of persistent cough on an acquired brittle bone linked to aging?

13.6.2.2 Subdural Hematoma (SDH)

SDH covers a large clinical scope in the elderly: when acute and massive it can be lethal whereas some chronic forms are almost asymptomatic or can be confused with neurological or even psychiatric diseases.

But our main concern is that through literature (and conversely to child abuse), it is almost never associated with EA.

Retrospective personal studies in hospital settings showed that SDH are quite frequent in patient over 65, 20% of them having no clear causal mechanism and none of them being considered as possible indicator of EA by the hospital teams [19]. Prospective studies in the same setting showed that elderly patients with SDH presented several risk factors of being EA, a possibility never raised by the hospital teams involved.

It is amazing to see that a SDH is an undisputed emergency alarm signal of abuse for pediatricians whereas there is absolutely no such forensic reflex in the elderly.

Anatomical conditions are however favorable to SDH in the elderly and in some ways comparable to young children: weak neck musculature, wide meningeal space and tension on bridge veins from brain atrophy in the elderly (same result as from asynchronous growth of skull and brain in babies); hemorrhagic diathesis due to widespread use of antiaggregant and anticoagulant is an additional risk factor, specific to the elderly (Figs. 13.8–13.10).

In some cases a "shaken granny syndrome" has even been hypothesized [20, 21].

13.7 Diagnosis of Elderly Abuses in the Dead

Far a large majority of people, dying when old is kind of normal! **Underreporting is therefore the rule**, as illustrated by our personal data: In Montpellier University Hospital (France) 25% of 601 forensic autopsies performed in 2016 concerned people 65 years or older whereas they represent almost 70% of deaths in this hospital.

The first and essential step is therefore to consider the possibility of EA, even when there is no clear evidence of foul play, and report to judicial authorities to initiate the process of an autopsy. This makes sense when one considers objectively the motivations to kill an elderly person (suffering, dependent, and acrimonious and, with heritage perspective…) in comparison to those for killing a child (a situation where forensic autopsy is the rule).

Considering the current performances and accessibility of postmortem CT SCAN for bone trauma and SDH, this exam should be done before autopsy, each time a suspicion of EA exists, to detect signs of repeated and unreported former traumas (Figs. 13.11 and 13.12).

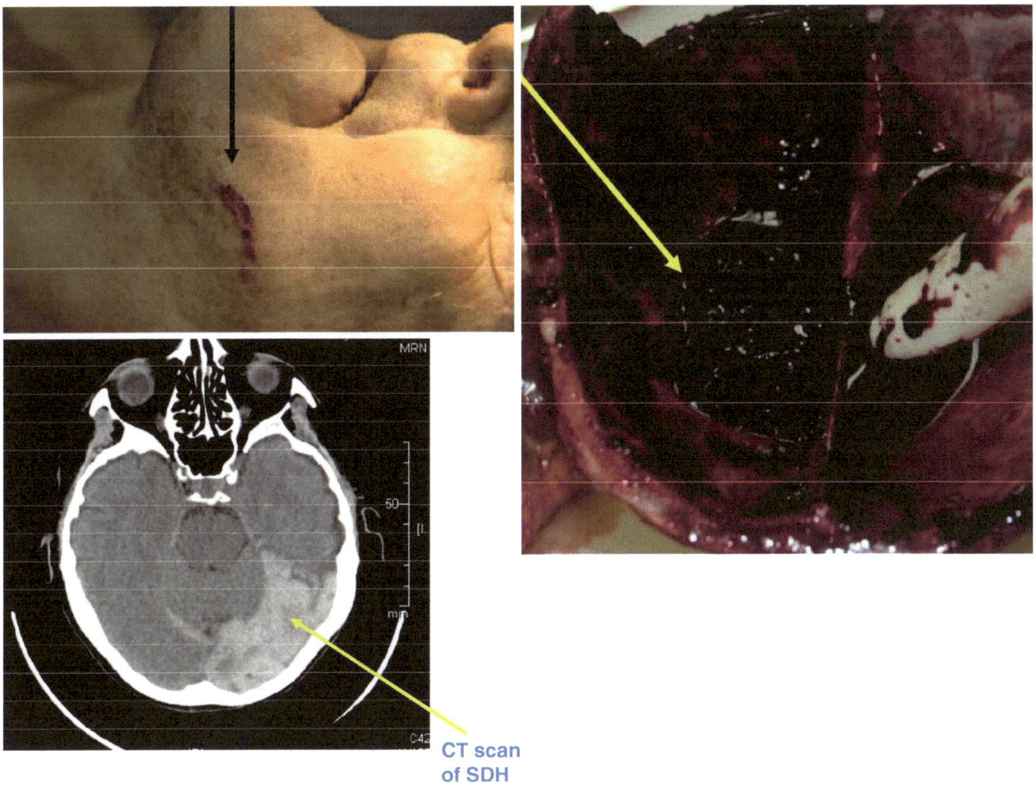

Figs. 13.8–13.10 Minor trauma to the face resulting in an acute, lethal SDH, and CT scan of SDH

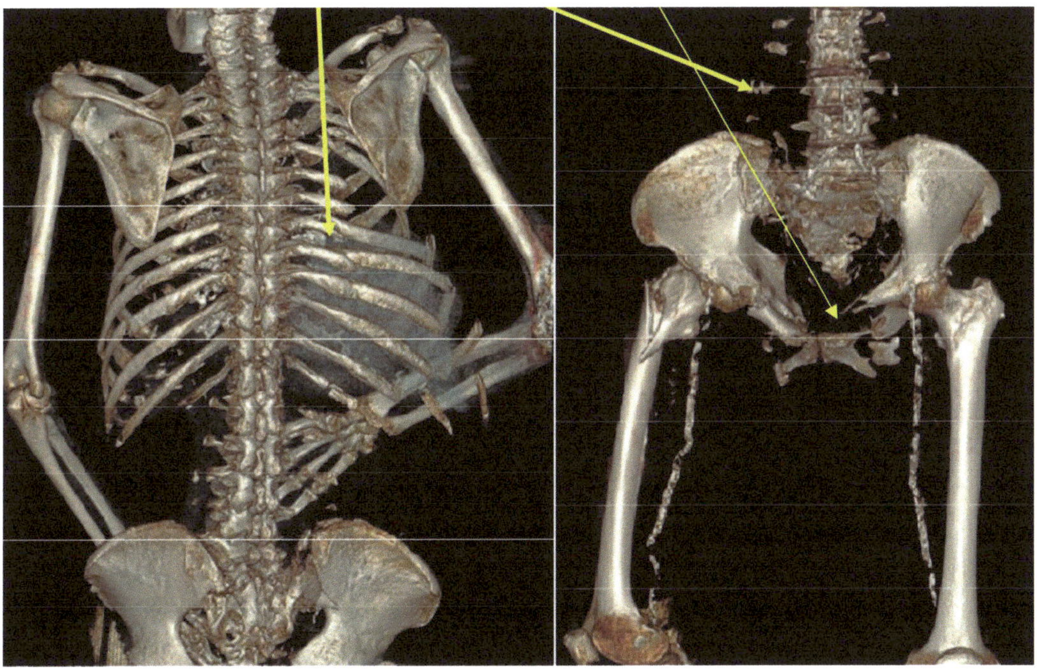

Fig. 13.11 Multiples fractures of ribs, transverse lumbar process and pelvis (3D-reconstructions): postmortem CT scan

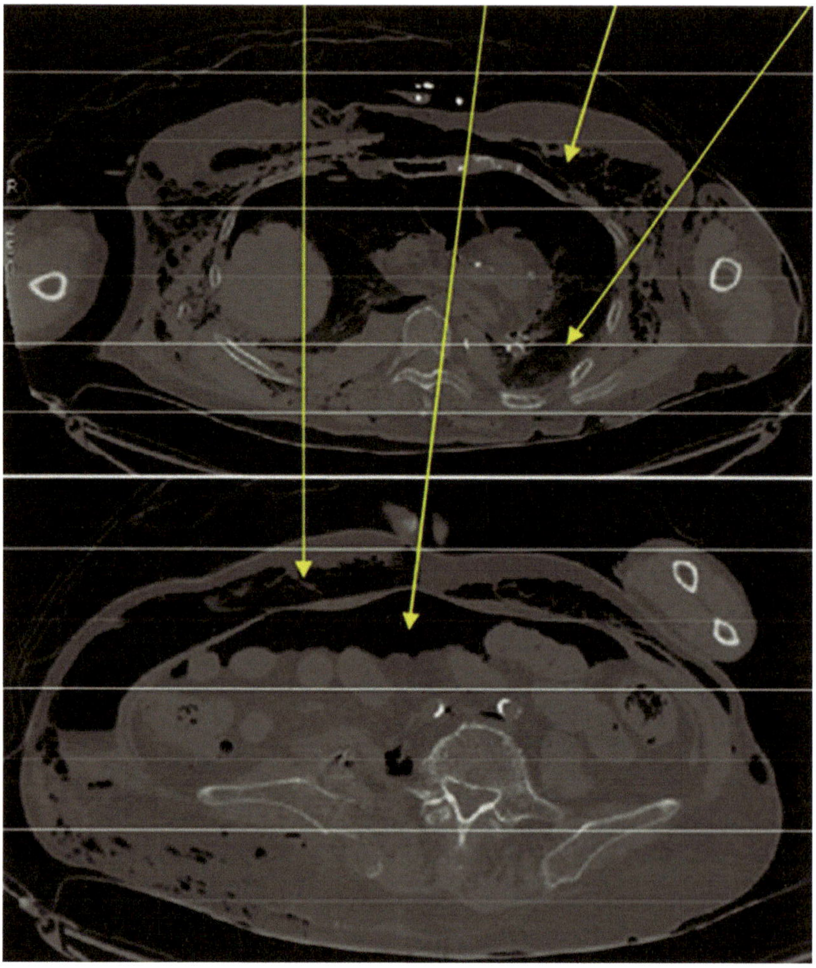

Fig. 13.12 Polytrauma with thoracic trauma (emphysema, hemopneumothorax, and pneumomediastinum) and abdominal trauma (emphysema and pneumoperitoneum)

13.8 Conclusion

Imaging should play a greater role in detecting and confirming EA.

Health professionals have their part of responsibility: they do not think enough of the possibility of EA, especially when compared to their behavior when there is a suspicion of child abuse and, at a lower degree, of battered women case. It is of course partly due to the insufficient training they get at the medical schools, which are not enough aware of this major and still growing problem.

We therefore share the conclusion of a recent radiology paper which was: "*we hope that radiologists consider elder abuse as a possibility on their differential diagnosis, or this mistreatment may continue to be unrecognized*" [10].

Large-scale radiologic studies are still desperately needed to characterize the imaging findings in elder abuse and provide a tool to correlate an individual radiography finding to EA.

But imaging alone will not be sufficient in addressing this major public health problem: an interprofessional-team approach including specialists in other disciplines (geriatricians, forensic doctors, psychiatrist…), social workers, law enforcement, and protective services professionals is absolutely necessary.

And from a larger point of view it is also the problem of our modern western societies which are so eager to take care (and talk) of all types of victims (of war, crime, occupational and domestic violence's, rape, sex exploitation, etc.) but remain blind (and silent) to EA.

Not necessary to refer to NIETZSCHE (or FREUD) to guess that this attitude takes its roots in the imbalance between the personal reward and egotist satisfaction one get by taking care of EA, on one side, and, on the other side, the anguish to face our common and inevitable future, i.e., aging and death…

References

1. Center for Disease Control and Prevention (CDC) (2003) Trends in aging—United States and worldwide. MMWR Morb Mortal Wkly Rep 52(6):101–104
2. Brock JN (1998) The evolution of aging population. State of Business Magazine XI:3
3. Ministère des Affaires sociales et de la Santé. http://social-sante.gouv.fr/
4. Burston GR (1975) Letter: Granny-battering. Br Med J 3(5983):592
5. House US (1987) Elder abuse and neglect. JAMA 257:966–971
6. Baccino E (2006) Médecine de la violence. Prise en charge des victimes et des agresseurs. Maltraitance envers les personnes âgées. Masson Ed, p 129–139
7. Lachs MS, Pillemer KA (2015) Elder abuse. N Engl J Med 373(20):1947–1956
8. Connolly M, Brandl B, Breckman R (2014) The elder justice roadmap: a stakeholder initiative to respond to an emerging health, justice, financial and social crisis. Department of Justice, Washington
9. Acierno R, Hernandez MA, Amstadter AB, Resnick HS, Steve K, Muzzy W et al (2010) Prevalence and correlates of emotional, physical, sexual, and financial abuse and potential neglect in the United States: The National Elder Mistreatment Study. Am J Public Health 100(2):292–297
10. Wong NZ, Rosen T, Sanchez AM, Bloemen EM, Mennitt KW, Hentel K et al (2017) Imaging findings in elder abuse: a role for radiologists in detection. Can Assoc Radiol J 68(1):16–20
11. Fraga S, Lindert J, Barros H, Torres-González F, Ioannidi-Kapolou E, Melchiorre MG et al (2014) Elder abuse and socioeconomic inequalities: a multilevel study in 7 European countries. Prev Med 61:42–47
12. Wiglesworth A, Austin R, Corona M, Schneider D, Liao S, Gibbs L et al (2009) Bruising as a marker of physical elder abuse. J Am Geriatr Soc 57(7):1191–1196
13. Murphy K, Waa S, Jaffer H, Sauter A, Chan A (2013) A literature review of findings in physical elder abuse. Can Assoc Radiol J 64(1):10–14
14. Rondepierre L, Galéa Y, Baccino É (2016) Approche médico-légale de l'hématome sous-dural de la personne âgée, étude prospective. Université Montpellier, Montpellier, p 1
15. Louvel J-P, Henry J, Aurengro A (2009) Imagerie médicale en gériatrie. In: Gériatrie, 2nd édn edn. Masson, Paris
16. Kempe CH, Silverman FN, Steele BF, Droegemueller W, Silver HK (1962) The battered-child syndrome. JAMA 181:17–24
17. Kleinman PK (1990) Diagnostic imaging in infant abuse. AJR Am J Roentgenol 155:703–712
18. Rosen T, Bloemen EM, Harpe J, Sanchez AM, Mennitt KW, McCarthy TJ et al (2016) Radiologists' training, experience, and attitudes about elder abuse detection. AJR Am J Roentgenol 207(6):1210–1214
19. Barbesier M, Baccino E (2015) Approche médico-légale de l'hématome sous-dural de la personne âgée. Étude préliminaire. Rev Médecine Légale 6(3–4):98–102
20. Pounder DJ (1997) Shaken adult syndrome. Am J Forensic Med Pathol 18(4):321–324
21. Azari AA, Kanavi MR, Saipe NB, Potter HD, Albert DM, Stier MA (2013) Shaken adult syndrome: report of 2 cases. JAMA Ophthalmol 131(11):1468–1470

14 Forensic Radiology: Penetrating Versus Non-penetrating Trauma

Giuseppe Bertozzi, Francesca Maglietta, Monica Salerno, and Francesco Pio Caffarelli

It is a grave disservice to confuse the performance of autopsies with the spark of insight which the autopsy may trigger. We want the insight; and autopsies alone, no matter how numerous, are not the equivalent.

L. King

With the advent of modern legal medicine, in the new scientific method era, and in the light of evidence-based medicine, systematization of knowledge is required to ensure that the evidence on which courts rely is not merely the personal opinion of medicolegal witnesses. To guarantee the best forensic practice, this initiative has benefited from the value of imaging in recent decades. This relationship is founded on the ability of radiology to provide evidence characterized not only by high diagnostic credibility but also by important documentary power.

The first time a radiological image was used in a court was in a case of attempted murder involving a gunshot wound in Montreal, Canada [1]. In the 1970s, Wüllenweber et al. introduced computed tomography (CT) to document gunshot injuries [2]. A milestone in the evolution of forensic imaging was the introduction of the Virtopsy project by Dirnhofer and Vock in Switzerland, with inclusion of three-dimensional (3D) photogrammetry and surface scanning, to document patterned injuries [3–5]. With a multidisciplinary approach, this project tried to provide a standardized method of radiological technology application in the forensic field. In 2002, the expression "virtual autopsy" was presented by Thali et al. [6, 7]. Nowadays, since autopsy is so often preceded by postmortem imaging as a routine practice in many forensic institutes, it has been suggested that the field of forensic radiology is evolving into an autonomous subspecialty between forensic medicine and radiology [8, 9]. This depends on the need to fully to understand each available technique and its advantages and limitations, as the value of the examination is strictly linked to the method used and the ascertainer's skills in performance and interpretation of the resulting imaging [10].

14.1 Role of Radiology

On the basis of evidence-based medicine, it is necessary to systematize current knowledge regarding the use of different imaging methods,

G. Bertozzi · F. Maglietta · M. Salerno
Department of Clinical and Experimental Medicine, University of Foggia, Foggia, Italy
e-mail: monica.salerno@unict.it

F. P. Cafarelli (✉)
Department of Radiology, University of Foggia, Foggia, Italy
e-mail: francesco.cafarelli@libero.it

G. Lo Re et al. (eds.), *Radiology in Forensic Medicine*,
https://doi.org/10.1007/978-3-319-96737-0_14

including the recent scientific literature. Indeed, in a recent review, Baglivo et al. analyzed 661 publications to categorize them, concluding that there were five fields of diagnostic imaging application to forensic pathology: documentation of injury or disease (51%, n = 340/661) and identification (22%, n = 143/661), followed by documentation of normal postmortem findings (16%, n = 109/661), educational articles on the role of imaging (8%, n = 55/661), and documentation of foreign objects (2%, n = 14/661). Going deeper, it is interesting to observe that documentation of injury or disease identified unnatural causes of death in 52% of cases (n = 176/340), natural causes of death in 45% (n = 152/340), and pathology affecting living subjects (such as cases of attempted murder and suicide) in 4% (n = 12/340). Among unnatural causes of death, blunt force trauma and gunshots were found more frequently (43%, n = 76/176, and 19%, n = 33/176, respectively), than penetrating trauma, drowning, strangulation, intoxication, thermal injuries, and mixed lesions (which together represented 38%). With regard to natural causes of death, cases in which central nervous and cardiovascular system diseases were involved accounted for 45% (n = 69/152) and 27% (n = 41/152), respectively; the remaining causes afflicted the musculoskeletal or respiratory system or were related to abdominal findings (together accounting for 28%). Furthermore, CT and magnetic resonance imaging (MRI) were used alone and mainly in cases of injury or disease (53%, n = 116/217, and 61%, n = 92/151, respectively) but with a precise and specific orientation: CT in cases of unnatural death (77%, n = 89/116) and MRI in cases of natural death (86%, n = 79/92). The cases related to unnatural causes of death in which CT was applied concerned, above all, gunshot injuries and trauma (97%, n = 86/89). Natural deaths in which MRI was applied mostly concerned cardiovascular or central nervous system diseases (95%, n = 75/79). On the other hand, radiograms were residually used in studies based on identification of human remains (79%; n = 31/39) [11].

This review and its data provide a coherent manifestation of the actual and usual uses of the different imaging techniques in cadaver examination, borrowed from clinical practice. Indeed, CT is suggested to be even more useful than autopsy in identification and localization of skeletal injuries (Fig. 14.1) [5]. The usefulness of MRI is in diagnosing causes of death other than skeletal diseases [12]. Although it is rarely used, postmortem CT angiography (PMCTA) is part of a validated protocol from the Technical Working Group Postmortem Angiography Methods (TWGPAM) to visualize vascular system injuries [13–15]; however, costs and body alterations caused by contrast media infusion, affecting subsequent autopsy, strongly limit its spread and usage. Conventional radiography retains its role in identification studies of human remains. Ultrasound plays a residual application in forensic evidence documentation—because of its operator-dependent subjectivity and image

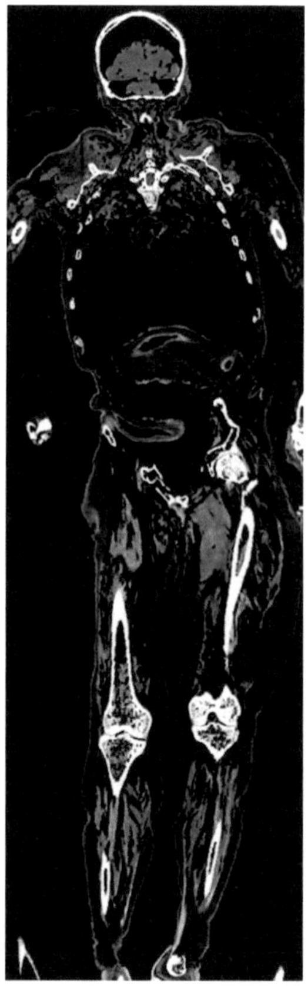

Fig. 14.1 Coronal noncontrast computed tomography (*CT*) scan showing multiple rib and pelvic fractures advanced post-mortal changes

alteration by postmortem gas—being employed, above all, in fetal studies [16].

In detail, the pivotal role that imaging plays in forensic investigation, which is strictly linked to technological advances and software implementation, depends on the ability to perform complex studies in a few seconds through multiplanar reconstructions, multiparametric analysis, and integration of different techniques (Fig. 14.2). In general, as in clinical radiology, the different techniques now used in forensic pathology can be classified as basic methods (such as conventional x-rays, CT, and MRI) and complementary methods (such as postmortem angiography).

14.1.1 Conventional X-Ray

Conventional x-ray is the oldest technique used in forensic pathology and was the most frequently used in the past, but now it has almost been replaced by CT in modern settings. Anyway, radiography permits us to visualize skeletal injuries, reveal the presence and localization of radio-opaque foreign bodies (such as in gunshot wounds), recognize anthropometric features by bone analysis, and aid identification of persons, mainly by means of orthopantomography.

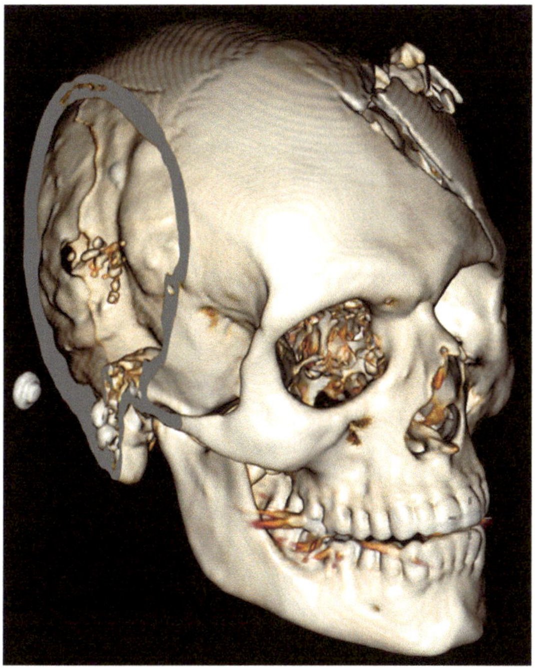

Fig. 14.2 Three-dimensional (*3D*) virtual reality (*VR*) reconstruction computed tomography (*CT*) scan showing fractures of the occipital bone (entrance) and frontal bone (exit) due to a gunshot

14.1.2 Computed Tomography

Nowadays, postmortem CT (PMCT) is the most frequently used imaging technique in the forensic field, thanks to its high resolution, its short examination time (scanning of a whole body in a short period of time, from a few seconds to minutes), and its abilities to adapt study parameters to each case and reconstruct images on multiple planes and in three dimensions (3D volume rendering) [17].

PMCT shows its immediate usefulness in examination of the skeletal system, without forgetting the possibility of detecting all types of foreign bodies, such as projectiles or surgical materials, making this technique the most helpful screening tool for subsequent conventional autopsy. As far as projectiles are concerned, PMCT can provide information about the number, form, dimensions, localization, and trajectory, visualizing either bone or metal fragments (Fig. 14.3).

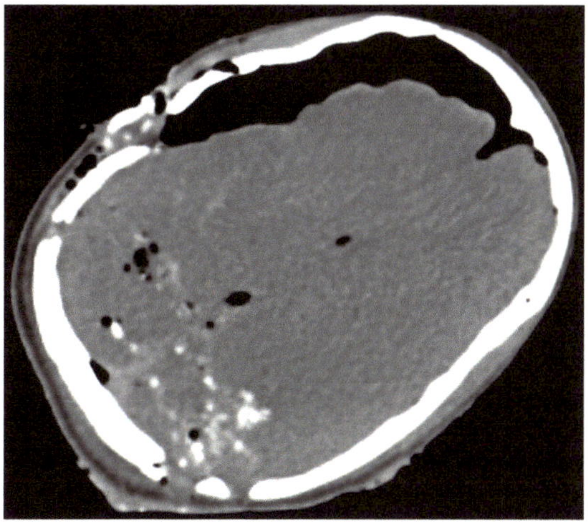

Fig. 14.3 Axial noncontrast computed tomography (*CT*) scan showing pneumocephalus and multiple temporal and parietal fractures with minute osseous fragments along the trajectory of the bullet

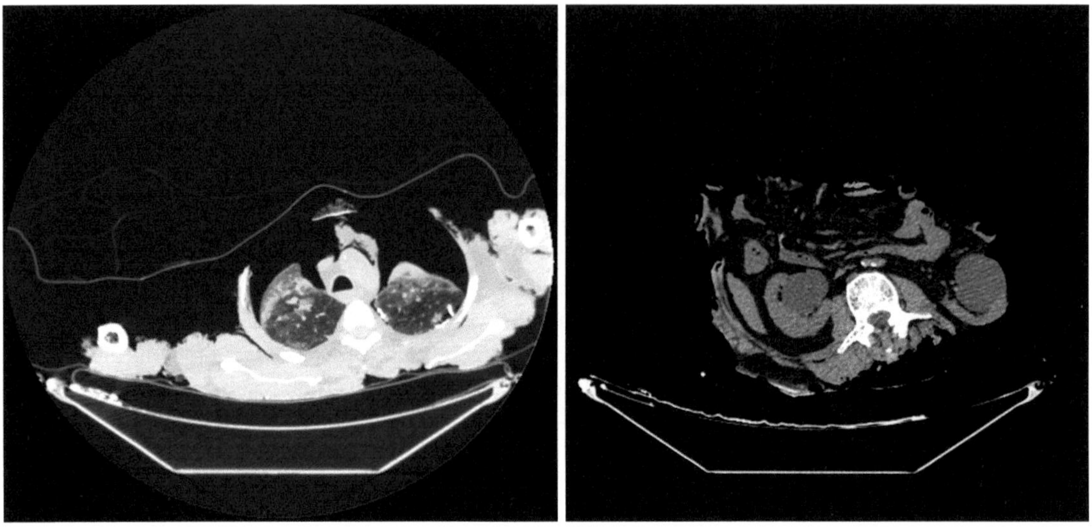

Fig. 14.4 Axial noncontrast computed tomography (*CT*) scans showing grave cutaneous and osseous losses due to burn lesions

Its shorter time of execution, allowing rapid internal inspection of the whole lesion pattern, makes this technique applicable to investigation of mass catastrophe victims, reporting even the presence of medical implants or peculiar body characteristics (anthropometric parameters for estimation of age and sex), which are useful in victim identification [18].

The main advantage of this method, which is extremely anatomical, is that it provides an immediate visual representation of the injurious pattern; such evidence is intuitively more understandable by the various judicial authorities. Its main limitation is its low sensitivity in analyzing parenchymal organs, because of its reduced capability in detecting organ findings. This is why this technique is frequently employed in investigation of traumatic death causes, such as gunshot cases and trauma with skeletal lesions or hyperdense bloody collections, but has limited utility in examination of natural death causes (Fig. 14.4) [19].

14.1.3 Magnetic Resonance Imaging

MRI can overcome PMCT limitations in soft tissue differentiation and characterization, helping forensic investigations to detect natural causes of death [20] or identifying traumatic soft tissue injuries [21]. Postmortem MRI (PMMRI) reveals subcutaneous lesions as well-defined liquid collections due to traumatic pathophysiological processes consisting of vessel injury, interstitial hemorrhage, and edema. For example, MRI allows elucidation of internal neck alterations [22] in strangulation cases.

A further application makes this imaging method capable of detecting suspected bone fractures by means of marrow edema, prompting forensic pathologists to seek them during conventional autopsy. Moreover, this technique can visualize parenchymal injuries (i.e., pulmonary contusions).

Fetal death cases are a developing field of PMMRI employment. Fineschi et al. demonstrated the utility of this technique in identifying organ pathologies to facilitate planning of the autopsy technique and subsequent sampling for histological investigations to clarify fetal death causes that would otherwise remain unknown.

14.1.4 Angiography

Although it has proved useful in detecting bone injuries and even injuries to large vessels, PMCT has obvious limitations in visualization of soft tissues and the vascular system. To overcome this limitation in clinical multidetector CT (MDCT), a contrast medium is injected. At the beginning of the new millennium, the same method was carried out in corpses; indeed, in 2005, Jackowski et al. reported preliminary results from a study of a minimally invasive technique of whole-body PMCTA, using cannulation of the right femoral artery and a meglumine ioxitalamate injection as a contrast medium [23].

This and other experiments, however, led to the conclusion that to perform useful PMCTA, the same conditions that apply in the living should be reproduced in the corpse. Starting from this hypothesis, the consequent conclusion was to establish postmortem circulation in the corpse that would allow whole-body perfusion. The resulting method, known as two-step postmortem angiography, consisted of establishing postmortem perfusion as the first step and injecting contrast media with capture of sequential images as the second step, using a heart–lung machine (modified for use as a perfusion instrument) and an injected oily liquid, introduced by Grabherr et al. [24].

In February 2012, TWGPAM was established, consisting of nine participating centers, six of them being in Europe, including the Department of Forensic Pathology of Foggia. The purpose of this international working group was to make PMCTA a technique accepted by the forensic scientific community and jurisprudence, by defining standardized and validated protocols. This multicenter research project has produced several techniques: multiphase PMCTA (MPMCTA); PMCTA using an aqueous contrast medium based on polyethylene glycol [25]; targeted coronary angiography (TCA), in England [26]; and PMCTA with cardiopulmonary resuscitation, in Japan [27]. Among these techniques, however, only one has attained the introduction of a standardized protocol: MPMCTA, introduced by the Medical Center of Lausanne, Switzerland.

The protocol consists of a native CT scan and three angiographic phases (arterial, venous, and dynamic) by injection of a specific contrast medium, Angiofil® (Fumedica AG, Muri, Switzerland), by means of femoral vessel cannulation on one side femoral vessels [28]. Perfusion is guaranteed by a heart–lung machine (Virtangio®, Fumedica AG), allowing visualization of the whole vascular system of the head, chest, and abdomen but not the vascular tree distal to the site of cannula insertion. Consequently, the anatomy, morphology, and functionality of the lower limb vascular system upstream of the venous incarnation site and downstream of the arterial site are not measurable. This is why at the Department of Forensic Pathology of Foggia, an axillary approach has been demonstrated that is useful to visualize the lower limb vascular axis, especially in cases where examination of such areas appears relevant, such as deaths suspected to be consequent upon pulmonary thromboembolism [29].

This technique has demonstrated its greatest ability in diagnosing causes of sudden cardiac death, guaranteeing visualization of coronary arteries and identification of vascular obstructions or the source sites of fatal hemorrhages. The use of the contrast medium also allows detection of damage to soft tissues or parenchymal organs.

The sensitivity of this method has been compared with that of conventional autopsy in all of these types of cases and even for characterization of stab and gunshot injuries. Furthermore, recently, with extravascular and external local application of contrast media, reconstruction of stab directions and documentation of the inflicted wound depth have been demonstrated [30, 31].

14.1.5 Microradiology

A developing new technique that will find its application in forensic settings is microradiology, which is a standard tool in qualitative and quantitative evaluation of bone structure (such as trabecular volume and thickness) but is also useful in identifying other than bone tissue, employing the higher diagnostic power of CT. This technique allows identification of lesions, fractures, and every other kind of alteration associated with bones or calcified tissues [32–35]—for example, information about the morphology of the tool used to damage the bone [36] or about the timing of a fracture. As previous stated with regard to CT, this technique is of interest in forensic anthropology and odontology for identification of unknown victims after disfiguring trauma, such as fire victims [37].

An experimental study conducted by Cecchetto et al. demonstrated that this nondestructive technique with 3D reconstruction was able to identify gunshot residue on the skin surface and in the epidermis and dermis layers around the entrance hole in fresh specimens, and in the dermis layer around the entrance hole in decomposed specimens [38]. A previous study had demonstrated the absence of these residues in each layer around the exit hole [39, 40]. These studies have highlighted the potential of this technique to locate and characterize entrance and exit lesions in fresh bodies or those altered by putrefaction, fire, or water [38, 41, 42].

Furthermore, a hypothetical application of this technique is the possibility to visualize the architecture of cardiac blood vessels, using its affinity for calcified tissues [43].

Micro-MRI imaging, which takes advantage of the sensitivity of MRI for parenchyma, could be employed in neuropathology to estimate neuronal loss or head injuries, and also in fetal pathology to document alterations affecting the whole body or a specific organ, such as isolated heart block, in order to plan a subsequent conventional autopsy or histopathological sampling [44].

14.2 Penetrating Versus Non-penetrating Traumas

Injuries can be caused by blunt or penetrating traumas. Blunt traumas are linked to the action of an object acting to contuse and, therefore, lacking cutting or pointed edges.

This type of instrument can cause specific types of lesions, such as contusions, abrasions, lacerations, and bone fractures. Most blunt traumas are due to motor vehicle accidents, but they can also be caused by accidental falls or work-related accidents. Conversely, penetrating traumas are injuries resulting from the action of an object with a cutting or pointed edge that causes an open wound affecting the skin and underlying layers, and thus also affecting internal organs. Among penetrating injuries, gunshots and stabbings represent the major causes. Gunshot injuries are often considered perforating injuries because of their extremely violent force, meaning they can pass through all body layers and leave entrance and exit holes.

14.2.1 Non-specific Findings

When the first Virtopsy postmortem examination was conducted in 2000 [45], no radiologist or forensic pathologist knew what a "normal" cadaver appearance was on radiological imaging and how postmortem changes, from autolysis to putrefaction, could influence radiological imaging. Nowadays, some non-specific and specific postmortem findings are known.

The first postmortem changes are *algor mortis*, *livor mortis*, and *rigor mortis*. Among these, *livor mortis* occurs after cessation of the circulation and subsequent failure of arterial propulsion and venous return. Because of gravity, blood passes through vessel walls, diffusing into the lowest noncompressed areas. Stagnant erythrocytes cause a bluish-red discoloration of the skin, called "hypostasis"; this phenomenon also happens in soft tissues and organs. During CT scans, hypostatic collection in soft tissue, lungs, or other solid organs could be misinterpreted as pathological findings, such as contusions, hematomas, or infective lung pathology [46].

Indeed, because of cardiovascular arrest and blood stasis, the brain starts to suffer hypoxic damage, resembling a stroke. This process results in brain edema and loss of corticomedullary differentiation. The first phenomenon is shown by an increase in the dimensions of the brain, obscuring sulci and reducing ventricle or cistern spaces. The second phenomenon is strictly linked to the edema and parenchymal autolysis, which cause attenuation of the border between grey and white matter. This lessening of the differentiation is early demonstrated in CT imaging, while in MRI studies this differentiation persists for much longer.

Moreover, as a normal putrefaction process, bacterial metabolism causes gas formation, usually beginning in the bowels before spreading throughout the whole body. However, a distinction has to be made between pathological premortem gas accumulation and postmortem decomposition gas. The first phenomenon is most frequently associated with fractures (for example, in the head after cranial trauma) or invasive surgical procedures (for example, in hepatobiliary ducts after endoscopic retrograde cholangiopancreatography (ERCP)) and appears to be focally localized, whereas the second phenomenon shows a diffuse gas presence in different body segments and in different locations not necessarily associated with traumatic injuries.

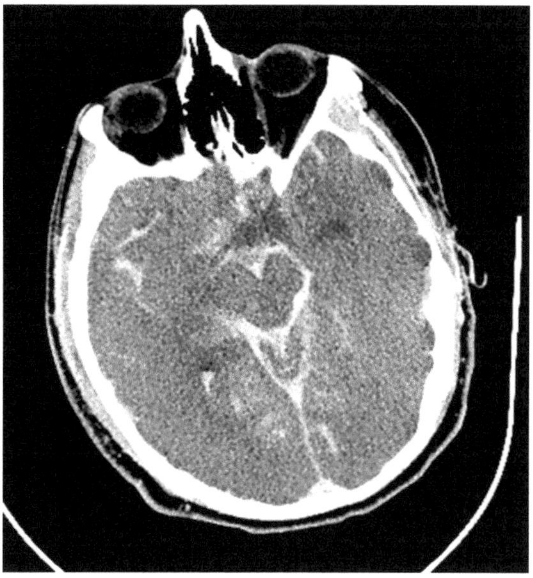

Fig. 14.5 Brain computed tomography (*CT*) axial scan showing a subarachnoid hemorrhage with subtentorial and ventricular involvement after blunt trauma

14.2.2 Specific Signs in Head Investigations

PMCT surpasses conventional radiology in allowing detection of neurocranial and facial fractures. Furthermore, this technique diagnoses intracranial hematomas as hyperdense collections in every localization: epidural, subdural, subarachnoid, or intraventricular hemorrhages, as well as intraocular hemorrhages associated with orbital or skull base fractures (Fig. 14.5).

PMCT imaging before autopsy, especially in cases of traumatic injury with open skull fractures, can find pneumocephalus and cerebral venous and arterial gas emboli, which are barely detectable during postmortem examination unless a modified technique is used in which the body is opened under water. In such cases, PMCT can provide information that is useful to plan the most suitable autopsy approach. A differential diagnosis is needed in cases of postmortem putrefactive gas accumulation, considering that subcutaneous emphysema and air in the left side of the heart are absent.

Penetrating gunshot injuries often affect the head segment, because of its vital content, in cases of suicide or homicide; for example, in the latter instance, a gunshot injury is often the so-called coup de grace. On CT imaging, bullets can be easily found as hyperdense foreign bodies, and they can thus be located and described in terms of their number, shape, dimensions, and integrity. Furthermore, thanks to the structure of cranial bone, the entrance hole can be identified or visualized by bone fragments going from the internal bone layer into the encephalic parenchyma as a wake following the channel excavated by the bullet trajectory. On CT imaging, a parenchymal laceration usually assumes a conical shape, with its base at the entrance wound. Similar considerations apply to the exit hole. Moreover, the entrance hole is characterized by an inner layer that is more comminuted than the outer layer, whereas an outer hole more comminuted than the inner layer characterizes the exit hole in cases of perforating injuries [47]. On the other hand, it is uncommon for this part of the body to suffer stab wounds, because of the natural protection and resistance that the cranial table provides against sharp instruments. However, as was learned from the famous stabbing of King Henry II of France by a broken shaft of a lance through the orbit [48], there are particular areas that allow nonmissile penetrating instruments to access and injure the central nervous system—for example, the orbit, temporal region, and nape.

Knives, screwdrivers, scissors, pencils, ice picks, and stilettoes are usually involved in casualties leading to death from vessel lacerations with massive intracranial hemorrhage, brain stem damage, or vital brain damage. The usefulness of PMCT in identifying fractures, hemorrhages, trajectories, and encephalic areas affected by these lesions is limited only by metal artifacts or high-density foreign material artifacts.

As far as other techniques are concerned, MRI has demonstrated high sensitivity in visualization of subarachnoid hematomas and less sensitivity for epidural and subdural hematomas. The highest sensitivity was shown in detection of galeal hematomas. Among traumatic brain injuries, a particular scenario in which MRI has demonstrated its utility is diagnosis of coup and countercoup trauma [49].

14.2.3 Specific Signs in Neck Investigations

Although they are rare, blunt and penetrating traumas of the neck are associated with high mortality, and this is not surprising if one considers the anatomical structures located here, such as the laryngotracheal axis, common carotid artery, internal jugular vein, vagus nerve, cervical vertebrae, and aerodigestive structures.

Strangulation injuries are associated with particular PMCT and PMMRI findings. Indeed, PMCT has high sensitivity in diagnosis of laryngohyoid fractures, providing easier visualization and better documentation than classical autopsy. Furthermore, skin hemorrhages, subcutaneous hemorrhages, and intramuscular hemorrhages can be detected with postmortem examination but even more with PMMR. Sternocleidomastoid and platysma muscle hemorrhages are frequently seen, as well as a perifocal hematoma surrounding fractured laryngeal structures, which, if present, are pathognomonic findings in strangulation. Moreover, venous congestion in these cases can cause an edematous process in the lymph nodes, which is revealed by PMMR.

PMCT also uncovers bony cervical injuries, which can result from blunt cervical trauma, such as a hyperextension injury. Atlanto-occipital or atlantoaxial fractures and dislocation can be easily detected, as can lower cervical vertebral fractures with spinal canal encroachment, allowing a hypothesis of medullar compression at this level as a possible cause of death; such compression can be caused by traumatic pneumorachis.

The usefulness of PMCT in neck study includes foreign body investigation. This technique, as stated in Sect. 2.2, allows localization and identification of foreign objects lodged just above the narrow cricopharyngeal sphincter, or gunshot wounds, which account for a considerable percentage of spinal cord injuries [50].

14.2.4 Specific Signs in Chest Investigations

Imaging provides some information in cases of suspected blunt or penetrating chest trauma, or trauma ascertained during external examination of a cadaver, including the possibility to diagnose chest wall injuries, pneumothorax, pneumopericardium, hemothorax, hemopericardium, and lung, cardiac, aortic, or vascular injuries (Fig. 14.6).

Fractures of the sternum, ribs, or vertebrae are easily recognized in PMCT, as well as their complications such as pneumothorax (tension pneumothorax is usually associated with chest wall trauma as the primary cause of death or with both pneumorachis and pneumocephalus as secondary

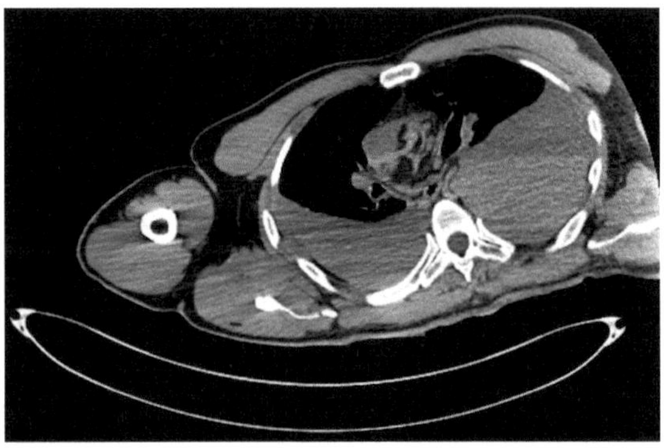

Fig. 14.6 Axial noncontrast computed tomography (*CT*) scan showing collapse of vascular structures (the heart and vessels) with pleural hyperdense effusion due to aortic rupture

causes of death) or pneumopericardium and hemothorax, which, if massive, represent well documented causes of death. This latter can be associated with a "vanishing aorta" [51]—a specific PMCT sign due to a fatal hemorrhage with bloody diversion to a extravasal location and subsequent vessel collapse, leading to the vanishing aorta and pulmonary arteries, caval veins, and even heart chambers that appear smaller than usual. The simultaneous presence of a massive hemothorax and a vanishing aorta sign is suggestive of aortic rupture.

Another specific PMCT sign is a "hyperdense armored heart," which suggests a condition of blood collection in the pericardial sac, leading to a hypothesis of cardiac tamponade from a cardiac rupture, following cardiac infarction or a penetrating injury.

Lung lacerations are also diagnosable with PMCT, although consolidation and ground-glass areas are ambiguous signs that are difficult to interpret, being connected to postmortem hypostasis (as stated above) or lung contusions, hemorrhages, infective pneumonia, or pulmonary edema due to fluid overload, cardiac failure, or even drowning. This is a clear example in which a multidisciplinary approach between legal medicine and radiology could provide the most appropriate interpretation.

On PMCT imaging, stab wounds and gunshot injuries show channels characterized by air inclusion linear defects in thoracic tissues associated with pneumothorax in ante- and postmortem imaging [52–56]. These wound channels can be identified by the presence of foreign bodies along their course, such as metal fragments from a gunshot.

Furthermore, blunt traumas such as car accidents can cause immediate or delayed intra-abdominal organ herniation into the pericardial sac or pleural space, leading to cardiac tamponade or failure with left ventricle compression or respiratory failure. PMCT can show diaphragm laceration and anomalous localization of the abdominal organs.

PMMRI, on the other hand, demonstrates the highest sensitivity in identifying pneumothorax but also allows detection of lung contusions and lacerations with higher specificity than PMCT (though with a similar limitation due to hypostasis). Myocardial rupture and associated pericardial effusion can be clearly diagnosed thanks to MRI, and pneumomediastinum can also be detected.

14.2.5 Specific Signs in Abdominal Investigations

Imaging applied to this body segment is useful in diagnosing intra-abdominal blood collection following blunt or penetrating traumas, such as perihepatic and perisplenic blood and perirenal fluid extending to the perirenal fat, or a massive hemoperitoneum. PMMRI demonstrates high sensitivity in identifying hepatic lesions and renal traumatic lesions, but has low sensitivity for splenic ruptures.

PMCT can reveal the presence of a significant pneumoperitoneum, raising suspicion of a bowel injury. Even in this segment, PMCT remains the best imaging technique to detect lumbar vertebral and pelvic fractures, even those associated with hemorrhage and PMCT signs of exsanguination sufficient to cause death—for example, an abdominal aorta laceration following blunt or penetrating trauma.

14.3 Conclusions

As in clinical radiology, deep knowledge of each technique, with its advantages and limitations, is mandatory to ensure the correct choice so that any relevant information can be obtained from each case to help in medicolegal investigations. In penetrating trauma, conventional x-ray (above all, in the past) and postmortem computed tomography (PMCT) (nowadays) are considered the most useful imaging modalities to reveal any hyperdense foreign bodies, helping to reconstruct their trajectories and to distinguish organ injuries, such as fractures and lacerations, even in putrefied, carbonized, or otherwise damaged bodies.

In cases of traumatic death, in general, PMCT has been shown to be the tool of choice, providing not only fracture documentation but also information concerning the biomechanical origins of it, contributing to forensic reconstruction of a case. In cases of fatal hemorrhage following sharp and gunshot trauma, PMCT and multiphase PMCT angiography (MPMCTA), in particular, allow identification of the source of bleeding and formulation of a hypothesis regarding the trajectories of knives, needles, and projectiles.

In blunt trauma cases, PMCT and/or postmortem magnetic resonance imaging (PMMRI)—which are better used in combination—can provide information about both bone and parenchymal lesions; indeed, these techniques allow detection of soft tissue involvement, intra- or extra-axial brain hemorrhages, and contusions of the lung, heart, and liver.

This high sensitivity of postmortem imaging applied to forensic cases, in combination with the heightened documentary power of these techniques—whether they are used individually or together—contribute to the establishment of a unique discipline. The so-called forensic radiology, with a multidisciplinary approach furnished by all subspecialties—such as radiologists, pathologists, anthropologists, and toxicologists—may provide high-quality evidence for medicolegal investigations and, above all, in jurisprudential courts.

References

1. Brogdon BG, Lichtenstein JE (2011) Forensic radiology in historical perspective. In: Thali MJ, Viner MD, Brogdon BG (eds) Brogdon's forensic radiology. 2. CRC Press, Boca Raton, pp 9–23
2. Wüllenweber R, Schneider V, Grumme T (1977) A computer-tomographical examination of cranial bullet wounds (author's transl) [article in German]. Z Rechtsmed 80:227–246
3. The Virtopsy Project (2012) www.virtopsy.com. Accessed 5 May 2019
4. Thali MJ, Braun M, Brüschweiler W, Dirnhofer R (2000) Matching tire tracks on the head using forensic photogrammetry. Forensic Sci Int 113:281–287
5. Thali MJ, Yen K, Schweitzer W, Vock P, Boesch C, Ozdoba C, Schroth G, Ith M, Sonnenschein M, Doernhoefer T, Scheurer E, Plattner T, Dirnhofer R (2003) Virtopsy a new imaging horizon in forensic pathology: virtual autopsy by postmortem multislice computed tomography (MSCT) and magnetic resonance imaging (MRI)—a feasibility study. J Forensic Sci 48:386–403
6. Bisset RA, Thomas NB, Turnbull IW, Lee S (2002) Postmortem examinations using magnetic resonance imaging: four year review of a working service. BMJ 324:1423–1424
7. Thali MJ, Kneubuehl BP, Vock P, Allmen G, Dirnhofer R (2002) High-speed documented experimental gunshot to a skull-brain model and radiologic virtual autopsy. Am J Forensic Med Pathol 23:223–228
8. Rutty GN, Morgan B, O'Donnell C, Leth PM, Thali M (2008) Forensic institutes across the world place CT or MRI scanners or both into their mortuaries. J Trauma 65:493–494
9. O'Donnell C, Woodford N (2008) Post-mortem radiology—a new sub-speciality? Clin Radiol 63:1189–1194
10. Meadowcroft WH (1986) The ABC of the x-rays. Simpkin, Marshall, Hamilton, Kent & Co, London
11. Baglivo M, Winklhofer S, Hatch GM, Ampanozi G, Thali MJ, Ruder TD (2013) The rise of forensic and post-mortem radiology—analysis of the literature between the year 2000 and 2011. J Forensic Radiol Imaging 1:3–9
12. Brant WE, Helms CA (eds) (2007) Fundamentals of diagnostic radiology, 3rd edn. Lippincott Williams & Wilkins, Philadelphia
13. Grabherr S, Djonov V, Yen K, Thali MJ, Dirnhofer R (2007) Postmortem angiography: review of former and current methods. AJR Am J Roentgenol 188:832–838
14. Saunders SL, Morgan B, Raj V, Rutty GN (2011) Post-mortem computed tomography angiography: past, present and future. Forensic Sci Med Pathol 7:271–277
15. Ruder TD, Hatch GM, Ebert LC, Flach PM, Ross S, Ampanozi G, Thali MJ (2012) Whole body postmortem magnetic resonance angiography. J Forensic Sci 57:778–782
16. Uchigasaki S, Oesterhelweg L, Gehl A, Sperhake JP, Püschel K, Oshida S, Nemoto N (2004) Application of compact ultrasound imaging device to postmortem diagnosis. Forensic Sci Int 140:33–41
17. Borowska-Solonynko A, Solonynko B (2015) The use of 3D computed tomography reconstruction in medico-legal testimony regarding injuries in living victims—risks and benefits. J Forensic Legal Med 30:9–13
18. Brough AL, Morgan B, Rutty GN (2015) Postmortem computed tomography (PMCT) and disaster victim identification. Radiol Med 120:866–873
19. Roberts IS, Benamore RE, Benbow EW et al (2012) Post-mortem imaging as an alternative to autopsy in the diagnosis of adult deaths: a validation study. Lancet 379:136–142
20. Ruder TD, Ebert LC, Khattab AA, Rieben R, Thali MJ, Kamat P (2013) Edema is a sign of early acute myocardial infarction on post-mortem magnetic resonance imaging. Forensic Sci Med Pathol 9:501–505

21. Yen K, Vock P, Tiefenthaler B et al (2004) Virtopsy: forensic traumatology of the subcutaneous fatty tissue; multislice computed tomography (MSCT) and magnetic resonance imaging (MRI) as diagnostic tools. J Forensic Sci 49:799–806
22. Christe A, Thoeny H, Ross S et al (2009) Life-threatening versus non life-threatening manual strangulation: are there appropriate criteria by MR Imaging of the neck? Eur Radiol 19(8):1882–1889
23. Jackowski C, Thali MJ, Sonnenschein M, Aghayev E, von Allmen G, Yen K et al (2005) Virtopsy: postmortem minimally invasive angiography using cross section techniques—implementation an preliminary results. J Forensic Sci 50:1175–1186
24. Grabherr S, Gygax E, Sollberger B, Ross S, Oesterhelweg L, Bolliger S et al (2008) Two step postmortem angiography with a modified heart-lung machine: preliminary results. AJR Am J Roentgenol 190:345–352. https://doi.org/10.2214/AJR.07.2261
25. Jackowski C, Persson A, Thali MJ (2008) Whole body postmortem angiography with a high viscosity contrast agent solution using polyethylene glycol as contrast agent dissolver. J Forensic Sci 53:465. https://doi.org/10.1111/j.1556-4029.2008.00673.x
26. Roberts IS, Benamore RE, Peebles C, Rooobottom C, Traill ZC (2011) Technical report: diagnosis of coronary artery diseases using minimally invasive autopsy: evaluation of a novel method of post-mortem coronary CT angiography. Clin Radiol 66:645–650. https://doi.org/10.1016/j.crad.2011.01.007
27. Lizuka K, Sakamoto N, Kawasaki H, Miyoshi T, Komatsuzaki A, Kikuchi S (2009) Usefullness of contrast-enhanced postmortem CT. InnerVision 24:89–92
28. Grabherr S, Doenz F, Steger B, Dinhofer R, Dominguez A, Sollberg B et al (2011) Multi-phase post-mortem CT angiography: development of a standardized protocol. Int J Legal Med 125:791–802. https://doi.org/10.1007/s00414-010-0526-5
29. Pomara C, Bello S, Grilli G, Guglielmi G, Turillazzi E (2015) Multi-phase postmortem CT angiography (MPMCTA): a new axillary approach suitable in fatal thromboembolism. Radiol Med. 120(7):670–673. https://doi.org/10.1007/s11547-014-0467-z
30. Bolliger SA, Ruder TD, Ketterer T, Glaser N, Thali MJ, Ampanozi G (2014) Comparison of stab wound probing versus radiological stab wound channel depiction with contrast medium. Forensic Sci Int 234:45–49
31. Fais P, Cecchetto G, Boscolo-Berto R et al (2016) Morphometric analysis of stab wounds by MSCT and MRI after the instillation of contrast medium. Radiol Med 121:494–501
32. Fais P, Giraudo C, Viero A et al (2016) Micro computed tomography features of laryngeal fractures in a case of fatal manual strangulation. Leg Med (Tokyo) 18:85–89
33. Chen T, Chodara AM, Sprecher AJ, Fang F, SongW TC, Jiang JJ (2012) A new method of reconstructing the human laryngeal architecture using micro-MRI. J Voice 26:555–562
34. Pelletti G, Viel G, Fais P, Viero A, Visentin S, Miotto D, Montisci M, Cecchetto G, Giraudo C (2017) Micro-computed tomography of false starts produced on bone by different hand-saws. Leg Med (Tokyo) 26:1–5
35. Kettner M, Potente S, Schulz B, Knauff P, Schmidt PH, Ramsthaler F (2014) Analysis of laryngeal fractures in decomposed bodies using microfocus computed tomography (mfCT). Forensic Sci Med Pathol 10:607–612
36. Thali MJ, Taubenreuther U, Karolczak M et al (2003) Forensic microradiology: micro-computed tomography (micro-CT) and analysis of patterned injuries inside of bone. J Forensic Sci 48:1336–1342
37. Sandholzer MA, Baron K, Heimel P, Metscher BD (2014) Volume analysis of heat-induced cracks in human molars: a preliminary study. J Forensic Dent Sci 6:139–144
38. Cecchetto G, Amagliani A, Giraudo C et al (2012) MicroCT detection of gunshot residue in fresh and decomposed firearm wounds. Int J Legal Med 126:377–383
39. Cecchetto G, Giraudo C, Amagliani A et al (2011) Estimation of the firing distance through micro-CT analysis of gunshot wounds. Int J Legal Med 125:245–251
40. Viero A, Giraudo C, Cecchetto G et al (2014) An unusual case of "dyadic-death" with a single gunshot. Forensic Sci Int 244:E1–E5
41. Fais P, Giraudo C, Boscolo-Berto R et al (2013) Micro-CT features of intermediate gunshot wounds severely damaged by fire. Int J Legal Med 127:419–425
42. Fais P, Viero A, Amagliani A, Viel G, Montisci M, Miotto D, Cecchetto G (2015) Identification of bullet entrance in different type of intermediate firearm wounds through micro-computed tomography analysis. J Forensic Radiol Imaging 3:147–152
43. Yu TY, Finney BH, Dehghani H, Claridge E, Thomas S (2013) Three dimensional analysis of cardiovascular development in mouse embryos using x-ray micro-computed tomography. Microsc Anal 27:12–13
44. Bertrand A, Pasquier A, Petiet A et al (2013) Micro-MRI study of cerebral aging: ex vivo detection of hippocampal subfield reorganization, microhemorrhages and amyloid plaques in mouse lemur primates. PLoS One 8:e56593
45. Thali MJ, Yen K, Schweitzer W et al (2003) Virtopsy, a new imaging horizon in forensic pathology: virtual autopsy by postmortem multislice computed tomography (MSCT) and magnetic resonance imaging (MRI)—a feasibility study. J Forensic Sci 48(2):386–403
46. Christe A, Flach P, Ross S, Spendlove D, Bolliger S, Vock P, Thali MJ (2010) Clinical radiology and postmortem imaging (Virtopsy) are not the same: specific and unspecific postmortem signs. Leg Med (Tokyo) 12:215–222

47. Offiah C et al Imaging assessment of penetrating craniocerebral and spinal trauma. Clin Radiol 64(12):1146–1157
48. Faria MA Jr (1992) The death of Henry II of France. Historical vignette. J Neurosurg 77:964–969
49. Besenski N (2002) Traumatic injuries: imaging of head injuries. Eur Radiol 12:1237–1252
50. Bono CM, Heary RF (2004) Gunshot wounds to the spine. Spine J 4:230–240
51. Aghayev E, Sonnenschein M, Jackowski C et al (2006) Postmortem radiology of fatal hemorrhage: measurements of cross-sectional areas of major blood vessels and volumes of aorta and spleen on MDCT and volumes of heart chambers on MRI. Am J Roentgenol 187(1):209–215
52. Ruder TD, Ross S, Preiss U, Thali MJ (2010) Minimally invasive post-mortem CT angiography in a case involving a gunshot wound. Leg Med (Tokyo) 12(2):57–112
53. Schnider J, Thali MJ, Ross S, Oesterhelweg L, Spendlove D, Bolliger SA (2009) Injuries due to sharp trauma detected by post-mortem multislice computed tomography (MSCT): a feasibility study. Leg Med (Tokyo) 11(1):4–9
54. Vullo A, Panebianco V, Cannavale G, Aromatario M, Cipolloni L, Frati P, Santurro A, Vullo F, Catalano C, Fineschi V (2016) Post-mortem magnetic resonance foetal imaging: a study of morphological correlation with conventional autopsy and histopathological findings. Radiol Med. 121(11):847–856
55. Cafarelli FP, Grilli G, Zizzo G, Bertozzi G, Giuliani N, Mahakkanukrauh P, Pinto A, Guglielmi G (2019) Postmortem imaging: an update. Semin Ultrasound CT MR 40(1):86–93
56. D'Errico S, Martelloni M, Cafarelli FP, Guglielmi G (2018) Neurofibromatosis 1 and massive hemothorax: a fatal combination. Forensic Sci Med Pathol 14(3):377–380

15 Imaging for Ballistic Trauma: Other Applications of Forensic Imaging in the Living

Salvatore Serraino, Livio Milone, Dario Picone, Antonina Argo, Sergio Salerno, and Massimo Midiri

15.1 Firearms

Firearms are mechanical instruments that allow launching remote specific bodies with mass (bullets) exploiting burst gas energy.

They generally can be classified into portable (guns, rifles, etc.) and stationary (cannons, mortar, etc.); the former are enormously spread and considered as the first homicidal lesion means.

Conventionally portable weapons have a caliber <20 mm.

Fire weapons are classified according to length, differentiating short gun barrel (guns) from rifles, and presence of grooves into the barrel, differentiating between smooth bore and rifled arms. According to firing mechanism, firearms are classified into manual repeating short or long barrel, semiautomatic (guns or rifles), and automatic (Tables 15.1 and 15.2).

S. Serraino (✉) · S. Salerno · M. Midiri
University of Palermo, Palermo, Italy
e-mail: sergio.salerno@unipa.it; midiri.massimo@unipa.it

L. Milone · A. Argo
Department of Sciences for the Promotion of Health and Maternal and Child Care "G. D'Alessandro", University of Palermo, Palermo, Italy
e-mail: livo.milone@unipa.it; antonella.argo@unipa.it

D. Picone
Department of Biopathology and Medical Biotechnologies, University of Palermo, Palermo, Italy

It must be pointed out that, in rifled guns (short or long barrel), "caliber" is defined as the inner diameter of the barrel measured between two opposite voids of the groove; from a conventional point of view, a weapon caliber consists of the caliber of the cartridge for which is, in fact, built (for example, 38-caliber revolver special).

In the smooth-bore weapons, the caliber is indicated by a number corresponding to the number of spherical lead balls, having a diameter equal to that of the barrel, which can be obtained from a pound of lead.

15.2 Terminal Ballistics Notions

15.2.1 General Characteristics of Gunshot Injuries

When the projectile achieves the target, it generates a series of events on the drawn region and on the body that classically are the study object of medicolegal discipline study.

The surface of the body and its coating (i.e., textiles and skin) may contain essential information for the investigation of gunshot wounds. The two superficial layers are therefore discussed separately.

Obviously, the most important object of study is the harmfulness on the body; the forensic diagnosis is often required even for the living, not only for medical purposes but also, mainly, for issues

G. Lo Re et al. (eds.), *Radiology in Forensic Medicine*, https://doi.org/10.1007/978-3-319-96737-0_15

Table 15.1 Main classification criteria for firearms

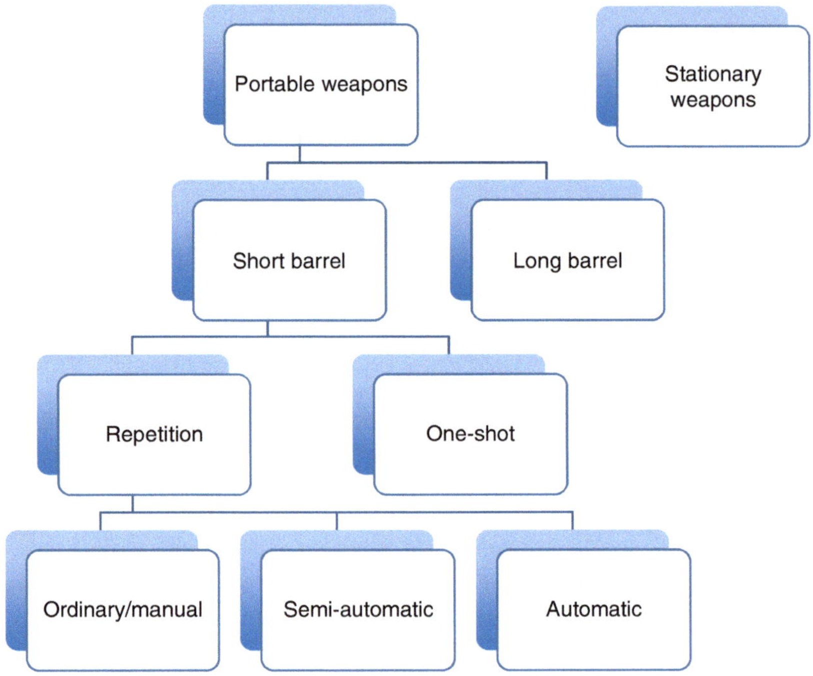

Table 15.2 Weapon discriminating features

• Functioning typology
• Caliber
• Brand and model
• Registration number
• Barrel (twist number and orientation)
• State of use, maintenance, efficiency

that are often encountered in the legal field with crime-survived victims, differential diagnosis of attempted murder and attempted suicide, etc.

The extent of body injury is obviously a function of the type of the bullet and of caliber and energy possessed when this achieves the body. These parameters moreover indirectly involve an assessment of the firing distance.

In the following discussion authors will differentiate the lesion's characteristics as those due to the use of a unique projectile weapon versus those due to the use of hunting weapons in multiple loading; though the physical principle underlying the two types of weapons is identical, difference appears in the harmfulness, both internally and externally, in the use of these different types of weapons and ammunition.

When the projectile (or projectiles) reaches the body surface, part of the energy is transferred because of the impact and a further amount of energy is spent in the crossing of the skin; ulterior progression through the body of the victim and the eventual ejection are linked to the residual energy of the projectile.

It must be considered, in fact, that along the body-crossing trajectory the projectile gives energy to the surrounding tissues, proportionally to the degree of deformation and the entity of the resistance of the crossed tissues.

15.3 Characters from the Single-Bullet Injuries

15.3.1 Entrance Wounds

15.3.1.1 Textiles

Many entrance and exit wounds are located in body regions commonly covered by garments; therefore, the clothing of every gunshot wound victim should be investigated closely. A textile perforation commonly produces one textile defect at the site but in case of folds there may be five or more defects originating from one gunshot. In a dressed body region, the outside surface of textiles but not the skin will show soot, powder remnants, or bullet wipe-off/ring of dirt.

A primary entrance defect in textiles is commonly circular in shape but the morphology also depends on the textile's own characteristics so that tears and oblong defects are possible. Exit wounds frequently are larger and more irregular because many bullets exit in a position diagonal to the longitudinal axis. However, there are a number of exceptions such as contact gunshots producing large stellate textile defects or slow projectiles producing small exit defects. The low temperature–time product of modern nitro powder allows scorching of superficial fibers in contact shots but commonly prevents relevant burning effects, which are typical for black powder.

15.3.1.2 Skin

After reaching the target, the projectile determines a blunt effect, with backing of the skin, and, overcoming its resistance, penetrates into the skin layers and in depth, where sufficient energy is provided. The perforation mechanism of skin is different in entry and exit wounds, resulting in various wound morphologies.

Typically, the entrance wound is a continuous round-shaped solution, slightly smaller than the projectile diameter because of the elastic retraction of the skin, which appears stretched and pushed forward during the penetration mechanism.

Because of the high velocity of the entering projectile and the backing of skin with tissue, the superficial area of the entrance region is *not* (contrary to common belief) indented or depressed in the shooting direction, as demonstrated by Madea and Karger et al. The dynamic multistep entrance mechanism results in the typical characteristics of skin entrance wounds from intermediate or distant range (Fig. 15.1):

1. The *central skin defect* of circular or oval shape: The bullet pushes the skin as a "glove finger"; the missing skin is destroyed by the tip of the projectile.
2. The *bullet wipe-off/ring of dirt* is a thin circular blackish discoloration directly around the skin defect. The projectile tends to "cleanse" all the impurities carried, such as gunshot residues, oil, dirt, and abrasions of the bullet and the barrel, and any foreign substances due to the previous impacts against secondary targets (traces of paint, wooden fragments, masonry debris, etc.). These debris are rubbed off the tip of the projectile onto the skin margins during initial penetration, leaving a residue of contaminants on the surface of the skin.

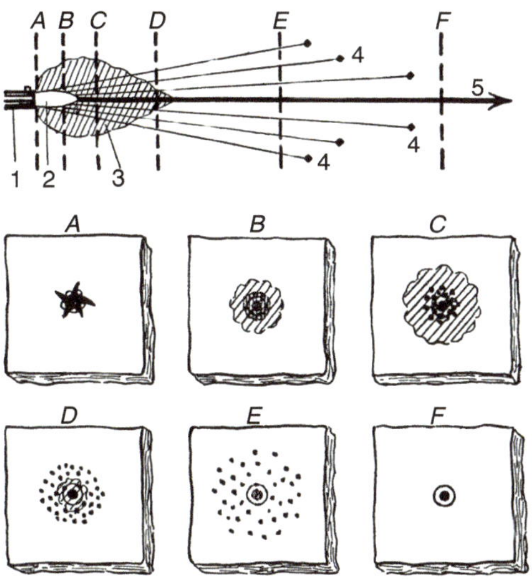

1	Fire mouth
2	Flame
3	Smoke
4	Gunpowder grains
A	**Star-shaped wound; vanishing ecchymotic-excoriated rim**
B	Bullet hole; ecchymotic-excoriated rim; burn halo; smoking halo
C	Bullet hole; ecchymotic-excoriated rim; tattoo; smoking halo
D	Bullet hole; ecchymotic-excoriated rim; smoking halo; tattoo
E	Bullet hole; ecchymotic-excoriated rim; tattoo
F	Bullet hole; ecchymotic-excoriated rim

Fig. 15.1 Scheme of the characteristics of inlet orifices for short-distance shots

3. The *abrasion ring or abrasion margin* develops symmetrically and concentrically in a zone 1–3 mm wide. It is due to massive temporary overstretching of the skin adjacent to the central defect, especially in the area of the outward bulge. This produces a loss of the superficial skin layer and epidermis, and the exposed corium dries up and later appears as a brownish or black margin. The production of the abrasion ring is probably supported by the tiny crushed skin particles moving tangentially to the skin wound margin but it cannot be produced by direct abrading contact with the bullet—neither the skin indents nor is there any contact with the projectile outside the zone of bullet wipe-off.
4. The contusion ring is also mainly due to the temporary overstretching of the skin around the central defect. The epidermis, however, is not lost but analogous to temporary cavitation in soft tissues there is bleeding beneath and inside the skin and possibly short skin tears. Consequently, the contusion ring appears as a thin circular reddish-bluish bruising of the skin.

The size of the ecchymotic-excoriated or wipe-off rim quite approximately reproduces the diameter (hence the caliber) of the projectile.

The entry orifice presents an everted appearance even in case of organic material (brain material, omentum, subcutaneous fat) spillage from the deep; leakage of blood from entrance orifices placed in gravitational sites may also cause margin eversion.

In some cases, subtle linear notches of the superficial skin layers, in radial disposition, may be noticed on the entrance orifice contour, due to epidermis slits after an abrupt distension under the perforating action of high-velocity projectiles; these findings do not have to be confused with the typical stellar figure of skin lesions for "contact" shots.

The circular shape of the entrance orifice, and surrounding flanges, is typical of shoots orthogonal to the skin, but these characteristics are not mandatory. This means that not every single component occurs in each entrance wound.

If the bullet hits skin with an oblique direction the resulting orifice and the related flanges have an elliptic, more or less accentuated, shape in relation to the angle of incidence on the skin. In this eventuality minor orifice axis and its ecchymotic-excoriated rim may be useful in the identification of the projectile diameter.

A graze wound occurs when the bullet strikes the skin at a shallow angle, producing a canal-like abrasion; in tangential wounds, the bullet enters the subcutaneous tissue. Both wound types can result in an elongated laceration of the skin, frequently including secondary skin tears running in the direction of fire. Reentry wounds occur if a bullet has perforated one part of a body, for example the arm, and then reenters in another part, for example the thorax. The body part initially perforated can be considered an intermediate target. Consequently, a reentry wound commonly presents as a large and irregular defect with ragged edges and a wide abrasion ring but no bullet wipe-off. Entrance wounds in the thick dermis of palms and soles can be stellate with short radiating tears, slit-like or H-shaped, and an abrasion ring is frequently missing.

Moreover, a variety of parameters such as ricochets/yawing bullets, deformed or slow projectiles, bony backing of the skin, or skin folds can produce atypical entrance wounds; if the projectile, rolling on itself in space (tumbling), reaches the target by the side or base, it tends to create an elliptical or a lockhole-shaped entry orifice (keyhole).

The bullets of smaller caliber and that are particularly sharp can produce abnormal orifices, such as linear slits recalling tip wound.

The entry orifice usually shows some secondary minor characteristics useful in determining firing distance.

In case of shots fired with the weapon mouth held in contact with the skin, the gases resulting from combustion tend to penetrate behind the projectile and expand into the wound, tearing and infiltrating the subcutaneous tissue; that's because lesion assumes a stellar radial aspect.

If weapon mouth is placed in close proximity to the skin surface, mold marks (figurative bruising) are produced after weapon recoiling and forward returning phenomena; they tend to reproduce the front plane of the weapon or some muzzle features (spring guide rod in the case of semiautomatic pistols, mouth of the other rod in the case of doublets, etc.).

When muzzle is a few centimeters distant from the skin, blaze produced by propellant combustion can produce hair burning, hence "*point-blank*," and a moderate epidermis superficial scald (*halo burn* or *burn*).

Carbonaceous residues of the fumes produced during gunpowder combustion tend to deposit around the entrance wound, so as to form a "halo of smoke," in case of shots from about 10 cm from the skin. These findings are more evident if weapons with black powder loading are used.

The halo of smoke can be easily removed cleaning the site of injury with water, also in order to better highlight the underlying cutaneous lesion characteristics.

During propellant explosion, not all of the powder granules undergo a complete combustion: the larger unburned or partially burned granules, with a certain kinetic energy, are projected forward behind the projectile and tend to deeply penetrate into the dermis and cannot be removed by simple washing; a "tattoo" halo is determined, whose amplitude and single element concentration are directly proportional to the firing distance.

All these described elements combine to formulate a fairly reliable diagnosis about the possible firing distance (Table 15.3).

Table 15.3 Firing distance determining features

• Shots fired in direct skin contact (starry input conformation).
• Blows with the muzzle slightly deviate from the skin (formation of an imprint mold).
• Shots fired at a very short distance (production of a halo of shots fired to burn within 5 cm of the weapon between the mouth and skin, the smoking alone for shots fired by the firearm 10 cm between the mouth and skin).
• Shots at short distance exploded (production of a halo of tattoo for shots fired within about 50 cm between the muzzle and skin; this distance may vary in relation to the weapon caliber and type of ammunition used).
• Over 50 cm is defined fail exploded "over short distances."

15.3.2 Intracorporeal Trajectory

After dermal penetration, the projectile typically continues its way inside the body, producing a channel, which tends to cross the body in a straight direction. Where there is the output of the projectile, the trajectory is called "complete" or "transfosso," if a large body cavity is crossed.

If the projectile, during body penetration, crosses tissues with different density and spends most of its residual energy, it is retained within the body, originating a "dead-end" track, which extends proportionally to projectile penetration capability and its energy.

An open loss of surface substance is caused by the projectile if skin is hit tangentially whereby the passage assumes "slither" or half-passage (glancing wound); in some cases, the passage may be superficial, connecting the entry and exit orifices after a short crossing of skin or muscle (seton trajectory).

When the projectile meets high-density tissues along the intracorporeal path, it may undergo deformation or even fragmentation with production of secondary transits detaching from the original trajectory.

In case of impact against bone, a number of fragments can form which behave as secondary projectiles.

Energy transfer when projectile passes through parenchymal or hollow organs may result in an outburst rupture, especially in case of high-velocity projectiles.

Inner trajectory does not always result straight; in case of low-energy bullet striking chest, it can be addressed along the ribs and ejected from the body without passing the thorax (circumnavigating route). Similarly, a projectile can be deflected after impacting a bony structure, and describes an angled track; in this case, the exit hole or retained projectile is discovered in an unexpected site.

15.3.3 Exit Wounds

Typically, the exit orifice is constituted by a circular shaped lack of substance with larger diameter than the entry one, whose margins are everted (following the shooting direction), often frayed or, otherwise, irregular often due to overturning phenomena inside the trajectory, and because there is no backing of the skin and the projectile velocity is commonly low.

The resulting exit wound morphology is variable; the wound margins are frequently irregular, torn, or slit-like, and any ecchymotic-excoriated flange is seen. In some particular conditions a pseudo-flange can be observed.

The main difference to entrance wounds is that the skin margins can be adapted. This means that there is no skin defect, so no skin is missing but the skin margins can be aligned properly.

Where the body surface where the exit hole is positioned leans against a certain consistency obstacle (wall, seats, belts, metal buckles, etc.), a sort of contusive rim may form because of against-resistance skin crushing; in this case the absence of the excoriated component on the orifice board allows a differential diagnosis. When the projectile goes to fragmentation along its track, exit wounds may appear irregularly linear and, in any case, show smaller diameter than the eventual corresponding exit orifice.

If the residual energy of the projectile does not allow its releasing, the projectile tends to remain under the skin; a subcutaneous bruising may demonstrate the presence, and local palpation helps in determining the exact site of retention, with the possibility to immediately retrieve after subcutaneous incision.

15.4 Characters from Multiple-Bullet Injuries

As already mentioned, in case of multiple-loading hunting weapons, cartridges carry a high number of ballistic elements (from a minimum of nine in the case of buckshot type 11/0 to several hundreds in the case of small shots).

At the time of the explosion, the ammunition leave the muzzle composed and compact, because of the gas pressure developed and of the boost created by the wad. Ammunition still remain compact and piled up to a certain distance from the muzzle (mass effect), but after 1–2 m air resistance tends to disperse the elements that assume a concentric conformation or "shot pattern," whose dimensions (diameter) are a direct function of the firing distance.

If the shots or pellets group intercepts an intermediate target, a number of individual orifices equal to the number of target elements will be identified on the body surface; there are thus multiple entry orifices corresponding to multiple trajectories inside the body, which create devastating effects on the organism, such as brain breaking-up in the case of shots to the head, or parenchymal destruction in the case of shots to the trunk.

Easier than single projectile, ballistic elements tend to remain retained in the body, as well as in some cases even wad elements (wads, pads, wad containers) whose study may provide useful information about ammunition and loading.

15.5 Radiological Reconstruction of a Gunshot Wound

To perform a radiological evaluation before autopsy is nowadays indicated.

A range of radiological methods may be applied in gunshot dead people postmortem evaluation; each technique shows, anyway, advantages and limitations or, in some cases, real and absolute contraindications.

Conventional radiography, yet a stronghold of medicolegal application of radiology, especially in forensic sciences, is widely represented on the territory, being not much expensive, reproducible, fast, and easy to perform. Another important quality is the very accurate spatial resolution in spite of a non-sufficient contrast resolution, in particular for soft tissues. A further significant limitation is the impossibility of obtaining adequate projection for an optimal exam execution (Fig. 15.2).

Multi-detector CT (MDCT) has revealed to be the more complete and accurate, first of all according to some intrinsic characteristics such as its panoramic and volumetric view, the possibility of manipulating and reconstructing images, its intrinsic elevated spatial resolution and a high contrast resolution between bullets (the value density number was higher than evaluation CT capacity ≥3071

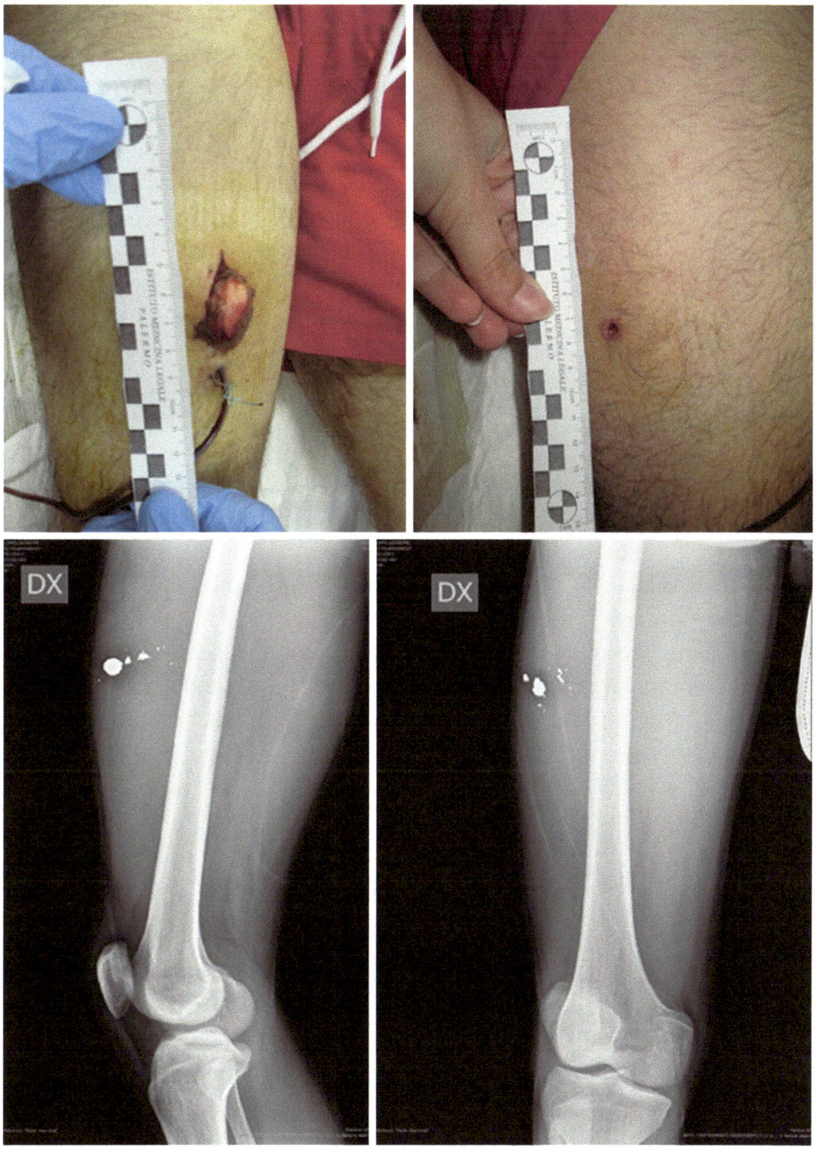

Fig. 15.2 Upwards are reported two photos showing the inlet orifice (on the left) and the outlet orifices (on the right) in a living individual. Downwards: Conventional radiographs in emergency department—before a surgical approach—accurately show the presence of metallic remains inside anterior-lateral thigh soft tissue. No bony lesions are seen

HU) and soft and hard tissues, and the possibility of performing a number of exams and storing obtained images perpetually, with the important implication of allowing any eventual re-evaluation when needed. Other advantages are the objectivity of the method, reproducibility, and availability on the territory. All of the described features, together with the speed of execution, noninvasiveness, and possibility of manipulation and reconstruction of the data acquired, make the MDCT a preferential technique in supporting investigation procedures and autopsy.

A great number of the known events a projectile may produce in human body are accurately identifiable and described with MDCT.

In CT images the ***projectile***, or its fragments, is visualized as a really spontaneous high-attenuation image (steadily higher than 3071, the maximum measurable value by CT scan), with non-identifiable contours because of the presence of surrounding beam-hardening artifact, most of the times showing a pinwheel shape in agreement with the helical acquisition. Our experience has shown the possibility to reduce the effect of the described artifacts on the final image thanks to post-processing procedure, in particular by increasing the screen width (CT-bone window) or by reconstructing images on sagittal–parasagittal plane.

The ***entry wound***, not always easily seen, appears as a superficial alteration of the skin profile presenting irregular margins and millimetric air bubbles into the underlying subcutaneous adipose tissue.

The ***exit wound***, where present, appears as a coarse irregularity of the skin profile, towards which multiple millimetric hyper-attenuating images generally converge, because of the presence of metal projectile remnants or, alternatively, bone fragments coming from the structure encountered by the bullet along its course; both air bubbles may also be present, especially in case of low-energy bullet (Fig. 15.3).

As regards the interaction a bullet may have with intracorporeal tissues, it is described below according to the different kinds of encountered tissue consistency.

The impact of the bullet with such a hard tissue as ***bone*** always generates a breaking, varying according to bullet energy, mass, and direction, and kind of the bone: simple or commingled fractures are more common in long or flat bone, with associated bone marrow spreading usually when long bones are involved; radial fractures are typical of flat bone involved in projectile entry; comminute or burst fractures are usually seen in short bones.

When a bullet, regardless of its size and conformation, hits ***cranial theca***, entry and exit orifices have a characteristic morphology that allows easy differentiation (Fig. 15.4).

In fact, entry orifice has a characteristic truncated cone-shaped conformation, with the smaller base on the external planking and larger diameter on the internal surface (Figs. 15.5 and 15.6), while the exit orifice shows similar morphology in an inverse arrangement (smaller base of the truncated cone on the internal side and the larger base outside) (Fig. 15.7).

A similar funnel-shaped or truncated cone aspect assumes the gunshot lesion on flat bones

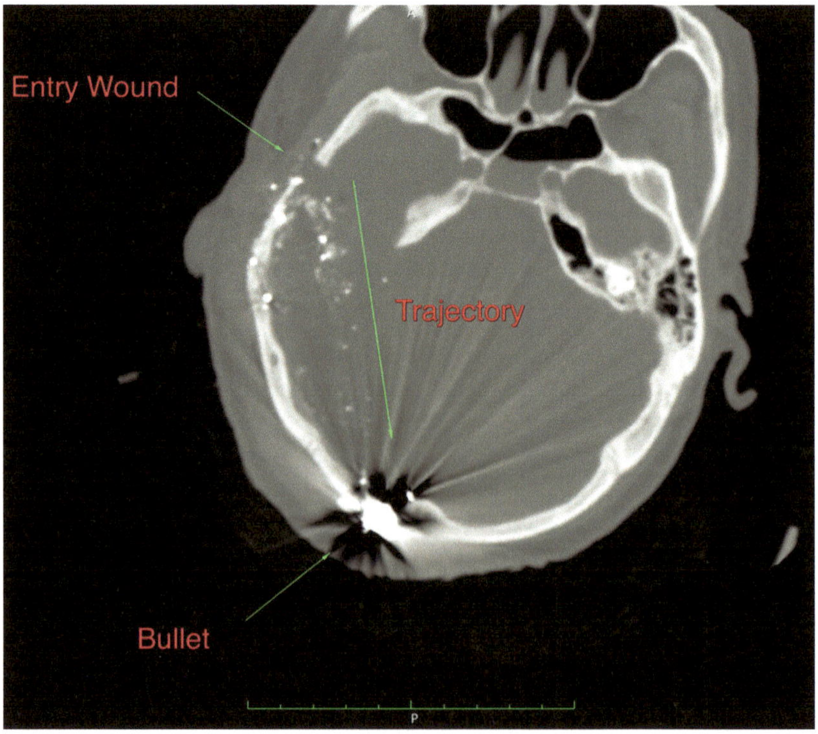

Fig. 15.3 Axial image filtered through bone window, with evidence of inlet orifice, with high-attenuation fragments around and along the trajectory of the bullet, retained on the inner side of the occipital skull. Findings are suggestive of low energetic projectile. Particularly evident are the beam-hardening artifacts around the bullet

such as the scapula or the pelvis, as well as the ribs.

Generally, fractured bone extremities tend to form an angle that is obtuse towards the bullet-escaping side.

Adipose tissue usually presents a fading hyperdensity because of micro-hemorrhage associated to edema due to the impact of the projectile.

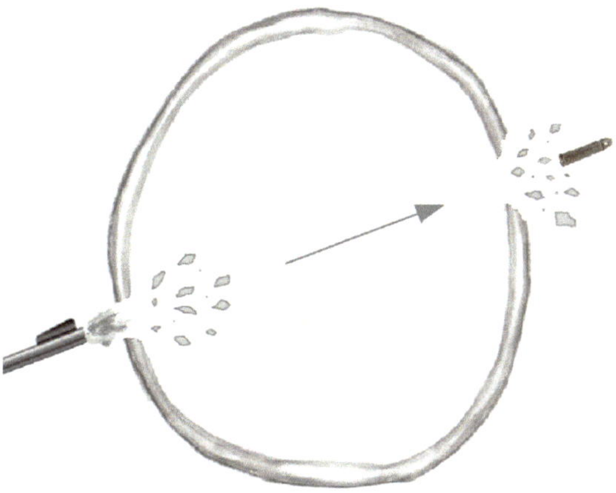

Fig. 15.4 Schematic representation of the projectile trajectory across the cranial theca; well shown are the effects of high velocity and energy impact between bullet and skull

Parenchymatous organs show very inhomogeneous density surrounding the projectile path because of tissue lacerations and consequent vessel hemorrhage; usually hypo-attenuating areas alternate with hyper-attenuating areas, both of them without clear margins. Hyperintense

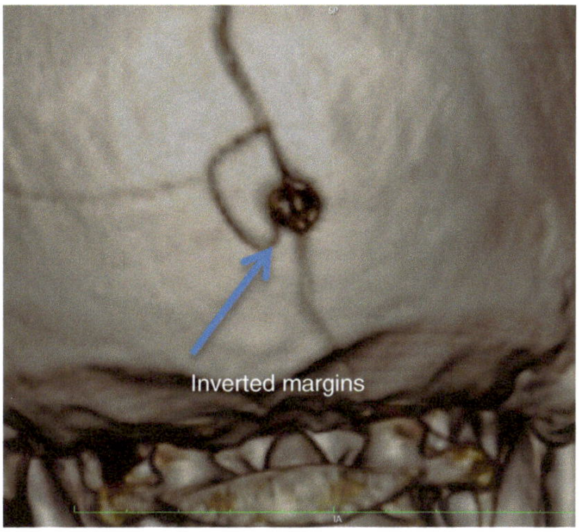

Fig. 15.6 3D volume rendering particularly of an inlet orifice, with visible inverted margins. Clear is a vertical fracture rim crossing the orifice, due to the impact with the bullet

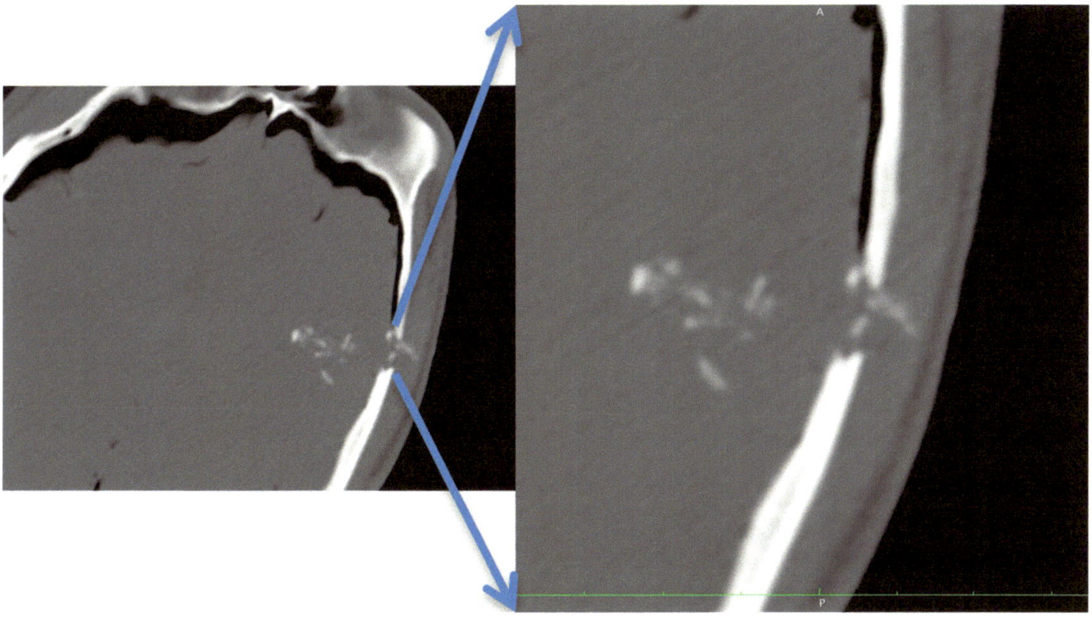

Fig. 15.5 Axial CT image, filtered with bone window, of a gunshot-wounded skull with the magnification of the inlet orifice, showing the typical truncated cone shape

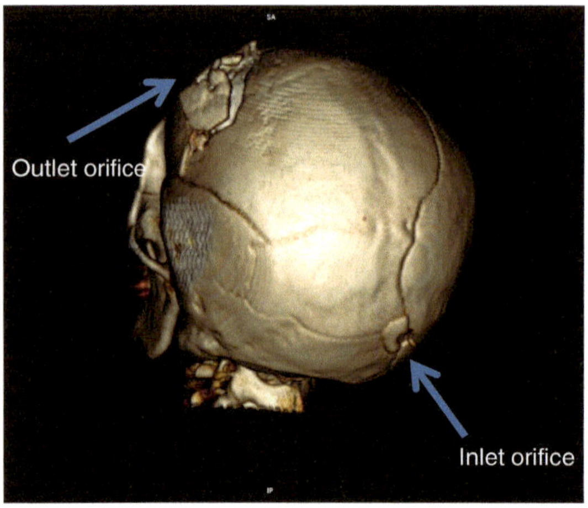

Fig. 15.7 3D VR of a complete skull showing inlet and outlet orifices; the former is a well-rounded wound, with clear margins, associated to a single skull fracture, while the latter presents multiple rims of fracture with commingled bone fragments, lifted up from unharmed bone

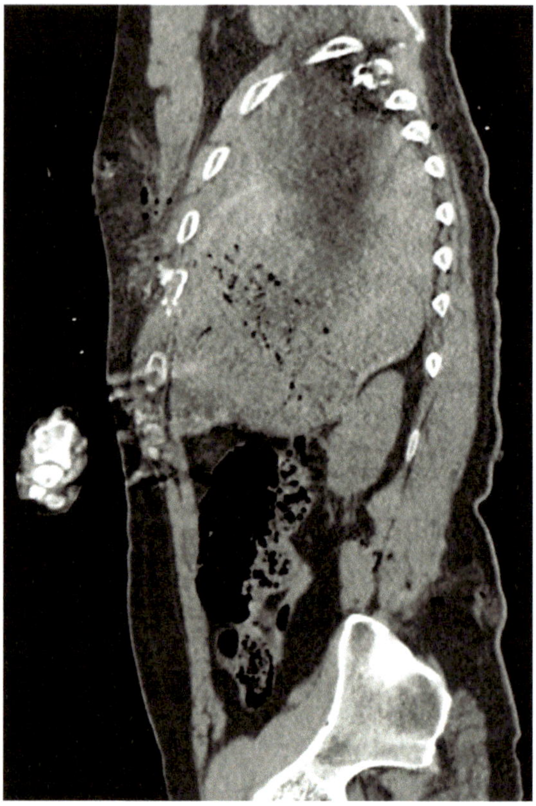

Fig. 15.8 Parasagittal MPR reconstruction of a whole bullet trajectory crossing abdominal cavity, involving soft subcutaneous tissues, kidney, liver, and ribbon

fragments (metallic or bony) may be found along the trajectory. Pneumothorax, pneumomediastinun, or pneumopericardium may be present when bullet, after piercing chest walls, involves these anatomical districts (Fig. 15.8).

As regards ***hollow organs***, mainly involved are intestinal loops, presenting wall interruption and thickening due to intramural edema and hemorrhage and concomitant edematous infarction of nearer mesenterium. Involvement of the gut may lead to a significant air spreading into the mesenteric fat, miming an intestinal perforation. Abnormal air quantity may also be seen in cardiac cavities if bullet transfixes it or upper airways together with great vessels.

Voluminous hemorrhages, seen as voluminous hyperintense collection with no clear margins, are present if the projectile damages main cardiovascular anatomical structures (heart; aorta; vena cava; pulmonary vessels; etc.).

15.6 Role of MDCT and Radiology in Medicolegal Investigation

As regards supporting autopsy and, in general, medicolegal investigations, PMCT is considered by a number of authors as a useful procedure that can elucidate patterns of injuries, providing strong medical evidence, especially useful in gunshot wound cases, allowing an easier location and retrieval of the bullet and/or its fragments inside the body.

As many studies report PMCT, completed by 3D MPR and VR reconstructions, has demonstrated to be really accurate in individuating the wound track discerning between entrance and exit wounds, the exact site of the bullet if retained, and the possible fragmentation and dispersion of the individual ballistic components (for example, separation on its way between jacket and lead core) and in identifying, quite accurately, the amount of visceral or bone lesions so as to define, with a high probability, the exact direction. PMCT therefore is considered absolutely reliable in correctly identifying all of the lethal wounds, and so the cause of death.

The same authors have, nevertheless, highlighted some limitations of the technique, such as the underestimation of the number of wounds if commingling paths occurred; the failure in helping identify specific sites of hemorrhage in case of chest wound; and even in case of craniofacial injury the path of the wound may not be clear. However a few cases of missed findings at autopsy (fracture of the cervical spine, bullet fragments in the posterior area of the neck), identified at MDCT, are reported. As reported by Filograna et al. another limitation consists of the radiologist's error, which however characterizes each radiological examination, both forensic and clinic.

Other conventional radiologic techniques have not still proved to be easily applicable and useful in supporting forensic evaluation in case of gunshot victims.

Some studies were carried out on postmortem MR (PMMR), e.g., to study bone marrow edema indirectly induced by a bullet, which barely missed the bone. PMMR is burdened by projectile metallic components that own magnetic susceptibility.

PMCT is desirable to become a standard in forensic practice as an aid to the traditional postmortem examination, aimed at obtaining as much information as possible in order to clarify the cause and manner of death.

The virtual autopsy, however, remains effective in identifying elements related to the circumstances of the death and in some specific case may enable the medical examiner not to perform an autopsy inspection (e.g.: single shot associated to certain victim history and circumstances of death, mass homicide).

Further Reading

Andenmatten MA, Thali MJ, Kneubuehl BP, Oesterhelweg L, Ross S, Spendlove D, Bolliger SA (2008) Gunshot injuries detected by post-mortem multi-slice computed tomography (MSCT): a feasibility study. Leg Med (Tokyo) 10(6):287–292

Berger N, Paula P, Gascho D, Flach PM, Thali MJ, Ross SG, Ampanozi G (2013) Bone marrow edema induced by a bullet after a self-inflicted accidental firing. Leg Med (Tokyo) 15(6):329–331

Bowen TE, Bellamy RF (1988) Emergency war surgery. In: Second United States revision of the emergency war surgery handbook. United States Department of Defense, Washington, DC, pp 74–82

DiMaio VJM (1999) Gunshot wounds. Practical aspects of firearms, ballistics, and forensic techniques. CRC Press, Boca Raton, FL

Donchin Y, Rivkind AI, Barziv J et al (1994) Utility of postmortem computed tomography in trauma victims. J Trauma 37(4):552–556

Dzieman AJ, Mendelson JA, Lindsey D (1961) Comparison of the wounding characteristics of some commonly encountered bullets. J Trauma 1:341–353

Fackler ML (1988) Wound ballistics. A review of common misconceptions. JAMA 259:2730–2736

Fackler ML, Malinowski JA (1985) The wound pro le: a visual method for quantifying gunshot wound components. J Trauma 25:522–529

Filograna L, Tartaglione T, Filograna E, Cittadini F, Oliva A, Pascali VL (2010) Computed tomography (CT) virtual autopsy and classical autopsy discrepancies: Radiologist's error or a demonstration of post-mortem multi-detector computed tomography limitation? Forensic Sci Int 195:e13–e17

Harcke HT, Levy AD, Abbott RM et al (2007) Autopsy radiography: digital radiographs (DR) vs. multidetector computed tomography (MDCT) in high-velocity gunshot wound victims. Am J Forensic Med Pathol 28:13–19

Heard BJ (2008) Handbook of firearms and ballistics. John Wiley, Chichester

Hollerman JJ, Fackler ML, Coldwell DM et al (1990) Gunshot wounds: 1. Bullets, ballistics, and mechanisms of injury. AJR Am J Roentgenol 155:685–690

Hollerman JJ, Fackler ML, Coldwell DM et al (1990) Gunshot wounds: 2. Radiology. AJR Am J Roentgenol 155:691–702

Jeffery AJ, Rutty GN, Robinson C, Morgan B (2008) Computed tomography of projectile injuries. Clin Radiol 63(10):1160–1166

Jeffery AJ (2010) The role of computed tomography in adult post-mortem examinations: an overview. Diagn Histopathol 16:546–551

Kahana T, Hiss J (1999) Forensic radiology. Br J Radiol 72:129–133

Karger B (2014) Handbook of forensic medicine. In: Madea B (ed) Forensic ballistics: injuries from gunshots, explosives and arrows, 1st edn. Wiley-Blackwell, Hoboken

Karger B (1995a) Penetrating gunshots to the head and lack of immediate incapacitation. I. Wound ballistics and mechanisms of incapacitation. Int J Leg Med 108:53–61

Karger B (1995b) Penetrating gunshots to the head and lack of immediate incapacitation. II. Review of case reports. Int J Leg Med 108:117–126

Karger B (2004) Schussverletzungen. In: Brinkmann B, Madea B (eds) Handbuch Gerichtliche Medizin. Springer, Berlin, pp 593–682

Karger B, Billeb E, Koops E, Brinkmann B (2002) Autopsy features relevant for discrimination between suicidal and homicidal gunshot injuries. Int J Leg Med 116:273–278

Karger B (2008) Forensic ballistics. In: Tsokos M (ed) Forensic pathology reviews, vol 5. Humana Press, Totowa, NJ, pp 139–174

Levy AD, Abbott RM, Mallak CT et al (2006) Virtual autopsy: preliminary experience in high-velocity gunshot wound victims. Radiology 240:522–528

MacPherson D (1994) Bullet penetration. Modeling the dynamics and the incapacitation resulting from wound trauma. Ballistic Publications, El Segundo, CA

Maiese A, Gitto L, De Matteis A, Panebianco V, Bolino G (2014) Post mortem computed tomography: useful or unnecessary in gunshot wounds deaths? Two case reports. Leg Med (Tokyo) 16(6):357–363

Milroy CM, Clark JC, Carter N et al (1998) Air weapon fatalities. J Clin Pathol 51:525–529

Oehmichen M, Meissner C, Konig HG et al (2004) Gunshot injuries to the head and brain caused by low-velocity handguns and rifles. A review. Forensic Sci Int 146:111–120

Peschel O, Szeimies U, Vollmar C, Kirchhoff S (2013) Postmortem 3-D reconstruction of skull gunshot injuries. Forensic Sci Int 233:45–50

Rutty GN, Boyce P, Robinson CE et al (2007) The role of computed tomography in terminal ballistic analysis. Int J Leg Med 122:1–5

Rutty GN (2007) Are autopsies necessary? The role of computed tomography as a possible alternative to invasive autopsies. Rechtsmedizin 17:21–28

Sellier K (1977) Schusswaffen und Schusswirkungen II. Schmidt-Römhild, Lübeck

Sellier K (1982) Schusswaffen und Schusswirkungen I. Schmidt-Römhild, Lübeck

Sellier K, Kneubuehl BP (1994) Wound ballistics and the scientific background. Elsevier, Amsterdam

Tartaglione T, Filograna L, Roiati S, Guglielmi G, Colosimo C, Bonomo L (2012) Importance of 3D-CT imaging in single-bullet cranioencephalic gunshot wounds. Radiol Med 117(3):461–470

Thali MJ, Viner MD, Brogdon BG (2011) Brogdon's forensic radiology, 2nd edn. CRC Press, Boca Raton, FL

Thali MJ, Yen K, Vock P et al (2003) Image-guided virtual autopsy findings of gunshot victims performed with multi-slice computed tomography and magnetic resonance imaging and subsequent correlation between radiology and autopsy findings. Forensic Sci Int 138:8–16

Wilson AJ (1999) Gunshot injuries: what does a radiologist need to know? Radiographics 19:1358–1368

Body Packing

16

Antonio Pinto, Alfonso Reginelli, Anna Russo, Giuseppina Fabozzi, Sabrina Giovine, and Luigia Romano

16.1 Introduction

Body packing is the ingestion or insertion of packed illicit substances in the human body. Dr. Deitel and Dr. Syed [1] illustrated first body packing in 1973, describing a patient with intestinal obstruction 2 weeks after ingesting hashish contained in a condom. Since then, drug smuggling has increased and new means of transport of narcotics have emerged. The most used regions of the body for this purpose are the components of the gastrointestinal tract: from mouth to anus, vagina, and ears. A wide range of illicit drugs may be transported using this way, including cocaine, heroin, marijuana, hashish, amphetamines, and "ecstasy" [2]. Cocaine is one of the most trafficked drugs, followed by heroin [3]. Condoms, latex gloves, and balloons are typically used as drug packets for retention in the body [4, 5]. While "*body packers*" transport packets of wrapped cocaine within their gastrointestinal tract by swallowing them, "*body pushers*" insert the packets into body cavities: vagina, rectum, or ears [6]. Body packers may also be named "*couriers*," "*internal carriers*," "*swallowers*," or "*mules*," whereas the term "*body stuffing*" refers to the swallowing of comparably small amounts of freely encased drug because of the scare of jailing and without planned attempt to carry the drugs across borders [7]. Body packers usually carry about 1 kg of narcotic, separated into 50–100 packets of 8–10 g each, even though more than 200 packets have been found in individual smugglers [8]. Radiological imaging methods are essential to diagnose body packing and to detect potential complications [9]. Increasing sophistication of traffickers and improvements in packaging add to the detection difficulty [10].

A. Pinto (✉) · L. Romano
Azienda Ospedaliera dei Colli,
Monaldi-Cotugno-CTO, Naples, Italy
e-mail: luigia.romano@aocardarelli.it

A. Reginelli · A. Russo
Department of Internal and Experimental Medicine,
University of Campania "Luigi Vanvitelli",
Naples, Italy
e-mail: alfonso.reginelli@unicampania.it;
anna.russo@unicampania.it

G. Fabozzi · S. Giovine
Department of Radiology, SG Moscati Hospital,
Aversa, Italy
e-mail: giuseppina.fabozzi@unicampania.it;
sabrina.giovine@unicampania.it

16.2 Drugs, Packets, and Body Packers

Usually, there are three main drugs smuggled using body packing: cocaine, heroin, and cannabis products. Synthetic drugs, such as ecstasy and lysergic acid, are uncommonly detected in body packers, probably because of the lower financial motivation associated with their transport and the

G. Lo Re et al. (eds.), *Radiology in Forensic Medicine*,
https://doi.org/10.1007/978-3-319-96737-0_16

easiness of synthesis closer to the end user [10]. The orally ingested packets are commonly round in shape, whereas the genitally inserted packets are usually oval, measuring 4–6 cm in length and 2–3 cm in width [11].

Three different types of cocaine packets have been described by McCarron and Wood [12]. Type I comprises roughly packed cocaine powder protected by two to four films of condoms: such a packet is particularly susceptible to leakage and rupture. Type II and type III include firmly packed cocaine powder or paste. The second type is strongly covered in several layers of tubular latex, while the third type has a layer of aluminum foil. Moreover, the type IV packet has been described by Pidoto et al. [13]: it is prepared by dissolving cocaine hydrochloride in a watery alcohol solution. The resultant dense cocaine paste is transferred into a processing apparatus and, when reinforced, is ready for packaging in tubular latex.

Body packers commonly ingest large bags (2–8 cm) containing drugs prior to crossing international borders, to recover them after arrival at their destination. Their drug bags are carefully packed and enveloped in containers expected to remain undamaged during the gastrointestinal tract transit [14].

The highest frequently involved drug is cocaine [15]. Each of these cocaine-filled packets measures 8–10 mm and consists of around 2–6 g of cocaine powder of variable cleanness (5–20%), mostly badly encased in several layers of packing material of changeable type, including glassine crack, plastic bags, cellophane paper, plastic wraps, aluminum foil, and condoms.

After swallowing the drugs, constipating agents such as diphenoxylate or loperamide may be used to extend the travel time. The travel time may alter from 24 h to 3 weeks [16]. After entering the destination section, the smugglers could use laxatives to get rid of their packets [17]. Under normal conditions, spontaneous passage of a drug-filled packet through the digestive system occurs within 30 h. However, in order to delay the bowel transit time, body packers may deliberately take anticholinergic agents to reduce bowel motility. Once they are at the point of arrival, they use laxatives, cathartics, or enemas to facilitate the passage of packets [18].

16.3 Radiological Methods to Investigate Body Packers

Imaging is essential in diagnosing body packing [19–22]. Plain abdominal radiography is the most common examination method [23–25]. Huge availability makes plain abdominal X-ray a relatively good screening tool to check out suspected body packers. Sensitivity for detection of drug packets by initial abdominal X-rays varies widely in the published literature with lower limits suggested to be 40% and upper limits over 90% in past decades [26–28]. Variability in detection depends on the type and purity of drugs (altering density), size and number of packets, packet material, location within intestines, and reader's experience. Densely packed heroin, hashish, and cocaine may have similar radiological appearances, being more radio-opaque than fecal balls on plain abdominal film. On plain abdominal radiographs, the common drug packet mimics are normal intestinal air, calcifications, scybala, and other foreign bodies [29–34].

Ultrasonography is infrequently used in the evaluation of suspected body packers. The disadvantages of US are its failure to identify the exact number of packages, to differentiate the types of drugs, and to be highly operator dependent [35]. Ultrasonography is a possible body-packing imaging method for pregnant women [36] even if it has a high sensitivity but a low specificity in suspected cases. Few studies have suggested that ultrasound represents a rather valuable diagnostic method in the assessment of ingested drug packages [37].

Magnetic resonance imaging (MRI) is rarely used as first-line emergency modality because of its high costs and limited availability. MRI is of limited value in detecting drug packets because of the lack of protons and motion artifacts caused by the bowel loops. The bowel must be immobilized with spasmolytic agents prior to MR study to reduce artifacts created by peristalsis [38, 39].

Currently, the management of drug packers is moving to rely more heavily on CT examination. Its sensitivity ranges from 95.6% to 100% [40]. It is commonly used for cases with negative abdominal plain films, which remain strongly suspicious of drug packing [12]. CT examination should be performed without oral or rectal contrast material administration, which may obscure concealed packages because of similarities in density. Before reading the CT examination, the scout CT view should be examined [41] especially in cases without a first plain radiograph. On CT examination, it is crucial to assess the entire gastrointestinal tract carefully, from the esophagus to the rectum [42]. Detection increases by viewing at lung settings—window width 1000 HU and window level 2700 HU—in addition to the common abdominal CT settings (window width 350 HU and window level 50 HU) [43].

Recently, some authors [44] reported that low-dose CT may be a practical alternative to abdominal radiography and will lead to improvements in the identification of illegal intra-abdominal packets. However, even CT is not infallible and there have been case reports of false-negative CT investigations [45, 46].

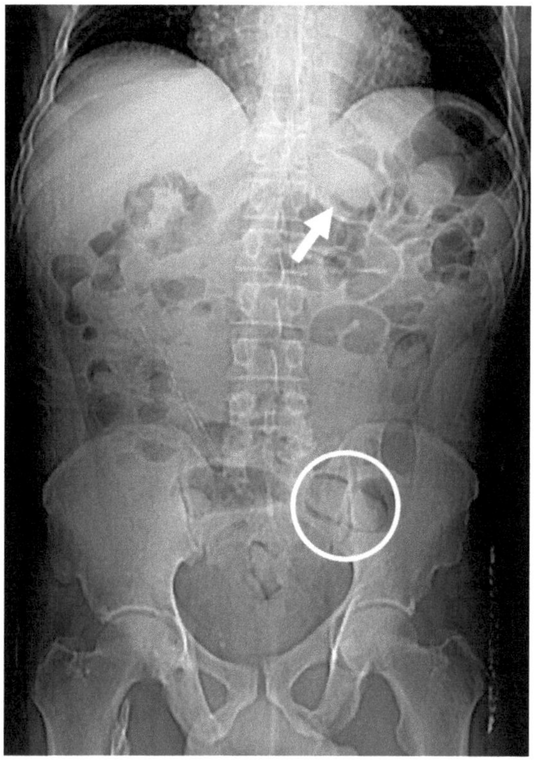

Fig. 16.1 Plain abdominal radiograph showing one well-defined opacity (white arrow) in the stomach not suggestive for alimentary content and the "double-condom sign" (white circle) defined as a clear crescent of air bordering an ovoid opacity

16.4 Radiological Appearance of Drug Packets

On plain abdominal radiographs, the radiologist should search for the presence of the following findings: (a) one or multiple well-defined opacities in the stomach, small bowel, or large bowel that are not suggestive of alimentary content [8]; (b) the "double-condom sign," defined as a clear crescent of air bordering an ovoid opacity [8]; (c) a smooth and uniformly shaped oblong structure, sometimes called the "tic-tac sign" [32]; and (d) the "parallelism sign," defined as firm packages aligning parallel to each other in the bowel lumen [32] (Figs. 16.1 and 16.2).

On ultrasonography, the packets appear as linear, oval or round, arcuate, smooth, and hyperechogenic structures, with posterior acoustic shadowing. They are better detected if the hollow viscus is filled with fluid [47].

As on plain abdominal film, the ingested packets appear on CT examination as round or oval dense foreign bodies located within the gastrointestinal tract, and classic appearances such as the "tic-tac sign" may be visible [48] (Fig. 16.3). The "rosette sign" is identified by the presence of air within the knot of the tied condom containing the drug in a manually wrapped packet: this sign is rarely observed nowadays because narcotic cartels are currently utilizing sophisticated packaging methods [11]. Other CT findings of drug packets are multiplicity of foreign bodies, double-condom sign, and parallelism sign [8]. Manipulation of CT may distinguish different types of drugs by estimating their HU [49] (Fig. 16.4).

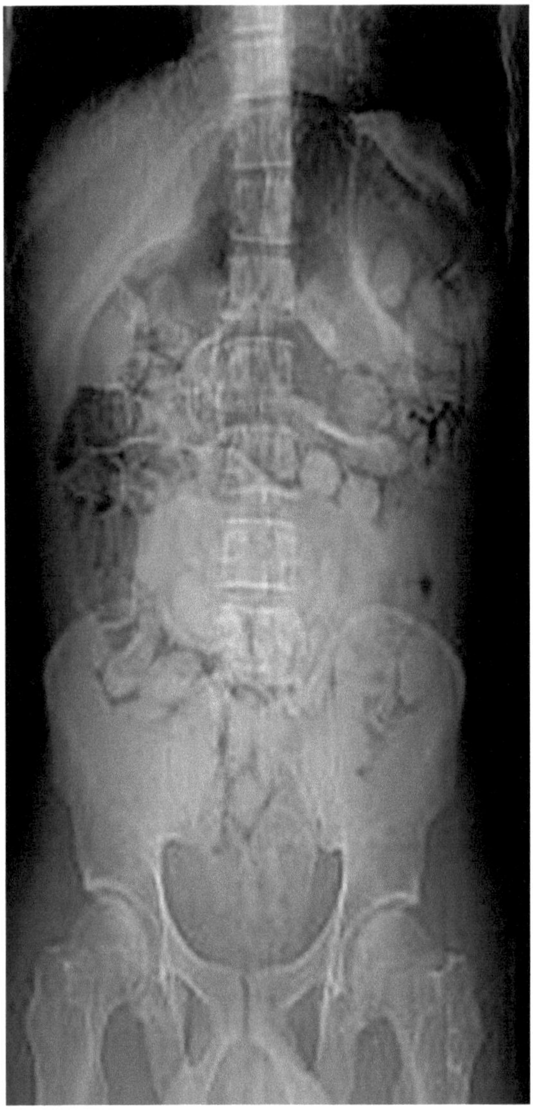

Fig. 16.2 Plain abdominal film shows a smooth and uniformly shaped oblong structure, sometimes called the "tic-tac sign" and the "parallelism sign," defined as firm packages aligning parallel to each other in the bowel lumen

16.5 Complications of Body Packing

Sophistication of the packaging methods used by drug smuggling organizations has reduced the morbidity of their "drug mules," although packet failure still represents a real risk and may cause poisoning in the country of origin, during flight or at their destination. The "body packer syndrome" occurs when packet rupture results in poisoning, usually after cocaine or heroin ingestion [50].

Body packers may present to healthcare providers in three ways: with signs and symptoms of drug toxicity owing to leaking or ruptured packets, with symptoms of gastrointestinal obstruction or perforation, or asymptomatic, either because they fear the consequences of packet rupture or because they are under arrest.

In the patient with "body packer syndrome" the symptoms should be promptly identifiable and point to the drug being carried. Cocaine may cause agitation, tachycardia, hypertension, sweating, dilated pupils, and hyperthermia. More serious effects are status epilepticus, seizures, myocardial infarction, and ventricular fibrillation. Heroin may produce a decreased level of consciousness, respiratory depression, and pinpoint pupils. Rupture or leakage may occur either by mechanical movement or by chemical digestion [51, 52].

Ingesting relatively large foreign bodies and slowing down passage can cause small- or large-bowel obstruction, possibly complicated by bowel perforation and subsequent peritonitis [53, 54]. Packet rupture will cause acute intoxication with the clinical outcome depending on the content of the packets, the amount spilled, and the timely intervention by medical staff.

Complications by intestinal obstruction and acute intoxication are now estimated to be below 5% [55].

16.6 Ethical and Medicolegal Issues

In the wake of the events of September 11, 2001, security at border crossings in the United States has increased dramatically. One of the unintended consequences of this action has been an increase in drug seizures. Faced with this increase in security, drug smugglers may begin using children, older people, and pregnant women as vehicles to transport their cargo [56, 57].

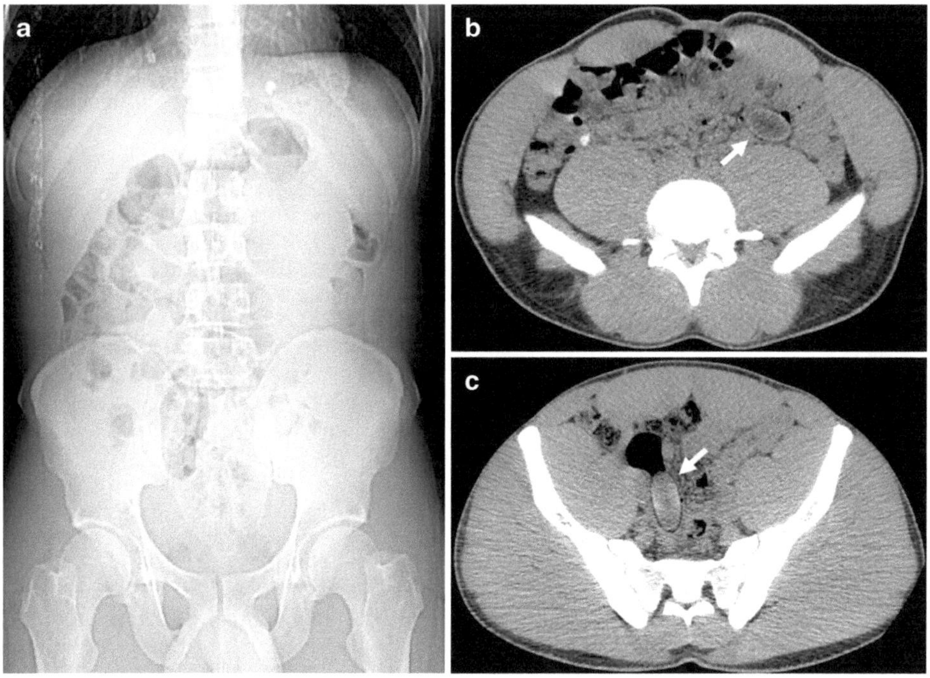

Fig. 16.3 CT examination: scout view (**a**) and axial scans (**b**, **c**). The ingested packets are detected as round or oval dense foreign bodies located within different portions of the gastrointestinal tract (white arrows) with classic appearance such as the "tic-tac sign"

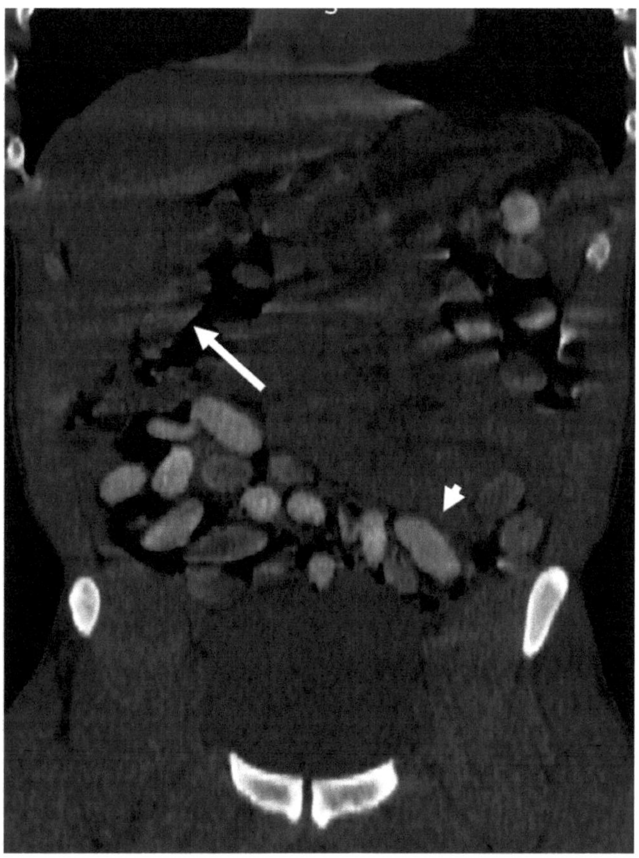

Fig. 16.4 CT examination (coronal reconstruction) shows different types of drugs by estimating their HU as low (white arrow) or high (white arrowhead) density

Pregnant women represent a challenge in management, particularly in the event of package rupture. In the pregnant body packer, a detailed medical history and physical examination are necessary before an appropriate treatment scheme is implemented, as treatment must address the anatomic and physiologic changes of pregnancy, essentially involving two patients.

People included in these illegal practices refer to the emergency department with multiple diagnostic, ethical, and legal issues. In addition to confirming the presence of concealed drugs, the radiologist must recognize and look for the signs of complications that these drug packages can cause. These include small-bowel or large-bowel obstruction, gastrointestinal perforation, and subsequent acute peritonitis [8].

Body packers usually know the exact amount of cargo they carry, but they have reasons to be deceitful, and the history may therefore be unreliable. Body packers in legal custody may refuse to undergo invasive (i.e., rectal) examinations and radiography, but they cannot insist on being medically cleared and discharged. Appropriate management is admission for observation.

16.7 Conclusions

Emergency departments face an increasing number of drug-related health problems, with difficult medicolegal and social consequences.

To minimize morbidity and mortality, imaging is increasingly being used, both for screening for the presence of packets and for investigating possible clinical complications once brought to medical attention. Radiologists should be aware of the imaging characteristics and test performances of radiography and CT to minimize false negatives and false positives and maintain good accuracy. CT with reduced radiation dose will likely be used more in the future.

References

1. Deitel M, Syed AK (1973) Intestinal obstruction by an unusual foreign body. Can Med Assoc J 109(3):211–212
2. Shahnazi M, Sanei Taheri M, Pourghorban R (2011) Body packing and its radiologic manifestations: a review article. Iran J Radiol 8(4):205–210
3. Utecht MJ, Stone AF, McCarron MM (1993) Heroin body packers. J Emerg Med 11(1):33–40
4. Kucukmetin NT, Gucyetmez B, Poyraz T, Yildirim S, Boztas G, Tozun N (2014) Foreign material in the gastrointestinal tract: cocaine packets. Case Rep Gastroenterol 8(1):56–60. (eCollection 2014)
5. Meyers MA (1995) The inside dope: cocaine, condoms, and computed tomography. Abdom Imaging 20(4):339–340
6. Schaper A, Hofmann R, Bargain P, Desel H, Ebbecke M, Langer C (2007) Surgical treatment in cocaine body packers and body pushers. Int J Color Dis 22(12):1531–1535
7. Reginelli A, Russo A, Urraro F, Maresca D, Martiniello C, D'Andrea A, Brunese L, Pinto A (2015) Imaging of body packing: errors and medico-legal issues. Abdom Imaging 40(7):2127–2142
8. Hergan K, Kofler K, Oser W (2004) Drug smuggling by body packing: what radiologists should know about it. Eur Radiol 14(4):736–742
9. Pinto A, Sparano A, Cinque T (2012) Foreign body ingestion and rectal foreign body insertion: diagnostic challenges. In: Romano L, Pinto A (eds) Errors in radiology. Springer Italia, Milan, pp 271–278
10. Pinto A, Reginelli A, Pinto F, Sica G, Scaglione M, Berger FH, Romano L, Brunese L (2014) Radiological and practical aspects of body packing. Br J Radiol 87(1036):20130500
11. Ab Hamid S, Abd Rashid SN, Mohd Saini S (2012) Characteristic imaging features of body packers: a pictorial essay. Jpn J Radiol 30(5):386–392
12. McCarron MM, Wood JD (1983) The cocaine "body packer" syndrome. Diagnosis and treatment. JAMA 250(11):1417–1420
13. Pidoto RR, Agliata AM, Bertolini R, Mainini A, Rossi G, Giani G (2002) A new method of packaging cocaine for international traffic and implications for the management of cocaine body packers. J Emerg Med 23(2):149–153
14. Traub SJ, Hoffman RS, Nelson LS (2003) Body packing—the internal concealment of illicit drugs. N Engl J Med 349(26):2519–2526
15. Fineschi V, Centini F, Monciotti F, Turillazzi E (2002) The cocaine "body stuffer" syndrome: a fatal case. Forensic Sci Int 126(1):7–10

16. Khan FY (2005) The cocaine 'body-packer' syndrome: diagnosis and treatment. Indian J Med Sci 59(10):457–458
17. Wetli CV, Mittlemann RE (1981) The "body packer syndrome"—toxicity following ingestion of illicit drugs packaged for transportation. J Forensic Sci 26(3):492–500
18. Booker RJ, Smith JE, Rodger MP (2009) Packers, pushers and stuffers—managing patients with concealed drugs in UK emergency departments: a clinical and medicolegal review. Emerg Med J 26(5):316–320
19. Algra PR, Brogdon BG, Marugg RC (2007) Role of radiology in a national initiative to interdict drug smuggling: the Dutch experience. AJR Am J Roentgenol 189(2):331–336
20. Beerman R, Nunez D Jr, Wetli CV (1986) Radiographic evaluation of the cocaine smuggler. Gastrointest Radiol 11(4):351–354
21. Grassi R, Di Mizio R, Pinto A, Romano L, Rotondo A (2004) Serial plain abdominal film findings in the assessment of acute abdomen: spastic ileus, hypotonic ileus, mechanical ileus and paralytic ileus. Radiol Med 108(1–2):56–70
22. Pinto A, Muzj C, Gagliardi N, Pinto F, Setola FR, Scaglione M, Romano L (2012) Role of imaging in the assessment of impacted foreign bodies in the hypopharynx and cervical esophagus. Semin Ultrasound CT MR 33(5):463–470
23. Horrocks AW (1992) Abdominal radiography in suspected "body packers". Clin Radiol 45(5):322–325
24. Krishnan A, Brown R (1999) Plain abdominal radiography in the diagnosis of the "body packer". J Accid Emerg Med 16(5):381
25. Lo Re G, Mantia FL, Picone D, Salerno S, Vernuccio F, Midiri M (2016) Small bowel perforations: what the radiologist needs to know. Semin Ultrasound CT MR 37(1):23–30
26. Flach PM, Ross SG, Ampanozi G, Ebert L, Germerott T, Hatch GM, Thali MJ, Patak MA (2012) "Drug mules" as a radiological challenge: sensitivity and specificity in identifying internal cocaine in body packers, body pushers and body stuffers by computed tomography, plain radiography and Lodox. Eur J Radiol 81(10):2518–2526
27. Hierholzer J, Cordes M, Tantow H, Keske U, Maurer J, Felix R (1995) Drug smuggling by ingested cocaine-filled packages: conventional x-ray and ultrasound. Abdom Imaging 20(4):333–338
28. Rousset P, Chaillot P, Audureau E, Rey-Salmon C, Becour B, Fitton I, Vadrot D, Revel MP (2013) Detection of residual packets in cocaine body packers: low accuracy of abdominal radiography-a prospective study. Eur Radiol 23(8):2146–2155
29. Caruana DS, Weinbach B, Goerg D, Gardner LB (1984) Cocaine-packet ingestion. Diagnosis, management, and natural history. Ann Intern Med 100(1):73–74
30. Grassi R, Pinto A, Valente T, Rossi G, Catalano O, Rotondo A, Landolfi V, Del Genio A (1997) Massive enterolithiasis associated with ileal dysgenesis. Br J Radiol 70:207–209
31. Lo Re G, De Luca R, Muscameri F, Dorangricchia P, Picone D, Vernuccio F, Salerno S, La Tona G, Pinto A, Midiri M, Russo A, Lagalla R, Cicero G (2016) Relationship between anxiety level and radiological investigation. Comparison among different diagnostic imaging exams in a prospective single-center study. Radiol Med 121(10):763–768
32. Niewiarowski S, Gogbashian A, Afaq A, Kantor R, Win Z (2010) Abdominal X-ray signs of intra-intestinal drug smuggling. J Forensic Legal Med 17:198–202
33. Pinto A, Reginelli A, Pinto F, Lo Re G, Midiri F, Muzj C, Romano L, Brunese L (2016) Errors in imaging patients in the emergency setting. Br J Radiol 89:20150914
34. Sica G, Guida F, Bocchini G, Iaselli F, Iadevito I, Scaglione M (2015) Imaging of drug smuggling by body packing. Semin Ultrasound CT MR 36(1):39–47
35. Meijer R, Bots ML (2003) Detection of intestinal drug containers by ultrasound scanning: an airport screening tool? Eur Radiol 13(6):1312–1315
36. Cordero DR, Medina C, Helfgott A (2006) Cocaine body packing in pregnancy. Ann Emerg Med 48(3):323–325
37. Cengel F, Bulakci M, Selcuk T, Savas Y, Ceyhan M, Kocak A, Bilgili CO (2015) The role of ultrasonography in the imaging of body packers comparison with CT: a prospective study. Abdom Imaging 40(7):2143–2151
38. Bulakci M, Ozbakir B, Kiris A (2013) Detection of body packing by magnetic resonance imaging: a new diagnostic tool? Abdom Imaging 38(3):436–441
39. Lo Re G, Tudisca C, Vernuccio F, Picone D, Cappello M, Agnello F, Galia M, Galfano MC, Biscaldi E, Salerno S, Pinto A, Midiri M, Lagalla R (2016) MR imaging of perianal fistulas in Crohn's disease: sensitivity and specificity of STIR sequences. Radiol Med 121(4):243–251
40. Lee K, Koehn M, Rastegar RF, van Hoorn F, Roy E, Berger FH, Nicolaou S (2012) Body packers: the ins and outs of imaging. Can Assoc Radiol J 63(4):318–322
41. Sengupta A, Page P (2008) Window manipulation in the diagnosis of body packing using computerized tomography. Emerg Radiol 15(3):203–205
42. Pinto A, Miele V, Pinto F, Di Mizio V, Panico MR, Muzj C, Romano L (2014) Rectal foreign bodies: imaging assessment and medicolegal aspects. Semin Ultrasound CT MRI 36(1):88–93

43. Ziegeler E, Grimm JM, Wirth S, Uhl M, Reiser MF, Scherr MK (2012) Computed tomography scout views vs. conventional radiography in body-packers—delineation of body-packs and radiation dose in a porcine model. Eur J Radiol 81(12):3883–3889
44. Poletti PA, Canel L, Becker CD, Wolff H, Elger B, Lock E, Sarasin F, Bonfanti MS, Dupuis-Lozeron E, Perneger T, Platon A (2012) Screening of illegal intracorporeal containers ("body packing"): is abdominal radiography sufficiently accurate ? A comparative study with low-dose CT. Radiology 265(3):772–779
45. Eng JG, Aks SE, Waldron R, Marcus C, Issleib S (1999) False-negative abdominal CT scan in a cocaine body stuffer. Am J Emerg Med 17(7):702–704
46. Hahn IH, Hoffman RS, Nelson LS (2004) Contrast CT scan fails to detect the last heroin packet. J Emerg Med 27(3):279–283
47. Chung CH, Fung WT (2006) Detection of gastric drug packet by ultrasound scanning. Eur J Emerg Med 13(5):302–303
48. Taheri MS, Hassanian-Moghaddam H, Birang S, Hemadi H, Shahnazi M, Jalali AH, Shakiba M, Nahvi V (2008) Swallowed opium packets: CT diagnosis. Abdom Imaging 33(3):262–266
49. Schmidt S, Hugli O, Rizzo E, Lepori D, Gudinchet F, Yersin B, Schnyder P, Meuwly JY (2008) Detection of ingested cocaine-filled packets—diagnostic value of unenhanced CT. Eur J Radiol 67(1):133–138
50. Greenberg R, Greenberg Y, Kaplan O (2000) 'Body packer' syndrome: characteristics and treatment—case report and review. Eur J Surg 166(1):89–91
51. Dorn T, Ceelen M, de Keijzer KJ, Buster MC, Luitse JS, Vandewalle E, Brouwer HJ, Das K (2013) Prevalence and medical risks of body packing in the Amsterdam area. J Forensic Legal Med 20(2):86–90
52. Mandava N, Chang RS, Wang JH, Bertocchi M, Yrad J, Allamaneni S, Aboian E, Lall MH, Mariano R, Richards N (2011) Establishment of a definitive protocol for the diagnosis and management of body packers (drug mules). Emerg Med J 28(2):98–101
53. Brown JA, Phang PT, Enns R, Butchart MK, Filipenko JD, Mason AC, Cooperberg PL (2002) Computed tomography to detect body packing: an unusual cause of small bowel obstruction. Can Assoc Radiol J 53(2):84–86
54. Cawich SO, Downes R, Martin AC, Evans NR, Mitchell DIS, Williams E (2010) Colonic perforation: a lethal consequence of cannabis body packing. J Forensic Legal Med 17(5):269–271
55. Berger FH, Nieboer KH, Goh GS, Pinto A, Scaglione M (2015) Body packing: a review of general background, clinical and imaging aspects. Radiol Med 120(1):118–132
56. Chakrabarty A, Hydros S, Puliyel JM (2006) Smuggling contraband drugs using paediatric "body packers". Arch Dis Child 91(1):51
57. Traub SJ, Kohn GL, Hoffman RS, Nelson LS (2003) Pediatric "body packing". Arch Pediatr Adolesc Med 157(2):174–177

17 Occupational Diseases: Asbestosis and Mesothelioma in Forensic Practice

Ambra Di Piazza, Antonina Argo, Edoardo Scalici, Antonio Guajana, Dario Picone, and Giuseppe Lo Re

In medicolegal [1] and forensic [2] observation occupational diseases have quite rare occurrence and are dealt with problems usually related to:

1. Causal chain reconstruction
2. Evidence of antemortem exposure
3. Relevance of incidental pathological findings at autopsy

To support the diagnosis, characteristic radiologic features and a combination of clinical features, related occupational history, literature supporting, and an association between the exposure and the disease process are requested. Further pathological findings emerging at biopsy or autopsy ancillary examination techniques may assist in the judgment related to causal chain reconstruction [3]; in this perspective the multidisciplinary (radiological, forensic, and clinical) approach is mandatory for medicolegal issues. To point out abovementioned key points of interest following cases will be illustrated to underline both autopsy and radiological features, essential to recognize and interpret for specific forensic field. Industrial injury benefits from occupational lung disease in most countries are currently referred to national or private work insurance, after medical causal recognition of time of work exposure. In Italy [4], all supposed or verified cases concerning asbestos exposure and mesotheliomas are considered by dedicated Work Medical Board Center [5]. In case of death of worker, as penal code refers to personal injuries and death, often medicolegal investigation is required by the court; causal effective role may be in conclusion defined as possible, or related to, or indemonstrable due to multiple exposure from environmental pollutant, which last denied the benefits for workers. In this context asbestos body/fiber demonstration plays a role in medicolegal context [6]. There are several ways to attempt to identify asbestos at postmortem. The easiest is to slice the lung parenchyma with a blade and to express pulmonary fluid onto several clean glass slides. A coverslip can be placed over this wet preparation and the slide examined microscopically for ferruginous asbestos bodies. Alternatively, the exposed lung tissue can be scraped with the blade and the material applied onto a clean glass slide and examined microscopically in the same way [2]. If asbestos bodies are seen then previous exposure is confirmed but the following methods may still be required for documentation and quantification of the degree of morphological abnormality. If asbestos is not identified then this does not exclude previous exposure and further sampling

A. Di Piazza (✉) · D. Picone · G. Lo Re
Department of Diagnostic Imaging, University of Palermo, Palermo, Italy

A. Argo · E. Scalici · A. Guajana
Department for Health Promotion, Maternal and Child Care, University of Palermo, Palermo, Italy
e-mail: antonella.argo@unipa.it; edoardo.scalici@unipa.it

G. Lo Re et al. (eds.), *Radiology in Forensic Medicine*,
https://doi.org/10.1007/978-3-319-96737-0_17

is necessary. Electron microscopy methods significantly underestimate the number of fibers that are present in a particular lung sample. If accurate quantification is required, then electron microscopical analysis is necessary. Measurements are made at around ×20,000 magnification. Some of the different types of asbestos fibers can also be distinguished using X-ray diffraction analysis [7].

17.1 Silicosis

Pneumoconiosis is a tissue reaction to the presence of an accumulation of dust in the lungs. One clinicopathologic form of this reaction is fibrosis, which can be focal and nodular (as in silicosis) or diffuse and reticular (as in asbestosis) [8]. The principal sources of industrial exposure to silica are free silica in mining, quarrying, tunneling, stonecutting, polishing, cleaning monumental masonry, sandblasting, and glass manufacturing and, in foundry work, pottery and porcelain manufacturing, brick lining, boiler scaling, and vitreous enameling. Coal miners are exposed to dusts that contain a mixture of coal, mica, kaolin, and silica in varying proportions [9]. Silicosis belongs to the group of pneumoconiosis and is caused by the inhalation of fine particles of crystalline silicon dioxide (silica). The evolution of the disease depends on quantity and time of exposure. High-resolution CT (HRCT) represents the gold standard in the evaluation of interstitial lung disease. Clinical presentation has always a late onset with an average time of 20 years after exposure. At the onset, mild forms could be asymptomatic; however dyspnea, cough, and expectoration are common symptoms in the late stage of the disease, especially when associated with tabagism or concurrent infections. Tubercular infection, moreover, can complicate silicosis and has to be suspected when symptoms as fever and weight loss are associated. Nodular silicosis or simple silicosis is not characterized by functional alterations; however in advanced forms an obstructive or a restricted or combined pattern can be present. Although there is no association between functional damage and radiological findings, functional tests can be altered before radiological alterations are seen [10]. Clinical presentation is characterized by two main forms: acute silicosis and classical one, which is divided into simple and complicated. Acute silicosis, also known as silicoproteinosis, is a rare condition related to heavy exposure to respirable free silica in enclosed spaces in which there is minimal or no protection from the silica. Radiological and clinical features are due to the filling of the airspace in the lung with proteinaceous material. Exposure times are frequently as short as 6–8 months. The disease is often rapidly progressive, with death caused by respiratory failure [9]. At chest radiographs a pattern of diffuse airspace or ground-glass disease in a peri-hilar distribution with air bronchograms is recognized [11]. HRCT shows bilateral centrilobular nodular ground-glass opacities, multifocal patchy ground-glass opacities, and consolidation, to refer to intra-alveolar accumulation of proteinaceous material. Sometimes a crazy-paving appearance, characterized by airspace filling and interlobular septal thickening, may be found [12]. The classical form, as suggested from the name, is more common and can be divided into two different forms according to radiological appearance. The first one is simple silicosis which is characterized by a pattern of small and round or irregular opacities. Nodular pattern represents the imaging standard. More common radiological findings are bilateral, symmetrical distributed small nodules (between 1 and 5 mm) both centrilobular and subpleural. The nodules are especially localized in the dorsal segments of the upper lobes and in the apical segments of the inferior lobes. In fact middle lung zone or peripheral one-third of the lung is more involved [13]. Smaller nodules can have more smooth margins than the bigger ones. Multifocal patchy ground-glass opacities can also be evidentiated [14]. In an overview, pulmonary volume can be normal or increased. Other radiological features are nodules localized in the subpleural zone which converge in agglomerations and seem to be pleural plaque, defined also pseudo-plaque [15]. Hilar and mediastinal adenopathy may precede the appearance of classical parenchymal lesions. Moreover, lymph node may calcificate, especially in the peripheral zone, configuring the eggshell calcification which is considered a highly suggestive pattern of silicosis.

Moreover big lesions are characterized by a progressive loss of regular margins and can configure consolidation, and configure the typical complicated form, which is a progressive massive fibrosis, developing through the expansion and confluence of silicotic nodules, in which focal necrosis can be present. At chest radiography it is possible to recognize large symmetrical bilateral opacities with a diameter of more than 1 cm with shaped margins. The coalescence of the nodule results in large opacities, more common in the middle lung zone or peripheral one-third of the lung [9]. HRCT highlights the presence of progressive massive fibrosis and emphysema. Calcifications may be present in the large opacities. Silicotuberculosis is a common complication in silicosis. It is characterized by asymmetric nodules or consolidation, cavitation, and rapid disease progression.

17.2 Asbestos-Related Pathologies

Exposure to asbestos is an important public health problem in all industrial societies. The term asbestos refers to several fibrous silicate minerals with the common feature of high resistance. They can be divided into two groups on the base of their form: serpentines and amphiboles. The most used type is chrysotile, belonging to serpentine group. The inhaled asbestos fiber penetrates deeply into the lung and pleura and starts a fibrogenic process. Asbestos-related disease can be divided into benign pleural diseases and parenchymal diseases both benign and malignant. Asbestos-related benign pleural diseases include pleural plaques, which are the most common presentation. They are more often asymptomatic and are detected at standard chest radiography, only 20 years after the exposure [16]. At HRCT it appears as discrete, focal irregular areas of pleural thickening of the parietal pleura along posterolateral and diaphragmatic contours of the lower thorax, often with sparing of the lung apices and costophrenic angles. Calcification is often associated. Asbestosis is rarely present without pleural plaques (Fig. 17.2). Pleural effusion is the earliest manifestation of previous asbestos exposure, making its first appearance 10 years after asbestos exposure. Diffuse pleural thickening is less frequent and less specific to asbestos exposure than pleural plaques. However it is more often associated with functional impairment [8].

The development of asbestosis has a definite dose-effect relationship. Fibrosis is the classic feature evolving in progressive reduction of both vital capacity and diffusing capacity. From the respiratory bronchioles and around them the fibrotic reaction starts and involves in a first phase the lower lobes adjacent to the visceral pleura. It also may begin with an intra-alveolar reaction, similar to desquamative interstitial pneumonitis [9].

Chest radiograph may show irregular opacities with a fine reticular pattern. Additional evidence of asbestos exposure such as calcified or noncalcified pleural plaques may be evident. HRCT findings are related to the duration and severity of the condition. The most common findings include centrilobular dot-like opacities, referable to peribronchial fibrosis; intralobular linear opacities, also known as reticulation; and subpleural lines (often curvilinear). In advanced phases of the disease it is possible to find parenchymal bands, traction bronchiectasis, patchy areas of ground-glass attenuation, small cystic airspaces, small areas of hypoattenuation, and honeycomb fibrosis in the end stage [17]. Pleural effusion and pleural plaques are common manifestations of asbestos exposure [18]. Nodal enlargement is not common, but, when present, has to be considered as a progression of the pathology to mesothelioma [19, 20] and bronchogenic carcinoma. Other benign parenchymal affection related to asbestos exposure includes rounded atelectasis which is due to a peripheral lobar collapse that develops in patients with pleural disease. It is more common to find in the subpleural, posterior, or basal region of the lower lobes. An important sign is "comet tail sign" produced by the crowding together of bronchi and blood vessels peripheral to the mass. Sometimes atelectasis can have wedge-shaped, lentiform, or irregular opacities or attenuation features.

Bronchogenic carcinoma can develop in 20–25% of asbestos-exposed population. Asbestos-related tumors are more common in the periphery of the lungs with a lower lobe distribution, where the fibers are present, in correlation with the usual distribution of asbestosis [8] (Figs. 17.1, 17.2, 17.3, 17.4, 17.5, 17.6, 17.7, 17.8, 17.9, and 17.10).

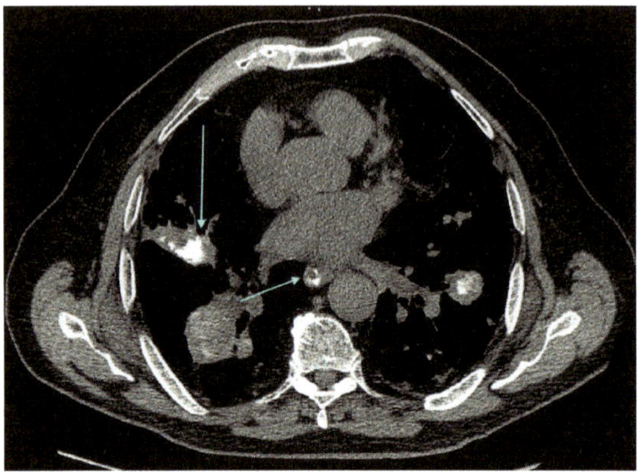

Fig. 17.1 Eggshell calcifications. Simple silicosis in an 80-year-old man who worked for 20 years in a coal mine. Thin-section unenhanced CT scan (1.0 mm thick) in mediastinal window settings at the level of the bronchus intermedius shows eggshell calcifications (arrows) in a subcarinal lymph node

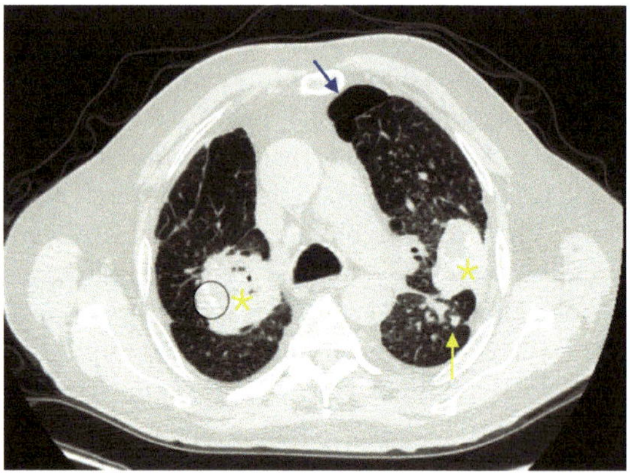

Fig. 17.2 Axial image from a thin-section unenhanced CT scan (1.0-mm-thick section) shows multiple nodules ranging between 5 mm and 4 cm (yellow arrow) with a perilymphatic (centrilobular plus subpleural) distribution in the upper lobe of both lungs (yellow arrow and star). They demonstrate a tendency toward coalescence of the nodules in the lung periphery (yellow arrow). It is possible to highlight the presence of coarse calcification of the biggest nodule (magnified). Paraseptal emphysema is also seen (blue arrow)

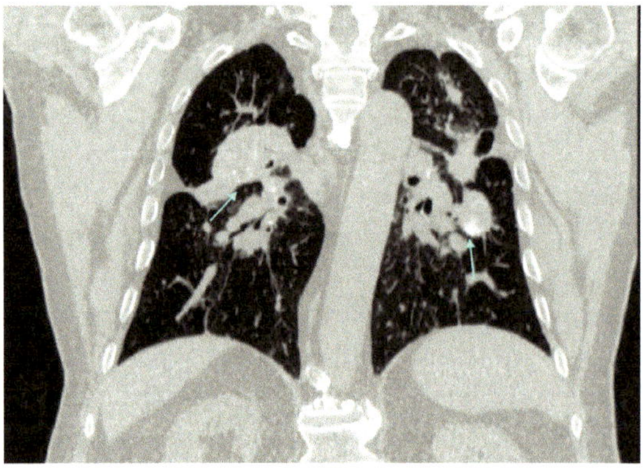

Fig. 17.3 Silicosis and progressive massive fibrosis in an 80-year-old male coal worker. Multi-planar reconstruction, coronally reconstructed image, (1.0-mm-thick section) obtained with mediastinal window settings showing bilateral conglomerate masses with calcifications (arrows), findings representing progressive massive fibrosis in the upper zone of both lungs

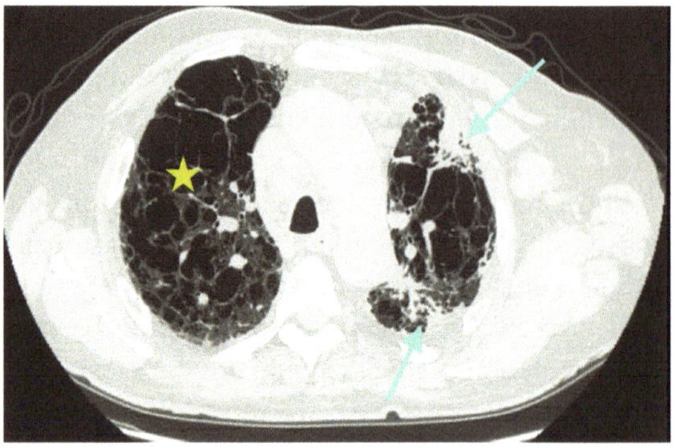

Fig. 17.4 Asbestosis in a 70-year-old man who worked for 30 years in a shipyard. Axial image from a thin-section unenhanced CT scan (1.0-mm-thick sections) in lung window settings shows subpleural consolidation (arrow) referred to mesothelioma in the upper left lobe, with reticulation, honeycombing, and advanced pattern of emphysema (yellow star)

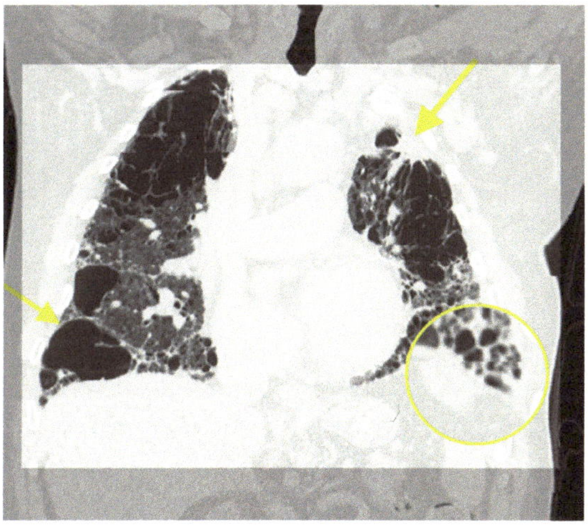

Fig. 17.5 Multi-planar reconstruction, coronal view (lung windowing), shows diffuse emphysema with cystic airspaces (yellow arrow in the right lung), subpleural consolidation with reduction of the global volume of the left lung (yellow arrow on the left lung), and honeycombing (magnified)

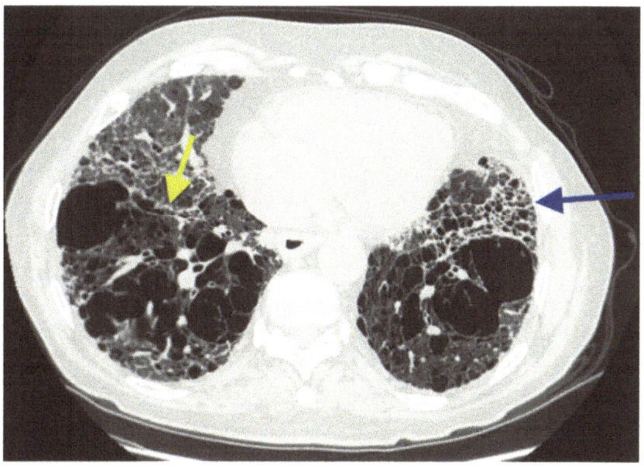

Fig. 17.6 High-resolution axial unenhanced CT image (lung windowing) at the level of the lung bases showing bilateral areas with cysts, reticular hyperattenuation, traction bronchiectasis (yellow arrow), and honeycombing (blue arrow) findings indicating a progressive pattern of fibrosis. This pattern also configures CPFE (combined pulmonary fibrosis and emphysema syndrome)

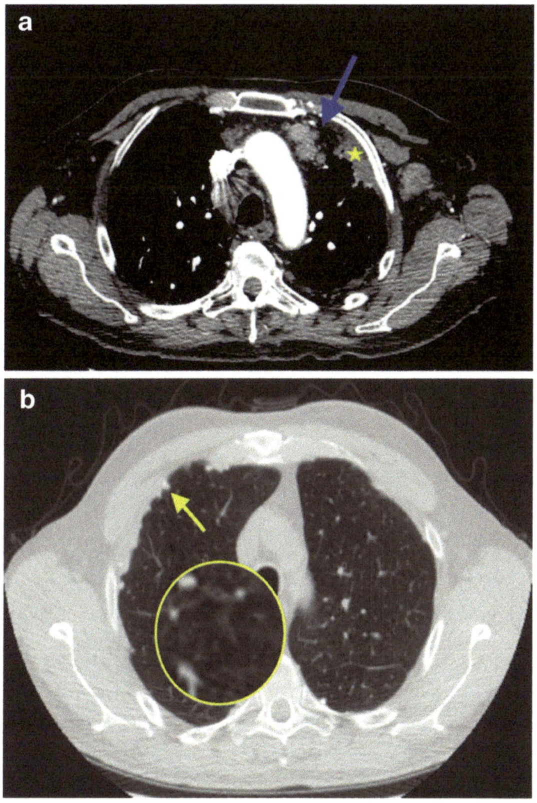

Fig. 17.7 (**a**, **b**) 70-Year-old man who worked for 30 years in a shipyard. High-resolution axial unenhanced CT image (lung windowing) highlighting multiple nodular pleural thickening (yellow arrow) and centrilobular (magnified)

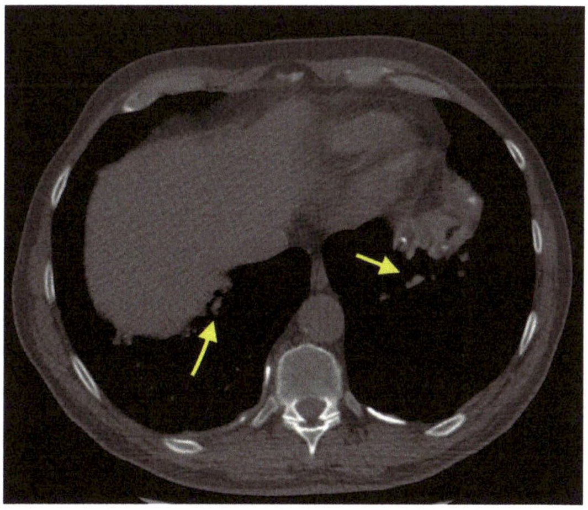

Fig. 17.8 Same patient, unenhanced high-resolution CT showing multiple nodular thickening of the diaphragmatic pleura (yellow arrow). **Malignant mesothelioma** is an uncommon and fatal neoplasm of the serosal lining of the pleural cavity, peritoneum, or both. The risk amount of mesothelioma in asbestos-exposed population is approximately 10% over their lifetime [21]. HRCT appearance is of a soft-tissue attenuation nodular mass which extends along pleural surfaces including into pleural fissures and often creating a pleural rind [22]. In 20% of cases calcifications are seen and usually represent engulfed calcified pleural plaques rather than true tumor calcification. It is possible to identify chest wall invasion through the identification of infiltration or direct extension in bone or muscle. Moreover advanced tumor invasion of the pericardium, diaphragm, and abdomen is a common finding

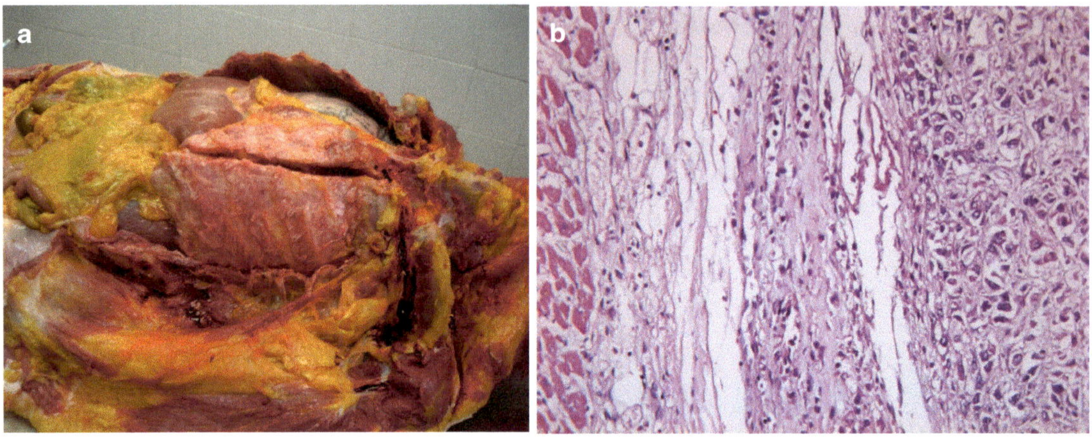

Fig. 17.9 Medical history: Man, 66 years, smoker, rail system worker as an electrician for 20 years (from 1970 to 1990) during which he referred extensive exposition to asbestos. Autopsy exam revealed widespread visceral pleural thickening of fibrotic consistency and greyish color, infiltrating left thoracic walls, diaphragm, and pericardium. Left lung was structurally subverted with multiple areas of fibrosis, bronchopneumonic foci, and edema. At histological examination multiple corpuscles and asbestos needles were found in neoplastic tissue. (**a**) Asbestosis as incidental findings at autopsy. (**b**) Histological stain of tissue lung: mainly polymorphic desmoplastic-sarcomatous aspects, infiltrating the lung parenchyma, with areas of septal fibrosis and multiple outbreaks of pneumonia and edema (H & H, ×20 magnification).

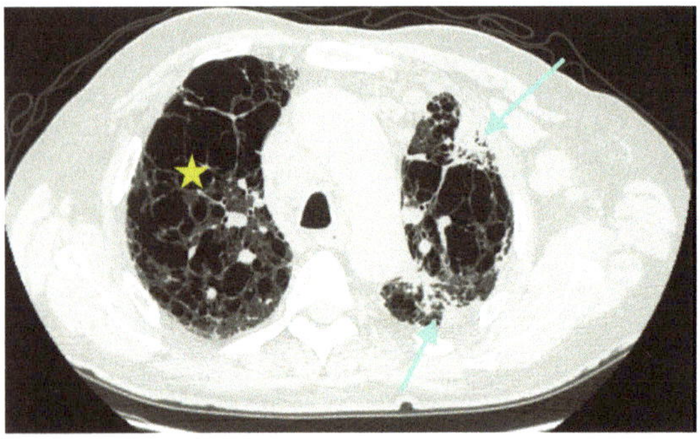

Fig. 17.10 Medical history: A 70-year-old man who worked for 30 years in a shipyard. Axial image from a thin-section unenhanced CT scan (1.0-mm-thick sections) in lung window settings shows subpleural consolidation (arrow) referred to as mesothelioma in the upper left lobe, with reticulation, honeycombing, and advanced pattern of emphysema (yellow star)

References

1. Samuels A (2015) Mesothelioma and law. Med Leg J 83(1):26–28
2. Sheaff MT, Hopster DJ (2005) Post mortem technique handbook, 2nd edn. Springer, London, pp 186–194
3. Crotty TB, Myers JL, Katzenstein AL, Tazelaar HD, Swensen SJ, Churg S (1994) Localized malignant mesothelioma. A clinicopathologic and flow cytometric study. Am J Surg Pathol 18(4):357–363
4. Verso MG, Zerbo S, Di Piazza A, Maresi E, Argo A (2018) Biphasic pleural mesothelioma in electrician working in a railway company: case report and current trends in mesotheliomas in Italy. G Ital Med Lav Erg 40(2):61–66
5. Comba P, Merler E, Pasetto R (2005) Asbestos related diseases in Italy: epidemiologic evidences and public health issues. Int J Occup Environ Health 11:36–44
6. Dawson A, Gibbs A, Browne K, Pooley F, Griffiths M (1992) Familial mesothelioma. Details of 17 cases with histopathologic findings and mineral analysis. Cancer 70(5):1183–1187
7. Capella S, Bellis D, Belluso E (2016) Diagnosis of asbestos-related diseases: the mineralogist and pathologist's role in medicolegal field. Am J Forensic Med Pathol 37(1):24–28
8. Kim KI, Kim CW, Lee MK, Lee KS, Park CK, Choi SJ, Kim JG (2001) Imaging of occupational lung disease. Radiographics 21(6):1371–1391
9. Chong S, Lee KS, Chung MJ, Han J, Kwon OJ, Kim TS (2006) Pneumoconiosis: comparison of imaging and pathologic findings. Radiographics 26(1):59–77
10. Bergin CJ, Müller NL, Vedal S, Chan-Yeung M (1986) CT in silicosis: correlation with plain films and pulmonary function tests. AJR Am J Roentgenol 146(3):477–483
11. Dee P, Suratt P, Winn W (1978) The radiographic findings in acute silicosis. Radiology 126(2):359–363
12. Marchiori E, Souza CA, Barbassa TG, Escuissato DL, Gasparetto EL, Souza AS Jr (2007) Silicoproteinosis: high-resolution CT findings in 13 patients. AJR 189(6):1402–1406

13. Grenier P, Chevret S, Beigelman C, Brauner MW, Chastang C, Valeyre D (1994) Chronic diffuse infiltrative lung disease: determination of the diagnostic value of clinical data, chest radiography, and CT and Bayesaian analysis. Radiology 191(2):383–390
14. Remy-Jardin M, Beuscart R, Sault MC, Marquette CH, Remy J (1990) Subpleural micronodules in diffuse infiltrative lung disease: evaluation with thin-section CT scans. Radiology 177(1):133–139
15. Arakawa H, Honma K, Saito Y, Shida H, Morikubo H, Suganuma N, Fujioka M (2005) Pleural disease in silicosis: pleural thickening, effusion, and invagination. Radiology 236(2):685–693
16. Roach HD, Davies GJ, Attanoos R, Crane M, Adams H, Phillips S (2002) Asbestos: when the dust settles an imaging review of asbestos-related disease. Radiographics 22 Spec No:S167–S184
17. Akira M, Yamamoto S, Inoue Y, Sakatani M (2003) High-resolution CT of asbestosis and idiopathic pulmonary fibrosis. AJR Am J Roentgenol 181(1):163–169
18. Battifora H, McHaughey WTE (1995) Tumor of the serosal membranes. Atlas of tumor pathology, 3rd series. AFIP, Washington, DC
19. Kane MJ, Chahinian P, Holland JF (1990) Malignant mesothelioma in young adults. Cancer 65(6):1449–1455
20. Pisani RJ, Colby TV, Williams DE (1998) Malignant mesothelioma of the pleura. Mayo Clin Proc 63:1234–1244
21. Wang ZJ, Reddy GP, Gotway MB, Higgins CB, Jablons DM, Ramaswamy M, Hawkins RA, Webb WR (2004) Malignant pleural mesothelioma: evaluation with CT, MR imaging, and PET. Radiographics 24(1):105–119
22. Zielinski M, Hauer J, Hauer L, Pankowski J, Nabialek T, Szlubowski A (2010) Staging algorithm for diffuse malignant pleural mesothelioma. Interact Cardiovasc Thorac Surg 10(2):185–189

Lie Detection: fMRI

18

Giuseppe La Tona, Maria Chiara Terranova,
Federica Vernuccio, Giuseppe Lo Re,
Sergio Salerno, Stefania Zerbo,
and Antonina Argo

From an evolutionary point of view, greater tactical deception is a feature that belongs to primates closer to humans, which have larger neocortices [1].

Detection indeed is a physiological ability that develops naturally during childhood in humans, and which is impaired among subjects with neurodevelopmental disorders (e.g., autism) or in patients with various psychopathy [1, 2]. Also in case of orbitofrontal lesions, deception seems to be impaired, since most of these individuals show social interaction problems which come from being notoriously tactless that in turn is due to total honesty and frankness [1, 2].

If deception is an absolute normal, although undesirable, condition in everyday life, in forensic practice, it plays a critical role, because of its detrimental implication in the judgement of guilt or innocence.

Humans are good at lying but very poor at lie detection; in face-to face interaction an average individual's ability to detect deception is slightly over 50%, the same rate that would be expected by chance [3].

That is the reason why over the past centuries, humans have developed many different methods to identify liars and to detect deception [4].

In ancient China, men who underwent an interrogatory were forced to fill their mouth with dry rice and then invited to spit it out. Deceiving was assessed if he/she took longer to spit the rice out of his/her mouth [4].

Even if this anecdotal method could seem old-fashioned and uncivilized, actually it has a scientific fundament, as sympathetic activation that is evoked in stressful conditions such as during deceiving suppresses salivation, and leads to a greater adhesion of the rice grains to liars' mouth, which are barely spitted out [4, 5].

The widely known lie detection machine—the polygraph—is based on the same neurophysiological concept, that is, the tendency for lies to be accompanied by activation of the sympathetic nervous system (SNS) [4]. Working principles of the polygraph machine consist of the measurement and recording of several physiological indices such as pulse, blood pressure, respiration, and skin galvanic conductivity, while the subject is asked and answers a series of questions [4, 6].

Even if polygraph has been widely used in the past, in 2003 American National Academy of

G. La Tona · M. C. Terranova · F. Vernuccio
G. Lo Re (✉) · S. Salerno
Department of Biopathology and Medical Biotechnologies, University of Palermo, Palermo, Italy
e-mail: giuseppe.latona@unipa.it; sergio.salerno@unipa.it

S. Zerbo · A. Argo
Department of Sciences for the Promotion of Health and Maternal and Child Care "G. D'Alessandro", University of Palermo, Palermo, Italy
e-mail: stefania.zerbo@unipa.it; antonella.argo@unipa.it

G. Lo Re et al. (eds.), *Radiology in Forensic Medicine*,
https://doi.org/10.1007/978-3-319-96737-0_18

Science reported high discrepancy on its accuracy, since while it could be up 99% it was often as low as 55%, depending on various conditions, on the setting (experimental vs. forensic), operator, examiner skills and attitude, questioning format, and response classification rules [7]. Thus considering most of the polygraph researches as "unscientific and biased," and concluding that polygraph testing is largely unreliable in the courtroom, it is outlawed—but widely used—for nongovernmental pre-employment screening [4, 6].

The issue is that the physiological data measured by polygraph reflect only the peripheral effects of SNS activation, and to overcome these limits scientists and forensics have studied other lie detector techniques, in order to identify more direct and impartial data [4, 8].

The appeal of this approach is that, instead of measuring emotional arousal resulting from deception, brain-based method evaluates central brain physiological changes associated directly with a cognitive process—deception or concealing information, for instance [4, 8].

Brain-based lie detection technology was pioneered using scalp-recorded electroencephalography (which is dated back to the 1920s), but fMRI (first applied in humans in 1992) is now the preferred modality, since it is able to localize blood flow in certain areas of the brain [8]. Although fMRI is widely superior to electroencephalography in localizing the source of the signal, it is more expensive and less mobile and it has a lower time resolution [8].

Magnetic resonance imaging (MRI) is a medical imaging technique that provides three-dimensional tomographic images of the body using high magnetic fields without ionizing radiation exposure [9].

The principles of functional MRI (fMRI) of the brain lie on the relationship between blood flow to the brain and brain demand for energy. So it is defined as a "correlational study" since it records brain state in parallel with ongoing mental activity or behavior, in order to define a correlation between these two parameters, but it is not able to establish a causal connection between brain activation and the kind of cognitive processes specifically [9, 10].

The brain needs energy to perform any task (thinking, perceiving, speaking, deceiving, and so on), so when an area of the brain is activated, the blood flow in that region increases, and oxygen level changes—this occurs rapidly (1–2 s) after neuron activation—bursting concentration of oxygenated hemoglobin in this area [9–12].

fMR technique is based on the difference in the magnetic properties of the blood vessel contents and the surrounding brain tissue, and relies on the different magnetic features of oxygenated and deoxygenated hemoglobin [9–12].

fMRI measures this difference, detecting changes in blood flow and oxygenated hemoglobin concentration—that is called blood oxygen level dependent (BOLD) effect—which is indirectly related to brain area activation [9–12].

The vast majority of fMRI in neuroscience relies on BOLD response, although it does not depict absolute regional brain activation, but relative changes in regional activity in a determined timeframe, as aforementioned [9–11].

Changes in BOLD signal are measured in a spatial volume. Every spatial volume, called voxel, reflects a small ($300 \times 300\ \mu m^2$ with a couple of millimeter slice thickness or $500 \times 500 \times 500\ \mu m^3$ isotropic) cube of brain tissue, which represents millions of brain cells. The active "illuminated" part of the brain on fMRI images represents the activation or deactivation of hundreds of clusters of voxel [9].

But, since blood incoming is not static, but flows rapidly, fMRI does not take "instant photo" of brain vascularization, but images come from the evaluation of the blood flow through a defined brain area over a short time (couple of seconds) [9–11].

These changes in blood oxygenation level occur as a part of the physiological brain activity, and since the pulse sequences used in fMRI do not alter neuronal firing or interfere with blood flow, fMRI is considered a noninvasive technique, and reveals how the brain works in real time [10].

In other terms, fMRI study is based on a dependent variable, that is, the brain activation, and an independent one, that is, a defined stimulus or task [9–12].

Once a brain area is activated due to a stimulus, oxygenated hemoglobin concentration in this area increases (relatively to the neutral/control condition) and BOLD signal is obtained [9–12].

Radiologically speaking, the dependent variable—the brain area activation—comes from a subtraction measure of blood paramagnetic behavior between the "rest/control" state and the stimulus/task state, which in turn represents the independent variable, which evokes an increase in blood flow and then in oxygenated hemoglobin [9–13].

At this point, it is essential to mention that even if fMRI is able to define brain state as a consequence of a cognitive process, it is not able to determine whether any specific pattern of brain activation is a necessary determinant of its associated behavior [9–12].

In other terms we can say that defined areas of the brain are activated during lying, but we cannot say that they are activated exclusively because of the cognitive process of lying.

Moreover, evaluating blood flow in specific brain areas is useful only if:

1. We know certain functional subunits of certain areas of the brain
2. We know the main blood flux in nonactivated situation

It has been demonstrated that, although there is not a single region of the brain that seems to be correlated to deception, recent meta-analysis found that certain areas are more active during deception versus truth conditions at a much higher statistical rate than chance: bilateral dorsolateral and ventrolateral prefrontal cortex, inferior parietal lobule, medial superior frontal cortex, and anterior insula [4, 11, 14, 15].

On the opposite, fMRI does not detect any region that is significantly more engaged in truth-telling conditions, suggesting that deception requires a greater effort than responding truthfully [4, 11, 14, 15].

Indeed, lying was demonstrated to come from "higher" cortical centers, such as the prefrontal cortex, that are essential to adaptive behaviors in brand new, difficult, or stressful situations, on the opposite to the posterior and subcortical regions, defined as "slave/lower" systems, which in turn may be sufficient to perform simple, routine, automated tasks [1].

But how does the fMRI work?

In order to define the difference between the active or non-active state, a widely standard maneuver in functional brain imaging is to isolate changes in a certain brain area associated with particular tasks.

This can be done by subtracting images taken in a control state from the images taken during the performance of the task which the researcher is interested in (target): images taken during truth-telling, and images taken during lie-telling [4, 9, 10].

But this implies the use of a standardized protocol that generates these behaviors, and this requires that these behaviors can be measured by fMRI.

These paradigms refer to the methods used to generate deceptive responses and appropriate controls, and the two basic ones are the comparison question test (CQT) and the guilty knowledge task (GKT), also known as the concealed information test (CIT). They are not unique for fMRI studies but they have been developed and used for forensic investigative use by the polygraph and the EEG [6, 8, 11, 13, 16, 17].

In CQT subject is invited to answer three kinds of questions: "relevant," "control," and "irrelevant."

The first one refers to the topic under investigation, and it presumes to evoke a lie: "Did you steal the car?"

The control one is instead used to elicit a strong response, correlated to a sympathetic arousal, but not about the topic of investigation: "Did you ever steal anything?"

The irrelevant one defines the baseline: "Are you sitting on a chair?" [8, 13].

Results come from the difference between the relevant and the control questions: a stronger physiological response (activated areas in fMRI) on the relevant question than on the control one is considered as an evidence of deception [8, 13].

There is a different type of "lie" that does not refer to "lie-telling" but to "not telling the truth, or concealing a part of it."

In GKT, subject is invited to answer a series of questions, created to evoke a fixed uniform response to multiple matters, including an "aspect of knowledge" that a guilty subject would try to conceal. Among these several neutral (control) questions, there is a relevant (target) alternative, for example a feature of a crime under investigation [8, 13].

Questions are chosen in a way that an innocent subject would not be able to discriminate the control ones from the relevant. For example, using the same aforementioned example, if the crime refers to a red stolen car, the question sequence would be "was the car white?" "was the car red?" "was the car blue?"

If the physiological response to the target question—"was the car red"—is widely larger than controls—"was the car white?" and " was the car blue?"—knowledge about the event is implied, and subject is presumed to be lying [8, 13].

It's interesting to notice that using GKT, physiological responses to simply hearing the relevant question, not necessary to answering deceptively, can be sufficient to determine whether the subject is concealing information or not [13].

In other terms, the CQT uses the measurement of physiological or psychophysical responses to define an answer as a lie, and the GKT implies such responses to indicate the presence of concealed knowledge.

The literature about fMRI in the lie detection field includes tasks that derive from these tests.

In 2002, in one of the earliest studies about the use of fMRI in deception detection, participants were given two play cards, and were instructed to deny the possession of one of them and confirm the possession of the other one. During fMRI examination patients were showed a series of cards, including the aforementioned ones, and they have to say if they have or do not have the cards they were seeing [18].

Images were acquired and compared between truth and lie states, and indicated the brain activity during deception and during truth-telling [4, 18].

In a similar experiment, the subject mentally picked a number between three and eight, and, under fMRI examination, while a series of numbers were shown on the screen, they have to deny to have picked the critical number (target) and denied having picked the other ones (controls) [19].

A more realistic experiment was conducted by Kozel et al., using a mock scenario, in which participants have to steal a ring or a watch, on their choice, and they have to put the item into a locker. Then, while undergoing fMRI, they have to deny possession of both items (deceive possession of stolen object: deception, TERGET; deceive possession of the other one: truth-telling, CONTROL). Then, in order to define a baseline, that is, the neutral state, they had to answer simple and meaningless questions such as "it is 2004?" or "do you live in US."

Comparing brain activation while answering different type of questions, researches tried to define the index of neural activity [4, 20].

Although this topic is of great forensic impact, nowadays the use of fMRI in lie detection is not yet widely allowed in the courtroom, because of a series of scientific, ethic, and legal motivations [8].

The main scientific issues of experimental deception-generating models are basically five:

- Endorsement: Subjects in the studies were endorsed to lie; in other terms lying was the target of the experiment, a desirable condition, for which participants were not only allowed, but also instructed, while in the real world deception is considered a despicable action that is usually hidden by the liar [8].
- Emotional impact on lying may modify fMRI findings in a real-world situation, where lying in a legal scenario may have potential impact on guilt or innocence sentences.
- Emotion can influence the neural circuitry of lying, of memory, of inhibition, and of cognitive control, leading to misinterpretation of truth about a highly emotional event, or what would be at stake if the lie were discovered [4, 21–24].
- Moreover, we must mention that anxiety, fear, or heightened emotional status leads to altered BOLD signal, not directly related to deception, in these cases [4].
- Role of memory: BOLD images indicate activation during lying, but it is not determined for sure if this activation occurs BECAUSE

OF the deception or as a consequence of other psychological processes, like memory, which may evoke the same pattern of activity [4, 25].

- Hakun et al. and Gamer et al. have tried to discern the memory issues from the deceiving pattern. In summary, patients were invited to mentally pick a selected number, and while undergoing fMRI they were showed a series of numbers. It has been demonstrated that both when subjects lied about the number they picked and when they simply saw this number, the same pattern of activation occurred, suggesting that it might be due to cognitive processes other than deception per se [4, 19, 25].
- This could be caused by the effort required by lie-telling that implies greater necessity of short-term (and long-term) memory and executive functions than truth-telling. Indeed, liars usually keep in mind two (or more) versions of the event in their working memory, and they force themselves to exhibit a natural behavior, and to inhibit the physiological instinct of answering in accordance with the reality [4].
- Countermeasures/practice: Studies have shown the impact of practice in prefrontal cortex activation, displaying that memorized lies result in a less BOLD activation when compared to unpracticed ones, in all regions (but in the one associated with memory retrieval) [4, 26–28].
- Similar efficacy has been shown in adopting simple countermeasures, like imperceptible finger or toe movements—that can reduce accuracy in detecting lies up to 33% [26]—or mental calculation during control sequences that arises cortical activation while defining the baseline state [4, 26–28].
- Individual neuroanatomy/neurophysiology variances may be the norm rather than the exception, thus leading to an extensive variability in brain area activation, especially in cortical regions which control higher brain functions, and which were subjected to a greater evolutionary development [11, 29].
- The individual variability is particularly important while examining criminals: a study of fMRI-based lie detection in criminal offenders affected by antisocial disorders found that a large majority of these participants did not show the typical prefrontal BOLD activation pattern during instructed deception [4, 30].
- Thus, considering that a relatively high portion of criminals meet the criteria for psychopathy, fMRI lie detection technique in this class of individuals may be unreliable [4, 30].
- Lying moreover can be a complex activity with various degrees and levels of prevarication, of different individuals of different health, age, sex, psychological tracts (for example, high anxiety and extraversion), and instruction, and the ability to detect simple deceptions in experimental setting may not translate into a forensic spendable technology in less controlled situations [4].

In other terms, nowadays fMRI can provide adequate accuracy in detecting deceptive behaviors in particular population and in particular circumstances that are far away from the real world.

Little is known about the accuracy of fMRI as a lie detector in real-world situations or in a legal scenario, in which no studies have yet defined its probative value (how many lies the tool misses and how often it identifies the truth as a lie).

Beyond the social, legal, and ethical issues, which fall outside the purpose of this chapter, it is undeniable that the main scientific shortcoming of the fMRI as a lie detection technology lies upon the sufficient degree of accuracy, specificity, and validity that a worldwide use of this method in such as delicate forensic field requires.

References

1. Spence SA, Hunter MD, Farrow TFD et al (2004) A cognitive neurobiological account of deception: evidence from functional neuroimaging. Philos Trans R Soc B Biol Sci 359(1451):1755–1762
2. Sodian B, Frith U (1992) Deception and sabotage in autistic, retarded and normal children. J Child Psychol Psychiatry 33(3):591–605
3. Ekman P, O'Sullivan M (1991) Who can catch a liar? Am Psychol 46:913–920

4. Farah MJ, Hutchinson J, Phelps EA, Wagner AD (2014) Functional MRI-based lie detection: scientific and societal challenges. Nat Rev Neurosci 15:123–131
5. Schafer ED (2008) In: Embar-Seddon A, Pass AD (eds) Forensic science. Salem Press, Ipswich, p 40
6. Ben-Shakhar G, Bar-Hillel M, Lieblich I (1986) Trial by polygraph: scientific and juridical issues in lie detection. Behav Sci Law 4:459–479
7. National Research Council (2003) The polygraph and lie detection. The National Academies, Washington, DC
8. Langleben DD, Moriarty JC (2013) Using brain imaging for lie detection: where science, law and research policy collide. Psychol Public Policy Law 19(2):222–234
9. Logothetis NK (2008) What we can do and what we cannot do with fMRI. Nature 453(7197):869–878
10. Rusconi E, Mitchener-Nissen T (2013) Prospects of functional magnetic resonance imaging as lie detector. Front Hum Neurosci 7:594
11. Shapiro ZE (2016) Truth, deceit, and neuroimaging: can functional magnetic resonance imaging serve as a technology-based method of lie detection? Harvard J Law Technol 29(2 Spring):528–549
12. Kwong KK, Belliveau JW, Chesler DA, Goldberg IE, Weisskoff RM, Poncelet BP et al (1992) Dynamic magnetic resonance imaging of human brain activity during primary sensory stimulation. PNAS 89:5675–5679
13. Wolpe PR, Foster KR, Langleben DD (2005) Emerging neurotechnologies for lie-detection: promises and perils. Am J Bioeth 5(2):39–49
14. Abe N (2011) How the brain shapes deception: an integrated review of the literature. Neuroscientist 17:560–574
15. Gamer M (2011) Detecting of deception and concealed information using neuroimaging techniques. In: Verschuere B, BenShakhar G, Meijer E (eds) Memory detection: theory and application of the concealed information test. Cambridge University Press, New York, NY, pp 90–113
16. Ben-Shakhar G (2001) A critical review of the controlled question test (CQT). In: Kleiner M (ed) Handbook of polygraph testing. Academic Press, London, San Diego, pp 103–127
17. Ben-Shakhar G, Bar-Hillel M, Kremnitzer M (2002) Trial by polygraph: reconsidering the use of the guilty knowledge technique in court. Law Hum Behav 26:527–541
18. Langleben DD et al (2002) Brain activity during simulated deception: an event-related functional magnetic resonance study. NeuroImage 15:727–732
19. Hakun JG, Seelig D, Ruparel K, Loughead JW, Busch E, Gur RC, Langleben DD (2008) fMRI investigation of the cognitive structure of the concealed information test. Neurocase 14(1):59–67
20. Kozel FA, Johnson KA, Mu Q, Grenesko EL, Laken SJ, George MS (2005) Detecting deception using functional magnetic resonance imaging. Biol Psychiatry 58(8):605–613
21. Phelps EA (2006) Emotion and cognition: insights from studies of the human amygdala. Annu Rev Psychol 57:27–53
22. Bush G, Luu P, Posner MI (2000) Cognitive and emotional influences in anterior cingulate cortex. Trends Cogn Sci 4:215–222
23. Levens SM, Phelps EA (2010) Insula and orbital frontal cortex activity underlying emotion interference resolution in working memory. J Cogn Neurosci 22:2790–2803
24. Lee TMC, Lee TMY, Raine A, Chan CCH (2010) Lying about the valence of affective pictures: an fMRI study. PLoS One 5:e12291
25. Gamer M, Klimecki O, Bauermann T, Stoeter P, Vossel G (2012) fMRI-activation patterns in the detection of concealed information rely on memory-related effects. Soc Cogn Affect Neurosci 7(5):506–515
26. Ganis G, Rosenfeld JP, Meixner J, Kievit RA, Schendan HE (2011) Lying in the scanner: covert countermeasures disrupt deception detection by functional magnetic resonance imaging. NeuroImage 55(1):312–319
27. Uncapher MR, Chow T, Rissman J, Eberhart J, Wagner AD (2012) Strategic influences on memory expression: effects of countermeasures and memory strength on the neural decoding of past experience. Soc Neurosci Abstr 905.13
28. Rissman J, Greely HT, Wagner AD (2010) Detecting individual memories through the neural decoding of memory states and past experience. Proc Natl Acad Sci U S A 107:9849–9854
29. Hamann S, Turhan C (2004) Individual differences in emotion processing. Curr Opin Neurobiol 14(2):233–238
30. Anderson NE, Kiehl KA (2012) The psychopath magnetized: insights from brain imaging. Trends Cogn Sci 16:52–60

Conventional Radiology for Postmortem Imaging

19

Stefano D'Errico, Diana Bonuccelli, Massimo Martelloni, and Giuseppe Guglielmi

19.1 Introduction

Immediately after its discovery in 1895, conventional radiography was used in the courts to document and illustrate gunshot wounds and for many years continued to represent the most widely used postmortem radiology technique in (1) determination of identity (when conventional methods such as fingerprinting or DNA analysis are not available or cannot be utilized), (2) traumatic injuries (road traffic fatalities, falls from heights, etc.), (3) gunshot wound fatalities, (4) child abuse, and (5) forensic anthropology.

One of the most famous cases that employed conventional radiography occurred in 1935 in Scotland. Human body parts were discovered in a river and subsequently identified as belonging to two women who were probably dismembered. At the same time, the nurse and the wife of a doctor in Lancaster were reported missing. Radiological examination of the body parts enabled rapid assessment of the age and size of the two victims. Identification was carried out by superposing X-ray images of the skulls with photographs of the alleged victims. The surgical precision used to dismember the two women as well as other information suggested that the perpetrator possessed medical skills.

Introduction of MDCT in forensic practice in the last decades allowed the opportunity to provide a two-dimensional multiplanar and three-dimensional anatomic survey prior to dissection that guides the forensic pathologist to specific abnormalities if necessary; however, due to the common availability of conventional radiography and the specific indications that justify its use, such as the examination of corpses and objects that cannot be examined by CT due to a large volume, conventional radiography still plays an important role in legal medicine and can be considered still useful because of its excellent resolution and absence of artifacts.

19.2 Conventional Radiology Before Autopsy: Where, How, When

For many years, forensic pathologists have used radiography to acquire a permanent record of part of a deceased person's anatomy and pathology before performing an autopsy. The images, which typically were obtained using conventional radiography or fluoroscopy, helped to document

S. D'Errico · D. Bonuccelli · M. Martelloni
Department of Legal Medicine, Azienda USL Toscana Nordovest, Lucca, Italy
e-mail: d.bonuccelli@usl2.toscana.it; m.martelloni@usl2.toscana.it

G. Guglielmi (✉)
Department of Radiology, University of Foggia, Foggia, Italy
e-mail: giuseppe.guglielmi@unifg.it

G. Lo Re et al. (eds.), *Radiology in Forensic Medicine*,
https://doi.org/10.1007/978-3-319-96737-0_19

Table 19.1 Imaging techniques in forensic radiology

	Advantages	Disadvantages	Field of application
Conventional radiography	Fast examination Easy to handle Simple data storage Relatively low maintenance costs Visualization of the skeletal system Detection of foreign bodies	Radiation (need for specific protection for the personnel) No 3D reconstructions Very limited visualization of soft tissue Superimposed image Quality strongly dependent on acquisition	Detection of foreign bodies Identification Age estimation Changes/lesions of the skeletal system

fractures, particularly in areas not easily seen during standard autopsy. Images also helped localize foreign material and collections of gases, prepare individual specimens, detect occult injuries, airplane and automobile parts, shrapnel and bomb fragments, etc.

Most forensic institutions possess their own X-ray devices; in other cases radiography can be performed with mobile units. If mobile units are employed and radiography is performed in the autopsy rooms, radiation protection measures should be strictly enforced to protect all personnel. Mobile units may also be used as backup when fixed units are nonoperational or as the primary unit for isolation or contamination cases and in field or temporary morgues.

Radiography is advantageous, as it is simple to perform, rapid, and cost efficient. Radiography is often implemented for infant corpses, for highly putrefied, charred, or otherwise altered bodies, and for bodies of unknown identity (Table 19.1).

Conventional radiology in forensic anthropology, identification, and child abuse are argumented in other chapters of this book.

19.2.1 Focus on Gunshot Wound Injuries

In 2006 the National Association of Medical Examiners recommended that radiographs be obtained as part of the investigation of any gunshot wound fatality and that recovery and documentation of foreign bodies be made for evidentiary purposes. Nowadays, in the investigation of gunshot wounds, conventional radiology is still universally used to locate the bullet, identify the type of ammunition and weapon used, document the path of the bullet, and assist in the retrieval of the bullet, even when MDCT is available as a complement of cross-sectional imaging. Orthogonal radiographic projections (frontal and lateral views) are the most optimal method of precise localization if radiography alone is being used. Lateral views can be added to the protocol to localize abnormalities in three dimensions as needed. Standard conventions for labeling of radiographs with identifying numbers or names and right- or left-sided body markers are necessary to avoid error.

The presence of a bullet is easily determined with conventional radiology by its characteristic shape and high radiographic attenuation. Measurement of its dimensions on radiography may be limited by inherent inaccuracies caused by geometric and physical factors. Radiographs show the borders of a metallic object very clearly but magnification always occurs because of the distance between the X-ray source and the body and bullet and the X-ray detector (Fig. 19.1). The shape and length of the object can be distorted when the object is not positioned perpendicular to the X-ray beam.

Bullets are composed of metals that have different composition and atomic number. Different metals may have unique visual and textural or tactile characteristics, but they are often indistinguishable in radiographic attention. Bullets are often encased in a copper or copper alloy jacket. They may also contain a steel perpetrator at the tip that is designed to enhance the bullet's ability to penetrate its target. The softer copper deforms more readily than the steel penetrator and even

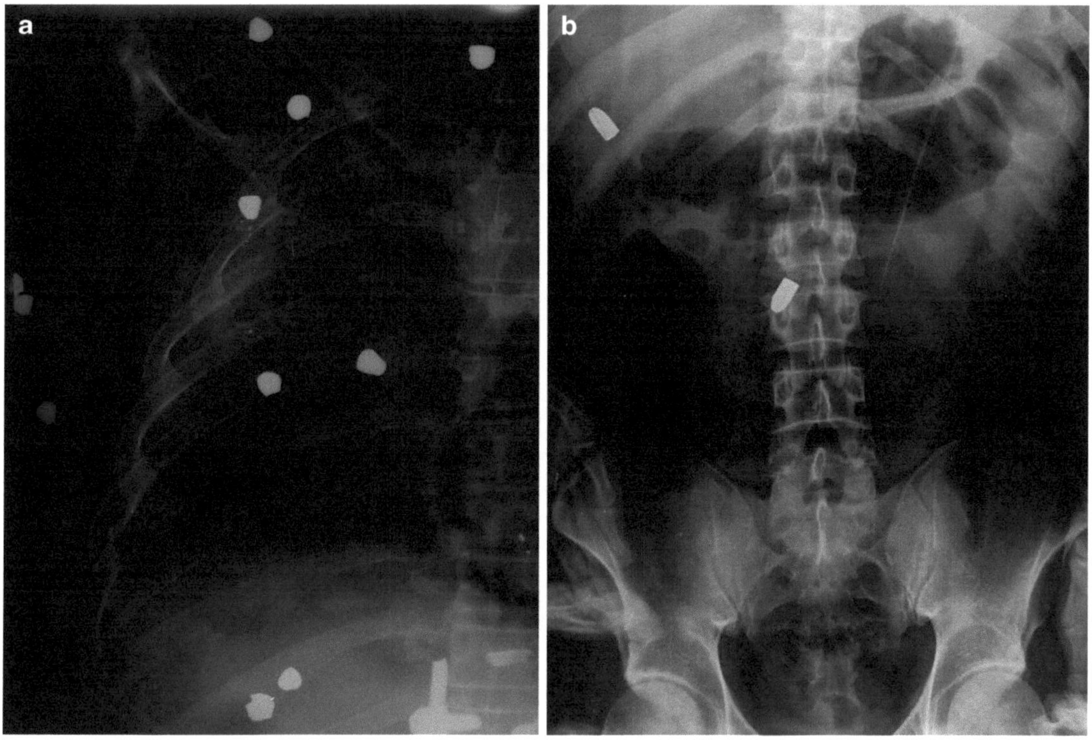

Fig. 19.1 (**a**) Digital radiograph shows 11 ovoid well-defined-in-shape metal pellets, similar in size. The pellets are grouped together, indicating that the shotgun was positioned at close range but did not have contact with the skin. (**b**) The shape and configuration of bullets are identical to the recovered

though they have the same radiographic attenuation, the shape may be a clue to the type of material. In cases where metal fragments exhibit a visible difference in attenuation, such as aluminum versus copper or steel, it is possible to see a difference on radiographs.

In *penetrating* gunshot injuries, bullets enter the body without exiting (Fig. 19.2a, b).

The bullet remains in the body as a single fragment or multiple fragments, depending on the bullet material and the interaction of the bullet with intermediate targets such as bone (Fig. 19.3a, b). If the bullet fragments along its course, metallic fragments will be deposited within the tissue along the course of the gunshot wound track.

In *perforating* gunshot wounds, if the bullet remains intact, there will be no residual metallic fragments in the body. In other cases a bullet may also fragment with portions remaining in the body and others exiting the body (Fig. 19.4).

The determination of the direction for perforating gunshot wounds relies on several features in addition to the characterization of entry and exit wounds. One of the most helpful features is the passage of the bullet through bone. When a bullet enters and exit bone, marginal fracturing creates beveling, with bevel occurring outward in the direction of travel.

Full-body radiography in case of gunshot wound fatalities is mandatory because it allows to document and locate all of the bullet fragments even when the bullet entered the body in one anatomic location; bullets often migrate to unexpected locations in the body and it is really confoundent in the determination of a wound track. This is particularly true when the bullet settles in a body cavity or tubular structure within the body such as the vasculature, trachea and bronchi, neural canal, and urinary and gastrointestinal tract. Bullets may travel to a location far from the wound path after entering a lumen or

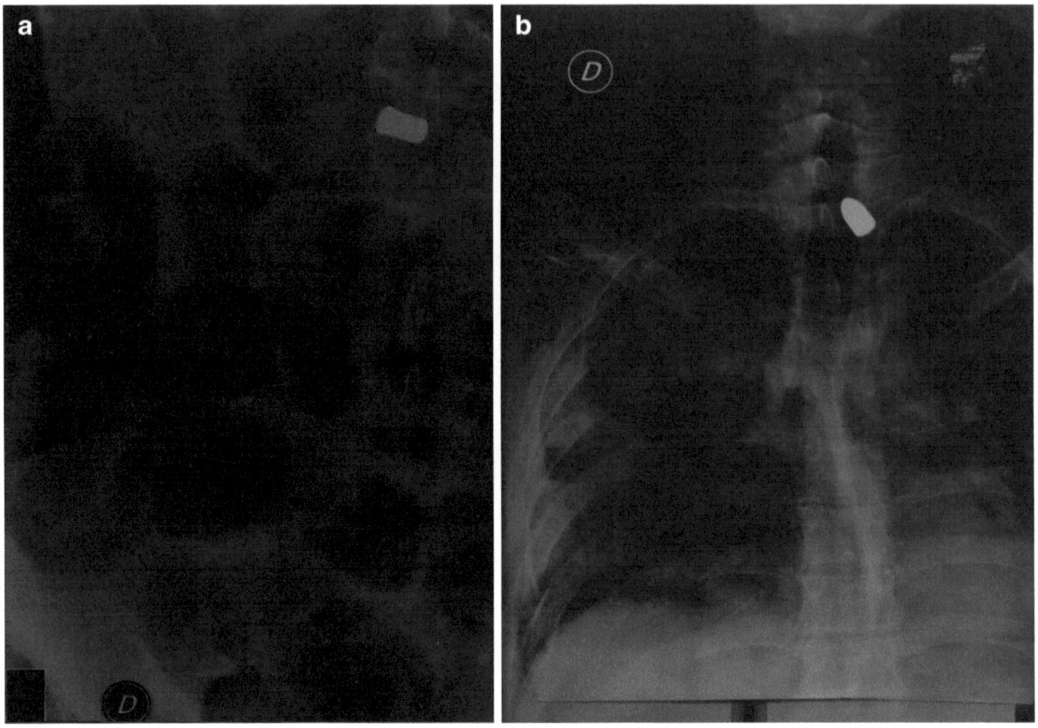

Fig. 19.2 Shotgun wound of the abdomen (**a**) and the thorax (**b**). Bullets with different shape and configuration

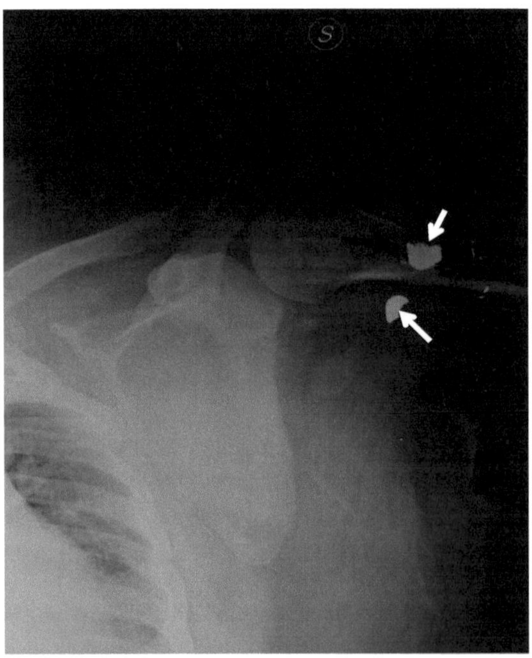

Fig. 19.3 Penetrating gunshot wound to the left arm. The bullet fragmented when impacted the humerus (white arrows). Comminute displaced fractures of the proximal third of the humerus are well documented (black arrow)

cavity. A variety of mechanisms, such as vascular flow, peristalsis, or simply gravity, may affect migration.

Multiple firearm wounds with overlapping anatomical trajectories may hamper individual projectile trajectory identification. These cases benefit from radiographic studies as it allows for identification of bone structure injuries as it traces a firearm projectile's possible trajectory; its most useful feature, however, is enabling the identification of shrapnel left by the projectile along its trajectory. Even if the caliber of the projectile found at the scene or victim is analyzed directly and thoroughly by a ballistics expert, this analysis may find further support in a radiographic study which also helps document evidence and preserve the chain of custody.

19.2.2 High-Energy Trauma

Adequate description and documentation of bone injuries in the study of traffic accident-related deaths are of major importance for the reconstruc-

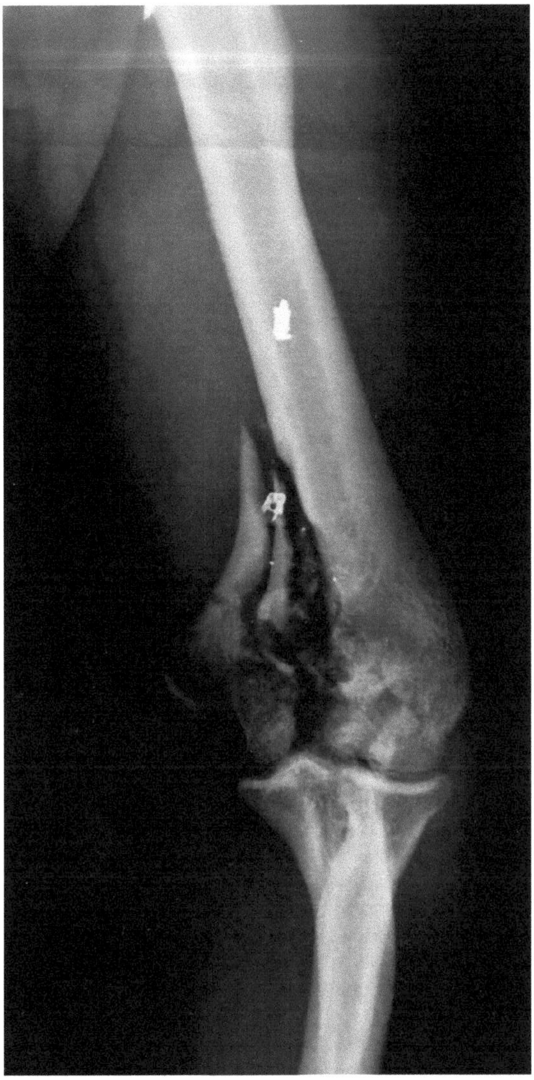

Fig. 19.4 Perforating gunshot wounds. Few little bullet fragments retained after impact with humerus while major part exited the body

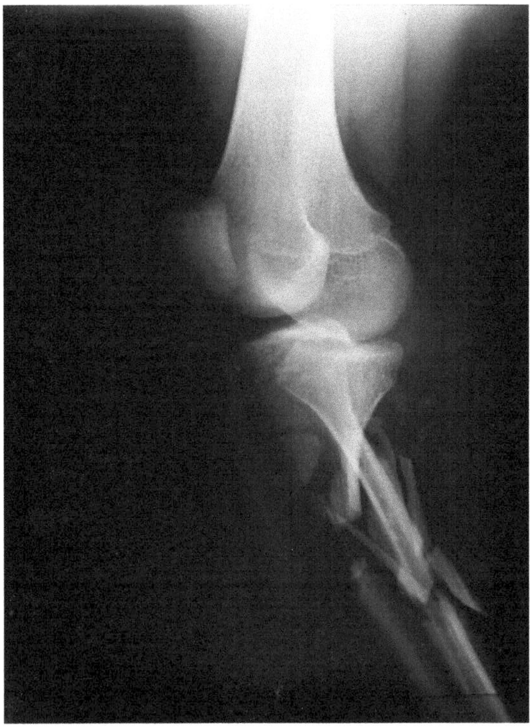

Fig. 19.5 Lower-leg X-Ray demonstrates high-energy injury

tion of the event. Pedestrians who are victims of traffic accidents frequently display fractures in lower limbs, commonly femur and tibia. The distance from the fracture site to the heel allows for estimation of the most prominent portion of the vehicle involved in the accident. Likewise, long-bone wedge fracture documentation enables to determine the primary impact direction by describing wedge-angle direction (Fig. 19.5).

In motorcycle accidents, cranial fracture description is essential; hinge fractures in particular are observed in motorcyclists after traffic accidents with lateral cranial impact. In car accidents, the driver usually suffers acetabulum fracture with femoral impact, whereas the copilot suffers cranial fractures following ejection through the windshield, with secondary cranio-encephalic trauma. Crushing lesions caused by motor vehicles frequently involve multiple costal fractures and pelvis fractures, as well as solid viscera bursting due to sudden increase in intra-abdominal and intrathoracic pressure. Traumatic diaphragmatic hernias occur along as well. All these lesions are easily documented via conventional radiology.

19.2.3 Pediatrics

Conventional radiology is the mainstay of postmortem imaging in forensic pediatrics. Emphasis is generally placed on skeletal development, both with regard to the gestational age and the presence of anomalies, such as skeletal dysplasias. In fetuses up to a gestational age of approximately 24 weeks, use of the mammography system is reported, as this has a high resolution and exquisitely depicts the fetal skeleton. In these cases a babygram, which visualizes developmental anomalies of the entire skeletal system in two or more views, is acceptable. In older fetuses and neonates a direct digital radiography system is preferably used. In babies and toddlers postmortem radiography is reserved for cases of sudden infant death syndrome (SIDS) or suspected child abuse. In these cases a full skeletal survey according to either the American College of Radiology or the Royal College of Radiologists should be performed, even if a whole-body CT is obtained. In older children (>4 years of age) postmortem conventional radiology plays a minor role and is only performed on special indications.

19.2.4 Miscellanea

Other applications of radiology in forensic medicine are possible, such as documenting bilateral pulmonary opacity in drowning cases and identifying radiopaque areas in the gastrointestinal tract of human drug couriers.

19.3 Conclusion

Technological advances in the last two decades led to revolutionary changes in imaging. Developments in multidetector computed tomography (MDCT) and magnetic resonance imaging (MRI) technology changed the practice of clinical medicine and radiology. The application of these technologies to forensic medicine changed traditional autoptical approach of pathologist and the use of conventional postmortem radiology which is now requested in few cases. Anyway, high availability and less expensivity make conventional radiology preferable in most situations (gunshot fatalities, high-energy trauma, highly putrefied, charred, or otherwise altered bodies, bodies of unknown identity).

Further Reading

Brogdon BG (1998) Forensic radiology. CRC Press, Boca Raton, FL

Cafarelli FP, Grilli G, Zizzo G, Bertozzi G, Giuliani N, Mahakkanukrauh P, Pinto A, Guglielmi G (2019) Postmortem imaging: an update. Semin Ultrasound CT MR 40(1):86–93

D'Errico S, Martelloni M, Cafarelli FP, Guglielmi G (2018) Neurofibromatosis 1 and massive hemothorax: a fatal combination. Forensic Sci Med Pathol 14(3):377–380

Di Maio VJM (1999) Gunshot wounds: practical aspects of firearms, ballistics and forensic techniques. CRC Press, Boca Raton, FL

Fatteh AH, Mann GT (1969) The role of radiology in forensic medicine. Sud Med Ekspert 19:16–18

Harcke HT, Levy AD, Abbott RM (2007) Autopsy radiography: digital radiographs (DR) vs. multidetector computed tomography (MDCT) in high velocity gunshot wound victims. Am J Forensic Med Pathol 28:13–19

Heinze S, Uebbing K, Schroder RJ, Urban R, Breitmeier D (2014) Conventional radiology versus the increasing importance of post mortem computed tomography. Arch Kriminol 234(3–4):127–133

Hoogeendoorn TS, van Rijn RR (2010) Current techniques in postmortem imaging with specific attention to paediatric applications. Pediatr Radiol 40:141–152

Levy AD, Harcke HT (2011) Essentials of forensic imaging. A text atlas. CRC Press, Boca Raton, FL

Peterson GF, Clark SC (2006) Forensic autopsy performance standards. In: National Association of Medical Examiners Annual Meeting (October 16, 2006), San Antonio, TX

Pomara C, Karch SV, Fineschi V (2010) Forensic autopsy. A handbook and atlas. CRC Press, Boca Raton, FL

Wilson AJ (1999) Gunshot injuries: what does a radiologist need to know? Radiographics 19:1358–1368

20 Postmortem Computed Tomography: From Acquisition to Reporting

Giuseppe Lo Re, Roberto Lagalla, Stefania Zerbo, Federica Vernuccio, Elvira Ventura, Sergio Salerno, Massimo Midiri, and Antonina Argo

20.1 PMCT Around the World

Since its first application performed in 1977 by Wüllenweber et al. [1] about a cranial bullet trajectory, CT imaging started to timidly appear in forensic scenery. It wasn't until multi-slice CT (MSCT) and 3D reconstructions that postmortem computed tomography (PMCT) gradually disclosed its full potential.

Its fast execution and relative affordability and the possibility to preserve body integrity and to reproduce and to store data recently granted PMCT a reliable space in forensic imaging. Lacking international guidelines on a still developing technique, every forensic institution, and then every country, developed its own approaches and procedures.

Usually PMCT is complementary and supplementary to conventional autopsy that still endures as gold standard in determining cause, manner, and mechanism of death.

In 2000 the Institutes of Forensic Medicine and of Diagnostic Radiology of the University of Bern, **Switzerland**, started a research project aimed to create scientific evidence to support new radiological techniques and their forensic application. The "Virtopsy" project (https://virtopsy.com/) is now an established reality in scientific community. As Thali et al. reported in 2007 [2], a large number of bodies underwent to both CT and MRI scans as standard procedure, giving an extended database to work on.

Similar experiences are reported by the Institute of Forensic Medicine of the University of Copenhagen and of the University of Southern **Denmark** [3, 4]. They conducted a study in which PMCT, if and when feasible, was part of forensic routine in cases selected for autopsy by the police authorities at medicolegal inquest.

As stated by Okuda et al. [5], because of low autopsy rate and extensive distribution of CT and MRI apparatus, **Japan** has been using since late 1990s postmortem imaging as an alternative to conventional autopsy, only to include the latter in a selected number of cases. Currently Japanese institutions tend to centralize postmortem imaging reports of exams performed all over the country to a specialized radiological center in Tokyo via remote network system, simultaneously

G. Lo Re (✉) · R. Lagalla · F. Vernuccio
S. Salerno · M. Midiri
Department of Biopathology and Medical Biotechnologies, University of Palermo, Palermo, Italy
e-mail: roberto.lagalla@unipa.it; segio.salerno@unipa.it; massimo.midiri@unipa.it

S. Zerbo · E. Ventura · A. Argo
Department of Sciences for the Promotion of Health and Maternal and Child Care "G. D'Alessandro", University of Palermo, Palermo, Italy
e-mail: stefania.zerbo@unipa.it; elvira.ventura@unipa.it; antonella.argo@unipa.it

G. Lo Re et al. (eds.), *Radiology in Forensic Medicine*,
https://doi.org/10.1007/978-3-319-96737-0_20

investing in specialists of forensic imaging training.

In **Italy** a PMCT could be requested only by coroners as a complementary exam to their evaluations. Italian Mortuary Police Guidelines state that every unnecessary mutilation or dissection of a dead body should be avoided. It appears clear that PMCT can hold an important role in forensic evaluation, leading to a rapid and selected focus of investigation process and postmortem examination. Moreover European Guidelines on legal autopsy suggest radiological examination if considered useful.

20.2 Application: When and Where

Keeping in mind that PMCT in a noninvasive, fast, and quite available method, it can be easily understood that coroners and forensic experts tend to rely on its application more and more frequently, especially when a crime is suspected. PMCT proved to be an excellent tool for detection and assessment of bone fractures [6, 7], injuries due to sharp trauma [8], and bullet trajectories [9] (Fig. 20.1).

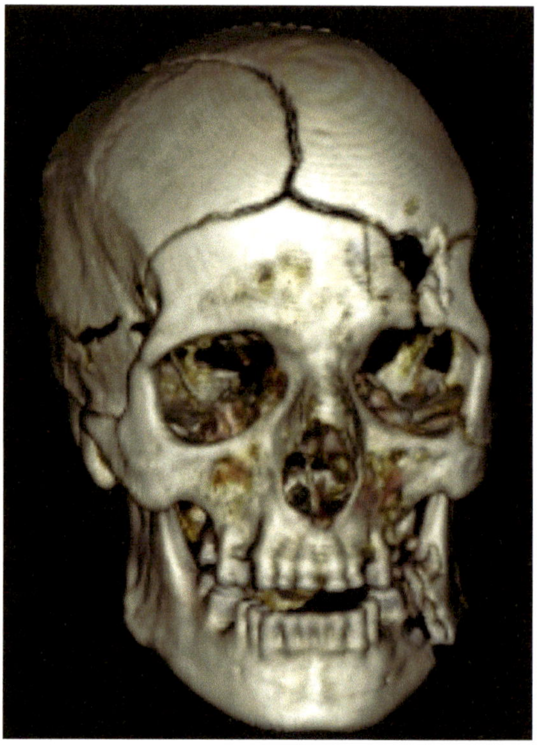

Fig. 20.1 3D volume rendering reconstruction of a skull, exit wound of a bullet trajectory, and fracture pattern can be noted

It has been used also in cases of drowning and asphyxiation, reaching a good correlation between CT findings and autoptic findings [10–13] (Fig. 20.2).

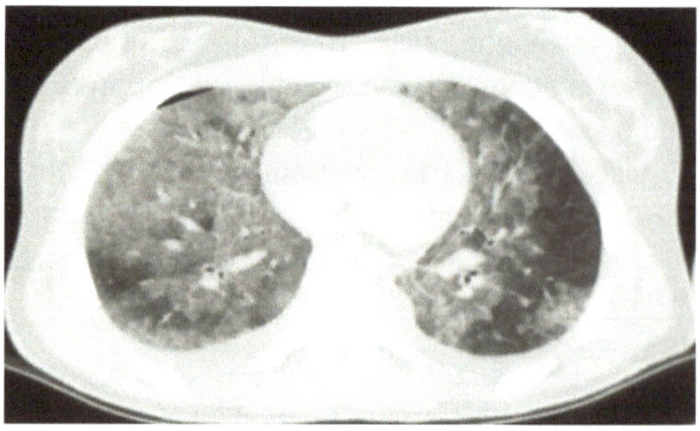

Fig. 20.2 PMCT axial section of lungs of a drowned victim of an airplane accident and diffuse ground-glass opacities can be noted

Because of its noninvasive nature, PMCT should be considered also in all cases where body is found in advanced state of decomposition or has been subjected to massive alterations, such as burning at high temperatures [14, 15]. Finally an important application of PMCT is certainly investigation following a mass disaster [16]. In this case all bodies could be scanned in site (through portable CT scanners, if feasible) or at a dedicated institution. Postmortem data (supposed cause of death, presence of medical devices, prosthesis, peculiar characteristics, previous fractures, etc.) could be gathered and used for identification [14, 17–19].

It's common opinion between forensic experts that PMCT could be used to gain as much preliminary data as possible to presume a cause of death and to better plan a regular autopsy that is an expensive and time-consuming method [20, 21]. It's our belief that a strict cooperation between forensic radiologist, coroner, and all forensic experts could be very rewarding. Both radiologists and coroners could focus their attention where needed and reach their purposes faster [22]. Even if autopsy is considered gold standard, we must note that in some cases PMCT proved to be sufficient to determine the cause of death. In our experience this was possible thanks to collaboration between all forensic figures that provided necessary preliminary observations to the radiologist who could be easily misled especially if not an expert in forensic imaging [23]. In sense the Japanese experience is very peculiar, as said above [24].

Unfortunately not all forensic radiologists have a forensic department available. If possible it's preferable to have dedicated scanners accessible at all times and appropriate structures, equipped for forensic exams, to reduce costs and to minimize delays from body recovery to radiological than autoptic examination. Our experience, as professionals involved in Italian and Sicilian background, concerns an academic institution, Policlinico "Paolo Giaccone" of University of Palermo. Coroners would bring bodies, always contained in a body bag, to our radiological department only after previous agreement with leading forensic radiologist. The majority of our exams are brought during evening hours, to avoid any contacts with patients who could be upset by the sight of a dead body, even if contained in a body bag. Our CT scanner performs regular activity during daytime and special cleaning is scheduled, if necessary, after forensic acquisition. Sharing regular activity of a CT section and forensic commitment leads to several problems in a radiologic department managing. First of all personnel need to be available at any time and often with little notice. No trained radiographers are generally available and forensic radiologists need to take extreme care of technical execution. Moreover, special transports need to be settled and, in order to gain state-of-the-art examinations, forensic equipment need to be acquired (e.g., contrast medium pump).

20.3 Acquisition: Protocols and Procedures

In our institution we perform basal scans of each body bag. First a 5 mm thick slice sequential scan of the head is performed, and then a spiral single scan is performed including all body volume (1.25- or 0.6-mm-thick slice acquisition, depending on if a more detailed representation of bones is required). If a single acquisition is not possible because of body positioning due to rigor mortis, scan would be repeated after repositioning [25]. Images are evaluated on dedicated workstation where 3D and multi-planar reconstructions are available. Reconstructions are particularly helpful to evaluate fracture patterns and bullet trajectories and to highlight any significant finding. We suggest to always perform multi-planar reconstruction (MPR) to evaluate general positioning of the body and to have a look at potential correlation between each finding (e.g., fracture patterns, distribution of hypostasis, fluid collection, and gas degeneration).

Extensive studies have been conducted about multiphasic angiography PMCT with contrast medium injection (MAPMCT). Contrast medium could be very useful in assessing organ-specific vascular patterns, vascular alteration under pathologic and physiologic conditions, and tissue changes induced by artificial and unnatural causes. Naturally trained personnel are essential. Giving up its peculiar noninvasive characteristic, PMCT acquires new spectrum of findings and new applications; postsurgical deaths and suspected cardiac failures are just two of them [26–28]. New techniques are approaching, such as postmortem ventilation, a procedure obtained through a special ventilator, aimed to better identify pulmonary pathologies [29].

We should remember that, especially if there's a crime investigation, this data need to be stored and displayed in court. Advanced 3D and MPR reconstruction could be very useful also for coroners and investigators. More than ever radiology is called to be as iconographic as ever, producing iconographic material to illustrate reports (Fig. 20.3).

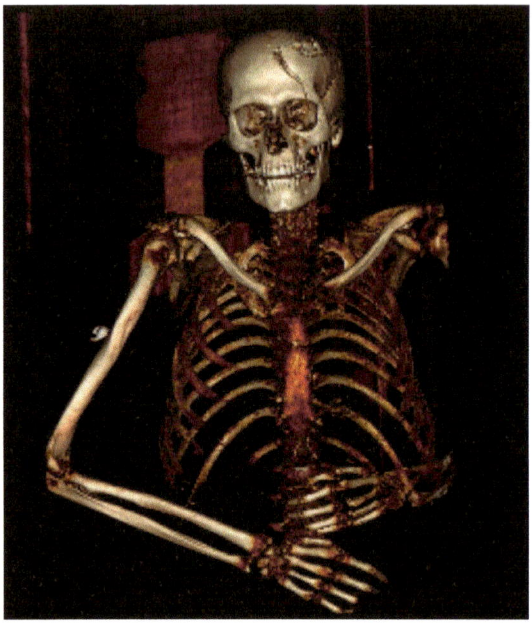

Fig. 20.3 3D volume rendering reconstruction, a retained bullet positioned at posterolateral left omerus is shown, later was found between victim's clothes

20.4 What to Search in PMCT and What to Ask to Forensic Radiologist

Postmortem findings hide numerous challenges for radiologists. Firstly they need to know precise sequence of cadaveric decomposition and transformation, than they need to identify those changes in CT findings [30]. Time between death, recovery of body, and execution of forensic exams is crucial. Evaluation of internal organs could be compromised by post-biotic changings. This is especially true for blood [31], lungs [32], and cerebral parenchyma [33, 34]. Natural disarticulation needs also to be held into account; differentiating it from traumatic dislocation can be tricky [35]. For these reasons, unless the cause and time of death are clear, a classic autopsy should be performed only after PMCT.

Coroners requesting a PMCT should have a clear suspicion for the cause of death and, as for clinical CTs, ask specific questions to the radiologist. It's necessary to provide details on the manner of first recovery and initial status of the body. Anamnesis and contest are vital to any radiological examination. Knowing that bone tissues are easily visualized, trauma victims are certainly excellent subjects to undergo a PMCT. Furthermore advanced techniques as multiphasic angiography PMCT and postmortem ventilation [29] expand the number of answers that can be found in a body, miming a normal CT acquired in living patients.

A strict collaboration with coroners should be obtained also in report drafting. Coroners are generally more accustomed to court reports. Every forensic institution could come up with a structured report, to better adjust to different realities in forensic and radiological contests.

Especially in criminal cases reports should be as inclusive as possible, but at the same time it should be kept in mind that it will be part of a court case and that it's going to be read by non-medical professionals (solicitors, judges, etc.) [36]. Extensive iconographic material should be provided. As some studies reported 3D reconstructions are better appreciated [37] (Fig. 20.1). Privacy of patients is always a main goal of every institution, but it can be easily understood how a forensic exam could oblige to extreme privacy between professionals. This is particularly true if PMCTs are acquired in non-dedicated institutions, where personnel are not necessarily involved in the acquisition but can easily reach examination room.

References

1. Wüllenweber R, Schneider V, Grumme T (1977) A computer-tomographical examination of cranial bullet wounds. Z Rechtsmed 80:227–246
2. Thali MJ, Jackowski C, Osterhelweg L, Ross SG, Dirnhofer R (2007) VIRTOPSY—the Swiss virtual approach. Legal Med 9:100–104
3. Poulsen K, Simonsen J (2007) Computed tomography as routine in connection with medico-legal autopsies. Forensic Sci Int 171:190–197
4. Leth PM, Thomsen J (2013) Experience with postmortem computer tomography in southern Denmark 2006–11. J Forensic Radiol Imaging 1:161–166
5. Okuda T, Shiotani S, Sakamoto N, Konayashi T (2013) Background and current status of postmortem imaging in Japan: short history of "autopsy imaging (Ai)". Forensic Sci Int 225:3–8

6. Wilemann Y, Thali MJ, Kneubuehl BP, Bollinger SA (2008) Correlation between skeletal trauma and energy in falls from great height detected by postmortem multislice computed tomography (MSCT). Forensic Sci Int 180:81–85
7. Leth PM, Struckmann H, Lauritsen J (2013) Interobserver agreement of the injury diagnoses obtained by postmortem computed tomography of traffic fatality victims and a comparison with autopsy results. Forensic Sci Int 225:15–19
8. Schnider J, Thali MJ, Ross S, Osterhelweg L, Spendlove D, Bollinger SA (2009) Injuries due to sharp trauma detected by post-mortem multislice computed tomography (MSCT): a feasibility study. Legal Med 11:4–9
9. Kirchhoff SM, Scaparra EF, Grimm J et al (2016) Postmortem computed tomography (PMCT) in deadly gunshot wounds. Int J Legal Med 130:819. https://doi.org/10.1007/s00414-015-1225-z
10. Plaetsen SV, De Letter E, Piette M, Van Parys G, Casselman JW, Verstraete K (2015) Post-mortem evaluation of drowning with whole body CT. Forensic Sci Int 249:35–41
11. Leth PM, Madsen BH (2017) Drowning investigated by post mortem computed tomography and autopsy. J Forensic Radiol Imaging 9:28–30
12. Aquila I, Falcone C, Di Nunzio C, Tamburrini O, Boca S, Ricci P (2013) Virtopsy versus autopsy in unusual case of asphyxia: case report. Forensic Sci Int 229:e1–e5
13. Ruder TD, Thali Y, Schindera ST, Dalla Torre SA, Zech W, Ross S, Hatch GM (2012) How reliable are Hounsfield units measurements in forensic radiology? Forensic Sci Int 220:219–223
14. Thali MJ, Yen K, Schweizer W, Vock P, Ozdoba C, Dirnhofer R (2003) Into the decomposed body—forensic digital autopsy using multislice-computed tomography. Forensic Sci Int 134:109–114
15. Murakami T, Akashi S, Uetani M, Murase T, Yamamoto T, Ikematsu K. Burned bodies: how do we evaluate the death in a fire on CT? EPOS Electronic Presentation Online System (105) ECR
16. O'Donnell C, Iino M, Mansharan K, Leditscke J, Woodford N (2011) Contribution of postmortem multidetector CT scanning to identification of the deceased in a mass disaster: experience gained from the 2009 Victorian bushfires. Forensic Sci Int 205:15–28
17. Ruder TD, Kneubuehl BP, Gotsmy WF, Mathier S, Ebert LC, Thali MJ, Hatch GM (2012) Radiologic identification of disaster victims: a simple and reliable method using CT of the paranasal sinuses. Eur J Radiol 81:e132–e138
18. Pfaeffli M, Vock P, Dirhofer R, Braun M, Bollinger SA, Thali MJ (2007) Post-mortem radiological CT identification based on classical ante-mortem X-ray examinations. Forensic Sci Int 171:111–117
19. Sidlerr m, Jackowski C, Dirnhoefer R, Vock P, Thali M (2007) Use of multislice computed tomography in disaster victim identification—advantages and limitations. Forensic Sci Int 169:118–128
20. Thomsen AH, Jurik AG, Uhurenholt L, Vesterby A (2009) An alternative approach to computerized tomography in forensic pathology. Forensic Sci Int 183:87–90
21. Kasahara S, Makino Y, Hayakawa M, Yajima Y (2012) Diagnosable and non-diagnosable causes of death by postmortem computed tomography: a review of 339 forensic cases. Legal Med 14:239–245
22. Roberts IAS, Benamore RE, Benbow EW, Lee SH, Harris JN, Jackson A, Mallett S, Patankar T, Peebles C, Roobottom C, Traill ZC (2012) Post-mortem imaging as an alternative to autopsy in the diagnosis of adults deaths: a validation study. Lancet 379:136–142
23. Filograna L, Tartaglione T, Filograna E, Cittadini F, Oliva A, Paascali V (2010) Computed tomography (CT) virtual autopsy and classical autopsy discrepancies: Radiologist's error or a demonstration of post-mortem multi-detector computed tomography (MDCT) limitation? Forensic Sci Int 195:e13–e17
24. Kaneko T, Hibi M, Nakatsuka A, Omori Y, Hatada T, Takei Y, Takeda K (2010) Postmortem computed tomography is an informative approach for prevention of sudden unexpected natural death in the elderly. Risk Manag Healthc Policy 3:13–20
25. Flach PM, Gascho D, Schweitzer W, Ruder TD, Berger N, Ross SG, Thali MJ, Ampanozi G (2014) Imaging in forensic radiology: an illustrated guide for postmortem computed tomography technique and protocols. Forensic Sci Med Pathol 10:583–606. https://doi.org/10.1007/s12024-014-9555-6
26. Grabherr S, Djonov V, Thali MJ, Dirnhofer R (2007) Postmortem angiography—review of former and current methods. AJR 188:832–838
27. Vogel B, Heinemann A, Gehl A, Hasegawa I, Hopker W-W, Poodendaen C, Tzikas A, Gulbins H, Reichenspurner H, Puschel K, Vogel H (2013) Postmortem computed tomography (PMCT) and PMCT-angiography after transvascular cardiac interventions. ARCH MED SĄD KRYMINOL LXIII:255–266
28. Grabher S, Grimm J, Dominguez A, Vanhaebost J, Mangin P (2014) Advances in post-mortem CT-angiography. Br J Radiol 87:20130488
29. Germerott T, Flach PM, Preiss US, Ross SG, Thali MJ (2012) Post-mortem ventilation a new method for improved detection of pulmonary pathologies in forensic imaging. Legal Med 14:223–228
30. Christe A, Flach P, Ross S, Spendlove D, Bollinger S, Vock P, Thali MJ (2010) Clinical radiology and postmortem imaging (Virtopsy) are not the same: specific and unspecific postmortem signs. Legal Med 12:215–222
31. Jackowski C, Thali M, Aghayev E, Yen K, Sonnenschein M, Zwygart K, Dirnhofer R, Vock P (2006) Postmortem imaging of blood and its characteristics using MSCT and MRI. Int J Legal Med 120:233–240

32. Shiotani S, Kohno M, Ohashi N, Yamazali K, Nakayama H, Ko W, Oyake Y, Itai Y (2004) Non-traumatic postmortem computer tomographic (PMCT) findings of the lung. Forensic Sci Int 139:39–48
33. Berger N, Ampanozi G, Schweitzer W, Ross SG, Gascho D, Ruder TD, Thali MJ, Flach PM (2015) Racking the brain: detection of cerebral edema on postmortem computed tomography compared with forensic autopsy. Eur J Radiol 84:643–651
34. Flach PM, Egli TC, Bollinger SA, Berger N, Ampanozi G, Thali MJ, Schweitzer W (2014) "Blind spots" in forensic autopsy: improved detection of retrobulbar hemorrhage and orbital lesions by post-mortem computed tomography (PMCT). Legal Med 16:274–282
35. Persson A, Falk J, Berge J, Jackowski C (2013) Atlanto-axial rotatory subluxations in post-mortem CT: radiologists be aware of a common pitfall. Forensic Sci Int 225:9–14
36. Ebert LC, Ruder TD, Martinez RM, Flach PM, Schweitzer W, Thali MJ, Ampanozi G (2015) Computer assisted virtual autopsy using surgical navigation techniques. AJR 204:W58–W62
37. Ampanozi G, Zimmermann D, Hatch GM, Ruder TD, Ross S, Flach PM, Thali MJ, Ebert LC (2012) Format preferences of district attorneys for post-mortem medical imaging reports: understandability, cost effectiveness, and suitability for the courtroom: a questionnaire based study. Legal Med 14:116–120

Images in Forensic Thanatology

21

Magdy Kharoshah, Dalia Alsaif, Marwa Al Bayat, Ghada Al Shamsi, and Kholoud Alsowayigh

21.1 Introduction

Imaging techniques are highly effective devices used extensively by forensic analysts, such as medical examiners, forensic pathologists, and anthropologists. They can be applied to aid the interpretation of results in medicolegal cases. Typically, radiologists have acquired expert knowledge in imaging procedures, and forensic investigation teams draw upon these vitally important skills when conducting forensic consultations. Therefore, radiological examinations perform a vital function in detecting foreign bodies (for example, bullets or air embolism), as well as providing evidence of fractures and other mechanical trauma-related injuries. A virtual alternative to traditional autopsy, known as virtopsy, adopts a new approach, where whole-body computed tomography (CT) and magnetic resonance imaging (MRI) scans can now be used to produce both two-dimensional and three-dimensional images. It presents another option for families averse to autopsies, as well as working in parallel with conventional procedures to produce enhanced visual representations of postmortem results. Globally, forensic laboratories typically compare antemortem and postmortem radiographic plates in order to establish the identity of unknown deceased persons. In addition, the extensive use of electronic databases nowadays, in the majority of hospitals, has significantly decreased the lead time required to retrieve specific X-rays. This has resulted in forensic pathologists and anthropologists frequently relying upon a comparative analysis of radiographic plates in order to confirm the identity of unknown deceased people. Furthermore, this has become a well-established practice both in routine identification processes and where mass fatality events have occurred. Radiographs are a rapid, efficient, and comparably straightforward tool when used to determine the identity of a person in a postmortem examination. Forensic age estimation of individuals who are either alive or dead is largely dependent on correlating radiographs with dental and skeletal developmental stages of growth. The primary purpose of this chapter is to outline the way in which radiology can be used effectively in investigation of death in specific circumstances [1].

M. Kharoshah (✉) · D. Alsaif · M. Al Bayat
G. Al Shamsi
Dammam Forensic Medicine Center,
Dammam, Kingdom of Saudi Arabia

K. Alsowayigh
Jeddah Forensic Medicine Center,
Jeddah, Kingdom of Saudi Arabia

21.2 Identification

Radiographic analysis of epiphyseal closure can be used to determine age at the time of

G. Lo Re et al. (eds.), *Radiology in Forensic Medicine*,
https://doi.org/10.1007/978-3-319-96737-0_21

death for unidentified bodies, in particular where it is not possible to conduct a postmortem (Fig. 21.1). Undertaking a comparative analysis of antemortem and postmortem radiographs generally produces positive identification results (Figs. 21.2 and 21.3). This can be achieved by matching previous and current indicators, for example, any historical evidence of orthopedic or general surgery that had been carried out.

Teeth are remarkably resilient, as they comprise extremely durable substances, such as enamel. Restorative materials used in dentistry have the capacity to withstand exposure to significant physical and chemical forces. Consequently, forensic dentistry is a very beneficial and robust technique, as a myriad of variations can occur to give every individual a unique identity. These include missing teeth, tooth crowns or root decay, fillings, and permanent or removable dental prosthesis, along with the usual differences in the shape and structure of dental crowns and roots (Fig. 21.4).

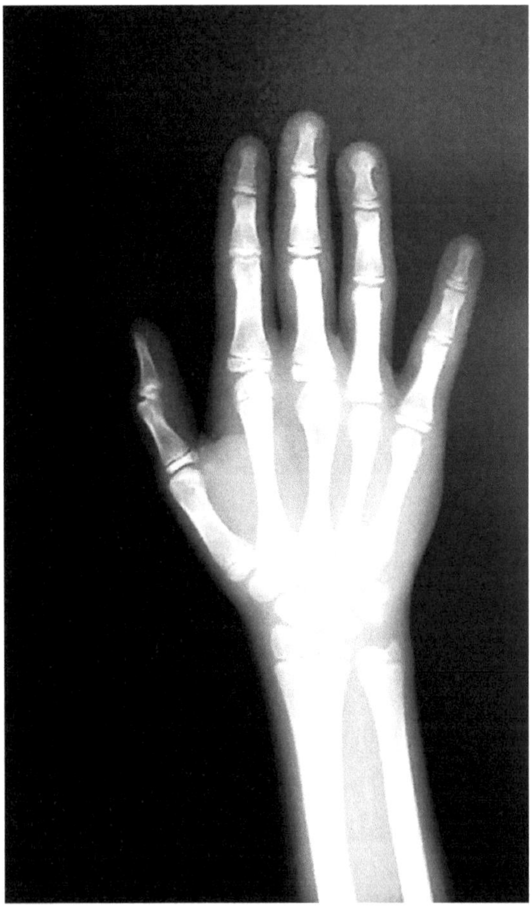

Fig. 21.1 Unfused metacarpal bones, distal end of radius, and ulna (less than 18 years in males)

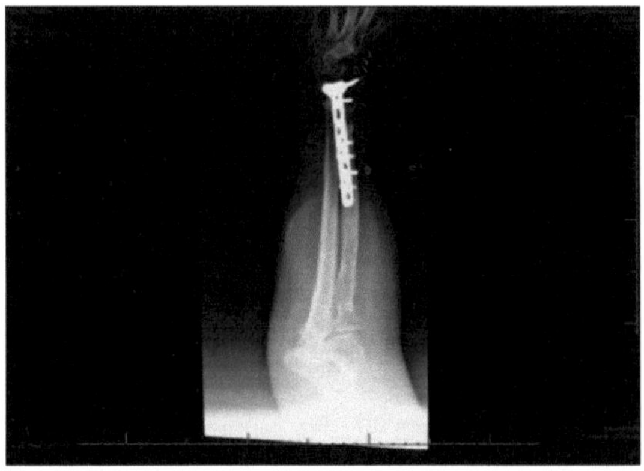

Fig. 21.2 X-ray of right forearm of unidentified female victim. Orthopedic surgery for fixation of radial fracture supports positive identification of her body

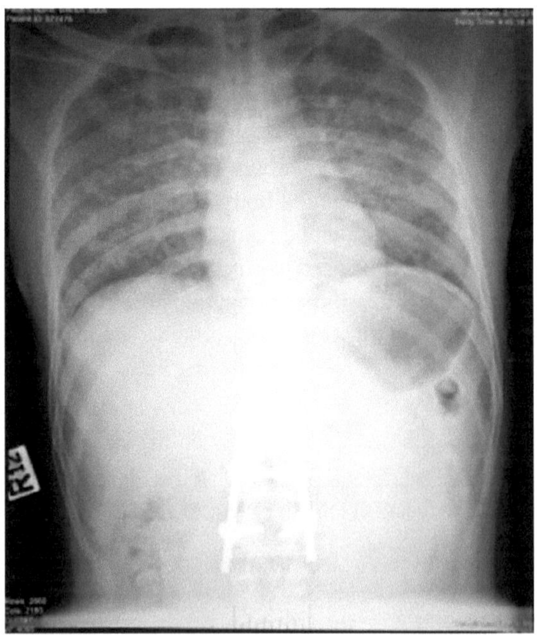

Fig. 21.3 Nails and plate fixation of vertebrae noticed during postmortem examination of unknown bodies

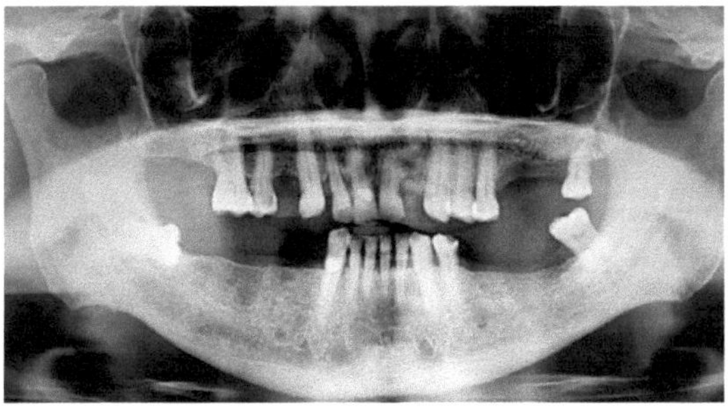

Fig. 21.4 Multiple missing teeth, multiple decayed teeth, multiple defective restorations

21.3 Asphyxia

Radiological findings are few in most of cases of asphyxial deaths. The purpose of postmortem radiological imaging is to assess the neck structures for findings that can guide the examiner at autopsy. The main aims are the detection of foreign body (Fig. 21.5) and skeletal fracture and the identification of congenital or natural diseases which could contribute to asphyxial death. By using this imaging, the examination of the soft tissues is limited and usually requires an autopsy and laboratory investigations. In some cases of the asphyxial death, the cause of death can't be determined even with autopsy and histological examination [2].

21.3.1 Suffocation

In the upper airway obstruction by foreign body, plain X-ray, multi-slice computed tomography (MSCT), and magnetic resonance imaging (MRI) can be used to aid in the identification of the type and location of foreign body. Imaging of the airway prior to any intervention is very useful as the foreign body material can be dislodged and the location changed during organ removal at autopsy. In the diagnosis of smothering and chemical asphyxia, there are no specific findings that can be detected by using this imaging [2, 3].

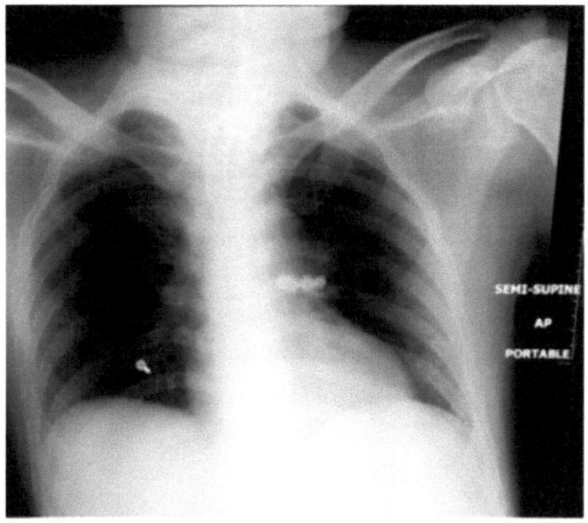

Fig. 21.5 Foreign body (artificial teeth) swallowed and impacted in left bronchus

21.3.2 Pressure on the Neck

Postmortem MSCT and MRI might be helpful to detect fractures that could be missed in autopsy of strangulation and hanging cases. The main findings are fractures of the greater horns of the hyoid bone, the superior horns of the thyroid cartilage, and less frequently the inferior horns and its lamina and the cricoid cartilage arch and rarely its lamina. Soft-tissue lesions such as subcutaneous, intramuscular, and lymph node hemorrhage could be detected by MSCT and MRI [4, 5].

MSCT in judicial hanging mainly shows fracture of the second cervical vertebra (C2) which is known as hangman's fracture. It is a fracture of neural arch of C2 vertebral body with fracture dislocation of C2 from C3 vertebra. Variation in C2 fracture may occur as well as fractures of other cervical vertebrae, thyroid cartilage, hyoid bone, and styloid processes. MSCT may also show interruption of the anterior and posterior longitudinal ligament with fracture dislocation or complete dissociation, and spinal cord transaction. Ligaments and spinal cord injuries are best showed with MRI. These findings can be missed in routine autopsy [6].

21.4 Motor Vehicle Accidents

Postmortem examination of causalities after motor vehicle accidents is conducted mainly to identify occupants, determine the cause of death, and exclude other factors that could lead to loss of control of the vehicle. However, determining the position of the occupants and who was in control of the vehicle if more than one was present could be the whole requirement of the investigative authorities. Reconstruction of the event can solve many questions that can't be answered by the autopsy alone.

While the external examination of the body can merely reveal deformity of the extremities that are not routinely dissected in autopsy, postmortem CT scans can show details of the fractures that can indicate the direction of the force and hence help with reconstructing the event. Messerer's wedge, for example, is a segment of fractured long bone that is displaced with the apex of the wedge indicating the direction of force (Fig. 21.6). This finding can be used to determine the position of the victim while he/she was hit by a vehicle [7].

In motor cycle accidents, the use of postmortem CT scan together with autopsy was found of significant importance in detecting fractures in the base of skull (fracture occipital condyles, ring and partial-ring fractures) and fractures of spinous and lateral processes of the spine; both can provide additive information about the cause and mechanism of death and are not detected easily by the autopsy alone. Also CT was found to be significant in detecting fractures of the shoulder part of the clavicle, lower limb fractures, and pneumothorax. All these are used in reconstruction of the accident and hence if it is accessible CT was found to be a mandatory technique in all cases of motorcycle fatalities [8]. Postmortem CT is superior to conventional autopsy in detecting serious injuries of abbreviation injury score (AIS) of three and more, especially if this involved skeletal injury, while it is less sensitive in detecting soft-tissue injuries [9].

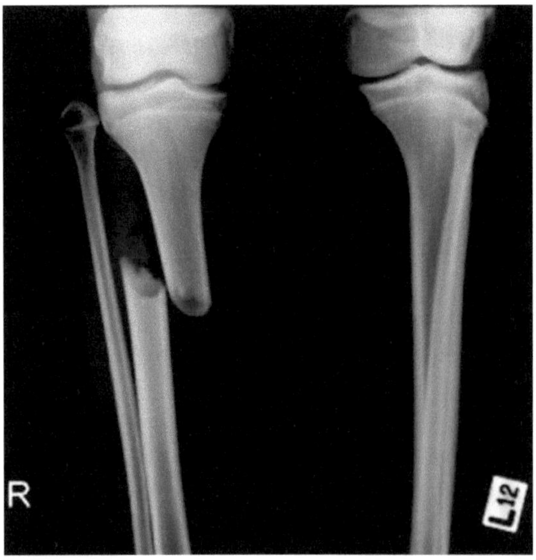

Fig. 21.6 Fractured tibia due to road traffic accident

In aviation accidents with small airplanes, anteroposterior and lateral X-rays are useful in detecting injuries of the upper and lower limbs that can be used to determine the position of the pilot. It was found that a higher number of right-sided hand injuries and left-side foot fractures can point that the person was in the control position. Interpretation of such findings requires full understanding of the controls of the airplane to correlate with findings [10]. CT scans can provide even more details of the fractures and displaced segments that can be used to determine the direction of force. 3D reconstruction of CT images provides better understanding of the event and is useful in reconstructing the accident [11].

21.5 Suspected Cases of Child Abuse

Autopsy in cases of child abuse mainly aims at determining the cause of death. Although the cause of death is required for the legal proceedings, the proof of abuse is of more importance in cases of suspected child abuse. It is significant to provide evidence that abuse has occurred by means of multiplicity of trauma that had occurred on different occasions. This can be shown by external examination of the body with skin injuries of different types and different ages. However, in some cases a radiological assessment is needed to be conducted to detect injuries that are not visible during autopsy or external examination and that can strongly indicate child abuse. Imaging modalities that are used in suspected cases of fatal child abuse include plain X-rays, CT scans, and MRI.

The findings of multiple fractures in different sites with different stages of healing are strongly associated with child abuse [12]. Healing of fractures is found as callus around the fracture site and can be detected about 14 days after the trauma. Plain X-rays can show callus but CT scans can detect earlier stages of healing at the edges of the fracture site in the form of osteosclerosis indicating different times of inflicted trauma [13].

Fractures that are indicative of child abuse include classical metaphyseal fractures. Metaphyseal fractures heal quickly without subperiosteal new bone formation and can be undetected in 4–8 weeks. Coned view of the long-bone metaphysis is needed to detect such fractures. Findings that are confused with classical metaphyseal fractures include lesions resulting from malnutrition in the form of defective osteoid matrix formation and collagen maturation of scurvy. This includes metaphyseal spur and lucent irregular dense metaphyseal margin [12].

Multiple rib fractures with different ages are strongly associated with abusive trauma and it is commonly found in the lateral or in the posterior part of the clavicle near its articulation with the spine. Skeletal surveys should include oblique chest X-rays to show rib fractures [14]. Occipital fractures are also suspicious of abuse therefore anteroposterior and lateral skull x-ray are needed to show such fractures.

It should be noted that birth trauma can lead to fractures that are detected later on radiography and could be confused with inflicted trauma. Fractures of birth trauma include clavicular fractures, diaphyseal humeral fractures, and proximal spiral or midshaft fractures of the femur [12].

CT and MRI detect injuries of internal organs that are common in child abuse as diffuse edema and loss of grey-white matter contrast indicative of head trauma and gaseous and fluid effusion in peritoneal cavity following traumatic intestinal perforation and liver laceration [13]. However, these organs are routinely examined during autopsy with injuries being more obvious.

Information from details of the incidents together with autopsy, radiological imaging, and laboratory results is needed in order to reach a diagnosis of child abuse.

21.6 Body Packers

Body packing is defined as the concealment of prepackaged drugs within the human body with the purpose of transporting the drugs from country to country. While body stuffing is also the concealment of drugs within the human body, it is usually of smaller amounts of drug packets and is for the purpose of hastily evading police detection in a sudden random search [15, 16].

The drugs are prepared into small packets made of condoms, latex gloves, or latex balloons, or they may even be wrapped in cellophane and then hidden anywhere inside the body such as in the GIT including the mouth and anus, or in the vagina and even sometimes in the ears [17, 18]. In cases where the drugs are inserted into the rectum or vagina it is referred to as body pushing [16, 19]. The most common drugs smuggled in this way are cocaine (regardless of its form), heroin, methamphetamine, and cannabis while hallucinogens, synthetic drugs, and ecstasy are not encountered as commonly [17–19].

The phenomenon of body packing can lead to a devastating medical emergency if the packets rupture, resulting in an acute intoxication or the so-called body packer syndrome. The signs of intoxication may vary depending on the type of drug in the packet and the amount of drug that has leaked into the patient's system. But such signs and symptoms may range from a change in pupil size, vomiting, constipation, abdominal pain, seizures, and even loss of consciousness [17, 18]. Body packing may also lead to bowel obstruction and perforation and even peritonitis, which is in itself a medical emergency. That is why proper imagining for the detection of body packing is very essential in order to treat the patient. In fatal cases of drug smuggling, the radiologist also plays an important role in detecting the exact location and number of drug packets for easy removal during autopsy.

Plain abdominal radiographs are the commonly used to detect body packers owing to their easy availability and low cost. In a standard ABX, the drug packets are typically seen as multiple, heterogeneously dense, uniformly shaped oval or rectangular objects found in a row or a cluster within the alimentary tract; this finding is referred to as the "tic-tac sign." Other commonly seen signs include the "double-condom sign" which is seen when there is air trapped between the multiple layers of the latex material used to package the drugs. The "rosette sign" is seen when there is air trapped within the knots where the packing material was tied [17, 18, 20]. The clarity of these signs is influenced by the number of packets ingested, the radiodensity of the packing material used, and the radiodensity of the drug itself (liquid cocaine has a density similar to that of feces, heroin is less dense than feces while cannabis is more dense than feces) [19, 20].

An unenhanced CT scan has a higher rate of sensitivity and specificity when compared to a standard ABX, owing to its better spiral resolution and better contrast [19]. This is why an unenhanced CT provides better more accurate information regarding the exact position and number of drug packets [21]. This is especially useful for some forensic centers which only open the stomach and duodenum and rectum but not the whole of the intestines on routine autopsy cases; in such scenarios a postmortem CT would provide enough reason to autopsy the intestines, and furthermore accurately locate the drug packages. One of the complications of body packing is that the packages are prone to leakage or even rupture, leading to bowel obstruction or even bowel perforation. In such cases a postmortem CT may assist the forensic pathologist in determining the cause of death prior to an autopsy, by properly identifying intact and ruptured packages, or perforated bowels [22]. It is important to keep in mind that a contrast-enhanced CT is not useful in determining the number and location of the drug packages; instead it can be used for the identification of a perforated bowl as a complication or a cause of death [17, 19, 23].

21.7 Firearm Injuries

Injury resulting from firearm use is a growing public health concern, and is a major cause of death in the United States [24]. This is one of the many reasons why gunshot injuries are considered to be a principal field of study in regards to postmortem forensic radiology. Postmortem forensic radiology is a useful noninvasive tool used to help identify the exact location of a missile within the body, identify the missal's track, and help identify the type of missile and possibly the weapon used. And of course, a postmortem radiograph is very essential in identifying whether or not a gunshot wound even exists in a severely decomposed body [25].

In cases of firearm fatalities, a postmortem plain radiograph is a very useful tool; it is usually the first step taken to help identify the projectiles in the body (Figs. 21.7 and 21.8). A postmortem radiograph essentially helps the forensic pathologist in retrieving the bullet or bullets; it saves time by giving an idea of the projectile's location, instead of having to blindly look for the bullet in body during autopsy, because it is common knowledge that a projectile can be seen at a site some distance from its entry point, especially if it collided with bone along its path. Recovering these projectiles counts as a crucial piece of evidence, because when retrieved they can be further

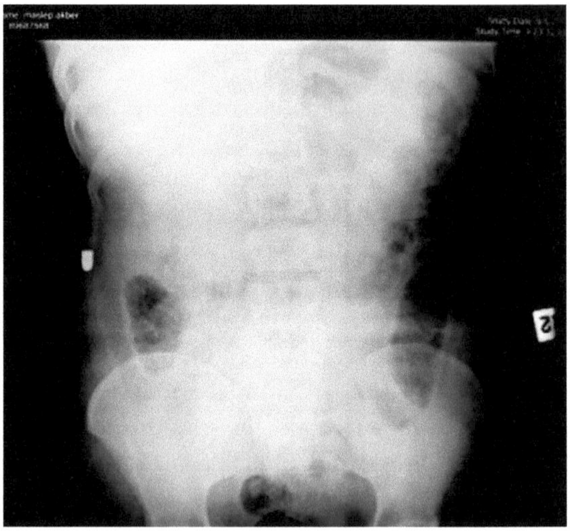

Fig. 21.7 Retained bullet in the abdomen

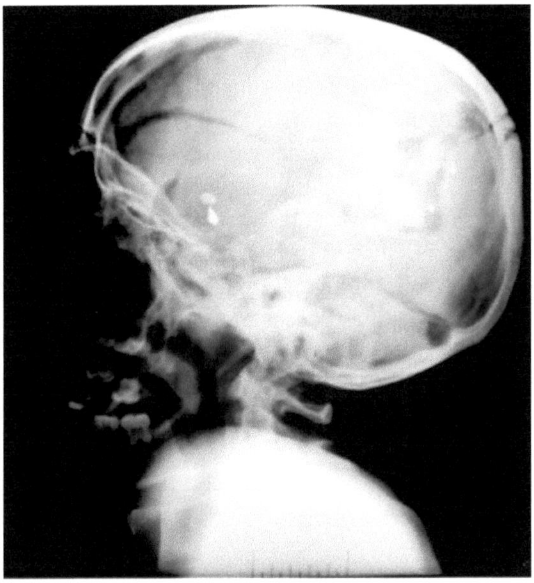

Fig. 21.8 Fragmented bullet in cranial cavity

examined for the presence of rifling class characteristics to help identify the weapon used. These radiographs also help in identifying the number of projectiles found within the body; it is essential to correlate between the number of entrance and exit points and the number of projectiles found inside the body and the number of projectiles found at the scene of death [25–27]. Despite this, postmortem plain radiographs are at a disadvantage, because they reduce the 3D human body into a 2D image [25, 28].

Where a plain postmortem radiograph provides a simple 2D image a postmortem CT provides a more accurate 3D image of the body, thereby allowing better interpretation in regards to the missile's track and better distinction between entrance and exit wounds, and above all aiding in the reconstruction of the crime scene [25, 28]. Postmortem CT is considered to be a highly efficient modality to identify the accurate location of a bullet and bullet fragments [27]. Postmortem CT is also beneficial in providing a comprehensive review of the damage imposed on the internal organs especially to the areas of the body that are harder to reach during autopsy such as the posterior neck region and the face; postmortem CTs are also beneficial in reconstructing images of skeletal injuries [28, 29].

21.8 Diving Accidents

Fatalities due to diving accidents rarely present to the forensic examiner. According to Divers Alert Network 2006, 1 in about 40,000 dives results in death. The cause of death is attributed mostly to drowning. However, drowning can be just the immediate cause of death with other factors acting as triggers. The role of the forensic examiner is to exclude violence, determine the cause of death, and detect the trigger that leads to drowning [30].

Among the causes of death in diving is pressure-related fatalities including barotrauma and arterial gas embolism. The presence of gas in certain body areas is fatal and the way by which it gets access to the body is explained by two physical laws of pressure. Barotrauma is best explained by Boyle's law stating that the volume of a gas is inversely proportionate to the pressure when the temperature is constant. Hence, during rapid ascent from deep water, the volume of air in lungs increases as the pressure decreases. Air that is entrapped in the lungs by a disease or breath holding will lead to rupture of alveoli and damage to lung tissue with air escaping to surrounding space causing pneumothorax and subcutaneous emphysema. Air can find its way to pulmonary veins and get to left heart and systemic circulation with arterial gas embolism. Death can occur due to stroke or cardiac ischemia due to air embolism [30, 31].

Another pressure-related fatality is due to decompression sickness, which occurs in water depth of 21–30 m and is explained by Henry's law stating that the mass of gas that is dissolved in a fluid is proportionate to the pressure of gas over the fluid. The longer and deeper the dive lasts, the more dissolved the inert gas. As the pressure decreases the gas will appear in the fluid as bubbles [30]. During rapid ascent, where there is no time for gradual expiration of air, bubbles appear in vessels and tissues. Pain due to the presence of air in ears and joint, although nonfatal, can lead to drowning accidents. Also air in these parts indicates that a gas decompression has occurred in the body [31]. Appearance of gas bubbles in blood vessels can lead to arterial gas embolism and death if it reaches vital organs. Collection of air in cardiac chambers can lead to pump failure and death. It must be acknowledged that gas in the body can result from other causes as resuscitation with intubation, venous cannula, putrefaction, and off-gassing (postmortem decompression).

Investigating deaths in pressure-related fatalities needs a team work of the police, technical experts to examine the diving apparatus, and forensic pathologists. While special procedures are needed during autopsy to detect gas in vessels or body cavities, radiological imaging can be of great help especially if a forensic pathologist is not available or if special autopsy procedures can't be conducted. Radiological imaging modalities that can be implied include X-ray and computed tomography scans.

X-ray films are the most useful imaging modalities in detecting air in the body and should be used routinely before autopsy [31]. Chest X-rays of barotrauma cases showed pneumothorax and diffuse alveolar shadowing. Gas was detected by X-rays in aorta, inferior vena cava, and arterial blood vessels including brachial, left common carotid, axillary, common and external iliac, profunda and superficial femoral, vertebral, basilar arteries, and circle of Willis. It was also reported in hepatic vessels and portal venous system, and in venous plexus around the base of bladder. Gaseous distention of small bowel, large bowel, and stomach and intramuscular gas in abdominal wall and leg muscles were also reported [32].

Computed tomography scans were found to be more sensitive in detecting gas and as little as 0.5 cm^3 of intracerebral gas [32]; however this sensitivity could be a drawback of this method as it can lead to confusion with gases developing in the body following putrefaction. Putrefactive gases can form in the body as early as 26 h following death but only in small amounts. It was reported in the heart as a small bubble and as trivial amount in hepatic vessels. The examiner should be cautious in the interpretation of these findings before referring them as a cause of death. Although CT scans are recommended by the Royal College of Pathologists in Australia [33], some investigators find X-rays superior to CTs because of the CT's high sensitivity. A CT of chest, neck, and head is recommended if possible. Together with MRI, CT can be superior in detecting bubbles in meningeal vessels and spinal artery [34]. CT findings include gas in cardiac and cerebral vessels, pleural cavities, coronaries, liver, and kidney vessels.

Routine radiological images should be part of the investigative process in cases of diving accidents together with autopsy. The radiological imaging can be the only way to detect gas in the body, which is used as a cause of death.

21.9 Drowning

Computed tomography (CT) of victims of drowning may show excessive fluid in the paranasal sinuses, maxillary sinuses, sphenoid sinuses, nasal pharynx, oropharynx, trachea, ground-glass opacities in the lung, pleural fluid, esophageal fluid, stomach fluid, and pericardial fluid. CT is better than autopsy in detecting fluid in the organs, because handling of the body during autopsy can lead to movement of the fluid [35]. These findings can be caused by different mechanisms other than drowning, and may be absent in some cases. Diagnosis of drowning is difficult and an exclusion of other causes is needed [36].

Using the density of sinus fluid to differentiate between saltwater and freshwater drowning by postmortem CT is better than using the sinus fluid volume. And it was found that the difference in density is much notable than differences in volume with higher density in saltwater drowning [37].

References

1. Thali MJ, Vock P (2003) Role and techniques in forensic imaging. In: Payne- James J, Busutil A, Smock W (eds) Forensic medicine: clinical and pathological aspect. Greenwich Medical Media, London, pp 731–746
2. Rutty GN, Jeffery AJ, Raj V, Morgan B (2010) The use of postmortem computed tomography in the investigation of intentional neonatal upper airway obstruction: an illustrated case. Int J Legal Med 124:641–645

3. Iino M, O'Donnell C (2010) Postmortem computed tomography findings of upper airway obstruction by food. J Forensic Sci 55:1251–1258
4. Kempter M, Ross S, Spendlove D, Flach PM, Preiss U, Thali MJ, Bolliger SA (2009) Post-mortem imaging of laryngohyoid fracture in strangulation incidents: first results. Legal Med 11:267–271
5. Yen K, Thali MJ, Aghayev E, Jackowski C, Schweitzer W, Boesch C, Vock P, Dirnhofer R, Sonnenschein M (2005) Strangulation signs: initial correlation of MRI, MSCT, and forensic neck findings. J Magn Reson Imaging 22:501–510
6. Hayashi T, Hartwig S, Tsokos M, Oesterhelweg L (2014) Postmortem multislice computed tomography (pmMSCT) imaging of hangman's fracture. Forensic Sci Med Pathol 10:3–8
7. Benali L, Gromb S, Bou C (2013) Post-mortem imaging in traffic fatalities: from autopsy to reconstruction of the scene using freely available software. Int J Legal Med 127:1045–1049
8. Moskała A, Woźniak K, Kluza P, Romaszko K, Lopatin O (2016) The importance of post-mortem computed tomography (PMCT) in confrontation with conventional forensic autopsy of victims of motorcycle accidents. Legal Med 18:25–30
9. Sochor MR, Trowbridge MJ, Boscak A, Maino JC, Maio RF (2008) Postmortem computed tomography as an adjunct to autopsy for analyzing fatal motor vehicle crash injuries: results of a pilot study. J Trauma 65:659–665
10. Kubat B, Korthout T, van Ingen G, Rietveld LAC, de Bakker HM (2014) Radiological analysis of hand and foot injuries after small aircraft crashes. Forensic Sci Med Pathol 10:351–356
11. Folio RL, Harcke HT, Luzi SA (2009) Aircraft mishap investigation with radiology-assisted autopsy: helicopter crash with control injury. Aviat Space Environ Med 80(4):400–404
12. Ross AH, Juarez CA (2016) Skeletal and radiological manifestations of child abuse: implications for study in past populations. Clin Anat 29:844–853
13. Dedouit F, Mallinger B, Guilbeau-Frugier C, Rougé D, Rousseau H, Telmon N (2011) Lethal visceral traumatic injuries secondary to child abuse: a case of practical application of autopsy, radiological and microscopic studies. Forensic Sci Int 206: e62–e66
14. Kempa AM, Butlerb A, Morrisb S, Mannc M, Kempa KW, Rolfea K, Siberta JR, Maguire S (2006) Which radiological investigations should be performed to identify fractures in suspected child abuse? Clin Radiol 61:723–736
15. Dolinak D, Matches E, Lew E (2005) Forensic pathology: principles and practice. Elsevier/Academic Press, Burlington, MA. ISBN: 0-12-219951-0
16. Flach PM, Ross SG, Ampanozi G, Ebert L, Germerott T, Hatch GM, Thali MJ, Patak MA (2012) "Drug mules" as a radiological challenge: sensitivity and specificity in identifying internal cocaine in body packers, body pushers and body stuffers by computed tomography, plain radiography and Lodox. Eur J Radiol 81:2518–2526
17. Reginelli A, Russo A, Urraro F, Maresca D, Martiniello C, D'Andrea A, Brunese L, Pinto A (2015) Imaging of body packing: errors and medicolegal issues. Abdom Imaging 40:2127–2142
18. Lee K, Koehn M, Rastegar RF, van Hoorn F, Roy E, Berger FH, Nicolaou S (2012) Body packers: the ins and outs of imaging. Can Assoc Radiol J 63:318–322
19. Berger FH, Nieboer KH, Goh GS, Pinto A, Scaglione M (2015) Body packing: a review of general background, clinical and imaging aspects. Radiol Med 120:118–132
20. Niewiarowski S, Gogbashian A, Afaq A, Kantor R, Win Z (2010) Abdominal X-ray signs of intraintestinal drug smuggling. J Forensic Legal Med 17:198–202
21. Schulz B, Grossbach A, Gruber-Rouh T, Zangos S, Vogl TJ, Eichler K (2014) Body packers on your examination table: how helpful are plain X-ray images? A definitive low-dose CT protocol as a diagnosis tool for body packers. Clin Radiol 69:525–530
22. Bin Abdul Rashid SN, Rahim ASA, Thali MJ, Flach PM (2013) Death by 'ice': fatal methamphetamine intoxication of a body packer case detected by postmortem computed tomography (PMCT) and validated by autopsy. Forensic Sci Med Pathol 9:82–87
23. Shahnazi M, Sanei Taheri M, Pourghorban R (2011) Body packing and its radiologic manifestations: a review article. Iran J Radiol 8(4):205–210
24. Cherry D, Runyan C, Butts J (2001) A population based study of unintentional firearm fatalities. Inj Prev 7:62–65
25. Andenmatten MA, Thali MJ, Kneubuehl BP, Oesterhelweg L, Ross S, Spendlove D, Bolliger SA (2008) Gunshot injuries detected by post-mortem multislice computed tomography (MSCT): a feasibility study. Legal Med 10:287–292
26. Brogdan BG (1998) Forensic radiology. CRC Press, Boca Raton. isbn:0-8493-8105-3
27. Kirchhoff SM, Scaparra EF, Grimm J, Scherr M, Graw M, Reiser MF, Peschel O (2016) Postmortem computed tomography (PMCT) and autopsy in deadly gunshot wounds—a comparative study. Int J Legal Med 130:819–826
28. Maiese A, Gitto L, De Matteis A, Panebianco V, Bolino G (2014) Post mortem computed tomography: useful or unnecessary in gunshot wounds deaths? Two case reports. Legal Med 16:357–363
29. Jeffery AJ, Rutty GN, Robinson C, Morgan B (2008) Computed tomography of projectile injuries. Clin Radiol 63(10):1160–1166
30. Lü Derwald S, Zinka B (2008) Fatal diving accidents: two case reports and an overview of the role of forensic examinations. Forensic Sci Int 180:e1–e5
31. Carson WK, Mecklenburg B (2005) The role of radiology in dive-related disorders. Mil Med 170(1):57–62
32. Wheen LC, Williams MP (2009) Post-mortems in recreational scuba diver deaths: the utility of radiology. J Forensic Legal Med 16:273–276

33. Oliver J, Lyons TJ, Harle R (1999) The role of computed tomography in the diagnosis of arterial gas embolism in fatal diving accidents in Tasmania. Australas Radiol 43:37–40
34. Ozdoba C, Weis J, Plattner T, Dirnhofer R, Yen K (2005) Fatal scuba diving incident with massive gas embolism in cerebral and spinal arteries. Neuroradiology 47:411–416
35. Plaetsen SV, De Letter E, Piette M, Van Parys G, Casselman JW, Verstraete K (2015) Post-mortem evaluation of drowning with whole body CT. Forensic Sci Int 249:35–41
36. Kawasumi Y, Kawabata T, Sugai Y, Usui A, Hosokai Y, Sato M, Saito H, Ishibashi T, Hayashizaki Y, Funayama M (2012) Assessment of the relationship between drowning and fluid accumulation in the paranasal sinuses on post-mortem computed tomography. Eur J Radiol 81:3953–3955
37. Kawasumi Y, Usui A, Sato Y, Sato Y, Daigaku N, Hosokai Y, Hayashizaki Y, Funayama M, Ishibashi T (2016) Distinction between salt water drowning and freshwater drowning by assessment of sinus fluid on postmortem computed tomography. Eur Soc Radiol 26:1186–1190

Postmortem Imaging in Mass Disasters

22

Antonina Argo, Salvatore Serraino, Federico Midiri, Giuseppe Lo Re, Stefania Zerbo, Angelo Iovane, and Roberto Lagalla

The term "mass casualty" in the forensic field refers to a sudden tragic event involving a large number of people; such an event determines the need to perform a large number of autopsy exams, possibly in a short time. The typology of disaster may be various, resulting in the necessity of analyzing a huge number of bodies, sometimes mutilated and particularly difficult to identify.

Precisely, these characteristics make the radiologist's role particularly important in defining individual bodies and mutilations, as well as helping to identify the causes of death of the individual involved.

Different kinds of disasters require processing and identification of multiple victims. Railroad and aircraft accidents are not so uncommon and immediately come to mind; natural disasters, such as earthquakes, floods, and hurricanes are likewise recurrent problems; Hurricane Katrina and the Southeast Asia Tsunami of 2004 are examples where radiology was a key component of the response. Mass casualties are unfortunately not restricted to natural occurring or accidental causes; terrorist attacks (Oklahoma City in 1995; 2001, 11th September events; London in 2005) are recent examples in which radiology played a significant role in both identification of the victims and investigations of the accidents.

Mass casualties tend to involve emergencies that are unexpected and result in stressful situation when even those with no or scarce interest or experience could be called to play a role. Radiology could be helpful in the task of identifying victims, in cooperation with a multidisciplinary team, usually headed by a forensic specialist.

Identification of victims of mass casualties is important for a number of reasons, some not immediately obvious. Usually, it will be known that certain groups of people are among the victims of an event, but the degree of confusion that can be found, for example, in passenger manifests and occupancy lists, is often surprising, because of their inaccuracy, even in a closed population.

Humanitarian and psychological reasons, moreover, drive efforts to return body remains to relatives, but only after reaching a highly accurate identification. Legal and insurance requirements for precise identification are clear. The scientific importance of accurate individual

A. Argo (✉) · S. Zerbo · A. Iovane
Department of Sciences for the Promotion of Health and Maternal and Child Care "G. D'Alessandro", University of Palermo, Palermo, Italy
e-mail: antonella.argo@unipa.it; stefania.zerbo@unipa.it; angelo.iovane@unipa.it

S. Serraino · G. Lo Re · R. Lagalla
Department of Biopathology and Medical Biotechnologies, University of Palermo, Palermo, Italy
e-mail: roberto.lagalla@unipa.it

F. Midiri
University of Palermo, Palermo, Italy
e-mail: radpa@unipa.it

G. Lo Re et al. (eds.), *Radiology in Forensic Medicine*,
https://doi.org/10.1007/978-3-319-96737-0_22

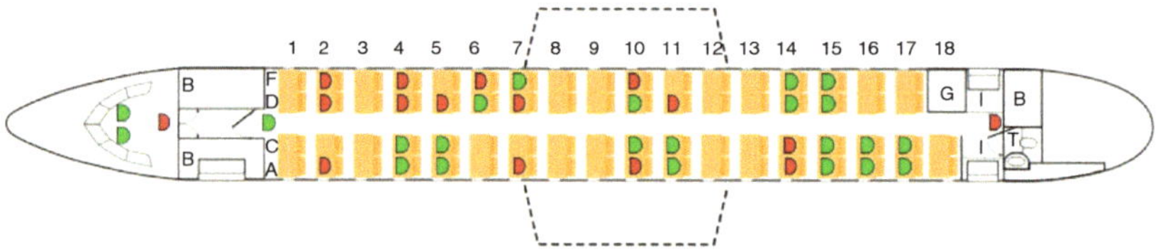

Fig. 22.1 Plan map of the ATR 72 Tuninter 1153 fallen in front of the Sicilian coast (Ustica, Palermo, 2005). In red are highlighted seats of deceased people, and in green seats of survived passengers

identification, not so obvious, can turn out to be very important: the role of scientific research in these accidents lies in the necessity to go back to the injury mechanism leading to death, and its relationship with the environment at the moment of the tragedy, particularly to try to prevent the event in the future by improving engineering and safety procedures, as well as a source of knowledge for uncommon mechanism of death (Fig. 22.1).

However, any guidelines considering radiology and its applications as a full, constant, and effective step during forensic procedures after a mass disaster have not already approved.

After mass casualties, a number of organized procedures are needed to take place in the attempt of listing and identifying body remnants so to define and possibly recognize victims.

22.1 Mass Disaster Victim Identification

Identification is the main goal in the inauspicious case of a mass disaster with a large number of unknown victims and possible survivors, becoming one of the biggest challenges for first responders, police, and forensic disciplines. One task after a mass fatality incident is the accurate identification of the victims, and it is interesting how different identification tools, like forensic autopsy, odontology, and dactyloscopy, have been developed in modern times.

In parallel, the need to establish permanent DVI organizations was recognized and several countries established DVI teams, which include forensic pathologists, dentists, anthropologists, molecular biologists, fingerprint experts, and other specialists. These teams developed their own effective protocols for the identification processes, which can be different from country to country (historical and political structures, nature of the incident, etc.).

Mass fatality incidents can be classified in different ways. One differentiates between natural disasters such as earthquakes, floods, or bushfires, versus man-made incidents like transportation (airline, train) accidents, terrorist attacks, and war.

From a more active point of view, an important distinction is between "open" and "closed" disaster (Table 22.1); in open disasters there are difficulties associated with people reported as missing (individuals could have been reported erroneously as missing; family and friends report the same person using variations of their name; etc.). Alternatively, some individuals do not have any social or family contacts and will not be reported missing at all. Estimating the victim count from the number of recovered human remains can lead to overestimating it. This means that after an open disaster the reported missing list, initially huge, has to be necessarily corrected. Depending on the circumstances, the discrepancy between the number of missing individuals and the truly deceased can be very high.

A closed disaster is a mass fatality event usually with a predetermined number of potential victims (e.g., an airline accident). The DVI process after a closed disaster has the advantage of more rapid availability of antemortem data, which will often lead to shorter identification timelines.

Aside from the type of disaster, the DVI effort is also strongly influenced by the degree of destruction affecting the human remains and by the postmortem interval before recognizing

Table 22.1 Classification of mass fatality accidents

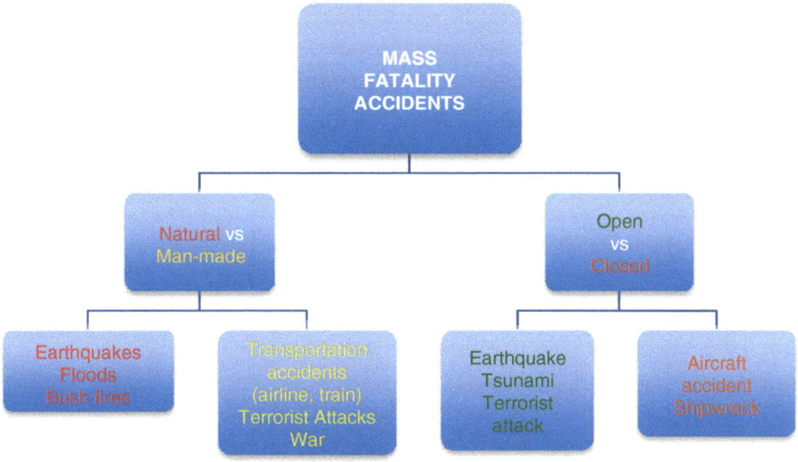

operations begin; extreme fragmentation and commingling of remains open the way to an almost exclusively DNA-based identification. In some cases, such as events with complete carbonization of bodies, even DNA profile study may not be feasible.

Mass fatality events with victims from more than one country require international cooperation of local forensic experts and national and international agencies (Solar Temple cult tragedy in Switzerland, with 48 victims belonging to five different nationalities, in 1994; 852 victims from 17 countries perished in the disaster of Finnish ferry MS *Estonia*, etc.); more than 30 international teams on the island of Phuket were involved after the 2004 tsunami.

In all cases, a successful identification effort is contingent on consistent nomenclature and labelling, adequate documentation, and standardized findings. Different approaches between DVI teams from various countries usually result in a certain mix-up; therefore it must be previously stated which nomenclature has to be used in all documentation.

In the context of the war crime victim identification, the DVI effort must adhere to strict forensic standards and aim at preserving evidence to be used in a possible trial against war criminals. International DVI standardization efforts date back to 1981 when the General Secretary of the international police agency Interpol formed a standing committee on victim identification after mass catastrophes [1, 2], thus resulting in the recommendation for the use of a standardized identification form for all unknown bodies (even with a single victim), so as to improve the flow of information and communication. A standardized form can also be considered a checklist with a consistent set of data recorded. Another advantage these forms bring is making the training faster and simpler for inexperienced personnel suddenly involved.

The quality of the available antemortem data has been shown to be critical for the accurate and timely identification of the missing; therefore the structure and staffing of the family assistance centers are an important component in a preparedness plan [3].

In order to make cooperation between different nationalities' DVI easier, digitalized standardized Interpol forms, facilitating the comparison between antemortem and postmortem information, in continuous updating, have been created.

22.2 DVI Team Structure

Mass fatality identification efforts are successful only where centralized data processing and effective information flow take place.

The structure of the victim identification teams may differ based on national differences. In most countries, as Interpol standards, mass fatality response is primarily a police function; here forensic pathologists and odontologists are involved in the DVI teams. Indispensable part of DVI team can be considered expert of dactyloscopy and forensic dentist, molecular biologist, pathologist, and anthropologist.

In DVI team, if necessary, can be involved the areas of psychological support, information technology (IT) infrastructure, criminal investigation, and hazardous material (chemical biological radioactive nuclear explosive or CBRNE) experts.

In some cases, there is also a major need for logistical support to provide power, freshwater, food, tents, and so on, to the first responders and DVI teams.

All specialists have defined roles within the team:

1. *Fingerprint experts* are responsible for the collection and comparison of fingerprints using different methods. This includes postmortem fingerprints, which may require specialized techniques [4].
2. *Forensic odontologists* examine the bodies to document the existing dental status. In addition, they have to add the missing person's dental scheme to the antemortem data collection. Finally, the tasks include the comparison of collected antemortem and postmortem findings to detect matches for possible identifications.
3. *Forensic molecular biologists* (DNA experts) advise on sample collection and receive DNA samples for typing. DNA samples must be obtained from investigated bodies, personal effects, and/or relatives of the deceased. Forensic biologists will use spreadsheets or specialized software to compare all DNA profiles and identify or rebind body parts, together with a biostatistical evaluation.
4. *Forensic pathologists* are responsible for the autopsy and documentation of the data collected for the missing persons. During the autopsy they will collect the postmortem DNA samples. The forensic pathologist will issue the death certificate and must thus be part of the identification process. If possible it is recommended to include a forensic pathologist as part of the body recovery group [5].
5. *Forensic anthropologists* can assist in incidents with high degrees of body fragmentation, or if skeletal remains are involved. Tracking the rebinding of body parts is critical and anthropologists have the expertise to check for data consistency prior to releasing a body [6].

The Interpol Standing Committee on DVI developed a guide for all aspects of the identification process [2]. This Committee includes three working groups: forensic odontology, forensic pathology, and a police working group, each with several subgroups.

Forensic odontostomatology, dactyloscopy, and forensic molecular biology belong to the primary identification methods; all others represent secondary identification methods.

The role of the forensic pathologist is multicentric and causes the need of participation in the different parts of the identification process: primarily, the forensic pathologist has to follow the Interpol Post-mortem Form for documentation of the findings, together with the collection of bodily fluids for toxicological investigations or DNA samples; whenever it is possible, the forensic pathologist should be included in the recovery team (sometimes the pathologist will be able to give important information about disaster circumstances).

Documentation of all collected information, antemortem and postmortem, is a very important component of the identification process. This includes the use of a standardized numbering form.

Following the rules suggested for international incidents, a strict separation between antemortem and postmortem information must exist for all documents; each set of information must be tagged with a country-specific identifier (normally corresponding to the international telephone country code).

Each set of human remains that is not attached and unambiguously connected to another larger part will receive a separate postmortem number.

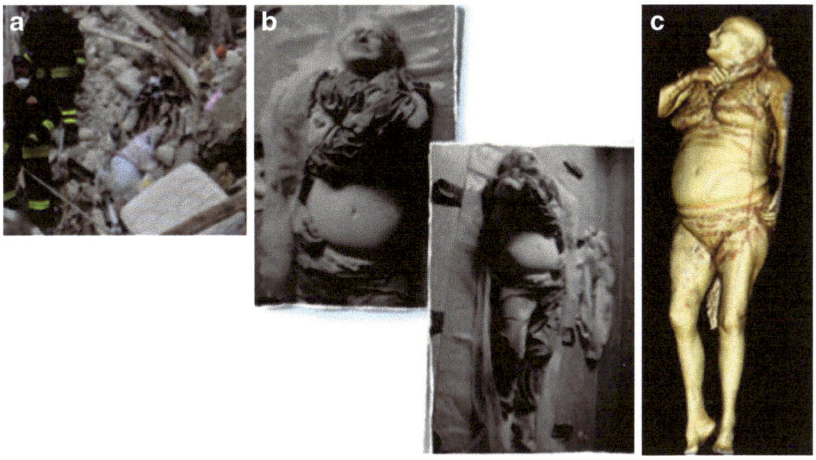

Fig. 22.2 Three main passages of corpse recovering in mass casualties, specifically the collapse of a building in Palermo, December 2012. (**a**) Rubbles of the collapse building, site of research and recover, where part of a body could be seen. (**b**) Corpse lying in a provisory morgue. (**c**) 3D VR reconstruction of the same body after CT-virtopsy

Photography is a critical part of documentation, because it objectively captures human remains, characteristic markings, and personal effects; high-quality photographs with a reference scale for size will allow for comparisons between antemortem and postmortem data (Fig. 22.2).

As in other areas of forensic science, quality management is an important part of DVI efforts; standardized operation procedures will ensure a consistent approach and rapid training of new team members, or a quick period of re-accustoming each time a team is called. Again, data verification and checks for consistency within a case can prevent sample mix-ups and mistakes [6].

22.3 Role of Radiology in "Mass Casualties" or "Disasters"

Mass disasters often require temporary morgues and improvised field X-ray (or CT) operations, because preexisting, permanent radiology facilities are not always available. Other requirements include using isolation garments or decontamination suits and make it logistically difficult to bring remains into working-class facilities, so it is important for radiologists and radiographers to be consulted in this kind of planning, to ensure the optimal organizational result. Usually police or military personnel will be required. Similar critical conditions were caused by Katrina hurricane (August 2005, USA) when the Central Medical Examiner (ME) facility was totally destroyed by flooding (Fig. 22.3a). A temporary ME office was set up in a disused mortuary without X-ray. However, all the bodies were first processed through DMORT, a federal program consisting of three complete mass casualty processing facilities including living quarters for staff, with excellent radiology services (Fig. 22.3b–d). Once deployed, which takes about 10 days, any pathologist can volunteer their services under the license of the local medical examiner and have immunity for malpractice. They do not themselves have to be licensed in the state. It is primarily used for ID and storage with autopsies done at the ME's office. It is clear that radiological team, hopefully in multidisciplinary ME team (Fig. 22.4a–c), may play a significant role in case of "mass casualty" situation.

Different imaging procedures have been considered standard in forensic pathology and have therefore an important role in DVI. Originally the only method used was X-ray but with continued development and the introduction of new technologies like CT or magnetic resonance imaging (MRI) antemortem reference images are increasingly based on these formats. This means that the same technologies are gaining importance for postmortem examinations.

Postmortem CT (CT-virtopsy or so-called *digital exhumation*) scans become predominant in situations where an autopsy is either not possible,

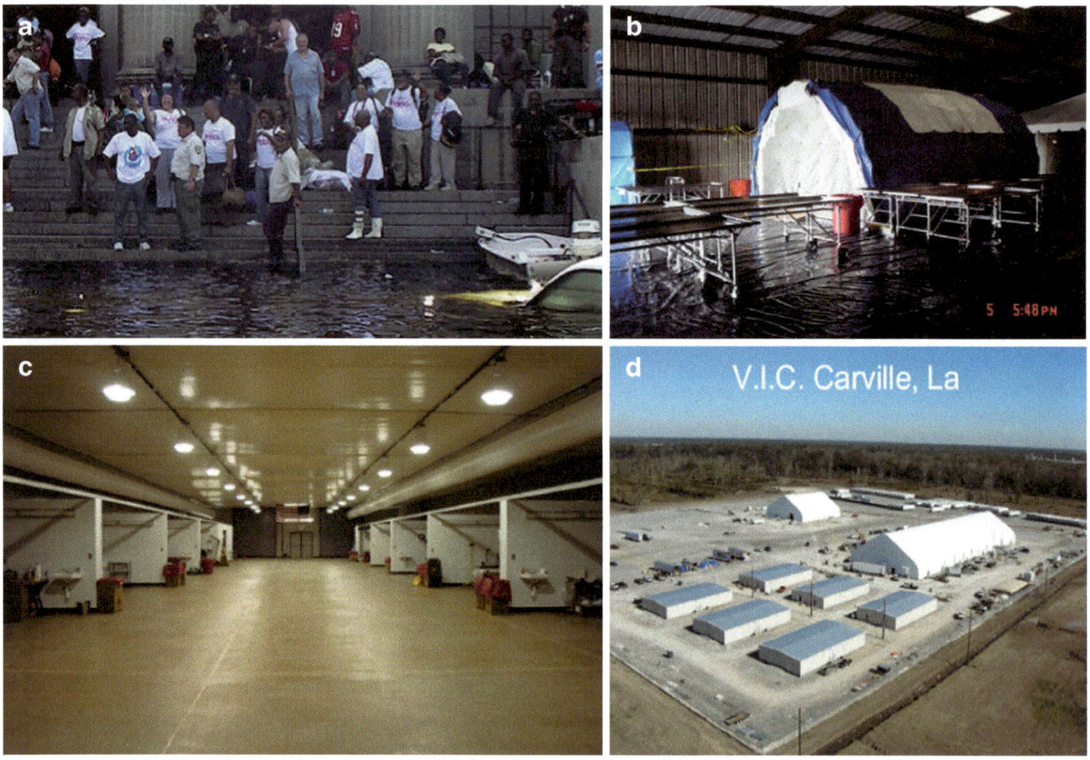

Fig. 22.3 (**a**) Flooded Downtown Medical Examiner office during Katrina disaster (courtesy of Steven B. Karch). (**b**) Equipment of body rescue and medicolegal examination during Katrina disaster in New Orleans (courtesy of Steven B. Karch). (**c**) Work environment. (**d**) Building area, top view

because of the characteristics of the disaster, or prohibited by religious objections or ethical concerns. It is expected that radiological equipment should be available for mass fatality incidents; sometimes it may be necessary to transport the equipment to the response site.

Availability of mobile trailer-mounted CT scanners provided of control area, reporting room, on-board generator, and cooling system is likely to be considered the gold standard in "mass casualties," even because a mobile CT scanner can be taken almost anywhere [7, 8]. Nevertheless, the possibility of having such an expensive resource continually available requires considerable economic and logistical planning, sometimes provided by agency/external for humanitarian reason (Fig. 22.4a).

In case of provisory radiological fields, a great attention must be paid on radiation exposition; workers, especially if constantly present, must be exposed to the minimum radiation dose as possible, within controlled areas, and adequately shielded. Dental X-rays are routinely used in dental practices and depending on the country of origin for the victims may be a good source of antemortem data. Postmortem X-rays that capture invisible treatments such as root canal work are now standard.

Equipment such as CT or MRI are already established as forensic pathology imaging tools and especially CT is well suited for postmortem diagnostics. In support of victim identification projects, it generates a complete set of findings, including stents, old fractures, or other anatomical aberrations that can be stored and visualized without additional preparation; main limitation for CT scan may be the potential "beam-hardening" artifacts caused by metal fillings. Even though currently a visual examination cannot yet be replaced, CT scans are a technology

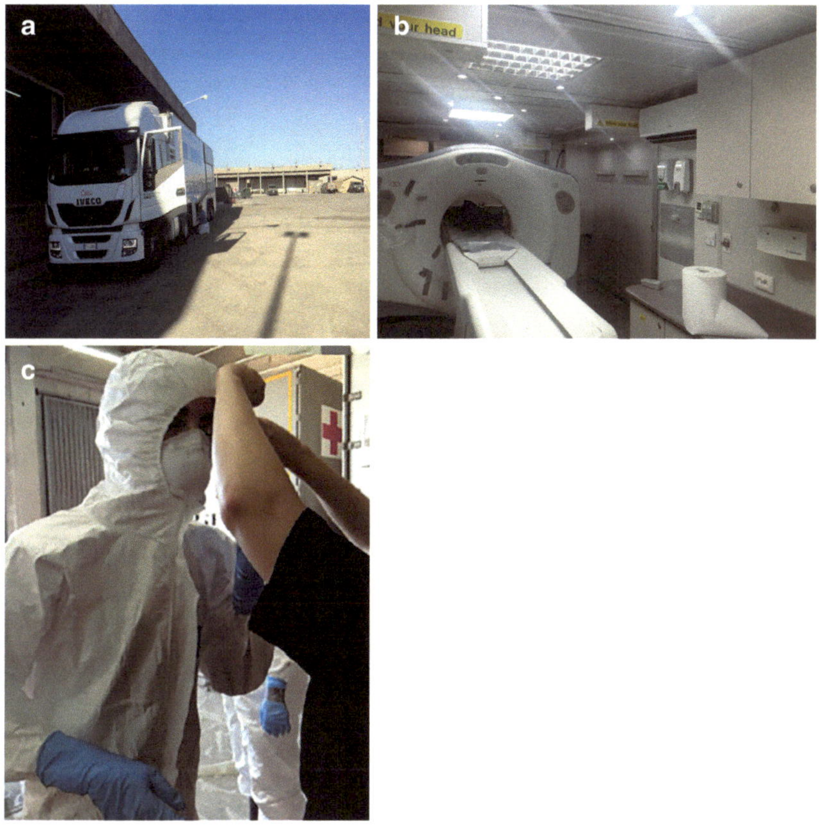

Fig. 22.4 (**a**) Mobile CT van in Sicilian military harbor; (**b**) interiors of mobile CT scan in operative theatre of humanitarian mission in Melilli, Sicily, 2016. (**c**) Forensic radiologists' team in mass disaster (migrants' rescue boat PMTC, Melilli Sicily, Italy)

that will allow for objective documentation [9, 10]. In 2007, the group of Thali had discussed the advantages and disadvantages of CT scans for DVI projects [11]. Especially under these circumstances where the material to be tested cannot be examined by other means, modern imaging technology provides an option that will still generate results [12, 13].

X-ray or CT scans are also a valuable tool for screening human remains for hidden explosive devices in war or terror attack situations, where such devices may be present on suicide bombers. CT scan has also the advantage that images can be re-examined every time it is necessary by the forensic pathologists or dentists, when searching for specific findings.

Up to now the main experience has been made using conventional radiology machinery, highly performing in studying tissues with elevated intrinsic contrast resolution (bones; lungs; external objects; etc.); now, with the advent and possible employment of mobile CT, a great improvement is expected both in quality of data collection (especially for soft tissues) and in making the body examination quicker.

Some and often complex logistical difficulties due to the implications of the radiological technology mast be considered, such as the transportation of expensive and bulky machinery, the creation of appropriate structures to carry out the investigation with minimized radiological environmental impact, and, more important, the involvement of dedicated professional figures such as, firstly, radiologists and technicians, and paramedical personnel, often without any specific experience and training.

Stronger becomes the need of a standardized procedure protocol in the case of "chain" work during the intersection with other professionals, so as to give more information, useful for investigation, in less time possible, making other specialist job faster and not hindering them.

Important decision must be stated about the role of radiology, in order to make cooperative work more effective as possible:

- When to use radiological technology (for all bodies or only in selected cases, such as those considered responsible of the event, or others; in all types of disasters or only closed/open).
- What kind of information is requested to radiologist in case of mass disasters: causes of death are often recognized and verified, and it is possibile to provide crucial informations by the post-mortem imaging of the deceased; collection of a number as large as possible of clues—elements useful in victim recognition, such as estimation of gender, age, height, condition of intracorporeal tissues, existing pathology or deformation, as well as information regarding extrinsic conditions like taphonomy and objects worn and previous medical intervention.

22.4 Methodology in Radiologic Examination

The main goal of medical investigation in "mass casualties" is the identification of the victims, rather than determining the cause of death that should be previously known; the more adequate forensic protocol should be adopted depending on the nature of the accident, and it needs to be agreed in consultation with the coroner, medical examiner, radiologist, and other involved specialists.

In time, the best approach to such a situation has been considered the same as for the major trauma; some authors report a protocol made up by three steps: primary survey, secondary survey, and tertiary examination. This approach could be effective where X-ray is the first radiological technique employed, because of its intrinsic limitation. Nowadays, with the advent of CT-virtopsy and mobile CT, just one examination is sufficient to promptly provide useful information to suggest to pathologist the correct approach to further investigations.

The main objectives of radiological examination, which in our opinion must be realized before any other research, are (Figs. 22.5 and 22.6):

- Recognition of body parts that can be used for identification, especially when particularly fragmented and decomposed.
- Indication of whether the remains of more than one victim are present in one body bag.
- The localization and, if possible, the nature of any dangerous material (unexploded device; metallic sharp fragments, etc.).
- Estimation of skeletal injuring and concomitant presence of perforating object (projectile or fragments; etc.).
- Presence of personal effects, paying attention to the not unlikely possibility of commingling.
- Presence of identifying feature that can be associated only to a few victims (prosthetic joint replacement, dental prosthesis, sign of previous surgery, etc.).

All these information should be fixed on radiological reports; they are likely to be different from those in clinical practice, and it is desirable to edit them according to multidisciplinary team so as to focus immediately on these useful and important findings.

Moreover, categorizing and filing images and findings according to observed anatomical fragments may facilitate rapid retrieval during further examinations, or comparison with antemortem data.

A possibly confounding factor may be the unnatural and random position of the corpse at the moment of recovering and successive radiological investigation; this issue was burdensome when X-ray was the only method used; nowadays the employment of CT reduces the possibility of this kind of mistake.

A more accurate review of some findings can be requested by other specialists, in specific cases, after their investigation, and it becomes easy thanks to the possibility of recording radiological exam with the advent of digital technology that allows a rapid and focused re-evaluation of the exam.

Such type of approach, as demonstrated, makes the job of the multidisciplinary team easier and faster because it facilitates the insertion of the radiological specialist in DVI and immediately focalizes the approaches of the other mem-

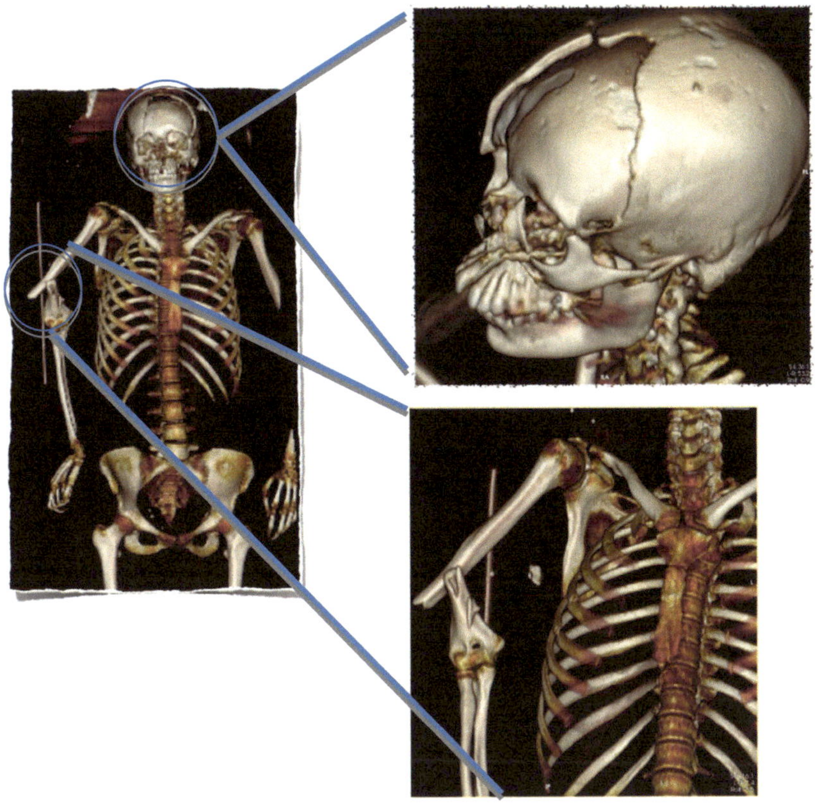

Fig. 22.5 3D volume rendering reconstruction of a victim of an air crash accident (ATR 72 Tuninter 1153 precipitation, Ustica, Palermo, August 2005) showing decomposed humerus fracture and, above all, embedded multi-fragmented frontal-parietal fracture, to be considered the most likely cause of death

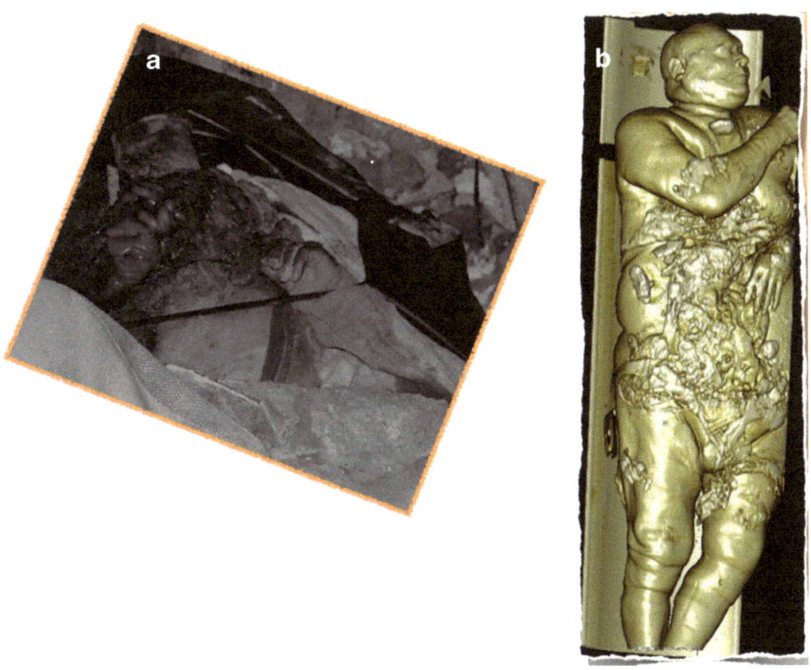

Fig. 22.6 (**a**) Photography of an eviscerated corpse on recovery site in building collapse in Palermo (Italy), December 2012. (**b**) 3D VR reconstruction of the whole-body CT scan of the same body

ber on findings that are fundamental for identification.

Radiology assumes a primary role, for example, when a visual identification is made difficult because of commingling of personal effects or body parts, or when corpses suffered from major trauma with disfigurement and dismemberment.

In association to what is described above, the presence of antemortem radiological examinations must not be underestimated, which lets a direct comparison with postmortem procedures, becoming a key point for identification.

Ultimately, final and precise identification process cannot be carried out if not after a detailed and accurate process of exclusion, especially when fragmented and commingled body parts are examined; a complete biostatistical system, supported by a wide and more accurate database, must be prepared to reach the goals; moreover, it must be pointed out that the quantity of matching characteristics required for a positive identification depends on the victim number.

CT-virtopsy should be performed trying to carry out less modification as possible to the corpse since it has been found that means with all clothing and personal effects in place, and in the same position of the retrieval. This approach should preserve evidences, but could be affected by the presence of generated artifacts on scans. Further examination, where needed, can be performed in a successive moment after disturbing object removal.

Generally a whole-body scan is performed through volumetric acquisition, soft tissue or bone filtered, with isotropic voxel (0.625 or 1 mm); this makes any post-processing protocol more accurate in spatial resolution such as three-dimensional multi-planar (3D-MPR) or volume rendering (3D-VR) reconstructions. All exams are recorded on the CT scanner, and all native or processed images are sent to and recorded on picture archiving and communication system (PACS) in a workstation.

The main limitation of CT, as previously mentioned, is the presence of "beam-hardening" artifacts caused by high-attenuation metallic objects (prosthesis, projectile, rings, necklaces, etc.); these are minimized or absent in conventional X-ray. In that sense, radiographs can be considered as a complement for CT examination. Moreover, a mobile C-arm fluoroscopy unit can be present in autopsy room in order to facilitate the retrieval of these objects.

The most important findings a radiologist must recognize and communicate in its report are the following modifications:

- Postmortem change and decomposition
- Blast injury
- Projectile injury
- Blunt-force injury
- Thermal injury
- Drowning

Another important focus point suggested by the most recent interdisciplinary discussion in forensic field is considering CT-virtopsy, and in general radiologic practises as autonomous and sufficient in a postmortem autopsy study; this has become a very debated as well as very interesting issue; however, according to our experience, the answer is that classic body-opening autopsy cannot be completely substituted by CT, or in general radiological, technique, which occipital should be an unmissable and helpful means of completion during postmortem evaluation, especially in "mass disasters," where a large number of human bodies and remains must be examined.

As conclusion, it can be stated that the execution of CT scans in these fatalities (in fact conventional radiology—as previously described—is not able to provide all the details needed and that a CT can give) is the radiology technique to be preferred in what can be considered as well as emergency situations.

Some authors state that the radiologist should set up a temporary workstation [Rutty et al.] at the morgue where supervising radiologic images and maintaining an immediate contact with other investigators. In order to ensure an effective working group, it is necessary to introduce the idea of a complete multidisciplinary forensic unit, where different specialists can work costantly, according to standardized protocols and procedures.

References

1. Interpol (1985) Resolution AGN/50/RES/3, 50th General Assembly, Nice. www.interpol.int (last accessed 26 March 2013). https://doi.org/10.17226/9984
2. Interpol (2009) Disaster victim identification guide. http://www.interpol.int/INTERPOL-expertise/Forensics/DVI (last accessed 26 March 2013)
3. Donkervoort S, Dolan SM, Beckwith M, Northrup TP, Sozer A (2008) Enhancing accurate data collection in mass fatality kinship identifications: lessons learned from Hurricane Katrina. Forensic Sci Int Genet 2:354–362. https://doi.org/10.1016/j.fsigen.2008.05.008
4. Kahana T, Grande A, Penalver J, Hiss J, Tancredi DM (2001) Fingerprinting the deceased: traditional and new techniques. J Forensic Sci 46:908–912
5. Lessig R, Rothschild M (2012) International standards in cases of mass disaster victim identification (DVI). Forensic Sci Med Pathol 8:197–199. https://doi.org/10.1007/s12024-011-9272-3
6. Budimlija ZM, Prinz MK, Zelson-Mundorff A et al (2003) World Trade Center Human Identification project: experiences with individual identification cases. Croat Med J 44(3):259–263
7. Rutty GN, Robinson CE, BouHaidar R, Jeffrey AJ, Morgan B (2007a) The role of mobile computed tomography in mass fatality incidents. J Forensic Sci 52(6):1343–1349
8. Rutty GN, Robinson C, Jeffrey A, Morgan B (2007b) Mobile computed tomography for mass fatality investigations. J Forensic Sci 3(2):138–145
9. Kirchhoff S, Fischer F, Lindemaier G et al (2008) Is post-mortem CT of the dentition adequate for correct forensic identification? Comparison of dental computed tomography and visual dental record. Int J Leg Med 122(6):471–479. https://doi.org/10.1007/s00414-008-0274-y
10. Thali MJ, Markwalder T, Jackowski C, Sonnenschein M, Dirnhofer R (2006) Dental CT imaging as a screening tool for dental profiling: advantages and limitations. J Forensic Sci 51(1):113–119. https://doi.org/10.1111/j.1556-4029.2005.00019.x
11. Sidler M, Jackowski C, Dirnhofer R, Vock P, Thali M (2007) Use of multislice computed tomography in disaster victim identification—advantages and limitations. Forensic Sci Int 169(2/3):118–128
12. Cordner SM, Woodford N, Bassed R (2011) Forensic aspects of the 2009 Victorian Bushfires Disaster. Forensic Sci Int 205(1–3):2–7
13. Leditschke J, Collett S, Ellen R (2011) Mortuary operations in the aftermath of the 2009 Victorian bushfires. Forensic Sci Int 205(1–3):8–14

Further Reading

Adams NS (2007) My life as a forensic radiographer. J Radiol Nurs 22(2):56–59

Blau S, Robertson S, Johnstone M (2008) Disaster victim identification: new applications for post-mortem computed tomography. J Forensic Sci 53(4):956–961. https://doi.org/10.1111/j.1556-4029.2008.00742.x

Bogen KT, Jones ED (2006) Risks of mortality and morbidity from worldwide terrorism: 1968–2004. Risk Anal 26(1):45–59. https://doi.org/10.1111/j.1539-6924.2006.00706.x

Bolster F, Linnau K, Mitchell S, Roberge E, Nguyen Q, Robinson J, Lehnert B, Gross J (2017) Emergency radiology and mass casualty incidents—report of a mass casualty incident at a level 1 trauma center. Emerg Radiol 24:47–53. https://doi.org/10.1007/s10140-016-1441-y

Brondolo E, Wellington R, Brady BAN, Libby BAD, Brondolo TJ (2008) Mechanism and strategies for preventing post-traumatic stress disorder in forensic workers responding to mass fatality incidents. J Forensic Leg Med 15:78–88. https://doi.org/10.1016/j.jflm.2007.04.007

Dawidson I (2007) Identification of the Swedish Tsunami victims in Thailand. Forensic Sci Int 169(1):S47–S48

Ferreira STG, Kuser HH, Garrido RG et al (2011) Floods and mudslides in the State of Rio de Janeiro and a plane crash in the Brazilian Amazon rain forest: a study of two different experiences in disaster victim identification (DVI). Forensic Sci Int Genet Suppl Ser 3:e156–e117

Fuhrmann A, Schreiner U, Lockemann U, Püschel K, Rother U (2001) Identifikation unbekannter Toter durch odontologische Untersuchungen. Dent Rec 11:37–41

Gill J (2006) 9/11 and the New York City Office of Chief Medical Examiner. Forensic Science and Medical Pathology 2:29–32

Harcke HT, Bifano JA, Koeller KK (2002) Forensic Radiology, response to the Pentagon attack on September 11, 2001. Radiology 223(1):7–8. https://doi.org/10.1148/radiol.2231011850

Interpol AFIS Expert Group (2010) Fingerprint standards. http://www.interpol.int/INTERPOL-expertise/Forensics/DVI (last accessed 26 March 2013). https://doi.org/10.3768/rtipress.2010.pb.0001.1005

Interpol Tsunami Evaluation Working Group (2010) The DVI response to the South East Asian Tsunami between December 2004 and February 2006. http://www.interpol.int/INTERPOL-expertise/Forensics/DVI (last accessed 26 March 2013). https://doi.org/10.3768/rtipress.2010.pb.0001.1005

James H, Ball J, Benthaus S et al (2005) Thai tsunami victim identification—overview to date. J Forensic Odontostomatol 23:1–18

Körner M, Geyer LL, Wirth S, Reiser MF, Linsenmaier U (2011) 64-MDCT in mass casualty incidents: volume image reading boosts radiological workflow. AJR 197(September):W399–W404

Krompecher T, Brandt-Casadevall C, Horisberger B, Perrier M, Zollinger U (2000) The challenge of identification following the tragedy of the Solar Temple (Cheiry/Salvan, Switzerland). Forensic Sci Int 110(3):215–226. https://doi.org/10.1016/S0379-0738(00)00176-6

Lessig R, Benthaus S (2003) Forensische Odonto-Stomatologie. Dent Rec 13:161–169
Lessig R, Prinz M. Mass disaster victim identification. In: Madea B (ed) Handbook of forensic medicine, 1st edn. https://doi.org/10.1364/OE.26.029769
Lessig R, Aspinall L, Bratzke H (2009) Identifizierungstätigkeit bei Massenunfällen und Katastrophen—Aktuelle Standards. Dent Rec 19:209–211
Levy AD, Harcke HT, Mallak CT (2010) Postmortem imaging MDCT features of postmortem change and decomposition. Am J Forensic Med Pathol 31:12–17. https://doi.org/10.1097/PAF.0b013e3181c65e1a
Lichtenstein JE, Madewell JE (1982) Role of radiology in the study and identification of casualty victims. Der Radiol 22:352
Meyer HJ (2003) The Kaprun cable car fire disaster—aspects of forensic organisation following a mass fatality with 155 victims. Forensic Sci Int 138:1–7. https://doi.org/10.1016/S0379-0738(03)00352-9
Morgan B, Adlam D, Phil D, Robinson C, Pakkal M, Rutty GN (2014) Adult post-mortem imaging in traumatic and cardiorespiratory death and its relation to clinical radiological imaging. Br J Radiol April 87(1036):20130662. https://doi.org/10.1259/bjr.20130662
Nye PJ, Tytle TL, Jarman RN, Eaton BG (1996) The role of radiology in the Oklahoma City bombing. Radiology 200:541. https://doi.org/10.1148/radiology.200.2.8685354
Peschel O, Lessig R, Grundmann C, Peter J, Tsokos M (2005) Tsunami 2004—Rechtsmedizinsche Erfahrungen aus dem Einsatz der Identifizierungskommission in den ersten Tagen in Thailand. Dent Rec 15:430–437
Prinz M, Carracedo A, Mayr WR et al (2007) ISFG: Recommendations regarding the role of forensic genetics for disaster victim identification (DVI). Forensic Sci Int Genet 1:3–12. https://doi.org/10.1016/j.fsigen.2006.10.003
Püschel K (2007) Schöne neue Welt von Virtopsy®, Autopsy Imaging, Radiosektion und Nekroradiologie. Dent Rec 17:5–6
Soomer H, Ranta H, Penttilä A (2001) Identification of victims from the M/S Estonia. Int J Leg Med 114(4–5):259–262
Thali MJ, Viner MD, Brogdon BG (2011) Brogdon's forensic radiology, 2nd edn. CRC Press, Boca Raton, FL. https://doi.org/10.1016/j.chom.2011.12.001
Tsokos M, Lessig R, Grundmann C, Benthaus S, Peschel O (2006) Experiences in tsunami victim identification. Int J Leg Med 120:185–187. https://doi.org/10.1007/s00414-005-0031-4
Viner MD, Rock C, Hunt N, Martin AW, MacKinnon G (2006) Forensic radiography, response to London suicide bombing on 7th July 2005. Proceedings of the American Academy of Forensic Sciences 58th Scientific Meetings, Seattle, WA, p 176
Virtopsy Team, Oesterhelweg L (2007) Atmosphere of departure in forensic medicine? Dent Rec 17:40–43
Walsh M, Reeves P, Scott S (2004) When disaster strikes; the role of the forensic radiographer. Radiography 10:33e43
Williamson HM (2011) Disaster management mobile protocols: a technology that will save lives. Am J Disaster Med 6(1):55–64

Postmortem Imaging in Drowning

23

Federica Vernuccio, Stefania Zerbo, Donatella Piscionieri, Federico Midiri, Giuseppe Lo Re, Massimo Midiri, and Antonina Argo

23.1 Introduction

The diagnosis of drowning is one of the most difficult in the field of forensic medicine since the autopsy findings are often not specific and the laboratory examinations are controversially appreciated by the scientific community. The main goal in this field is to determine whether the victim died due to "true" drowning or not. Concerning the cause of death, this can be unintentional, natural, due to suicide or homicide, or undetermined [1–3].

In a body recovered from water, we first need to determine if death occurred before or after entering the water; in case of death occurred after immersion in water, the cause may be exposure to hypothermia in the water, injuries occurred after entering the water, submersion, or to true drowning as a result of aspiration of water into the lungs.

In order to fully understand the time and cause of death in drowning cases, many features have to be considered including the evaluation of any previous victim's disease (i.e. ischemic heart disease, cerebrovascular disease, epilepsy, cardiac arrhythmias), autopsy findings, chemical and biological tests (i.e. diatoms test), and lesions encountered in the cadaver since fatal fractures may be responsible and explain some cases of postmortem drowning.

For these reasons, the study of cadavers recovered out of water comprises many medicolegal issues that are not easily solved by conventional autopsy and biological/thanato-chemical methods. Postmortem imaging performed prior to conventional autopsy may be a useful tool for the diagnosis of drowning-related deaths [4].

23.2 Pathophysiology of Drowning Effect on Respiratory System

Imaging findings can be fully understood after an adequate knowledge pathophysiology mechanisms of drowning.

Death by drowning is a form of asphyxia due to hampering of respiration by obstruction of mouth and nose by inhalation of fluids into the respiratory airways. In sudden immersion into cold water, the victim may take a deep breath and

F. Vernuccio (✉) · G. Lo Re · M. Midiri
Dipartimento di Biomedicina, Neuroscienze, Diagnostica Avanzata (BIND), University of Palermo, Palermo, Italy
e-mail: massimo.midiri@unipa.it

S. Zerbo · D. Piscionieri · A. Argo
Department of Sciences for the Promotion of Health and Maternal and Child Care "G. D'Alessandro", University of Palermo, Palermo, Italy
e-mail: stefania.zerbo@unipa.it; antonella.argo@unipa.it

F. Midiri
Dipartimento di Biomedicina, Neuroscienze, Diagnostica Avanzata (BIND), University of Palermo, Palermo, Italy

Department of Sciences for the Promotion of Health and Maternal and Child Care "G. D'Alessandro", University of Palermo, Palermo, Italy

G. Lo Re et al. (eds.), *Radiology in Forensic Medicine*,
https://doi.org/10.1007/978-3-319-96737-0_23

inhale water due to reflex induced by stimulation of the skin. Another possible scenario may be an increase of the CO2 level in the blood which stimulates the respiratory center, causing inhalation of the fluid into respiratory airways, and this fluid goes into the alveoli [5]. The pulmonary alveolar lining is semipermeable, thus allowing an exchange between the fluid entered in the alveoli and the blood.

Considering that blood normally contains 0.9% P/V of NaCl, when drowning occurs in freshwater (0.6% NaCl), water passes from the lungs into the blood (even more than 30–50% of the water sucked in after a few minutes) causing an increase of its volume, hemodilution, and, thus, hemolysis [6, 7]; moreover, the alveolar membrane is denatured by freshwater, with consequent alveolar collapse [8, 9]. These blood volume overload and reduced oxygen alveolar exchange will turn into anoxic brain damage and cardiac hypoxia, ventricular tachycardia/fibrillation, and death [9].

Conversely, when drowning occurs in saltwater drowning (about 3.5% NaCl), water will pass from the blood into the alveoli, causing alveolar/interstitial edema and hemoconcentration, hypovolemia, and consequential hypoxia; on the other hand, salt will pass from the alveoli to the blood, causing hypernatremia. In addition, in saltwater drowning, water dilutes alveolar surfactant [6, 7]. For these reasons, lungs are usually heavier in saltwater drowning than in freshwater one and the Ca^{2+}, Cl^-, Mg^{2+}, and Na^+ levels in left heart blood are increased in saltwater versus freshwater drowning [10].

The alteration of the alveolar membrane in antemortem drowning is an important physiopathological key to understand the well-known diatom test: in antemortem drowning (alive entry in water), the victim breathes in water, and diatoms enter along with water into lungs, and, after the rupture (denaturation/dilution) of the alveolar membrane, diatoms may be pushed into pulmonary veins and right heart and pumped into peripheral organs and body fluids. In postmortem drowning, the victim does not breathe, the alveolar membrane is not ruptured, and diatoms remain in the lungs but are not demonstrated in peripheral organs or body fluids. Identification of significant numbers of diatoms in the peripheral tissues, particularly bone marrow, indicates that death occurred after immersion in the water [11, 12].

The lungs should be examined first because if no diatoms are present in the lungs, it is very likely that there will not be diatoms in other organs.

A close cooperation and communication is needed between autopsy and the laboratory performing diatoms test because obtaining appropriate samples is of utmost importance [13]. In addition, data interpretation is not always concluding; the object is to compare the diatom profile of the water in which the body has been discovered with the presence (if any) of similar diatoms in the tissue samples. In the absence of standardized protocols and reliable cut-off values for diatoms between control and drowning cases, the diatom method cannot be accepted for the definitive diagnosis of drowning in a courtroom, but it represents a useful supportive tool for the diagnosis of death by drowning [1].

The macroscopic findings in the airways after drowning include the following:

- In the upper airways, the mixture of drowning liquid with edema liquid, bronchial secretions, and pulmonary surfactant produces a frothy fluid that, due to respiratory efforts during drowning, may reach nostrils and mouth, appearing as a "mushroomlike" foam [1]; however, this finding is also detectable in cardiogenic pulmonary edema, epilepsy, drug intoxication, and electrical shock [1].
- Concerning lungs, they appear—at gross examination—waterlogged and overdistended, also known as "emphysema aquosum," and their surfaces are pale and mottled, with red and grey areas, and occupy pleural cavities causing imprints of ribs on pleural surfaces; in 5–60% of drowning cases, subpleural hemorrhages, also known as Paltauf's spots, are encountered (Fig. 23.1) [1].

Immunohistochemistry staining, in addition to routine examination in E&E, may significantly

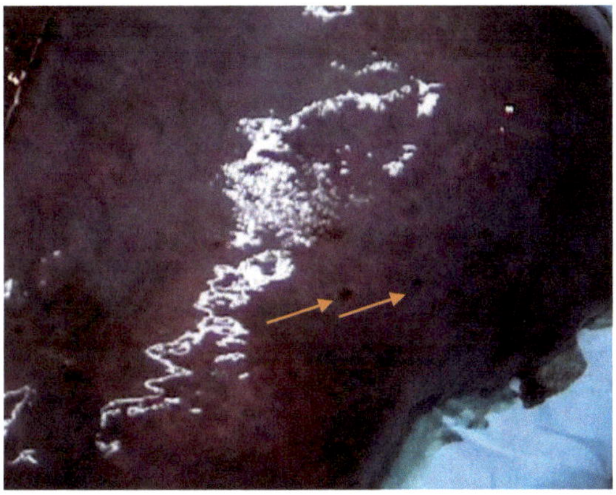

Fig. 23.1 Paltauf's spots (arrows) at postmortem lung inspection in drowning

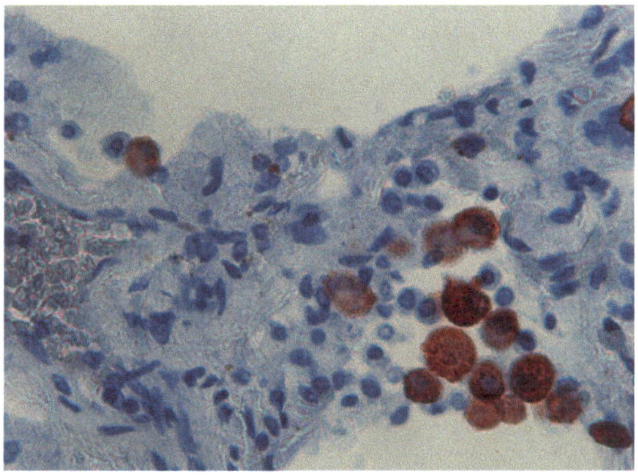

Fig. 23.2 Histological specimen (magnification ×40) in an accidental drowning of a 37-year-old man; lung tissue stained with CD68 shows macrophages (brown) at alveolar septa; terminal over insufflation of parenchyma can be appreciated

improve diagnosis [14–17] (Figs. 23.2 and 23.3, respectively).

23.3 Dry Drowning Versus Wet Drowning

In order to fully understand the pathophysiology of drowning, we need to differentiate dry drowning versus wet drowning.

Dry drowning represents 15% of all drownings and occurs when lungs becomes unable to extract oxygen from the air; this is due to an immediate and sustained laryngospasm due to

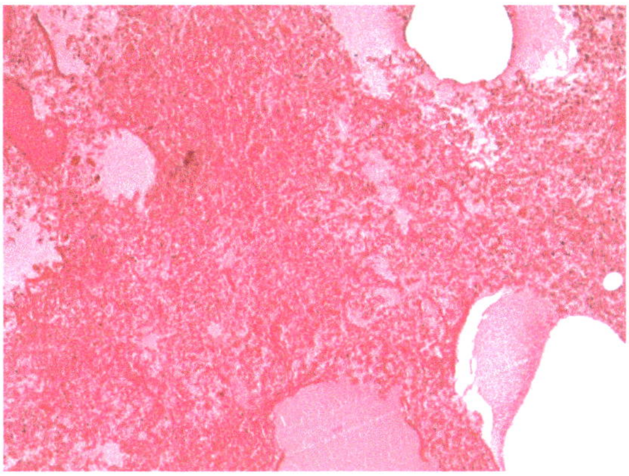

Fig. 23.3 In the same patient of Fig. 23.3, histological specimen (magnification ×20) shows pulmonary edema at E&E: Parenchyma has architectural disarray with consistent edema partially filling in the alveolar spaces

inflow of water into larynx that leads the victim to breathe deeper in the attempt to force air in the spasmed larynx; thus, in dry drowning there is no significant presence of fluid in the lungs [10].

Wet drowning or classical drowning is characterized by the inhalation of enormous quantities of liquid into lungs, with the above-seen consequences depending on the type of inhaled fluid.

Other less common types of drowning are the following [10]:

- Secondary drowning (2–5% of all drownings) which generally follows near drowning (an initial survival at least beyond 24 h after asphyxiation due to submersion) after a period of relative well-being
- Hydrocution or immersion syndrome (1–2% of all drownings) when death is due to cardiac arrest caused by a vagal inhibition due to stimulation of nerve at the surface of the body or at mucosal surfaces following immersion in cold fluid

23.3.1 Body Changes in Drowning Death: What Else Beyond Lungs

The diagnosis of drowning is not only done with the evaluation of lungs but other features are also taken into account.

23.3.2 Skin Changes: Decomposition of the Body

Depending on how long a body has been in the water, the body may have different aspects. If the deceased has been in the water for more than 1–2 h, the hands and soles typically show a "washerwoman" appearance (Fig. 23.4) [1].

When a body floats, tissues exposed to air may show destruction and mummification changes, while immersed body parts show adipocere transformation, which is a waxy decomposition due to bacterial hydrolysis and hydrogenation of adipose tissue [18]. The presence of marine scavenger organisms may quicken body's disarticulation and skeletonization, while algae colonization and exposure may lead to a greenish or blackish discoloration (Fig. 23.5) [1, 19–22].

In case of advanced decomposition, postmortem imaging through CT may help in the recognition and partial evaluation of internal organs (Fig. 23.6).

Concerning the *cardiovascular system*, inhalation of fluid results in obstruction of the pulmonary circulation and, consequently, right heart and great veins are dilated [23]. On the other hand the acute hypoxemia leads to catecholamine release and thus tachycardia and hypertension first, and bradycardia and hypotension thereafter [1, 24]. Finally, the study of the bacterioplankton in the blood of drowned cadavers appears to reflect the type of water aspirated [25]; coaxial cutting needle biopsy guided by postmortem CT used to sample internal body tissue for bacterioplankton PCR has been reported [26].

Concerning the *gastrointestinal tract*, fluid and foreign material like sand, mud, or weeds is encountered in the stomach in 3/4th and in bowel in 1/4th of all cases [10]. However, considering the possibility of an antemortem ingestion of liquid by the victim, the evaluation of the presence of fluid in the GI tract should include the comparison of the nature of this fluid with that of the water in which drowning occurred [10].

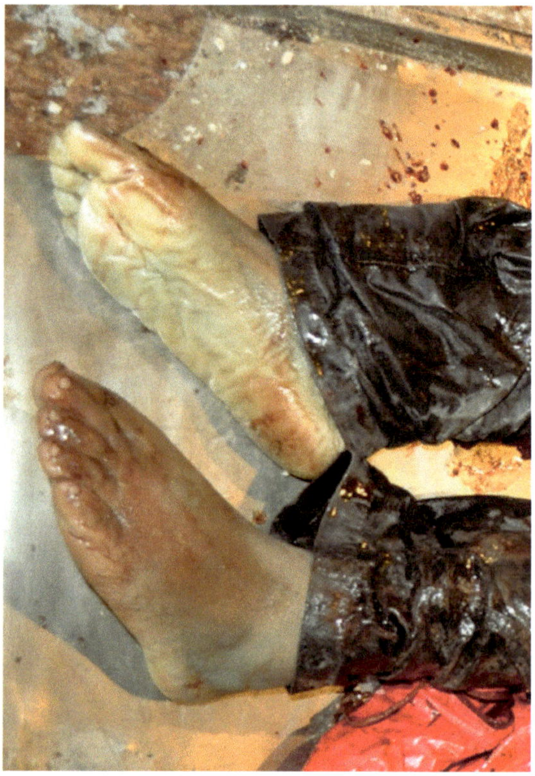

Fig. 23.4 Appearance of washerwoman feet about 1 week after drowning, in summer hot weather (personal observation)

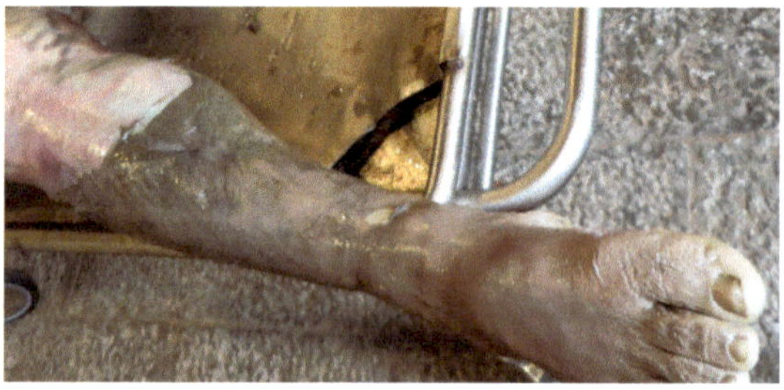

Fig. 23.5 Red-black skin discoloration in a cadaver recovered from seawater in summer hot weather, about 1 week after drowning (personal observation, Argo)

Concerning *central nervous system*, when the brain is deprived of oxygen for more than approximately 3 minutes, ischemic damage can occur, while a window of up to 4–6 min is estimated before irreversible neuronal damage occurs [1, 27].

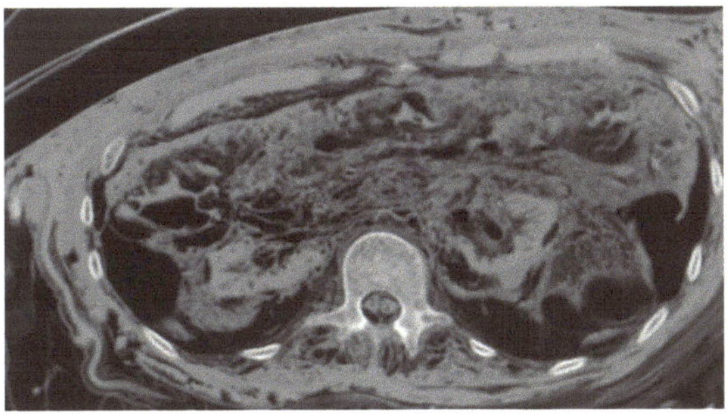

Fig. 23.6 Axial CT scan shows maceration of the posterior skin of the body in a victim recovered some months after shipwreck, mainly visible on the right with adipocere at the torso; although with the advanced decomposition both are detectable

23.4 Forensic Radiology in the Diagnosis of Drowning: A Systematic Approach

A systematic approach to CT evaluation is mandatory in order to encounter multiple different signs that may lead to the correct diagnosis [28]: on the one hand it allows to evaluate if there are fatal body injuries that could be responsible for postmortem drowning; on the other hand, it allows to assess many features that may help in the diagnosis of antemortem drowning (Fig. 23.7), with the differentiation of freshwater versus saltwater drowning. These features of antemortem drowning are discussed below.

23.4.1 Head-Respiratory System

Drowning victims have fluid in the maxillary, sphenoidal, ethmoidal, and frontal sinuses, although this finding may be just considered indicative and not diagnostic for drowning [29–31]. As demonstrated by Kawasumi et al. [32] sinus fluid volume is significantly greater and sinus fluid density is significantly lower in drowning cases than in non-drowning cases. Moreover, while the sinus fluid volume does not significantly differ comparing saltwater and freshwater drowning, the density of the sinus fluid is significantly higher in saltwater drowning than that of freshwater, with a candidate cutoff of 37.77 UH (77% sensitivity, 72% specificity) [33]. However, when considering the differentiation of wet or dry drowning and not drowning cadavers, the absence of significant differences between the fluid densities in the sinuses has been demonstrated, even if the average density is slightly lower in the wet drowning cadavers compared to dry drowning and non-drowning ones [34].

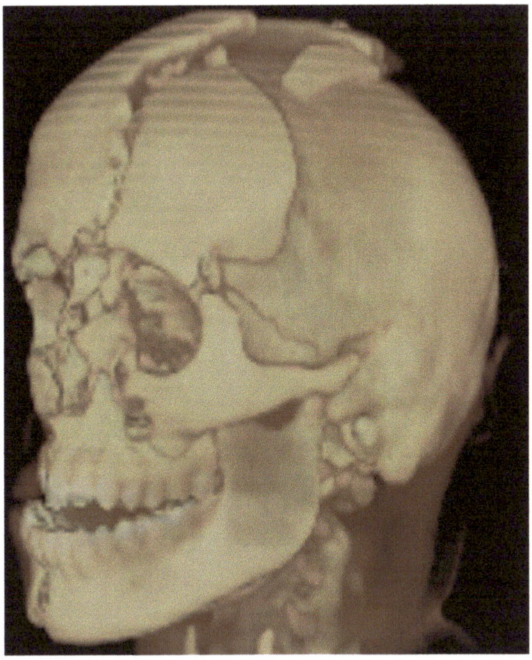

Fig. 23.7 Fatal *infra vitae* fractures of the skull in drowning

Concerning the temporal bone, hemorrhages in the mucosa of the middle ear and mastoid cells are encountered in 50% of all cases and it is generally bilateral; this is due to barotrauma and penetration of inhaled fluid into middle ear through the eustachian tube [1]. However, these hemorrhages in the temporal bone are not specific of drowning since they can also be encountered in case of hanging, strangulation, CO poisoning, drug overdose, and head injury [10].

Fluid is also encountered in all the upper airways, from the nasal cavity to the second-order bronchi, in most of the drowned

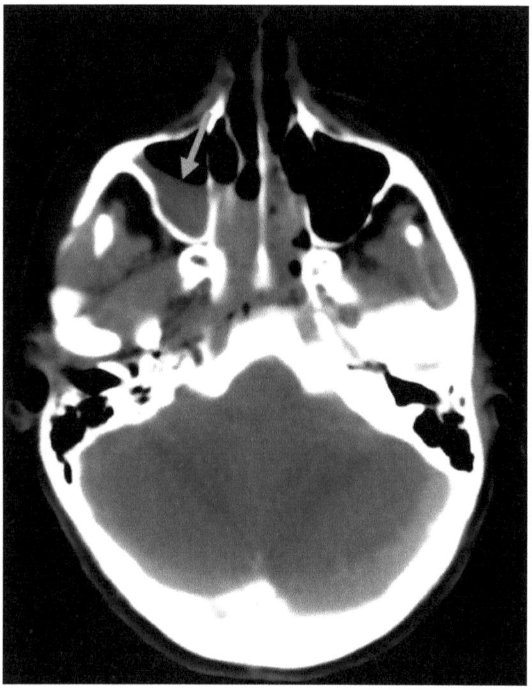

Fig. 23.8 Axial head CT scan with soft-tissue window shows an air-fluid level in the right maxillary sinus (arrow) in a drowned cadaver

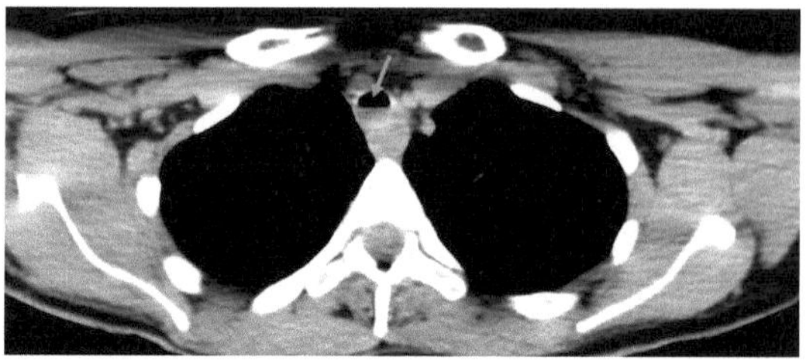

Fig. 23.9 Axial CT scan shows air-fluid level in the trachea (arrow); fluid is also detectable in the esophagus in a drowned cadaver

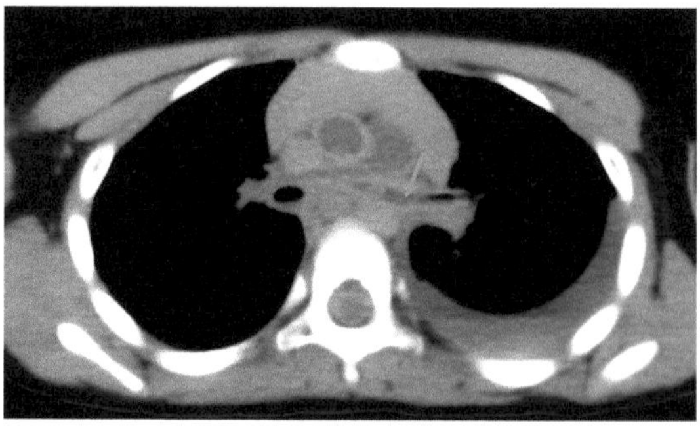

Fig. 23.10 Axial chest CT scan shows fluid in the left main bronchus (arrow) in a drowned cadaver

cadavers (Figs. 23.8, 23.9, and 23.10). Moreover, shell fragment in the airways may be sometimes encountered, also in the peripheral bronchi; this latter finding may suggest an active aspiration of water and shell fragments, thus leading to the conclusion of an antemortem drowning [35, 36].

The next step in the evaluation of the respiratory system is the study of the parenchymal changes observed in drowning. Parenchymal patterns that can be encountered are distinguished into two subcategories: ground-glass opacities and consolidations. Ground-glass opacities, which are the more commonly encountered in drowning cadavers, appear as hazy increased opacity of lung, with preservation of bronchial and vascular margins [37]. The typical mosaic pattern is due to the mismatch between perfusion and ventilation: the areas of ground-glass opacity correspond to hyperperfused areas, and the mosaic appearance to the alternance of hyperperfused and hypoperfused areas where more lucent areas correspond to emphysematous lung [38]. Consolidations, which are less frequently encountered, appear as a homogeneous increase in parenchymal attenuation without preservation of the margins of vessels and airway wall [37]. Another parameter that can be assessed is the bronchial-arterial coefficient that is calculated as the fraction between the diameter of the bronchus and the diameter of pulmonary artery: this parameter is significantly lower in drowning cadavers due to the bronchospasm [38].

Thus, at chest CT classic radiological findings consist of pan sinusal fluid, mastoid cell fluid, subglottic tracheal and bronchial fluid, and ground-glass opacity with septal lines within the lung, mainly mild with apical and perihilar distribution, with extensive "fluffy" areas of increased opacity that tend to coalesce (Fig. 23.11) [4, 29, 39, 40]. The appearance and the advancement of pulmonary congestion and edema change after a certain lapse of time

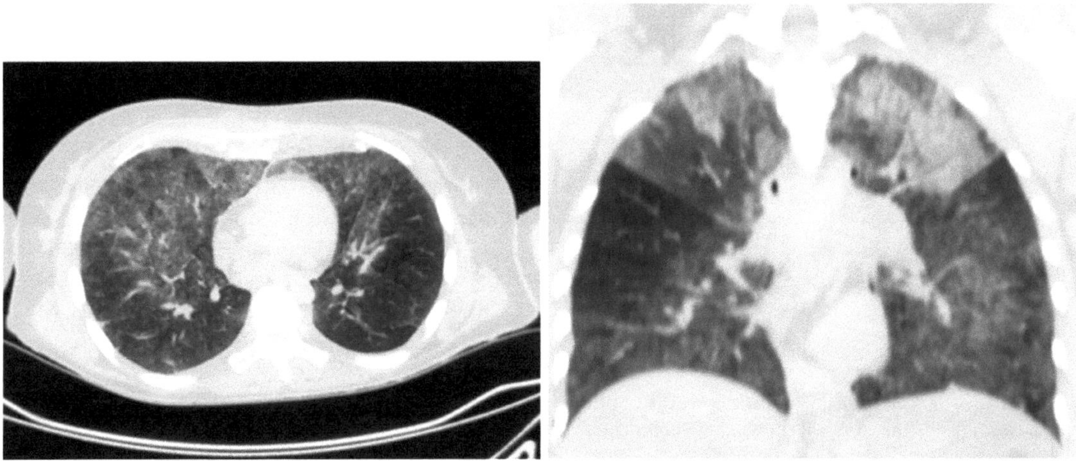

Fig. 23.11 Axial and coronal pulmonary CT performed in a woman victim of an air disaster, showing bilateral patchy "ground-glass" areas in the lung parenchyma due to drowning after air crash

due to the natural postmortem changes of the corpse [41].

Finally, pleural fluid is often present in drowning death, mainly in saltwater drowning compared to freshwater one [37]. The electrolyte analysis of pleural effusion, mainly of sodium, potassium, and chloride ions, may be used as an indicator for determining whether drowning occurred in seawater or freshwater [29, 42, 43].

23.4.2 The Thoracic Cavity, Beyond the Respiratory System

Hyperexpansion of the lungs may result in a lower position of the diaphragm, and this is assessed evaluating the rib level of diaphragm dome, mainly the right hemidiaphragm because its position is less flexible than the left [37]. Considering the vascular structures, the above-described hemodilution following freshwater drowning results in reduction of the mean density in the inferior vena cava and in the right atrium, and a blood density in the right atrium below 55 is indicative of hemodilution [37, 38]. Finally, excessive pericardial fluid, mainly located anteriorly, is found in freshwater drowning victims [37].

23.4.3 The Digestive System

Drowning often induces active swallowing or occasionally passive inflow of water into the upper gastrointestinal, although the latter is extremely rare. The presence of fluid in the esophagus, stomach, and duodenum is more commonly encountered in drowning victims than non-drowning ones [37, 38]. The absence of water in the digestive tract may suggest either rapid death by drowning or death prior to submersion [26], and it should lead to the investigation of a possible postmortem drowning.

In the CT evaluation of the fluid content in the stomach it is possible to encounter the "Wydler's sign" that is well known by the pathologist: collecting the entire gastric content in a beaker and allowing it to stand for an hour, the content divides into three layers, foam on the top, liquid in the middle, and solid component at the bottom [10]. These multiple layers of the stomach content, with different CT appearance and density, can be encountered also on CT in some cases of drowning; in particular, it is possible to recognize air on the top, froth as second layer, fluid as third layer, and debris at the bottom (Fig. 23.12) [37].

Finally, as an additional sign of hemodilution, the dimension and density of the spleen are

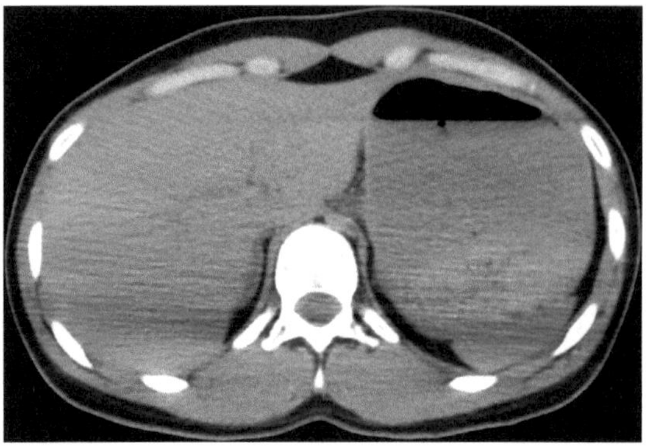

Fig. 23.12 Axial abdominal CT scan shows the multilayered content inside the stomach showing different density: higher density in the fundus and air on the top

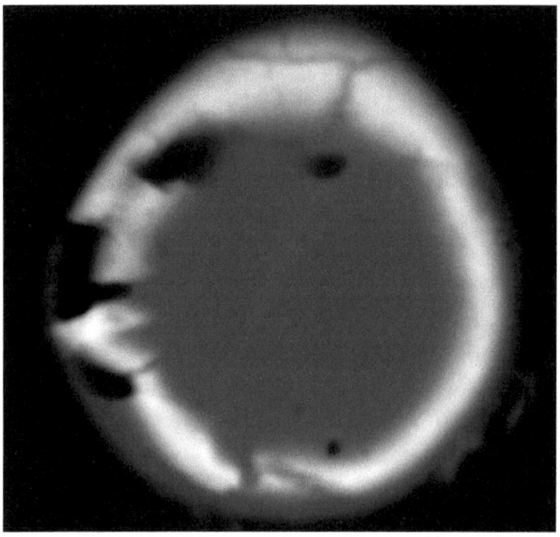

Fig. 23.13 Axial head CT scan performed in a child victim of an air crash. Bone window allows to recognize the multiple head fractures and to differentiate them from the normal cranial sutures; pneumocephalus is also evident

significantly lower in drowning victims compared to non-drowning ones, although a cutoff value has not been established yet [37].

23.5 Antemortem Versus Postmortem Injuries

Bodies recovered from water may show different antemortem or postmortem injuries, and their recognition and differentiation may be decisive for identifying the cause and manner of death [44].

Antemortem injuries due to falling into water (due to direct impact on the water surface or by striking fixed objects such as rock, cliffs, bridge, or boat) may be isolated or concur to drowning before the victim reaches the water. These types of injuries may range from severe head and neck injuries to skin lesions, muscle tears, bone fractures (Fig. 23.13), or internal organ laceration [1]. Postmortem injuries occur once the victim has fallen into the water or while in the water, and may range from injuries due to impact against any material or the bottom to those due to attack by marine predators [1].

23.6 Conclusion

In 2003 a group of international experts agreed on guidelines for unified drowning-related definitions and reporting at autopsy [45]. Since then, forensic radiology has become increasingly used and popular in the diagnosis and evaluation of drowning using postmortem CT. However, the postmortem findings must be related to the possible pathophysiological mechanism of drowning and a multidisciplinary approach is mandatory in order to compare and fit the autopsy and the CT findings.

References

1. Tsokos M (2005) Forensic pathology reviews, vol 3. Humana Press, Totowa. (Macroscopical, Microscopical, and Laboratory Findings in Drowning Victims. A Comprehensive Review. Philippe Lunetta, MD and Jerome H. Modell, MD, DSc (Hon) Forensic Pathology Reviews, Vol. 3 Edited by: M. Tsokos © Humana Press Inc., Totowa, NJ)
2. Asl N, Taftachi F, Memarian A, Kordrostami R, Zavareh F, Mehrpisheh S (2016) A 37-year-old woman found dead in a Jacuzzi: a case report. Med Leg J 84(3):159–161
3. Murayama M, Takahashi Y, R S, Watanabe K, Takahashi K, Kubo R, Kuninaka H, Kominato Y (2015) Characterization of five cases of suspected bathtub suicide. Leg Med (Tokyo) 17(6):576–578
4. Levy AD, Harcke HT, Getz JM, Mallak CT, Caruso JL, Pearse L, Frazier AA, Galvin JR (2007) Virtual autopsy: two- and three-dimensional multidetector CT findings in drowning with autopsy comparison. Radiology 243(3):862–868

5. Pearn J (1985) Pathophysiology of drowning. Med J Australia 142:586–588
6. Swann HG, Brucer M, Moore C, Vezien BL (1947) Fresh water and sea water drowning: a study of the terminal cardiac and biochemical events. Tex Rep Biol Med 5:423–437
7. Swann HG, Brucer M (1949) The cardiorespiratory and biochemical events during rapid anoxic death. VI. Fresh water and sea water drowning. Tex Rep Biol Med 7:604–618
8. Lawler W (1992) J Clin Pathol 45:654–659
9. Prahlow JA, Byard RW (2012) Atlas of forensic pathology: for police. Forensic Scientists, Attorneys, and Death Investigators
10. Aggrawal A (2016) APC forensic medicine and toxicology for MBBS. Avichal, New Delhi. ISBN: 978-81-7739-491-7
11. Zhao J, Ma Y, Liu C, Wen J, Hu S, Shi H, Zhu L (2016) A quantitative comparison analysis of diatoms in the lung tissues and the drowning medium as an indicator of drowning. J Forensic Legal Med 42:75–78
12. Rácz E, Könczöl F, Tóth D, Patonai Z, Porpáczy Z, Kozma Z, Poór VS, Sipos K (2016) PCR-based identification of drowning: four case reports. Int J Legal Med 130(5):1303–1307
13. Sheaff MY, Hopster DJ (2005) Post mortem technique handbook, 2nd edn. Springer, London
14. Du Chesne A, Cecchi Mureani R, Puschel K, Brinkmann B (1996) Macrophage subtype patterns in protracted asphyxiation. Int J Legal Med 109:163e6
15. Vacchiano G, D'Armiento F, Torino R (2001) Is the appearance of macrophages in pulmonary tissue related to time of asphyxia? Forensic Sci Int 115:9–14
16. Strunk T, Homaker D, Schulz R, Brinkmann B (2010) Reaction patterns of pulmonary macrophages in protracted asphyxiation. Int J Legal Med 124:559e68
17. Dettmeyer RB (2011) Forensic histopathology: fundamentals and perspectives. Springer, Berlin
18. Byard RW (2016) Adipocere-the fat of graveyards. Am J Forensic Med Pathol 37(3):208–210
19. Gotouda H, Takatori T, Terazawa K, Nagao M, Tarao H (1988) The mechanism of experimental adipocere formation: hydration and dehydrogenation in microbial synthesis of hydroxy and oxo fatty acids. Forensic Sci Int 37:249–257
20. Sorg MH, Dearborn JH, Monahan EI, Ryan HF, Sweeney KG, David E (1997) Forensic taphonomy in a marine context. In: Haglund WD, Sorg MH (eds) Forensic taphonomy. The postmortem fate of human remains. CRC Press, Boca Raton, FL, pp 567–604
21. Haglund WD, Sorg MH (2002) Human remains in aquatic environment. In: Haglund WD, Sorg MH (eds) Advances in forensic taphonomy. Method, theory, and archeological perspectives. CRC Press, Boca Raton, pp 201–218
22. Takatori T (2001) The mechanism of human adipocere formation. Legal Med (Tokyo) 3:193–204
23. Vij K. Textbook of forensic medicine & toxicology: principles & practice, 5th Ebook. ISBN: 9788131236239. Imprint: Elsevier India
24. Omar HR, Mirsaeidi M, Bosco G, Morgan K, Dalvi P, Helal E, Mangar D, Camporesi EM (2017) Cardiovascular complications and mortality determinants in near drowning victims: a 5-year retrospective analysis. J Crit Care 37:237–239
25. Kakizaki E, Kozawa S, Imamura N, Uchiyama T, Nishida S, Sakai M, Yukawa N (2011) Detection of marine and freshwater bacterioplankton in immersed victims: post-mortem bacterial invasion does not readily occur. Forensic Sci Int 211(1–3):9–18
26. Rutty GN, Johnson C, Amoroso J, Robinson C, Bradley CJ, Morgan B (2017) Post-mortem computed tomography coaxial cutting needle biopsy to facilitate the detection of bacterioplankton using PCR probes as a diagnostic indicator for drowning. Int J Legal Med 131(1):211–216
27. Nucci MP, Lukasova K, Sato JR, Amaro E (2017) Brain injury after moderate drowning: subtle alterations detected by functional magnetic resonance imaging. Brain Imaging Behav 11(5):1412–1421
28. Iino M, Aoki Y (2016) The use of radiology in the Japanese tsunami DVI process. JFRI 4:20–26
29. Lo Re G, Vernuccio F, Galfano MC, Picone D, Milone L, La Tona G, Argo A, Zerbo S, Salerno S, Procaccianti P, Midiri M, Lagalla R (2015) Role of virtopsy in the post-mortem diagnosis of drowning. Radiol Med 120:304–308
30. Kawasumi Y, Kawabata T, Sugai Y, Usui A, Hosokai Y, Sato M, Saito H, Ishibashi T, Hayashizaki Y, Funayama M (2012) Assessment of the relationship between drowning and fluid accumulation in the paranasal sinuses on post-mortem computed tomography. Eur J Radiol 81(12):3953–3955
31. Biljardta S, Brummela A, Tijhuisa R, Sieswerda-Hoogendoornb T, Beenenb LF, van Rijnb RR (2015) Post-mortem fluid stasis in the sinus, trachea and mainstem bronchi; a computed tomography study in adults and children. J Forensic Radiol Imaging 3:162–166
32. Kawasumi Y, Kawabata T, Sugai Y, Usui A, Hosokai Y, Sato M, Saito H, Ishibashi T, Hayashizaki Y, Funayama M (2013) Diagnosis of drowning using post-mortem computed tomography based on the volume and density of fluid accumulation in the maxillary and sphenoid sinuses. Eur J Radiol 82(10):e562–e566
33. Kawasumi Y, Usui A, Sato Y, Sato Y, Daigaku N, Hosokai Y, Hayashizaki Y, Funayama M, Ishibashi T (2016) Distinction between saltwater drowning and freshwater drowning by assessment of sinus fluid on post-mortem computed tomography. Eur Radiol 26(4):1186–1190
34. Lundermose SB, Jacobsen C, Jakobsen LS, Lynnerup N (2015) Exact volumetric determination of fluid in the paranasal sinuses after drowning. J Forensic Radiol Imaging 3:111–116
35. Bolliger S, Ross S, Marino L, Thali MJ, Schweitzer W (2015) Shell fragment aspiration seen at post-mortem computed tomography indicating drowning. J Forensic Radiol Imaging 3:87–90

36. Arun Babu T, Ananthakrishnan S (2013) Unusual presentation of sand aspiration in a 14-mo-old child. Indian J Pediatr 80(9):786–788
37. Vander Plaetsen S, De Letter E, Piette M, Van Parys G, Casselman JW, Verstraete K (2015) Post-mortem evaluation of drowning with whole body CT. Forensic Sci Int 249:35–41
38. Christe A, Aghayev E, Jackowski C, Thali MJ, Vock P (2008) Drowning—post-mortem imaging findings by computed tomography. Eur Radiol 18(2):283–290
39. Hyodoh H, Terashima R, Rokukawa M, Shimizu J, Okazaki S, Mizuo K, Watanabe S (2016) Experimental drowning lung images on postmortem CT—difference between sea water and fresh water. Leg Med (Tokyo) 19:11–15
40. Usui A, Kawasumi Y, Funayama M, Saito H (2014) Postmortem lung features in drowning cases on computed tomography. Jpn J Radiol 32(7):414–420
41. Shiotani S, Kobayashi T, Hayakawa H, Kikuchi K, Kohno M (2011) Postmortem pulmonary edema: a comparison between immediate and delayed postmortem computed tomography. Leg Med (Tokyo) 13(3):151–155
42. Usumoto Y, Sameshima N, Hikiji W, Tsuji A, Kudo K, Inoue H, Ikeda N (2009) Electrolyte analysis of pleural effusion as an indicator of drowning in seawater and freshwater. J Forensic Legal Med 16(6):321–324
43. Yajima D, Saito H, Sato K, Hayakawa M, Iwase H (2013) Diagnosis of drowning by summation of sodium, potassium and chloride ion levels in pleural effusion: differentiating between freshwater and seawater drowning and application to bathtub deaths. Forensic Sci Int 233(1–3):167–173
44. Szeremeta M, Janica JR, Niemcunowicz-Janica A, Pepinski W (2013) Fatal drowning as a result of an airplane crash—case report. Forensic Sci Int 226(1–3):e12–e15
45. Idris AH, Berg RA, Bierens J, Bossaert L, Branche CM, Gabrielli A, Graves SA, Handley AJ, Hoelle R, Morley PT, Papa L, Pepe PE, Quan L, Szpilman D, Wigginton JG, Modell JH (2003) American Heart Association. Recommended guidelines for uniform reporting of data from drowning: the "Utstein style". Circulation 108(20):2565–2574

Postmortem Imaging in Sudden Adult Death

24

Stefania Zerbo, Ambra Di Piazza, Antonio Pinto, Antonio Guajana, Antonietta Lanzarone, Elvira Ventura Spagnolo, Antonina Argo, and Massimo Midiri

24.1 Coronary Pathology

Coronary artery anomalies are found in 1% of the healthy population [1].

The most common abnormalities include a coronary artery that arises from the opposite sinus of Valsalva or the opposite coronary artery and takes a retroaortic, interarterial, prepulmonic, intramural, or trans-septal course; a coronary artery with a high takeoff point from the aorta; coronary artery fistulas; and coronary artery duplication. The hemodynamical significance is not so frequent, although these anomalies are the second most common cause of sudden death among young adults [1–4].

Common abnormalities which lead to sudden death are origin from pulmonary artery, from the opposite sinus of Valsalva or opposite coronary artery with intramural or interarterial course, and fistulas.

In vivo CTA represents a useful imaging technique which leads to best evaluation of the morphology and course of the coronary artery.

Most common cause of sudden death in adults is related to cardiovascular pathologies. Both conventional autopsy and postmortem imaging give a static information about tissue morphology, also after luminal examination of the coronary arteries with PMCT angiography (PMCTA), which has been demonstrated to be equivalent to autopsy [5–8].

However PMCTA doesn't provide any information about intraplaque pathology as rupture or hemorrhage [9].

Moreover it is difficult to attribute the cause of death to coronary artery disease during autopsy considering also that arrhythmia can be the immediate cause, even if there is a stenosis or thrombus [10].

Performing PMCTA when coronary syndrome is suspected as the cause of death can be useful because it can demonstrate the luminal patency in regions of calcification, thanks to the contrast injection under pressure. The same part can be defined as critical stenosis at autopsy [6].

S. Zerbo (✉) · A. Di Piazza · A. Lanzarone
E. Ventura Spagnolo · A. Argo
Department of Sciences for the Promotion of Health and Maternal and Child Care "G. D'Alessandro", University of Palermo, Palermo, Italy
e-mail: stefania.zerbo@unipa.it; elvira.ventura@unipa.it; antonella.argo@unipa.it

A. Pinto
Department of Radiology, Cardarelli Hospital, Naples, Italy

A. Guajana
Department of Radiology, Policlinic Hospital, Palermo, Italy

M. Midiri
Department of Biopathology and Medical Biotechnologies, University of Palermo, Palermo, Italy
e-mail: massimo.midiri@unipa.it

G. Lo Re et al. (eds.), *Radiology in Forensic Medicine*,
https://doi.org/10.1007/978-3-319-96737-0_24

Also if compared with the alive, qualitative assessment of stenoses cannot correlate with clinical significance [11] and severe coronary artery disease is not always associated with coronary occlusion [12].

Recently, direct measurements of pressure changes across a stenosis are used to understand if it is significant or not. This is obtained through the use of a "pressure wire" which helps to define the fractional flow reserve [13].

It has been reported in literature that through the insertion of catheters into the coronary arteries in cadavers, including a "pressure wire" to measure intraluminal pressure and an optical coherence tomography (OCT) catheter to provide high-resolution "virtual histology" images, it is possible to obtain the same kind of analysis [14].

PMCTA is very useful when a purely vascular information is required, but it is important to focus on two related problems related. The first one is the dispersal occurring during the time required to pump the contrast around the body that can reduce the contrast of the image. The second problem is related to the osmolality alterations of the interstitial space which may develop edema and histological changes, which may affect autopsy results [10].

At PMMR, information on coronary arteries is obtained without angiography, only using the absence of "chemical shift" artifact as a sign of stenosed vessel [15].

However, the diagnosis must be confirmed visually and/or histologically in order to rule out postmortem artifact [9].

24.2 Ischemic Heart Disease

In a recent published study Vanhaebost et al. demonstrated in a series of 40 cases that, however in forensic pathology, the identification of myocardial infarction is based on morphological findings (obtained through autopsy, histology, and immunohistochemistry) and biochemical investigations results; images obtained from multiphase PMCTA may identify myocardial infarction areas. As discussed before, PMCTA is very useful in the coronary artery imaging and in the evaluation of luminal narrowing, but in this study the authors demonstrate that myocardial areas characterized by contrast enhancement within the myocardium (increased radiopacity from contrast medium more than 95 Hounsfield units) can be suggestive of a myocardial infarction. In this study the enhancement of the myocardium correlated with the localization of the ischemia in 37 of 40 patients. In the other 3 patients, the enhancement of the myocardium correlated with increased levels of troponin T and I and myocardial ischemia, but in these cases it was related to other causes of death such as septic shock, pulmonary embolism, and trauma in patients with a severe coronaropathy [16].

The use of PMMR in the evaluation of cardiac ischemia can be very useful thanks to the intrinsic features.

As reported by Jackowski et al. in a study focused on eight cases with myocardial infarction as cause of death, unenhanced PMMR is a useful way to classify myocardial infarction [17].

Hyperacute ischemia that leads to death does not permit to develop alterations of the myocardial tissue, so it is possible only to recognize a fresh coronary occlusion. Moreover, both autopsy and unenhanced PMMR may fail in the identification of the myocardial changes, due to the short time between coronary occlusion and death.

On the other hand, **acute ischemia** is characterized by histological central necrosis, peripheral edema, and cellular reactions, which lead to different signal behavior. Necrosis is characterized by a low signal on T2-weighted, STIR, and FLAIR sequences. On the other hand, postinfarction hemorrhage has a high signal on T1-weighted sequences. Subepicardial involvement is recognizable through the evidence of increased signal in T2-weighted, STIR, and FLAIR sequences, while it is not significative on T1-weighted sequences. This effect is due to edema and cellular reactions of the peripheral regions.

Subacute ischemia shows high signal on T2-weighted, STIR, and FLAIR sequences, while the signal is not altered on T1-weighted sequences in these regions.

Chronic infarction shows signal loss on all the sequences with a characteristic decreasing from T2 to STIR and FLAIR to T1.

Subacute and chronic infarctions can be considered a cause of death when leading to acute cardiac insufficiency or generating lethal ventricular tachycardia [17].

Both PMCTA and PMMR are associated with a risk of thrombi dislodgement. Moreover they can't differentiate between vital and artifactual postmortem thrombi [9].

24.3 Pulmonary Thromboembolism

The differentiation between true pulmonary thromboembolism (PTE) and postmortem clotting is very challenging. To understand the real nature of the clot it is always necessary to perform a minimally invasive procedure, as a postmortem biopsy based on PMCT and PMCTA findings [18].

It has also been reported in literature the possibility to detect PTE through PMMR imaging [19].

In a recent study it has been reported that in 11 of 12 PTE cases, a characteristic morphology of the pulmonary trunk was identified and not depicted in the case–control group. In particular it was evidentiated the presence of an irregular-shaped filling defects in the pulmonary arteries with an absence of sedimentation of blood particles and only detectable plasma within the pulmonary trunk and arteries of the 11/12 confirmed PTE cases [20].

The presence of vessel congestion, although representing a marker of right heart failure, does not allow to differentiate between PTE and myocardial infarction [21].

Moreover the continuous filling defects from the right ventricle on PMCT images may suggest postmortem clotting [22].

24.4 Bleeding and Hemorrhages

Identifying the source of bleeding in acute bleedings and hemorrhages with a fatal evolution can be very challenging for forensic pathologists.

Both in traumatic or nontraumatic causes of bleeding, PMCT and PMCTA can really help the pathologists in the identification of the cause of death and bleeding.

24.5 Hemopericardium

Hemopericardium (cardiac tamponade) is one of the most common natural causes of death. The diagnosis of a hemopericardium is usually not difficult on PMCT and it is characterized by an expanded pericardial sac with high-density fluid. It can occur from a rupture due to myocardial infarction or dissecting aneurysm of the aorta; moreover it can have a traumatic origin such as blunt, penetrating trauma or iatrogenic manipulation to the chest. It often leads to sudden and unexpected death.

As reported by Watanabe et al., blood-containing pericardium showed three patterns of appearance: double band, single band, and horizontal level [23].

The cardiac motion selectively induces coagulation on the epicardial surface; on the other hand, the outer band is attributed to defibrination [24].

The double-band appearance is due to coagulated blood surrounded by non-coagulated hemorrhage. Thus the double band (consistent with armored heart) is a diagnostic sign of hemopericardial cardiac tamponade as the cause of death.

The presence of hemothorax has been reported to result from iatrogenic rupture of the pericardial sac during attempts at resuscitation and cardiopulmonary resuscitation has been reported to induce cardiopulmonary injury [25].

A single-band hemopericardium is associated with a modification of double-band hemopericardium: in fact the outer isodense band leaked into the pleural cavity due to cardiopulmonary resuscitation or other manipulation.

The horizontal level doesn't show a cardiac death; in fact it can be associated with high levels of stress factors in the blood often seen in cases of sudden death. The fluid level in the pericardium is due to the gravity and sedimentation which blood is subjected and represents only a postmortem change, not suitable for the diagnosis of cardiac tamponade [26].

As reported in the study of Watanabe et al., the measurement of pericardial fluid, compared to autopsy, showed lower volume in PMCT. This phenomenon is due to a leakage after incision and clotted blood is not entirely removed at autopsy. In other cases the pericardial fluid can redistribute in other thoracic spaces, such as pleural cavity or mediastinum, and pericardial volume can reduce during conventional autopsy compared with PMCT value. Moreover in this study, the pleural space fluid volume showed no significant difference between the PMCT volumetry and autopsy measurements [23].

24.6 Aortic Rupture

In clinical practice, CT and MRI, with or without contrast administration, are widely used as cross-sectional imaging techniques in the evaluation of aortic pathologies, thanks to their high diagnostic accuracy, which helps to identify the aneurism and to define sizes and relationships to organs and aortic branches [27, 28].

However, both techniques can be very useful to diagnose, as postmortem imaging, cases of a ruptured aneurysm which determines a pericardial effusion.

At PMCT it is possible to recognize the presence of the aneurysm, the size, and both asymmetrical pericardial and left pleural high-density effusion, with high suggestive of coagula.

PMMR can add an important diagnostic value through the demonstration of a pericardial defect, confirming aneurysm, mediastinal hematoma, pericardial enlargement, and left pleural effusion [29].

In these cases differential diagnosis includes iatrogenic or traumatic rupture of the pericardium, but it has to be associated with rib fractures, or congenital origin.

24.7 Cardiomyopathy

24.7.1 Hypertrophic Cardiomyopathy

Hypertrophic cardiomyopathy is characterized by hypertrophy of the left ventricular myocardium with a subsequent decrease in size of the left ventricular cavity [30].

Differential diagnosis includes both hypertensive heart disease and physiological remodeling in athletes.

At MR examination it is defined by the presence of 15 mm or more unexplained left ventricular hypertrophy; however 12–14 mm of hypertrophy may be seen in the initial phase of the pathology [31].

Asymmetric septal hypertrophy is the most common finding and is defined as hypertrophy with a ratio of septal to inferolateral wall thickness of 1.3 or more. Apical, midventricular, focal masslike, and right ventricular hypertrophy are other forms also seen.

At MR systolic anterior motion of the mitral valve (SAM), dynamic left ventricular outflow tract (LVOT) obstruction, and jet from mitral valve regurgitation are well seen on 2D SSFP cine images.

Another important tool of hypertrophic cardiomyopathy is delayed myocardial enhancement, seen in 50–80% of patients. Moreover if an apical aneurysm is present, it can increase the risk of sudden cardiac death [32].

No postmortem radiological observations have been reported for HCM, but PMMR alone or in conjunction with PMCTA should be considered, as previously suggested by Jackowski et al. [33]

24.7.2 Arrhythmogenic Right Ventricular Cardiomyopathy (ARVC)

Structural and functional abnormalities, mostly of the right ventricle, are the features of the pathology. The presence of a fibrofatty replacement of the right ventricular myocardium, starting from the epicardium, is the physiopathological mechanism which leads to wall thinning and aneurysm formation, typical of the inferior, apical, and infundibular walls.

Usually, it is localized to the in inflow tract, right ventricular outflow tract, and right ventricular apex, the so-called triangle of dysplasia [32].

Different diagnostic criteria allow to define the pathology as right ventricular functional and

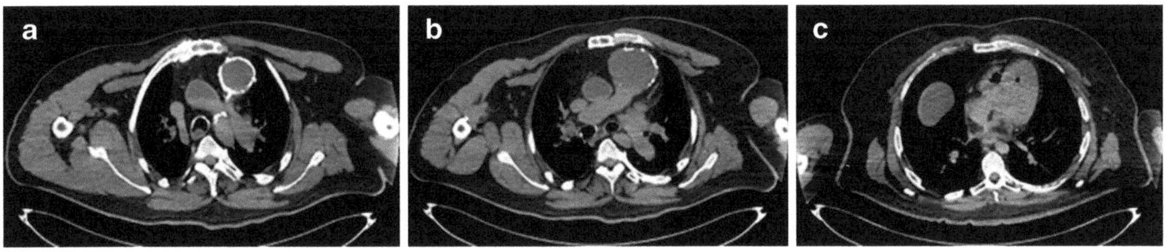

Fig. 24.1 (a–c) Relevant findings of previous surgical treatment for Fallot's tetralogy, at PMCT (18 h after death), in a case of suspected nonnatural death, before conventional autopsy

structural changes, electrocardiographical depolarization and repolarization abnormalities, ventricular arrhythmias, fibrofatty replacement of the myocardium, and a positive family history.

MRI permits to detect regional and diastolic ventricular dysfunctions related to intramyocardial fibrosis.

Differential diagnosis includes coronary artery disease [34].

Fatty infiltration and right ventricular dilation can also be seen at PMCTA [9].

As reported by Jackowski et al., the radiological aspects of ARVC in the postmortem setting have not been evaluated in comparative studies; however a case has been reported with fatty infiltration of the free right ventricular wall and thinning of the apical right ventricular wall visualized by PMMR, which was suggestive of ARVC [33].

24.7.3 Dilated Cardiomyopathy

The most common cause of congestive heart failure in young is dilated cardiomyopathy. It can be idiopathic or due to myocardial injury, such as coronary artery disease, viral myocarditis, systemic disease, nutritional deficiency, or alcohol related [32].

Characteristic features of the pathology include ventricular dilatation, decreased ventricular wall thickness with an increase in myocardial mass, and left ventricular or biventricular contractile dysfunction. Moreover mitral or tricuspid regurgitation, atrial enlargement, and intracardiac thrombus can be highlighted at imaging.

In some cases, a linear area of delayed enhancement in the midwall can represent midwall fibrosis [35].

Differential diagnosis includes coronary artery disease, myocarditis, and cardiac sarcoidosis [32].

As a personal experience we managed a case of sudden death in a patient who underwent heart surgery in his childhood for congenital heart dysmorphism (Fallot's tetralogy). Images of PMCT (Fig. 24.1) showed signs of surgical treatment of cardiac gross vessels and findings of dilated cardiomyopathy; this approach (PMCT before conventional autopsy) leads to "digital evidence" of natural disease significantly contributing to way of death explication in a male of sixth decade of life.

24.7.4 Noncompaction Cardiomyopathy

It is a rare congenital myocardial disorder in which embryonic myocardium persists.

It primarily affects the left ventricle, with the concomitant involvement of the right ventricle in 41% of cases, with an impairment of both diastolic and systolic ventricular function [36].

It may extend from the apical part along the lateral and inferior wall to the midportion of the ventricle. Patients are often asymptomatic.

An overall increased myocardial thickness with a two-layer appearance is the imaging hallmark. It consists of a thin compacted subepicardial layer (compacted myocardium) and a subendocardial thicker layer (noncompacted myocardium).

A NC:C ratio of more than 2.3 in end diastole is the threshold for diagnosing noncompaction cardiomyopathy [32].

References

1. Yildiz A, Okcun B, Peker T, Arslan C, Olcay A, Bulent Vatan M (2010) Prevalence of coronary artery anomalies in 12,457 adult patients who underwent coronary angiography. Clin Cardiol 33(12):E60–E64
2. Van der Werf C, Van Langen IM, Wilde AA (2010) Sudden death in the young: what do we know about it and how to prevent? Circ Arrhythm Electrophysiol 3:96–104
3. Eckart RE, Scoville SL, Campbell CL, Shry EA, Stajduhar KC, Potter RN, Pearse LA, Virmani R (2004) Sudden death in young adults: a 25-year review of autopsies in military recruits. Ann Intern Med 141:829–834
4. Doolan A, Langlois N, Semsarian C (2004) Causes of sudden cardiac death in young Australians. Med J Aust 180:110–112
5. Michaud K, Grabherr S, Doenz F, Mangin P (2012) Evaluation of postmortem MDCT and MDCT-angiography for the investigation of sudden cardiac death related to atherosclerotic coronary artery disease. Int J Cardiovasc Imaging 28:1807–1822
6. Morgan B, Biggs MJ, Barber J, Raj V, Amoroso J, Hollingbury FE et al (2013) Accuracy of targeted post-mortem computed tomography coronary angiography compared to assessment of serial histological sections. Int J Legal Med 127:809–817
7. Roberts IS, Benamore RE, Peebles C, Roobottom C, Traill ZC (2011) Diagnosis of coronary artery disease using minimally invasive autopsy: evaluation of a novel method of post-mortem coronary CT angiography. Clin Radiol 66(7):645–650
8. Saunders SL, Morgan B, Raj V, Robinson CE, Rutty GN (2011) Targeted post-mortem computed tomography cardiac angiography: proof of concept. Int J Legal Med 125(4):609–616
9. Michaud K, Grabherr S, Jackowski C, Bollmann MD, Doenz F, Mangin P (Jan 2014) Postmortem imaging of sudden cardiac death. Int J Legal Med 128(1):127–137
10. Morgan B, Adlam D, Robinson C, Pakkal M, Rutty GN (2014) Adult post-mortem imaging in traumatic and cardiorespiratory death and its relation to clinical radiological imaging. Br J Radiol 87:20130662
11. Topol EJ, Nissen SE (1995) Our preoccupation with coronary luminology. The dissociation between clinical and angiographic findings in ischemic heart disease. Circulation 92:2333–2342
12. Moise A, Lesperance J, Theroux P, Taeymans Y, Goulet C, Bourassa MG (1984) Clinical and angiographic predictors of new total coronary occlusion in coronary artery disease: analysis of 313 nonoperated patients. Am J Cardiol 54:1176–1181
13. Tonino PA, Fearon WF, De BB, Oldroyd KG, Leesar MA, Ver Lee PN et al (2010) Angiographic versus functional severity of coronary artery stenoses in the FAME study fractional flow reserve versus angiography in multivessel evaluation. J Am Coll Cardiol 55:2816–2821
14. Adlam D, Joseph S, Robinson C, Rousseau C, Barber J, Biggs M et al (2013) Coronary optical coherence tomography: minimally invasive virtual histology as part of targeted post-mortem computed tomography angiography. Int J Legal Med 127:991–996
15. Ruder TD, Bauer-Kreutz R, Ampanozi G, Rosskopf AB, Pilgrim TM, Weber OM et al (2012) Assessment of coronary artery disease by post-mortem cardiac MR. Eur J Radiol 81:2208–2214
16. Vanhaebost J, Ducrot K, de Froidmont S, Scarpelli MP, Egger C, Baumann P, Schmit G, Grabherr S, Palmiere C (2017) Diagnosis of myocardial ischemia combining multiphase postmortem CT-angiography, histology, and postmortem biochemistry. Radiol Med 122:95–105
17. Jackowski C, Christe A, Sonnenschein M, Aghayev A, Thali MJ (2006) Postmortem unenhanced magnetic resonance imaging of myocardial infarction in correlation to histological infarction age characterization. Eur Heart J 27:2459–2467
18. Ross SG, Thali MJ, Bolliger S, Germerott T, Ruder TD, Flach PM (2012) Sudden death after chest pain: feasibility of virtual autopsy with postmortem CT angiography and biopsy. Radiology 264(1):250–259
19. Jackowski C, Grabherr S, Schwendener N (2013) Pulmonary thromboembolism as cause of death on unenhanced postmortem 3T MRI. Eur Radiol 23(5):1266–1270
20. Ampanozi G, Held U, Ruder TD, Ross SG, Schweitzer W, Fornaro J, Franckenberg S, Thali MJ, Flach PM (2016) Pulmonary thromboembolism on unenhanced postmortem computed tomography: feasibility and findings. Legal Med 20:68–74
21. Mueller Y, Thali GA et al (2015) Distended diameter of the inferior vena cava is suggestive of pulmonary thromboembolism on unenhanced post-mortem CT. J Forensic Radiol Imaging 3(1):38–42
22. Burke MP, Bedford P, Baber Y (2014) Can forensic pathologists diagnose pulmonary thromboembolism on postmortem computed tomography pulmonary angiography? Am J Forensic Med Pathol 35:124–131
23. Watanabe S, Hyodoh H, Shimizu J, Okazaki S, Mizuo K, Rokukawa M (2015) Classification of hemopericardium on postmortem CT. Legal Med 17:376–380
24. Shiotani S, Watanabe K, Kohno M, Ohashi N, Yamazaki K, Nakayama H (2004) Postmortem computed tomographic (PMCT) findings of pericardial effusion due to acute aortic dissection. Radiat Med 22:405–407
25. Miller AC, Rosati SF, Suffredini AF, Schrump DS (2014) A systematic review and pooled analysis of CPR-associated cardiovascular and thoracic injuries. Resuscitation 85:724–731
26. Jackowski C, Thali M, Aghayev E, Yen K, Sonnenschein M, Zwygart K et al (2006) Postmortem imaging of blood and its characteristics using MSCT and MRI. Int J Legal Med 120:233–240

27. Gurney JW, Part II (2006) Section 2, Aorta and great vessels. In: Gurney JW, Stern EJ (eds) Diagnostic imaging: chest. Amirsys, Salt Lake City, pp 40–43
28. Rousseau H, Chabbert V, Maracher MA, El Aassar O, Auriol J, Massabuau P, Morenol R (2009) The importance of imaging assessment before endovascular repair of thoracic aorta. Eur J Vasc Endovasc Surg 38:408–421
29. Filograna L, Hatch G, Ruder T, Ross SG, Bolliger SA, Thali MJ (2013) The role of post-mortem imaging in a case of sudden death due to ascending aorta aneurysm rupture. Forensic Sci Int 228:76–80
30. Chun EJ, Choi SI, Jin KN et al (2010) Hypertrophic cardiomyopathy: assessment with MR imaging and multidetector CT. Radiographics 30(5):1309–1328
31. Gersh BJ, Maron BJ, Bonow RO et al (2011) ACCF/AHA guideline for the diagnosis and treatment of hypertrophic cardiomyopathy: executive summary—a report of the American College of Cardiology Foundation/American Heart Association Task Force on Practice Guidelines. Circulation 124(24):2761–2796
32. Stojanovska F, Garg A, Patel S, Melville DM, Kazerooni EA, Mueller GC (2013) Congenital and hereditary causes of sudden cardiac death in young adults: diagnosis, differential diagnosis and risk stratification. Radiographics 33:1977–2001
33. Jackowski C, Schweitzer W, Thali M, Yen K, Aghayev E, Sonnenschein M, Vock P, Dirnhofer R (2005) Virtopsy: postmortem imaging of the human heart in situ using MSCT and MRI. Forensic Sci Int 149(1):11–23
34. Zidan M, Nicoll R, Schmermund A, Henein M (2009) Cardiac multi-detector CT: its unique contribution to cardiology practice. Int J Cardiol 132(1):25–29
35. Assomull RG, Prasad SK, Lyne J et al (2006) Cardiovascular magnetic resonance, brosis, and prognosis in dilated cardiomyopathy. J Am Coll Cardiol 48(10):1977–1985
36. Weiford BC, Subbarao VD, Mulhern KM (2004) Noncompaction of the ventricular myocardium. Circulation 109(24):2965–2971

Post-mortem Foetal Imaging

25

Sergio Salerno, Filippo Alberghina, Maria Chiara Terranova, Giuseppe Lo Re, Emiliano Maresi, and Roberto Lagalla

25.1 Introduction

The gold standard for the diagnosis of foetal death is known to be the autopsy examination, which is sometimes supplemented by chromosomal and/or genetic studies [1–4].

Autopsy results are also of great value for genetic counselling for implementation of strategies for prevention of unnecessary risks in future pregnancies, but autopsy rates are continuously declining [5].

The reason for the decline in autopsies is multifactorial and complex [6, 7]. The impact of the perception and acceptance by the general public, clinicians and pathologists of autopsies is significant.

S. Salerno (✉) · M. C. Terranova · G. Lo Re
R. Lagalla
Department of Biopathology and Medical Biotechnologies, University of Palermo, Palermo, Italy
e-mail: sergio.salerno@unipa.it; roberto.lagalla@unipa.it

F. Alberghina
Ospedale "R.Guzzardi" Vittoria—ASP RAGUSA, Palermo, Italy

E. Maresi
Department of Sciences for the Promotion of Health and Maternal and Child Care "G. D'Alessandro", University of Palermo, Palermo, Italy
e-mail: emiliano.maresi@unipa.it

The low public consent rate is one of the most important reasons for the observed decline. The consent rate seems to depend on religion, ethnic origin, cultural attitude and public perceptions [8].

In addition, there are major practical problems associated with performing autopsy on central nervous system structures without formalin fixation. The foetal or stillborn brain is difficult to handle even with adequate fixation, even after modest post-mortem delay [9, 10]. This is due, in part, to the high water content of the immature brain compared with that of the adult brain [8].

Parental concerns about organ retention have resulted in requests of not removing the brain for fixation (which can take weeks); therefore, many brain studies are being performed on non-fixed tissue [9, 10].

Similar problems are found with the spinal cord, but these are compounded by the small size of the cord and structural disruption caused by dissection. These problems are major when dealing with unfixed tissue [11].

The considerable delays between foetal demise and autopsy probably contribute to the difficulty in handling the brain, as autolysis makes the tissue even more fluid-like.

Furthermore, cellular autolysis phenomenon is one of the main problems associated with performing autopsy after in utero retention of dead foetus. Autolysis usually affects the foetus after an intrauterine foetal death or stillborn baby most severely but is also seen in termination of

G. Lo Re et al. (eds.), *Radiology in Forensic Medicine*,
https://doi.org/10.1007/978-3-319-96737-0_25

pregnancy for foetal abnormality, as death frequently occurs before delivery [11].

Therefore, it is important to explore and develop alternative post-mortem diagnostic techniques.

Today post-mortem imaging has become an increasingly important part of the examination of deceased foetuses and neonates. Several studies demonstrate that imaging techniques are able to offer diagnostic indications comparable to those obtainable with conventional autopsy [11–14]. In some situations, MR imaging revealed to be superior to autopsy of an unfixed brain; the ability to image the brain in situ is also a particular advantage [11, 12].

A new task force on post-mortem imaging was established at the annual meeting of the European Society of Paediatric Radiology (ESPR) in Graz, Austria, in 2015. The main focus of the task force is the guidance and standardisation of non-radiographic post-mortem imaging, particularly post-mortem CT and post-mortem MRI to establish the cases in which post-mortem imaging should be used, the best imaging modality and optimal timing of imaging, the best and most appropriate imaging investigations according to the clinical scenario [15].

The majority of centres provide some post-mortem imaging service, most of which is performed within an imaging department and reported by a paediatric radiologist. However, the populations imaged as well as the details of the services offered are highly variable among institutions and lack standardisation. The use of post-mortem imaging, including skeletal radiography, CT and MRI, is increasing, providing a minimally invasive alternative to conventional autopsy techniques. The development of clinical guidelines and national standards is being encouraged, particularly for cross-sectional techniques [16].

25.2 Foetal Death

Several causes of foetal death were considered, but the most frequent causes were grouped into four types of disease: maternal, placental, foetal and external. Foetal deaths with an unexplained cause were classified as sudden intrauterine unexplained death (SIUD) [12].

Table 25.1 Definition of paediatric death [14]

Term	Definition
Late foetal loss	Delivered showing no signs of life between 20 and 24 weeks of pregnancy
Stillbirth	Delivered showing no signs of life after 24 weeks of pregnancy
Perinatal death	Stillbirths and early neonatal deaths
Early neonatal death	Death of a live born baby occurring within 7 days of birth
Neonatal death	Death of a live born baby occurring within 28 days of birth

Modified from Arthurs OJ et al. (2015) Paediatric and perinatal post-mortem imaging: the need for a subspecialty approach. Pediatr Radiol.; 45(4):483–90. https://doi.org/10.1007/s00247-014-3132-8

According to the 2003 revision of the Procedures for Coding Cause of Foetal Death Under ICD-10, the National Centre for Health Statistics defines foetal death (Table 25.1) as "death prior to the complete expulsion or extraction from its mother of a product of human conception, irrespective of the duration of pregnancy and which is not an induced termination of pregnancy. The death is indicated by the fact that after such expulsion or extraction, the foetus does not breathe or show any other evidence of life, such as beating of the heart, pulsation of the umbilical cord, or definite movement of voluntary muscles. Heartbeats are to be distinguished from transient cardiac contractions; respirations are to be distinguished from fleeting respiratory efforts or gasps".

The worldwide stillbirth rate declined by 14.5% from 22.1 stillbirths per 1000 births in 1995 to 18.9 stillbirths per 1000 births in 2009 [17].

25.3 Imaging Techniques and Findings

On 22nd November 2014, the Italian Ministry of Health approved a diagnostic protocol on foetus death, which considers not only autopsy but also other non-conventional investigations such as CT and genetic, cytogenetic, infectious disease tests and toxicological investigations [18]. Currently a number of post-mortem imaging techniques are available.

Obviously, informed consent has to be obtained from the parents and/or judgement authorisation, underlining that the examination is non-invasive and that the integrity of the body is respected.

Parents should be informed that post-mortem imaging techniques cannot replace a complete autopsy and they could complete post-mortem evaluation.

In second-trimester foetuses, most abnormalities are developmental and often have obvious macroscopic manifestations, which can easily be detected by imaging techniques, in particular by MRI. Examples include pathologies of the kidneys, liver, gut, abdominal wall and central nervous system [8].

25.3.1 Conventional Radiology

Radiograms (Figs. 25.1 and 25.2) are reported by a paediatric radiologist and emphasis is placed on skeletal development, with regard to both the gestational age and the presence of anomalies, such as skeletal dysplasia [13].

Skeletal ossification begins at 8 weeks. The clavicles are the first bones to ossify, shortly followed by the basi-occiput and face and the long-bone diaphyses. The ribs appear at about 10 weeks. Vertebral ossification begins at 11–12 weeks, with the neural arches ossifying cranio-caudally from C1, whilst the vertebral bodies progress cranially and caudally from the thoraco-lumbar junction. Later ossification landmarks include the ischium, which appears at 16–17 weeks, and the pubis, calcaneum, odontoid and manubrium, which appear at 22–25 weeks. In early-gestation foetuses, there is the potential to mistake normal lack of ossification with a skeletal dysplasia [19].

However, radiographs are limited for more advanced diagnoses and may not be cost effective [15].

25.3.2 Ultrasonography

The use of ultrasonography in post-mortem imaging, to date, has been limited [20, 21]. Implementation is hindered by a relative lack of knowledge about the possibilities of US by (forensic) pathologists. Not only can ultrasonography be used as an inexpensive imaging method in

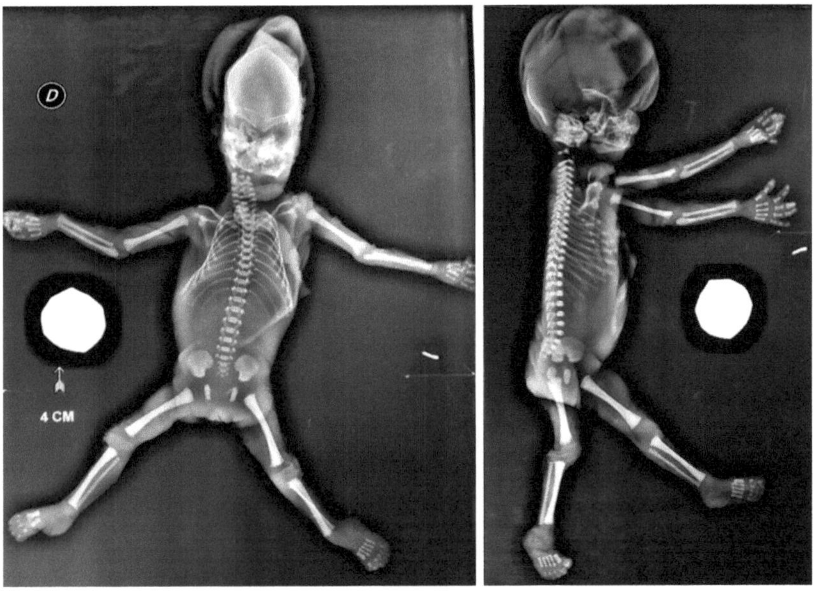

Fig. 25.1 Plain radiograph of a 27-week-old foetus

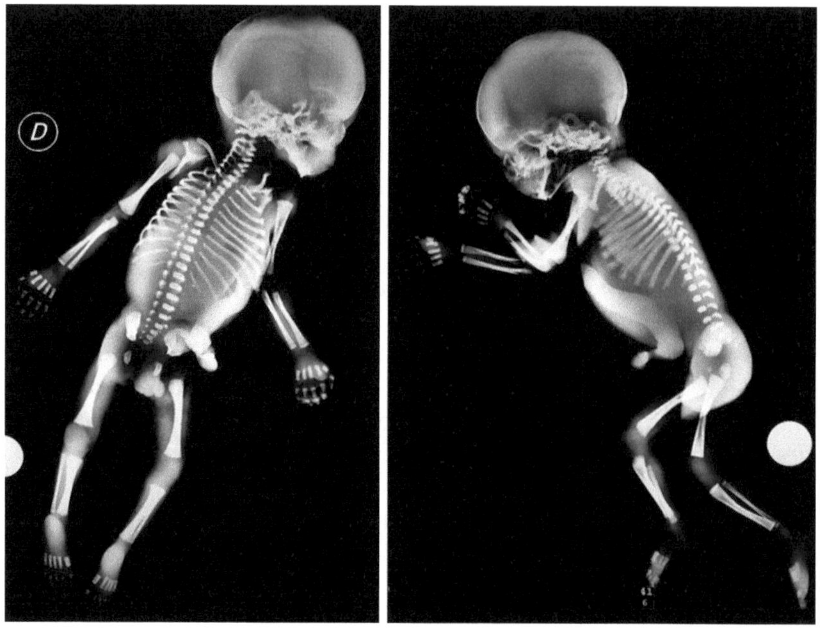

Fig. 25.2 Plain radiograph of a 27-week-old foetus. High-resolution radiography, performed on a mammography system, shows a normal skeleton depicted in minute detail

the absence of CT and/or MRI, but it can also be used to guide biopsy procedures in case of a minimal invasive autopsy.

25.3.3 Computed Tomography (CT)

Post-mortem CT is a fast technique that allows imaging of the whole body inside a body bag or coffin.

Compared to autopsy CT is superior in detecting bone anomalies or lesions; it is very useful to evaluate skeletal development (Fig. 25.3) and to detect the presence of haemorrhage and gas [22].

Some authors describe the use of micro-CT to evaluate the presence of heart diseases with encouraging results [23].

Furthermore, 3D reconstructions can be made (Figs. 25.4 and 25.5), which can be helpful in demonstrating anomalies.

Unenhanced post-mortem CT will give excellent bony detail and provide good diagnostic quality images in suspected skeletal dysplasias, with possible additional benefits from 3D reconstructions [24].

The main disadvantage of post-mortem CT compared to post-mortem MRI in foetuses is reduced soft-tissue contrast, due to reduced abdominal and subcutaneous fat; poor soft-tissue contrast is also problematic for evaluating brain parenchyma [15].

Some studies report addition of intravenous contrast (via femoral or umbilical vessels, or direct intra-cardiac injection) for angiography with initial promising results [24, 25].

25.3.4 Magnetic Resonance Imaging (MRI)

MRI should be performed as soon as possible after foetal death due to tissue degeneration.

More recent studies show that post-mortem MRI can also be used to perform other activities usually performed during autopsy, such as organ weight or volume estimation; limitations of this study include subspecialist reporting for individual organ systems and a lengthy comprehensive MR protocol, both of which are difficult to achieve in clinical practice [24].

Most post-mortem MR imaging is performed on 1.5-T scanners because of their wide availability; the selection of the coils depends on the size of the foetus.

The MRI protocol is divided into two separate parts. First of all, the neurocranium, then the tho-

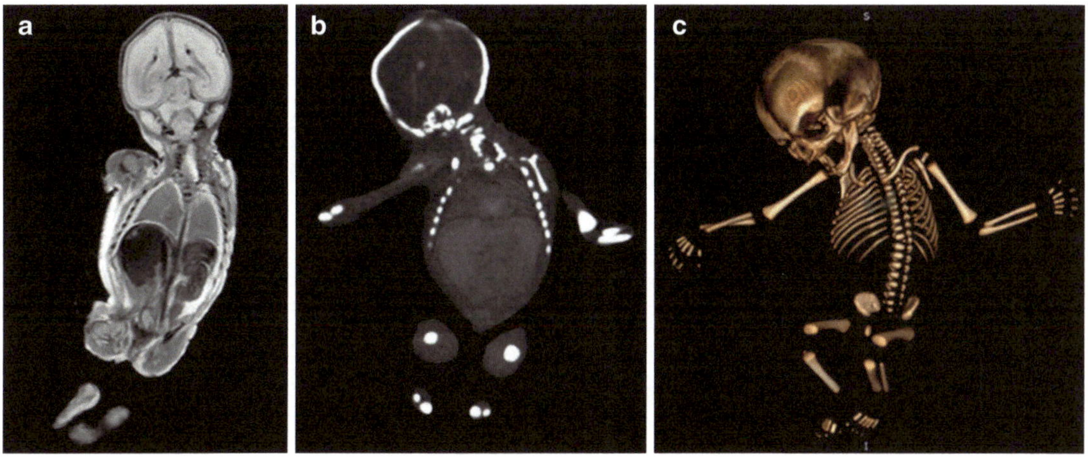

Fig. 25.3 Comparison of post-mortem MRI (**a**) and post-mortem CT (**b**) of a 20-week-old foetus. Visceral organs are not clearly seen on post-mortem CT, whilst the bony skeleton is clearly displayed on reconstruction of the CT image (**c**)

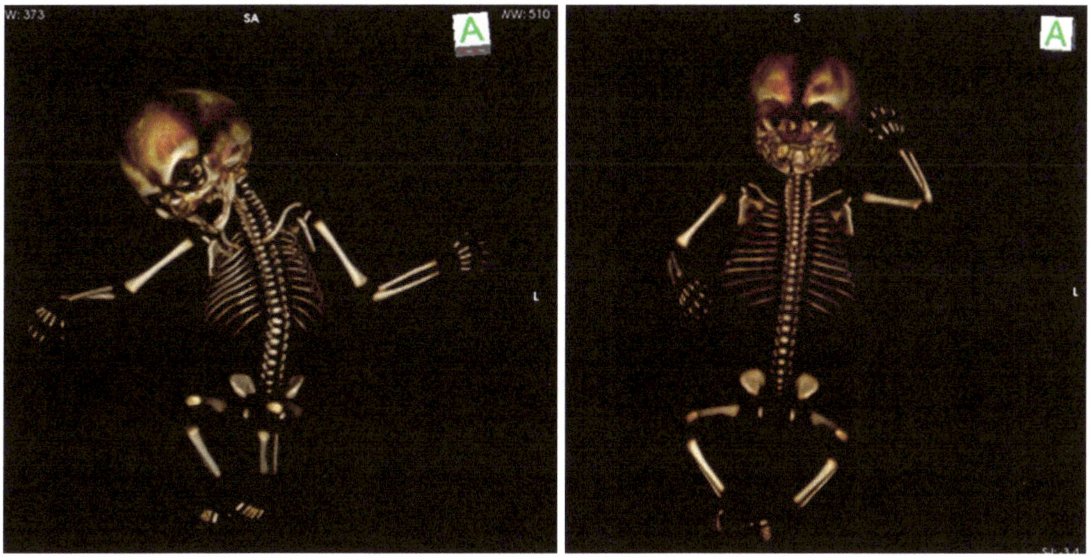

Fig. 25.4 Volume rendering (VR) whole-body reconstructions in two different foetuses. The use of 3D reconstructions can be very illustrative in comparison with plain radiography

rax and abdomen are imaged separately. The extremities are only imaged upon special request.

In most reports the imaging protocol consists of fast spin-echo T2 sequences in three orthogonal planes. In some reports, additional T2 spin density-weighted sequence is suggested to increase the contrast between cerebral grey and white matter [8].

Sometimes, DWI/DTI for the brain can be performed in selected cases (b-value 1000 s/mm^2).

Many experts in post-mortem MRI believe that T1-weighted sequences add little valuable information, so they should also be acquired [26].

Several studies demonstrate that MRI provided important information when compared with autopsy [27].

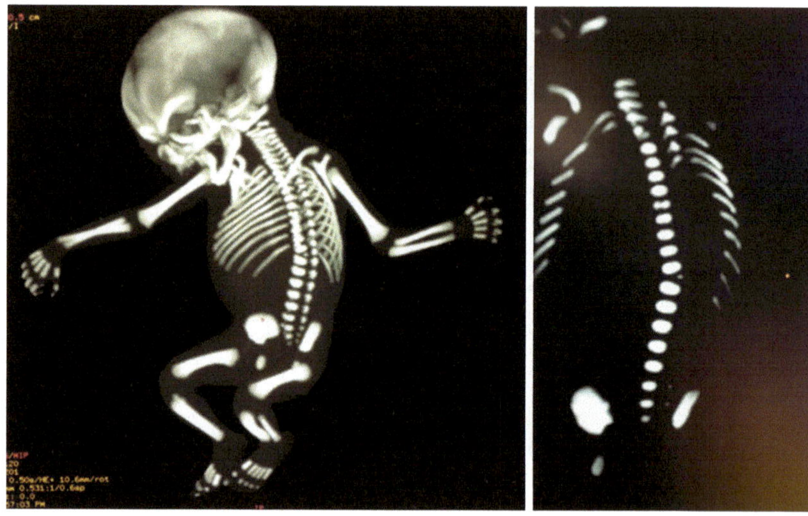

Fig. 25.5 CT reconstruction. Three-quarter MIP reconstructions centred on the trunk and on the spine of a 20-week-old foetus. CT reconstruction shows a small paraspinal calcification on the left compatible with accessory ossicle. A sagittal cleft of eighth thoracic vertebra is also visible (butterfly vertebra)

25.3.4.1 Central Nervous System

MRI could be a useful tool to provide more details on brain diseases than conventional autopsy [28, 29].

The major difference in the brains of foetuses or stillborns when compared with that of the adult is the virtual complete absence of myelin. This means that the water content and lipid content of grey and "white" matter are very similar. In this situation, it would be expected that the tissue contrast should be poor. The second trimester is an exceptionally active period of neuronal proliferation and migration; the developing neurons are situated in the immediate, periventricular germinal matrices, which were shown to have low signal intensity [30].

The major difference between post-mortem and in utero foetal brains is in the size of the extra-axial spaces. These are smaller in the post-mortem brain, presumably because of loss of CSF pressure [11].

MRI is particularly useful in the abnormalities of the central nervous system that is one of the most difficult areas to investigate at autopsy. Otherwise MRI, having the capability to evaluate the anatomy of the brain (Fig. 25.6), clearly shows normal cerebral structure and the development of the sulci and gyri [12].

MRI is more effective in identifying intraparenchymal blood components due to the alteration of signals compared to surrounding healthy brain tissue, this event being very frequent in foetuses or very infrequent in the case of maceration [12].

Furthermore, MRI detects abnormalities in the extra-axial compartment with a surprisingly higher frequency than autopsy [11].

Otherwise, the evaluation of the lungs and of the cardiac anatomy is more difficult.

25.3.4.2 Thorax

With regard to mediastinal structures, MRI investigation is reliable with particular reference to the abnormal position of the organs and of the heart chambers, although for greater definition of some cardiac abnormalities (such as atrial septal defect or ventricular septal defect) or infectious diseases such as myocarditis, dedicated sequences relating to the heart are required [31–33].

Lung imaging is difficult with MRI because lung parenchyma is mostly collapsed and does not contain air in stillborns, for the absence of the foetal first breath. Collapsed appearance of both lungs hampered, for example an accurate evaluation of eventual pneumonia or other infectious processes. However, MRI of the lungs allows the diagnosis of major structural lesions, as for example in the case with diaphragmatic hernia, and the evaluation of normal anatomical structure appearance (Fig. 25.7). MRI enables the distinction between pleural effusion from post-mortem

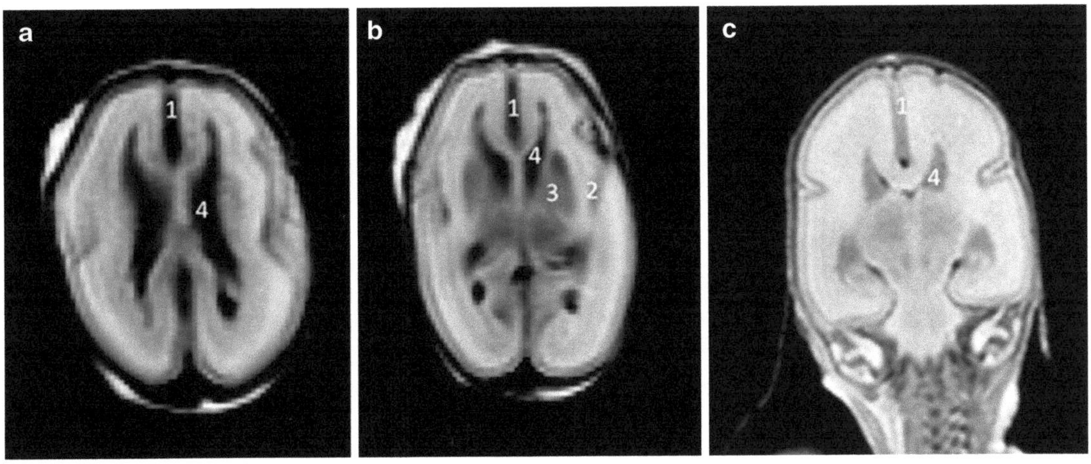

Fig. 25.6 Post-mortem MRI axial (**a**, **b**) and coronal (**c**) T2w TSE of a 20-week-old foetus; in these planes are clearly visible interhemispheric fissure (*1*), Sylvian fissures (*2*), basal ganglia (*3*) and lateral ventricles (*4*)

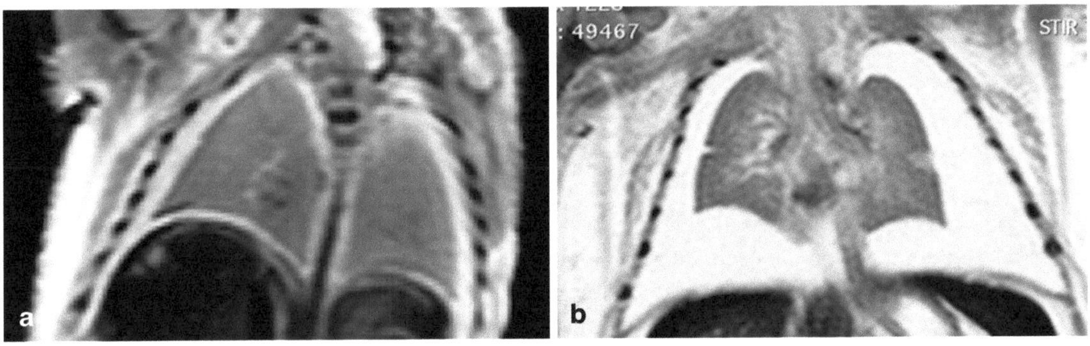

Fig. 25.7 Post-mortem MRI coronal T2w TSE. Comparison of two different foetuses centred on the thorax. In (**b**) is clearly visible partial collapse of both lungs associated with pleural effusion

phenomena through the use of T2-weighted sequences that signal static liquid [12].

Diagnosing lung hypoplasia is in most cases possible but exact assessment of the pulmonary lobulation is nearly impossible [26].

25.3.4.3 Abdomen

For the abdominal area (Fig. 25.8), MRI is a reliable examination in the case of anomalies and/or severe abdominal diseases and allows better classification of the disease even if unspecified [34].

Diaphragmatic hernias and herniated organs could be accurately diagnosed.

Renal anomalies are common major abnormalities. Normal kidneys have a low-signal-intensity cortex and a high-signal-intensity medulla on T2-weighted images. Cystic diseases of the kidneys could be classified by the morphologic appearance of the cysts; in particular autosomal recessive polycystic kidney disease has symmetrically enlarged kidneys with small uniform cysts, whereas multicystic dysplastic kidneys have large variably sized cysts with asymmetric kidneys [35].

MRI allows also a good evaluation of liver and spleen and associated diseases [8]. Ascites is easily detected.

In older foetuses, gastrointestinal tract could be evaluated. Bowel atresia could be suggested by abnormal dilatation, even if the exact site of atresia may be sometimes difficult to discern [35].

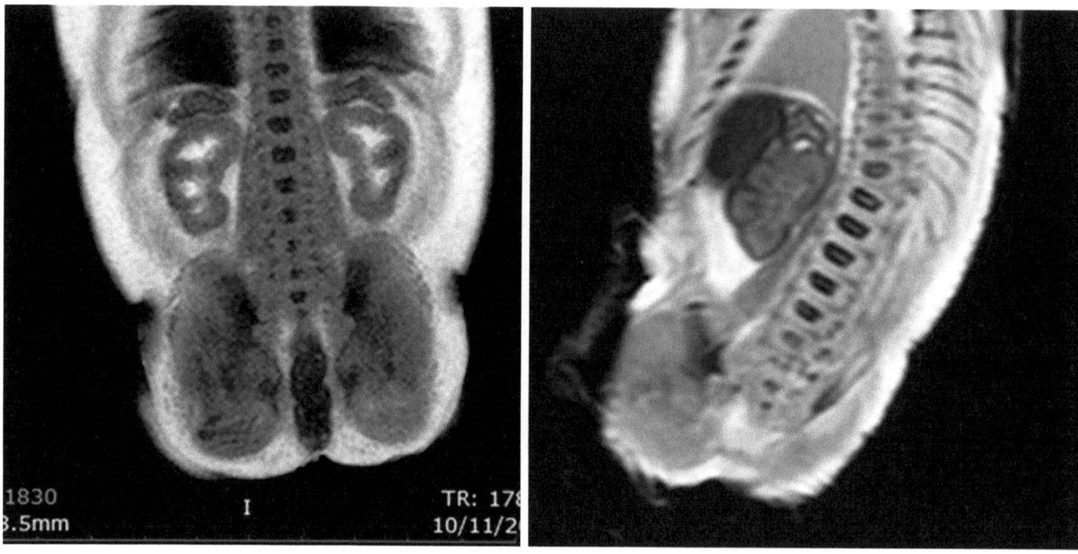

Fig. 25.8 Post-mortem MRI coronal T2w TSE in two different foetuses shows normal kidney with its lobes and the adrenal glands

25.4 Conclusion

By combining these clinical skill sets and recognising the contribution of each imaging and other modality to the final diagnosis, the optimal approach to the investigation after death can be determined for each case.

The integrated foetal post-mortem imaging service will include a multidisciplinary group of obstetricians, foetal medicine specialists, paediatric radiologists, perinatal pathologists and geneticists, to name but a few, who might be involved in the ongoing care and counselling of bereaved parents. Skeletal radiographs are to be performed where clinically indicated, followed by a post-mortem MRI in all cases in whom it may direct a full standard autopsy or in whom the parents decline traditional autopsy examination. Post-mortem CT and post-mortem US should be used to address specific issues, and on the basis of all the imaging (antenatal and post-mortem) targeted biopsy or full autopsy can be performed [36].

References

1. Bonetti LR et al (2011) The role of fetal autopsy and placental examination in the causes of fetal death: a retrospective study of 132 cases of stillbirths. Arch Gynecol Obstet 283:231–241
2. Miller ES et al (2016) Stillbirth evaluation: a stepwise assessment of placental pathology and autopsy. Am J Obstet Gynecol 214:115e1–115e6
3. Heller DS, Faye-Petersen OM (2015) Pathology of the still- born infant for the general pathologist: part 1. Adv Anat Pathol 22:1–28
4. Gordijn SJ et al (2002) Value of the perinatal autopsy: critique. Pediatr Dev Pathol 5(5):480–488
5. Brodlie M et al (2002) Ten years of neonatal autopsies in tertiary referral Centre: retrospective study. BMJ 324(7340):761–763
6. Burton JL, Underwood J (2007) Clinical, educational, and epidemiological value of autopsy. Lancet 369(9571):1471–1480
7. Griffiths PD et al (2005) Post-mortem MRI as an adjunct to fetal or neonatal autopsy. Lancet 365(9466):1271–1273
8. Lequin MH, Huisman TA (2012) Postmortem MR imaging in the fetal and neonatal period. Magn Reson Imaging Clin N Am 20(1):129–143. https://doi.org/10.1016/j.mric.2011.08.008
9. Cartlidge PHT et al (1995) Value and quality of perinatal and infant post mortem examinations:

cohort analysis of 400 consecutive cases. BMJ 310: 155–158
10. Vujanic GM et al (1995) Perinatal and infant postmortem examinations: how well are we doing? J Clin Pathol 48:998–1001
11. Griffiths PD et al (2003) Postmortem MR imaging of the fetal and stillborn central nervous system. AJNR Am J Neuroradiol 24(1):22–27
12. Vullo A et al (2016) Post-mortem magnetic resonance foetal imaging: a study of morphological correlation with conventional autopsy and histopathological findings. Radiol Med 121(11):847–856
13. Sieswerda-Hoogendoorn T and van Rijn RR(2010) Current techniques in postmortem imaging with specific attention to paediatric applications. Pediatr Radiol 40(2):141–152; quiz 259. https://doi.org/10.1007/s00247-009-1486-0
14. Arthurs OJ et al (2015) Paediatric and perinatal postmortem imaging: the need for a subspecialty approach. Pediatr Radiol 45(4):483–490. https://doi.org/10.1007/s00247-014-3132-8
15. Arthurs OJ et al (2016) ESPR postmortem imaging task force: where we begin. Pediatr Radiol 46(9):1363–1369. https://doi.org/10.1007/s00247-016-3639-2
16. Arthurs OJ et al (2014) Current status of paediatric post-mortem imaging: an ESPR questionnaire-based survey. Pediatr Radiol 44(3):244–251. https://doi.org/10.1007/s00247-013-2827-6
17. Cousens S et al (2011) National, regional, and worldwide estimates of stillbirth rates in 2009 with trends since 1995: a systematic analysis. Lancet 377(9774):1319–1330
18. Italian Ministry of Health (2014) Decree October 7. www.gazzettaufficiale.it/eli/id/2014/11/22/14A08847/sg
19. Calder AD, Offiah AC (2015) Foetal radiography for suspected skeletal dysplasia: technique, normal appearances, diagnostic approach. Pediatr Radiol 45(4):536–548. https://doi.org/10.1007/s00247-014-3130-x
20. Farina J et al (2002) Ultrasonographic autopsy (echopsy): a new autopsy technique. Virchows Arch 440:635–639
21. Uchigasaki S et al (2004) Application of compact ultrasound imaging device to postmortem diagnosis. Forensic Sci Int 140:33–41
22. Bolliger SA et al (2008) Virtual autopsy using imaging: bridging radiologic and forensic sciences. A review of the Virtopsy and similar projects. Eur Radiol 18:273–282
23. Lombardi CM et al (2014) Postmortem microcomputed tomography (micro-CT) of small fetuses and hearts. Ultrasound Obstet Gynecol 44(5):600–609. https://doi.org/10.1002/uog.13330
24. Sarda-Quarello L et al (2016) Whole-body perinatal postmortem CT angiography. Diagn Interv Imaging 97(1):121–124. https://doi.org/10.1016/j.diii.2014.11.002
25. Gorincour G et al (2015) The future of pediatric and perinatal postmortem imaging. Pediatr Radiol 45(4):509–516. https://doi.org/10.1007/s00247-014-3266-8
26. Breeze AC et al (2006) Use of a confidence scale in reporting postmortem fetal magnetic resonance imaging. Ultrasound Obstet Gynecol 28(7):918–924
27. Thayyil S et al (2011) Post mortem magnetic resonance imaging in the fetus, infant and child: a comparative study with conventional autopsy (MaRIAS Protocol). BMC Pediatr 11:120. https://doi.org/10.1186/1471-2431-11-120
28. Arthurs OJ et al (2015) Magnetic Resonance Imaging Autopsy Study (MARIAS) Collaborative Group. Diagnostic accuracy and limitations of post-mortem MRI for neurological abnormalities in fetuses and children. Clin Radiol 70:872–880
29. Orasanu E et al (2014) Brain volume estimation from post-mortem newborn and fetal MRI. Neuroimage Clin 6:438–444
30. Whitby E et al (2001) Ultrafast MR assessment of CNS abnormalities in third trimester pregnancy: methodology and early experience. Br J Obstet Gynaecol 108:519–526
31. Arthurs OJ et al (2014) Magnetic Resonance Imaging Autopsy Study (MARIAS) Collaborative Group (2014) Diagnostic accuracy of post-mortem MRI for thoracic abnormalities in fetuses and children. Eur Radiol 24:2876–2884
32. Thayyil S et al (2009) Post-mortem examination of human fetuses: a comparison of whole-body high-field MRI at 9.4 T with conventional MRI and invasive autopsy. Lancet 374:467–475
33. Sarikouch S et al (2008) Value of postmortem magnetic resonance imaging for fatal neonatal congenital heart disease: a case report. Pediatr Cardiol 29:667–669
34. Arthurs OJ et al (2015) Magnetic Resonance Imaging Autopsy Study (MaRIAS) Collaborative Group (2015) Diagnostic accuracy of post mortem MRI for abdominal abnormalities in foetuses and children. Eur J Radiol 84:474–481
35. Woodward PJ et al (1997) Postmortem fetal MR imaging: comparison with findings at autopsy. AJR Am J Roentgenol 168(1):41–46
36. Arthurs OJ, Taylor AM, Sebire NJ (2015) Indications, advantages and limitations of perinatal postmortem imaging in clinical practice. Pediatr Radiol 45(4):491–500. https://doi.org/10.1007/s00247-014-3165-z

Radiology for Postmortem

26

Stefania Zerbo, Laura Scopelliti,
Federica Vernuccio, Giuseppe Lo Re,
Antonina Argo, and Magdy Kharoshah

26.1 Introduction

When cardiac activity stops beating early postmortem signs of death became evident. The early changes include algor mortis, rigor mortis, and livor mortis while late postmortem changes involve the progressive breakdown of soft tissue and organs including the autolysis and putrefaction. These normal postmortem changes depend on internal and external factors, such as body temperature, preexisting conditions, underlying disease, medications (antibiotics), and postmortem interval.

Radiologic methods, such as computed tomography (CT) and magnetic resonance imaging (MRI), open new perspectives for exploring the inside of bodies and may contribute to the understanding of thanatology.

S. Zerbo (✉) · A. Argo
Department for Health Promotion, Maternal and Child Care, University of Palermo, Palermo, Italy
e-mail: stefania.zerbo@unipa.it; antonella.argo@unipa.it

L. Scopelliti · F. Vernuccio · G. Lo Re
Department of Radiology, Policlinic Hospital Palermo, Palermo, Italy

M. Kharoshah
Dammam Forensic Medicine Center, Dammam, Kingdom of Saudi Arabia

Jeddah Forensic Medicine Center, Jeddah, Kingdom of Saudi Arabia

26.2 Early Postmortem Changes

26.2.1 Hypostasis or Postmortem Lividity

Hypostasis reveals important information for forensic pathologists as indications to the cause of death and the position of the body after death.

Hypostasis occurs when the circulation has stopped and the plasma and all cellular component subjected to gravitation force sediment within the vascular system. This phenomenon leads to livores in the skin and in all muscles and organs.

Livor mortis usually appears as a blue-purple coloration of skin in the dependent areas of the body due to accumulation of blood in the capillaries within the dermis except the areas that are adhering to rigid supporting surface.

This discoloration is the resulting formation of deoxyhemoglobin due to oxygen dissociation from the hemoglobin of erythrocytes and continuous oxygen consumption from cells that initially survive after the cessation of cardiovascular function.

The color of hypostasis depends on the state of oxygenation at death: it is visible as cherry-pinkish in deaths due to intoxication by carbon monoxide and cyanides, after exposure of a body to cold temperatures; pink coloration is observed in drowning or is due to storage in a refrigerator. The hypostasis may appear as a brownish red

G. Lo Re et al. (eds.), *Radiology in Forensic Medicine*,
https://doi.org/10.1007/978-3-319-96737-0_26

when the death is due to ingestion of nitrates, in case of methemoglobin intoxication. Livores will spread green under the influence of putrefaction processes due to conversion of hemoglobin into sulfhemoglobin.

Lividity is difficult to identify in a dark-skinned individual and is poor in anemic [1].

The distribution of hypostasis depends on the posture of the body after death. If the body remains in supine or prone position after death livor mortis will be marked, respectively, posteriorly on the back or in the anterior surface of the body; if the body is discovered in vertical position (i.e., hanging) the hypostasis will be evident in the feet and distal part of the arms and hands (Fig. 26.1).

According to Madea, hypostasis is usually evident within 20–30 min after death; complete shifting livor occurs from 2 to 6 h and incomplete shifting is possible from 6 to 12 h; after 12 h the livor is fixed [2].

The capability of livores to shift is assumed to depend on a prevailing number of intact erythrocytes within the vascular system (sedimentation of blood); the fixation of livor mortis occurs as a result of the breakdown of erythrocyte membranes during autolysis when the erythrocytes become pervious for hemoglobin and its derivates with subsequent diffusion of hemolytic blood serum through the walls of the vessels.

The knowledge of these phenomena is important to distinguish the common early signs of death from antemortem lesions. The livores in the posterior wall of the left ventricle can be confused by an inexpert pathologist as early infarction; the livores in the dependent loop of intestine may mimic an intestinal infarction and hypostasis in dependent lung edema, congestion, and hemorrhages but histological examination is useful to differentiate the hypostasis from underlying antemortem diseases.

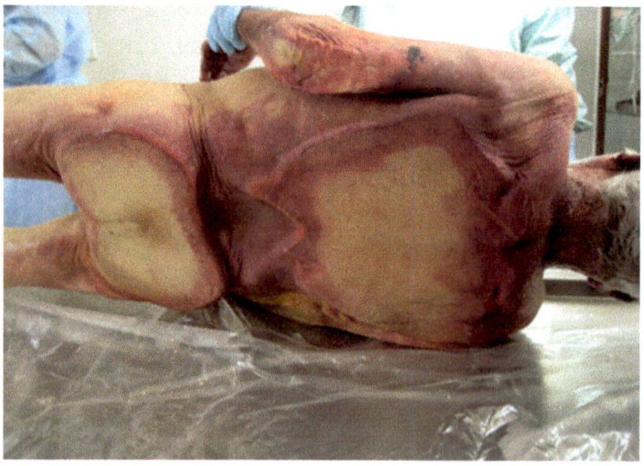

Fig. 26.1 Postmortem hypostasis on the back. The pale areas are the result of pressure against a hard supporting surface

26.2.2 Rigor Mortis

Rigor mortis is the stiffening of the body after death doe to a loss of adenosine triphosphate (ATP) from the body's muscles. It is a well-known phenomenon which sets on about 2–4 h after death.

After death generation of ATP is stopped and actin and myosin are arranged in interdigitating filaments that form a loose physicochemical combination called actomyosin that remains until decomposition occurs.

Rigor mortis does not appear contemporaneously in all muscles but following the "Nysten's rule."

Rigor mortis begins to appear in the mandibular joints (at earliest approximately 20 min postmortem), facial muscles, and neck; after 12–24 h postmortem rigidity affects muscles of the trunk and later the upper extremities and persists for 36–48 h. Usually rigor mortis disappears 72–80 h after death in the same order in which it has appeared; nevertheless gross variation of time course of cadaveric rigidity is reported in the literature [2].

Numerous intrinsic and extrinsic factors affect the development of rigor mortis. Factors accelerating the time of onset of rigor mortis are represented by physical exhaustion prior to death, exposure to high body temperature/fever at the time of death, convulsions prior to death, i.e., hanging and suffocation, and high ambient temperatures. On the other hand the main factors that delay the time of onset of rigor mortis are debilitating diseases, cachexia, exposure to cool/cold ambient temperatures, and death after a short agonal period.

Rigor mortis, also, is found in internal organs such as the myocardium, uterus, gallbladder, and urinary bladder.

In the heart, rigor causes the ventricles to contract, which may be misinterpreted by the inexperienced pathologist for left ventricular hypertrophy.

26.3 Later Postmortem Changes

Decomposition is a mixed process of autolysis and putrefaction. Autolysis is the breakdown of cells and organs through an aseptic chemical process caused by intracellular enzymes. Putrefaction of human tissue is due to bacterial degradation of soft tissue.

Decomposition may differ from body to body, from environment to environment, and even from one part of the same corpse to another. The onset of putrefaction depends on two main factors: the environment and the body. This process can be accelerated by high temperature, this process can be accelerated and on the other hand the cool temperature delays or stops the putrefaction.

Decomposition is also accelerated by obesity and heavy clothing, and in subjects who died of infectious diseases or penetrating injuries. Decomposition is delayed by tight clothing in cases of administration of antibiotics before death and in individuals with a considerable loss of blood prior to death.

The putrefaction is characterized by a sequence of events. The earliest signs of putrefaction, usually in the first 24–36 h, are a greenish discoloration of the lower quadrants of the abdomen followed by greenish discoloration of the head, neck, and shoulders; swelling of the face due to bacterial gas formation; and the abdomen becoming bloated and as a result of bacteria proliferation the evidence of "marbling" of the skin in the veins of the subcutaneous tissues. During putrefaction the body undergoes generalized bloating (60–72 h) followed by vesicle formation, skin slippage, and hair slippage. The last event of putrefaction is the skeletonization of a body. The time of skeletonization depends on local environment and usually occurs from few weeks to few years.

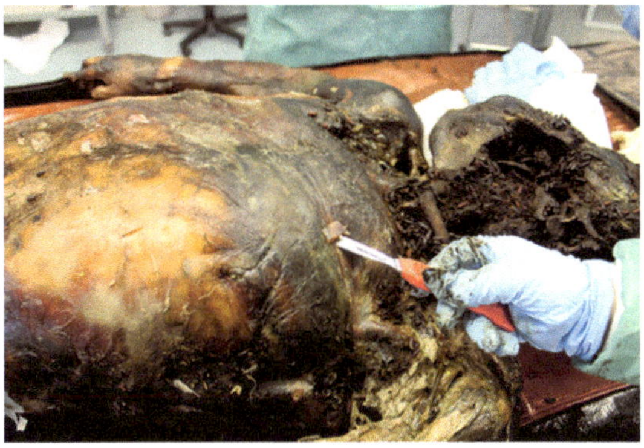

Fig. 26.2 Postmortem decomposition showing partial skeleton of face and putrefactive changes in the arms and trunk after 3 months of death. In these cases we observed also a postmortem damage on the neck by predators

Animal predators such us mice, rats, dogs, maggots, and mammals can be included in the range of destruction.

In addition, the timescale for decomposition may vary greatly in different circumstances and climates, and even in the same corpse: the head and arms may be skeletalized, while the legs and trunk, perhaps protected by clothing or other covering, may be moderately intact (Fig. 26.2).

26.3.1 Maceration and Adipocere Formation

Within a few hours after a stay of a corpse in the water maceration of the skin occurs on the palmar surface of the hands and the plantar surface of the foot. The terms of maceration of the skin depend on water temperature (Fig. 26.3).

Adipocere is a waxy decomposition product formed from bacterial hydrolysis and hydrogenation of adipose tissue, which generally occurs in bodies under prolonged submersion (prolunged submersion in water or in moist soil) and in anaerobic environment. The product the maceration of in.

The accurate determination of postmortem interval (PMI) using the formation of adipocere is very complicated. Adipocere formation has

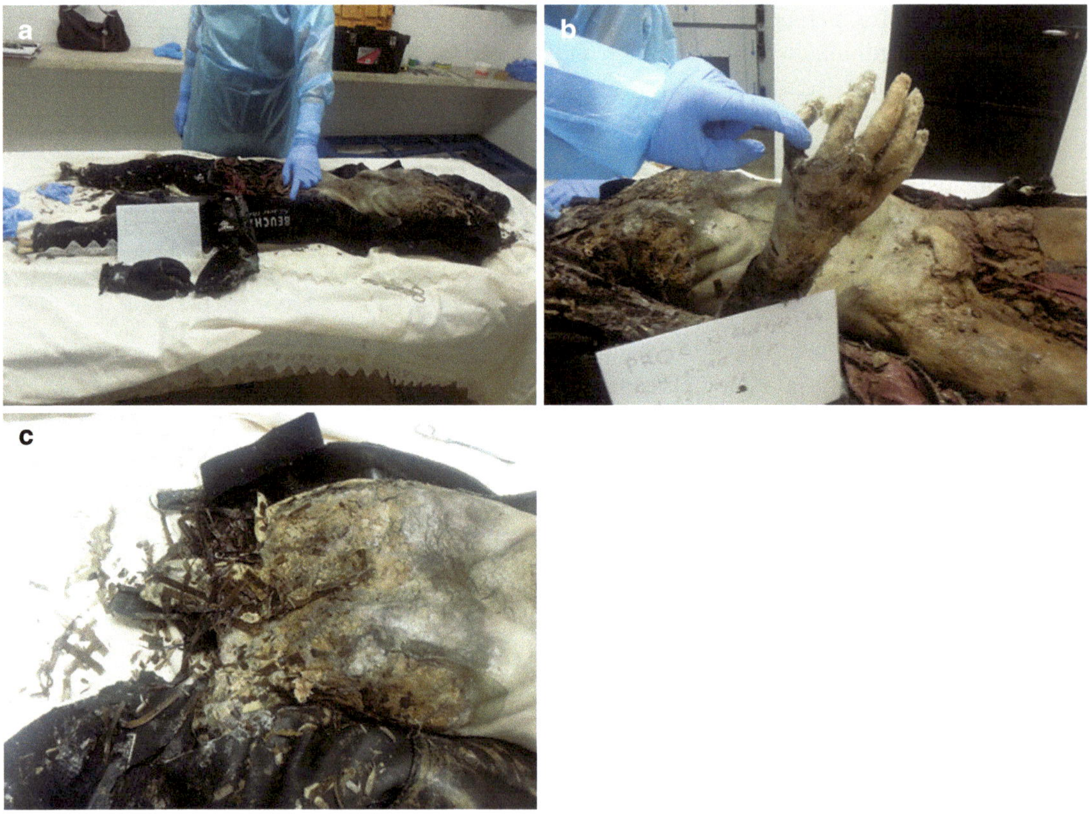

Fig. 26.3 (**a–c**) Unidentified human body (winter 2012, Trapani, Sicily) of male subject wearing scuba diving dress; the torso is preserved, showing maceration due to floating in marine seawater; head, upper limbs, and feet are lost due to maceration and microfauna action

been extensively investigated. At first time triglycerides composed of neutral fats are degraded by endogenous lipases and then bacterial enzymes convert neutral fats into fatty acids; successively these are converted to hydroxy-fatty acids, with oleic acid being the primary source of 10-hydroxystearic acid which is the main component of adipocere [3–6]. Its formation depends on the amount of body fat and on the temperature and depth of the water in which the body was situated. It may persist for many months or decades. Warm temperatures, mildly alkaline pH, and anaerobic conditions accelerate adipocere formation by providing a fertile environment for bacterial growth (*Clostridium perfringens*). A complete adipocere formation occurs after many years [7].

Adipocere provides good preservation of organs, tissues, and organs [8] (Fig. 26.4).

26.4 Postmortem Imaging in Forensic Thanatology

Postmortem imaging has been validated to be a reasonable alternative to conventional autopsy and has become a useful tool to detect potential causes and manner of death in trauma cases, acts of violence or abuse, and human identification of deceased [9–12].

The use of computed tomography (CT) and magnetic resonance imaging (MRI) is recently becoming a potential tool to investigate the early and later postmortem changes in internal organs

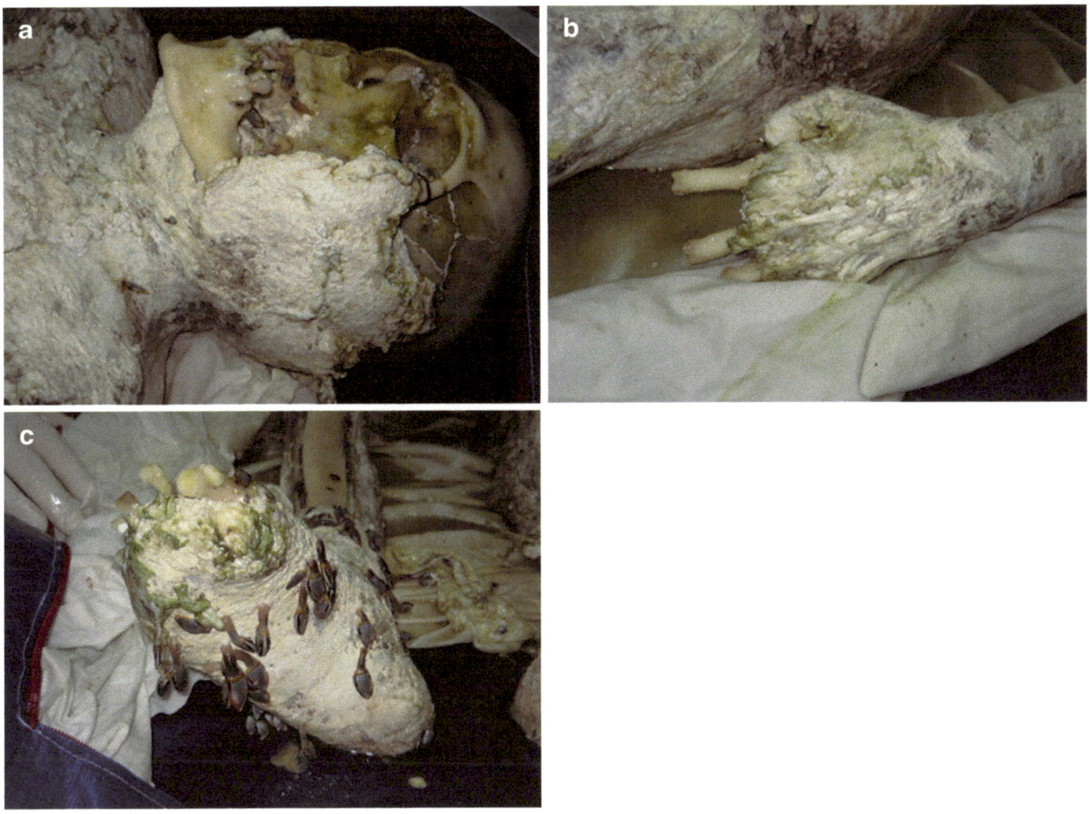

Fig. 26.4 (a–c) Adipocere formation at head, hands, and feet, with detachment of finger (male, unidentified, year 2009)

but they cannot be used for the estimation of the PMI [13–15].

Among the early postmortem changes, livor mortis is the earliest to set in and can be detected on imaging, whereas rigor mortis and algor mortis do not affect CT findings [9]. The mechanism of appearance of the hypostasis depends on postmortem changes of blood after cessation of the circulation, such as sedimentation, postmortem clotting, and internal livores [13].

Immediately after cessation of circulation, position-dependent fluid sedimentation develops and these phenomena are well detected by PMCT and PMMR (Figs. 26.5, 26.6, and 26.7).

Knowledge of these phenomena is an important component of postmortem imaging interpretation in order to distinguish the physiological postmortem changes from underlying disease and pathological findings [13]. As recommended by O'Donnel a program of quality audit should be instituted in order to contrast the main error in diagnostic image such as nonrecognized finding and incorrect interpretation of findings [16].

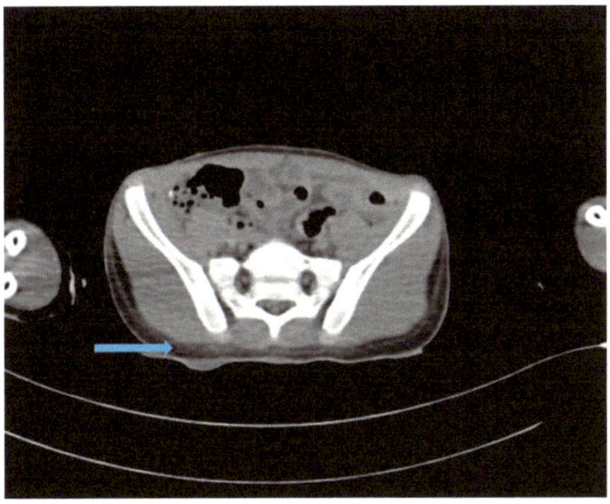

Fig. 26.5 Dorsal gravitational hypostasis (arrow) with fluid collection at CT scan image

The hypostasis is detected at postmortem MR images as a dark hypointense layer [17].

Jackowski et al. in the virtopsy project describe in 44 cases the imaging appearance of early postmortem alterations and conclude that sedimentation of blood, internal livores, and postmortem clotting are well detected in lungs and heart predominantly by MRI while are nonvisualized in liver and spleen. The MSCT imaging is superior than RMI to detect livores in the lungs because it is able to discriminate between air and blood accumulation [13, 14].

The typical sign of livor mortis of the lung is characterized by a diffuse ground-glass opacity in the dependent lower posterior lobes of with a horizontal demarcation line to the anterior nonaffected lung which may be interpreted like an air-blood level. The livores of lungs can be confused with aspiration or contusion but in these cases a focal pattern of airspace disease is more common [18].

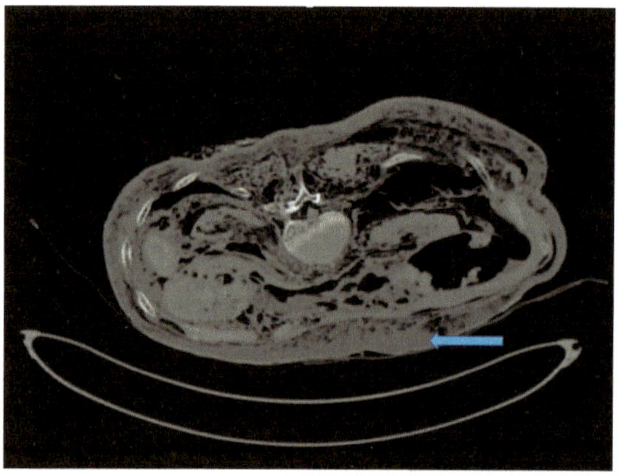

Fig. 26.6 CT imaging of abdominal wall hypostasis (arrow) on a putrefactive corpse

Decomposition through autolysis, putrefaction, and insect and animal predation produces dramatic alterations in the appearance of the body on PMCT and MRI.

MCST is the most used technique to investigate a small collection of gas in the bodies that cannot be detected on conventional autopsy. It is also able to use a contrast method to differentiate gas formed during early stage of decomposition from a vital air embolism.

The earliest changes due to decomposition on postmortem imaging are usually in the brain. At MCST the cerebral autolysis is well detected as loss of grey–white matter differentiation and decreased attenuation and loss of sulcal definition [19] (Fig. 26.8).

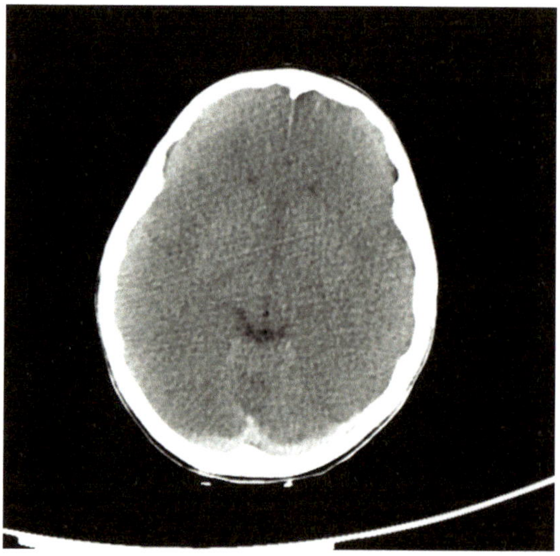

Fig. 26.8 Cerebral autolysis at CT scan image

Fig. 26.7 (**a**, **b**) Hypostasis on subcutaneous fat on left side (**a**) with a magnification (**b**) at CT scan image

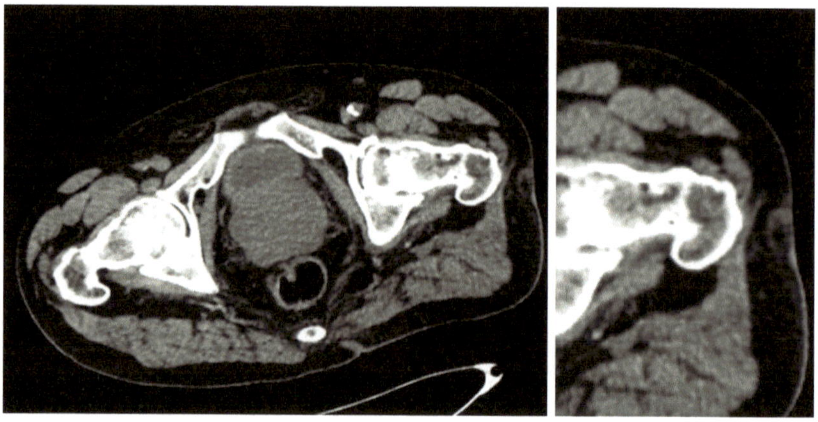

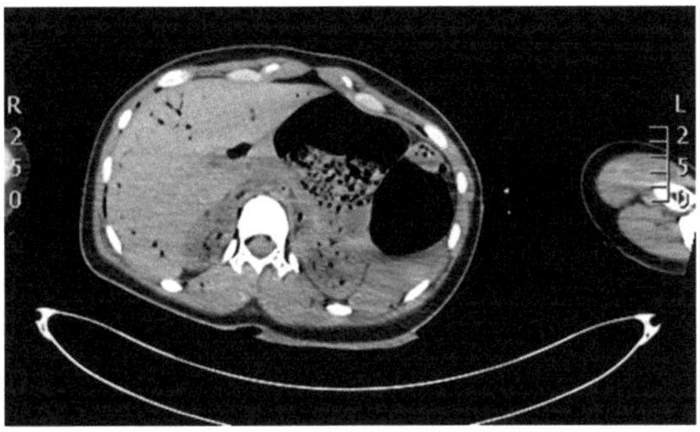

Fig. 26.9 Air bubbles in hepatic portal system

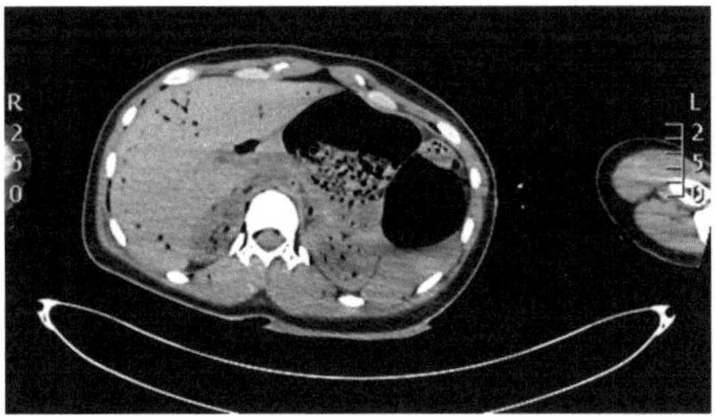

Fig. 26.10 Diffuse putrefactive air bubbles in soft tissues of abdomen in CT scan image

Later gas appearing in the intracranial vessels and finally the brain liquefies and becomes water attenuation [20].

The intra-abdominal compartment is the first region to exhibit putrefactive changes of decomposition with gas evident in the intestinal wall and the mesenteric vessels and portal venous system as described for the first time by Yamazaki et al. in 190 cases of nontraumatic death with a mean interval of 2 h after death [21] (Fig. 26.9).

In the later stage the putrefaction affects whole body and we can observe on MCST and MRI diffuse distribution of gas bubbles [18, 19] (Fig. 26.10).

Although gas collection is a normal finding in the decomposed corpse it must be distinguished from pathological findings and radiologist must be informed about peri- and postmortem circumstances. For example the evidence of gas in the mesenteric and hepatic veins may occur in death following infection diseases but in those cases gas is found anywhere; gas accumulation is associated to resuscitation procedures or mucosal damage of the bowel. In the advanced stage of putrefaction the gas accumulation in small and large bowel should be misinterpreted by radiologist—without experience or specific knowledge on CT appearances of common postmortem changes—such as embolism, pneumoperitoneum, and aerobilia but the putrefactive gas is usually symmetrically distributed in the body.

Further evaluations are necessary with a longer postmortem time MCTS examination to identify the typical later changes of postmortem decomposition and detect the distribution of putrefactive gas in all organs.

In the literature only few cases report on application of virtopsy to identify the appearance of adipocere. As reported by Jackowski et al. the distribution of adipocere formation could be documented using MSCT data while MRI cannot detect the adipocere [22].

References

1. Knight's (2016) Forensic pathology, 4th edn. CRC Press, Boca Raton
2. Madea B, Henssge C, Reibe S, Tsokos M, Kernbach-Wighton G (2014) Postmortem changes and time since death (Chapter 7). In: Madea B (ed) Handbook of forensic medicine. Wiley Blackwell, Hoboken, pp 77–98
3. Pfeiffer S, Milne S, Stevenson RM (1998) The natural decomposition of adipocere. J Forensic Sci 43:368–370
4. Cotton GE, Aufderheide AC, Goldschmidt VG (1987) Preservation of human issue immersed for five years in fresh water of known temperature. J Forensic Sci 32:1125–1130
5. Takatori T (1996) Investigations on the mechanism of adipocere formation and its relation to other biochemical reactions. Forensic Sci Int 80:49–61
6. Takatori T (2001) The mechanism of human adipocere formation. Legal Med 3:193–204
7. Kasuda S, Kudo R, Yuui K, Imai H, Nakata M, Hatake K (2016) An autopsy case of complete adipocere formation. A case report. Legal Med 18:49–51
8. Yan F, McNally R, Kontanis EJ, Sadik OA (2001) Preliminary quantitative investigation of postmortem adipocere formation. J Forensic Sci 46:609–614
9. Panda A, Kumar A, Gamanagatti S, Mishra B (2005) Virtopsy computed tomography in trauma: normal postmortem changes and pathologic spectrum of findings. Curr Probl Diagn Radiol 44:391–406
10. Daly B, Abboud S, Ali Z et al (2013) Comparison of whole-body post mortem 3D CT and autopsy evalu-

ation in accidental blunt force traumatic death using the abbreviated injury scale classification. Forensic Sci Int 225:20–26
11. Jacobsen C, Lynnerup N (2010) Craniocerebral trauma—congruence between post-mortem computed tomography diagnoses and autopsy results: a 2-year retrospective study. Forensic Sci Int 194:9–14
12. Jalalzadeh H, Giannakopoulos GF, Berger FH, Fronczek J, Van de Goot FRW, Reijnders UJ, Zuidema WP (2015) Post-mortem imaging compared with autopsy in trauma victims—a systematic review. Forensic Sci Int 257:29–48
13. Jackowski C, Thali M, Aghayev E, Yen K, Sonnenschein M, Zwygart K, Dirnhofer R, Vock P (2006) Postmortem imaging of blood and its characteristics using MSCT and MRI. Int J Legal Med 120:233–240
14. Jackowsk C, Schweizer W, Thali M, Yen K, Aghayev E, Sonnenschein M, Vock P, Dirnhofer R (2005) Virtopsy: postmortem imaging of the human heart in situ using MSCT and MRI. Forensic Sci Int 149:11–23
15. Thali MJ, Yen K, Schweitzer W, Vock P, Ozdobac C, Dirnhofer R (2003) Into the decomposed body: forensic digital autopsy using multislice-computed tomography. Forensic Sci Int 134:109–114
16. O'Donnell C (2010) An image of sudden death: utility of routine post-mortem computed tomography scanning in medico-legal autopsy practice. Diagn Histopathol 16:552
17. Thali MJ, Yen K, Schweitzer W, Vock P, Boesch C, Ozdoba C (2003) Virtopsy, a new imaging horizon in forensic pathology: virtual autopsy by postmortem multislice computed tomography (MSCT) and magnetic resonance imaging (MRI)—a feasibility study. J Forensic Sci 48:386–403
18. Christe A, Flach P, Ross S, Spendlove D, Bolliger S, Vock P, Thali MJ (2010) Clinical radiology and postmortem imaging (Virtopsy) are not the same: specific and unspecific postmortem signs. Legal Med 12:215–222
19. Levy AD, Harck HT, Mallak CT (2010) Postmortem imaging: MDCT features of postmortem change and decomposition. Am J Forensic Med Pathol 31(1):12–17
20. Offiah CE, Dean J (2016) Post-mortem CT and MRI: appropriate post-mortem imaging appearances and changes related to cardiopulmonary resuscitation. Br J Radiol 89:20150851
21. Yamazaki K, Shiotani S, Ohashi N, Honda MDK (2003) Hepatic portal venous gas and hyperdense aortic wall as post-mortem computed tomography findings. Legal Med 5:338–341
22. Jackowski C, Thali MJ, Sonnenschein M, Aghayev E, Yen K, Dirnhofer R (2005) Adipocere in postmortem imaging using multislice computed tomography (MSCT) and magnetic resonance imaging (MRI). Case report. Am J Forensic Med Pathol 26:360–364

27 Pitfalls on Postmortem Imaging: The Need of Blending Conventional and Virtual Autopsy on Burnt-Charred Body

Giuseppe Lo Re, Antonina Argo, Salvatore Serraino, Stefania Zerbo, Elvira Ventura Spagnolo, and Massimo Midiri

27.1 Introduction

Evaluation of criminal burning is often a difficult challenge in the view of misinterpretation of wound/fracture victims and usually poor case history of this criminal offense. When assisting the courts in similar case of inquiry, jointly forensic traditional autopsy and CT-MR postmortem virtual approach may assist forensic experts in adequate reconstruction of cause, manner, and way of death, significantly to find evidence of found wound/fracture and relative interpretation.

27.2 Heat-Related Modification on Human Bones and Postmortem Imaging

The burned human remains in crime scenes are typically difficult to identify, recover, and manage [1]. All of the burned material at the scene, including body tissues, is often modified to a similar appearance. In particular, even though bone is certainly the most resistant to high temperature exposure, at temperatures above 700 °C it presents a complete combustion of the organic substances with incineration and recrystallization of the inorganic matter; this phenomenon is defined as "calcination." A charred or calcinated bone is known to be more fragile. The perimortem or postmortem fracturing, fragmentation, and bone loss resulting from recovery techniques add to the difficult task of autopsy and laboratory analysis of burned human remains. This is especially problematic for bone trauma analysis, as its most immediate goal is distinguishing perimortem trauma from postmortem alteration, and shape lesion from heat-related traumatic lesion. With regard to burning-related changes, as shrinkage, literature reported that [2] low temperatures (less than 800 °C) of minimal duration produce minimal shrinkage. However, temperatures as low as 300 °C can lead to loss of human albumin. When only minimal heat has been applied, the effects of evidence for burning can be difficult to detect. The ultimate skeletal effects are determined not just by the temperature of the heat applied but also by the duration of the heat event, oxygen supply, and extent of flesh or other protective materials in contact with the skeletal remains. The extent of protective materials present represents an important factor since they maximize differ-

G. Lo Re (✉) · S. Serraino · M. Midiri
Department of Biopathology and Medical Biotechnologies, University of Palermo, Palermo, Italy
e-mail: massimo.midiri@unipa.it

A. Argo · S. Zerbo · E. Ventura Spagnolo
Department of Sciences for the Promotion of Health and Maternal and Child Care "G. D'Alessandro", University of Palermo, Palermo, Italy
e-mail: antonella.argo@unipa.it; stefania.zerbo@unipa.it; elvira.ventura@unipa.it

G. Lo Re et al. (eds.), *Radiology in Forensic Medicine*,
https://doi.org/10.1007/978-3-319-96737-0_27

ences in the temperature of the heat source and the temperature of the affected skeletal remains. Since temperature of the heat source can differ extensively from bone temperature, the duration of the heat becomes important.

Experimental studies on animal model (sheep humeri) reported by Ubelaker indicate that between 150 and 1150 °C heat temperature effects on bone structures were not apparent. Holden et al. documented that the organic component of bone survived until temperatures of 400 °C. Beginning at 600 °C the bone mineral recrystallized. Melting of bone mineral occurred at 1600 °C. Calcination is closely linked to contact with live coals.

The accurate interpretation of perimortem bone trauma is crucial to anthropological [3] and pathological analyses. In this scenario of complex evaluation of gross and microscopic human bone structure, Rx traditional approach (usually on-site morgue facilities or with portable apparels) contributes to essential findings [4] (Fig. 27.1); the postmortem computed tomography (CT) and MR can significantly help to identify human body and contextual relationships of remains as well as other physical evidences at the scene like the foreign bodies and bullets that have a potential forensic meaning [5]. Aim of several studies is focused to evaluate the role of postmortem CT-MR in the identification of the sequence of perimortem and postmortem events and the typical findings in burned bodies.

The relationship to severely heat-damaged areas of tissue usually is obvious and well known in forensic practice, but fractures may be worrying in interpretation. In cases involving extreme exposure to fire, burned skeletal elements typically exhibit severe fragmentation and fracturing limiting interpretation and distinction of antemortem and perimortem trauma. In experimentally burned bone, heat causes dehydration of the bone collagen, leading to shrinkage, distortion, cracking, fragmentation, and destruction of bone [6, 7]. Potentially this may simulate blunt injury but not sharp force injury (Herrmann 1999). Heat-induced fractures and traumatic fractures may be difficult or impossible to distinguish, and scanning electron microscopy is reported to be useful (Herrmann 1999) (Fig. 27.2). CT scan analysis may consistently help to distinguish different sharp fracture patterns [8], in accord with experimental studies which demonstrated that all sharp force traumas remained visible and recognizable following incineration [9]. More recently, Thali et al. [10] demonstrated also the role of virtual autopsy with multi-slice computed tomography and magnetic resonance imaging in diagnostic findings of charred body, limited to distinction about premortem and vital signs.

Characteristic alterations of proper burned bone depend on temperature and time of exposure, as follows:

- Cortical thinning and loss of matter
- Smoothing of the sharp edges, especially in case of previous exposed fractures
- Various alterations of bone marrow density, associated to the presence of air

The main difference noticed by literature between bones directly destroyed by fire and bones previously fractured and after exposed to flames is that in the latter one the presence of sharp rounded edges is always accompanied by the almost complete substitution of bone marrow with air, after tissue combustion (Fig. 27.2). However, our evaluation of corpses undergone to different times of exposure to fire literature observed different kind of alterations associated to different kind of bones.

In some cases involvement of thoracic cage is documented. Especially if sternum and ribs were mostly exposed to fire, CT postmortem was able to identify cortical thinning and erosion involving bones from external to internal surface and diagonally, with homogenous bone marrow involvement following a linear progression. Also complete burning of chondrocostal cartilage was detected.

Findings similar to those we described for skull and thoracic cage can be recognized in other flat bones. Main characteristic of **long bone** involvement in prolonged burning process is disarticulation with unaltered articular surfaces. Moreover, it is essential to identify bone marrow loss from exposed surface and air with distal fragments.

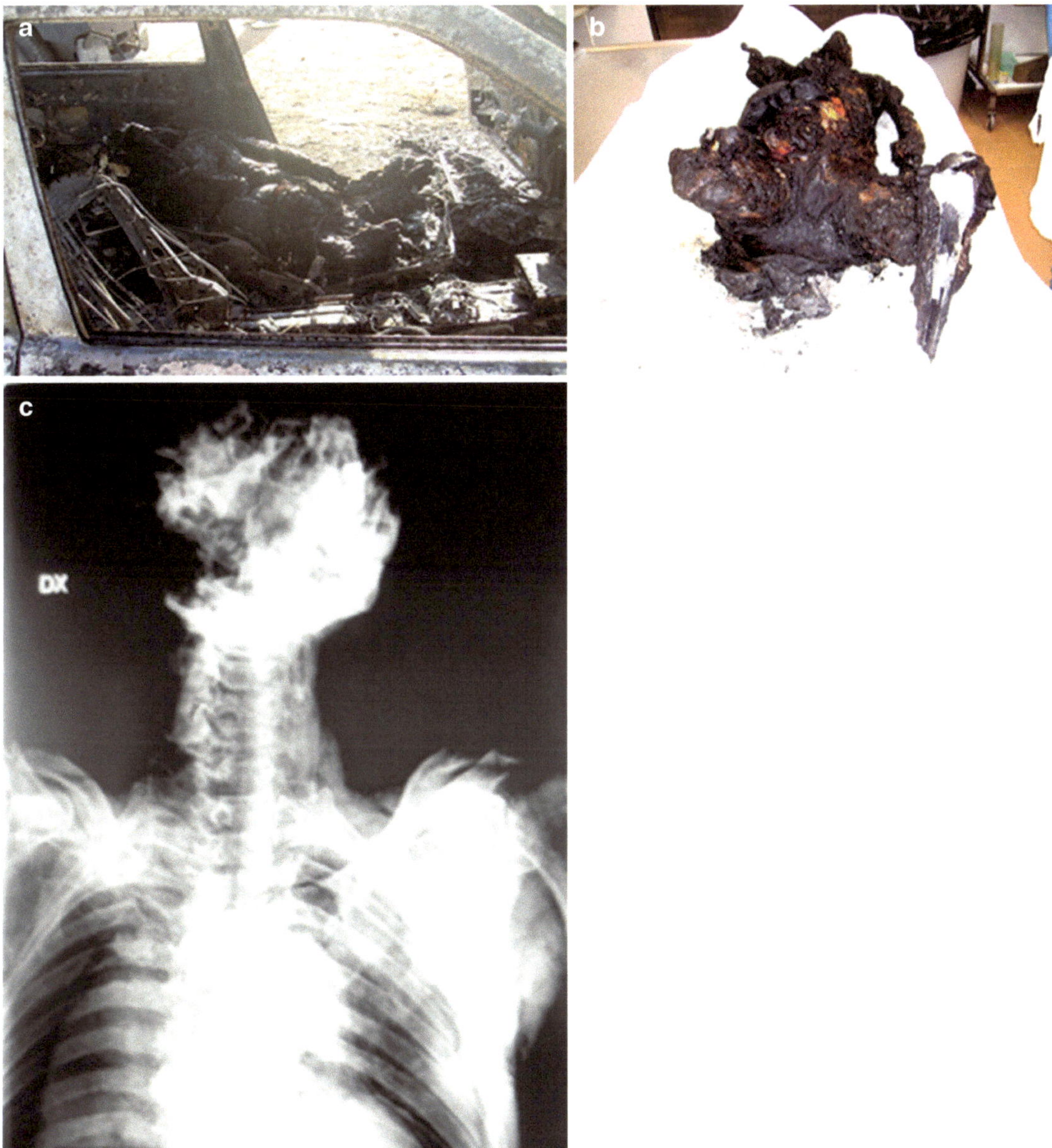

Fig. 27.1 Charred body found in an old burnt car, placed in the driver's seat. External examination showed complete carbonization (**a**); there was heat dismemberment of all four limbs, with partial left-side saving. (**b**) Trachea showed soot traces. The other organs had a "cooked meat" appearance. (**c**) Total body Rx excluded the presence of bullet or metallic fragments into the carbonized body

In our "case report" body we found bilateral complete fractures of both ulnar and radial medial diaphysis. In this case we were able to detect sharp and rounded edges and severe bone marrow loss from exposed surface to proximal diaphysis, giving to the bones a "cavitating" aspect (Fig. 27.2). Neat appearance of these edges suggests amputation with a sharp and heavy blade before burning; moreover, characteristics of bone marrow involvement and rounded edges suggest a prolonged exposure to fire. Distal fragments and hands were not found near victim remains. We could assume that they underwent charring or, most probably, that they were removed and dis-

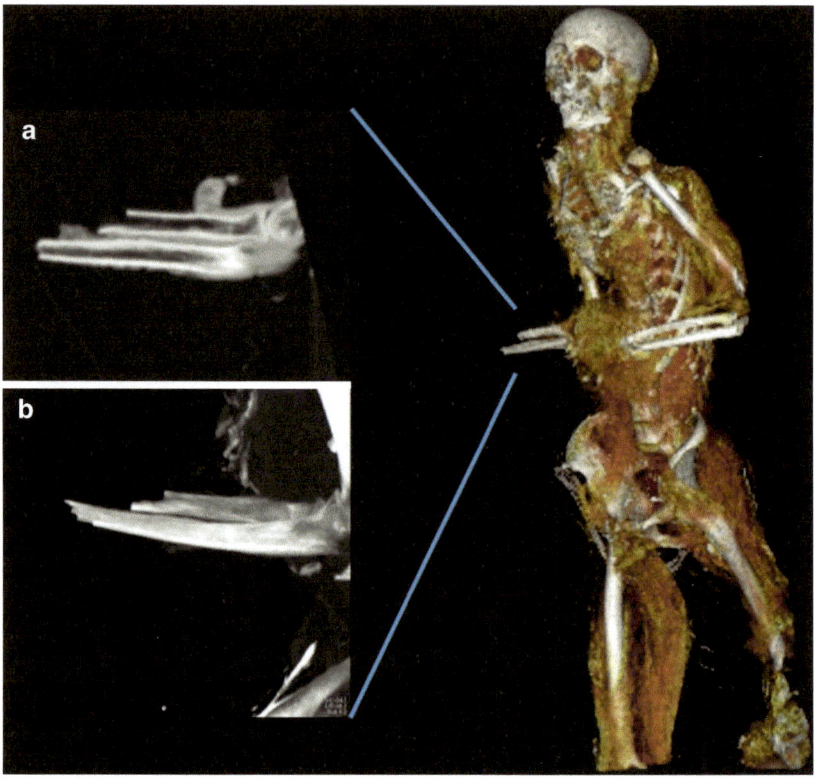

Fig. 27.2 Burned corpse with truncated-like upper extremities; in (**a**) notice the absence of bone marrow; in (**b**) a MIP reconstruction stressing sharp bone edges

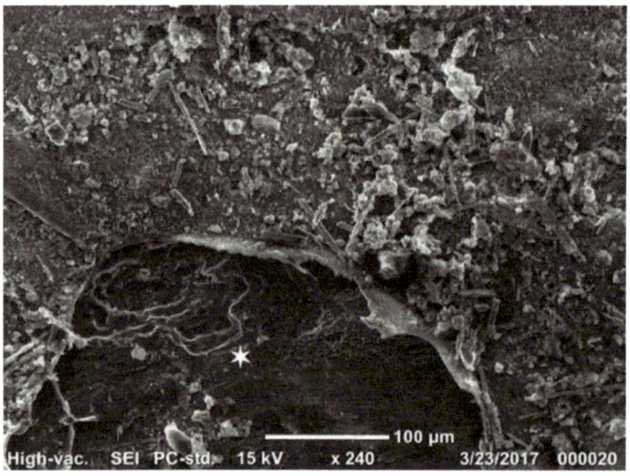

Fig. 27.3 Microphotographs of electron microscopy. A scanning electron microscopy image of charred human humeri, at ×240 magnification, with evidence of detached periosteum (star) and cavity produced by lost lamellae

missed before fire started. Microphotographs of electron microscopy lead to a significant contribution (Fig. 27.3). With regard to flat bones, PMCT may help in distinguishing before premortem and postmortem alteration of the skull (Fig. 27.4), additionally to stereomicroscope examination [11]. This appearance is justified by direct fire action on a previously fractured, composed of skull. Fire would gradually burn the skull, acting from skin and periosteum surface to endosteum, finally charring the whole bone. The presence of a fracture occurred before death is suggested by the identification of multiple subtle hypo-attenuating lines going through the whole bone.

We, however, have to state that in corpses exposed to fire for a very long time, the description of bone rests is quite prohibitive, especially if there is any modification that occurred in life or immediately after death but before burning.

Postmortem CT could implement and improve postmortem findings in burned bodies, especially if performed in corpses exposed to fire for not such a long time, before incineration, by describing each bone alteration, finalized not only at body recognition, but also in order to understand if there are any bone lesions that occurred before burning. This kind of statements could also modify the legal action results [12–29].

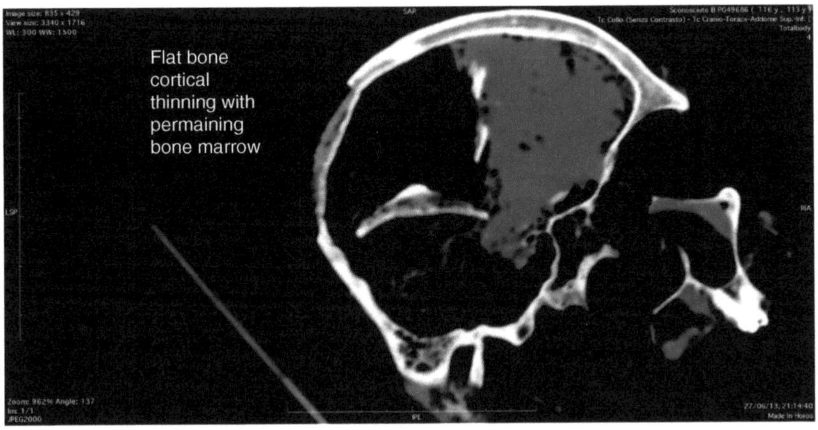

Fig. 27.4 Particular of a burned skull, with thinning or disappearance of cortical bone

References

1. Ubelaker D (2009) The forensic evaluation of burned skeletal remains: a synthesis. Forensic Sci Int 183:1–5
2. Thompson TJU (2005) Heat-induced dimensional changes in bone and their consequences for forensic anthropology. J Forensic Sci 50(5):1–8
3. Stuckert CM, Kricun ME (2011) A case of bilateral forefoot amputation from the Romano-British cemetery of Lankhills, Winchester, UK. Int J Paleopathol 1(2):111–116
4. Averna L, Argo A, Cascino FM, Nicosia A, D'Anna T, Procaccianti P (2012) Suspected child abuse: unusual death in western country. Suicide or homicide? EMBJ 7(11):52–54
5. Carcione P, Lo Re G, Argo A, Carcione G, Picone D, Zerbo S, Scopelliti L, Sortino C, Procaccianti P (2014) Role of MDCT virtopsy in valuation of burned bodies and its comparison with traditional autopsy Conference Paper, January 2014, European Society of Radiology, Wien
6. Fanton L, Jdeed K, Tilhet S, Malicier D (2006) Criminal burning. Forensic Sci Int 158:87–93
7. Grabherr S, Baumann P, Minoiu C, Fahrni S, Mangin P (2016) Post-mortem imaging in forensic investigations: current utility, limitations, and ongoing developments. Res Rep Forensic Med Sci 2016(6):25–37
8. Bohnert M, Rost T, Faller-Marquardt M, Ropohl D, Pollak S (1997) Fractures of the base of the skull in charred bodies: post-mortem heat injuries or signs of mechanical traumatization? Forensic Sci Int 87:55–62
9. Iwase H, Yamada Y, Ootani S, Sasaki Y, Nagao M, Iwadate K, Takatori T (1998) Evidence for an antemortem injury of a burned head dissected from a burned body. Forensic Sci Int 94:9–14
10. Thali M, Yen K, Plattner T, Schweitzer W, Vock P, Ozdoba C, Dirnhofer R (2002) Charred body: virtual autopsy with multi-slice computed tomography and magnetic resonance imaging. J Forensic Sci 47(6):1326–1331
11. Marella GL, Perfetti E, Arcudi G (2012) Differential diagnosis between cranial fractures of traumatic origin and explosion fractures in burned cadavers. J Forensic Legal Med 19:175–178
12. Adair TW, DeLong L, Dobersen MJ, Sanamo S, Young R, Oliver B, Rotter T (2003) Suicide by fire in a car trunk: a case with potential pitfalls. J Forensic Sci 48(5):1113–1116
13. Amadasi A, Borgonovo S, Brandone A, Di Giancamillo M, Cattaneo C (2014) A comparison between digital radiography, computed tomography, and magnetic resonance in the detection of gunshot residues in burnt tissues and bone. J Forensic Sci 59(3):712–717
14. Amadasi A, Brandone A, Rizzi A, Mazzarelli D, Cattaneo C (2012) The survival of metallic residues from gunshot wounds in cremated bone: a SEM-EDX study. Int J Legal Med 126(4):525–531
15. Bohnert M, Werner CR, Pollak S (2003) Problems associated with the diagnosis of vitality in burned bodies. Forensic Sci Int 135:197–205
16. Bohnert M, Schmidt U, Große Perdekamp M, Pollak S (2002) Diagnosis of a captive-bolt injury in a skull extremely destroyed by fire. Forensic Sci Int 127:192–197
17. Nigel CP (2006) Burn injury. In: Rutty GN (ed) Essential of autopsy practice. Current methods and modern trends. Springer, London
18. de Gruchy S, Rogers TL (2002) Identifying chop marks on cremated bone: a preliminary study. J Forensic Sci 47(5):1–4
19. Eckert WG, James S, Katchis S (1988) Investigation of cremations and severely burned bodies. Am J Forensic Med Pathol 9(3):188–200
20. Glassmann DM, Crow RM (1996) Standardization model for describing the extent of burn injury to human remains. J Forensic Sci 41(1):152–154

21. Gruenthal A, Moffatt C, Simmons T (2012) Differential decomposition patterns in charred versus un-charred remains. J Forensic Sci 57:12–18
22. Holden JL, Phakey PP, Clement JG (1995) Scanning electron microscope observations of heat-treated human bone. Forensic Sci Int 74:29–45
23. Marciniak SA (2009) A preliminary assessment of the identification of saw marks on burned bone. J Forensic Sci 54(4):779–785
24. Peuntes K, Cardoso HFV (2013) Reliability of cut mark analysis in human cartilage: the effects of blade penetration angle and intra- and interindividual differences. Forensic Sci Int 231:244–248
25. Robbins SC, Fairgrieve SI, Oost TS (2015) Interpreting the effects of burning on pre-incineration saw marks in bone. J Forensic Sci 60:S1
26. Rotschild MA, Raatschen HJ, Schneider V (2001) Suicide by self-immolation in Berlin from 1990 to 2000. Forensic Sci Int 124:163–166
27. Quatrehomme G, Bolla M, Muller M, Rocca JP, Grevin G, Bailet P, Ollier A (1998) Experimental single controlled study of burned bones: contribution of scanning electron microscopy. J Forensic Sci 43(2):417–422
28. Saukko P, Knight B (2016) Knight's forensic pathology, 4th edn. CRC Press, Taylor and Francis Group, New York, pp 475–495
29. Shkrum MJ, Johnston KA (1992) Fire and suicide: a three-year study of self-immolation deaths. J Forensic Sci 37(1):208–221

Brain Imaging in Postmortem Forensic Radiology

28

Yohsuke Makino, Maiko Yoshida, Daisuke Yajima, and Hirotaro Iwase

28.1 Introduction

The importance of brain postmortem imaging is roughly twofold. Firstly, brain postmortem imaging can assist autopsy in cause of death determination, in personal identification, and in various other forensic tasks. By knowing brain information in advance, pathologists and assistants who would perform irreversible and destructive investigations of the head of cadavers could prepare to search for the lesions suggested by imaging prior to the autopsy. Furthermore, it is advantageous that postmortem imaging provides highly reproducible information that can be investigated again even after dissection, burial, or cremation has been performed.

Secondly, postmortem imaging is useful for "triage" of autopsies. Much research effort has been made over the past 20 years to establish whether CT can be used as a screening tool for autopsies [1–10]. Through these efforts, some countries already decide on the necessity of autopsy based on postmortem CT in combination with or without toxicological screening. In the cranium, there are many fatal lesions and injuries that can be evaluated using postmortem imaging, which has the potential to reduce unnecessary autopsies. At the same time, since postmortem imaging cannot be a perfect substitute for autopsies, there are various pitfalls and limitations for investigating the cause of death based on postmortem imaging.

In this chapter, we introduce the main points of postmortem imaging of the brain in the context of these two points. We also describe our recommended protocol and the basic postmortem changes observed in CT to facilitate an accurate understanding of the imaging findings. In many areas, unfortunately, insufficient evidence is obtained. To some extent, this chapter describes the authors' experience-based opinions, arising from a daily comparison with autopsy results, and from applying the imaging diagnostics established in clinical radiology.

Y. Makino (✉) · H. Iwase
Department of Forensic Medicine, Graduate School of Medicine, The University of Tokyo, Tokyo, Japan

Department of Legal Medicine, Graduate School of Medicine, Chiba University, Chiba, Japan
e-mail: ymakino-tky@umin.ac.jp; iwase@faculty.chiba-u.jp

M. Yoshida
Department of Legal Medicine, Graduate School of Medicine, Chiba University, Chiba, Japan

D. Yajima
Department of Legal Medicine, Graduate School of Medicine, Chiba University, Chiba, Japan

Department of Forensic Medicine, School of Medicine, International University of Health and Welfare, Narita, Japan
e-mail: yajima.d@iuhw.ac.jp

G. Lo Re et al. (eds.), *Radiology in Forensic Medicine*,
https://doi.org/10.1007/978-3-319-96737-0_28

28.2 Protocol for Cranial Postmortem CT

Detailed CT imaging principles will be discussed in other chapters. Here, we describe the example of a protocol for cranial postmortem CT. However, fundamentally, each protocol should be set up together with forensic pathologists, radiologists, and radiographers in each facility.

The more detector rows are used, the shorter time is required to capture a wider image range. In postmortem imaging, it is unnecessary to pursue speed as much as in a clinical context. However, as whole-body imaging is performed, in CT with a small number of detector rows, it is possible that the load on the tube would become excessive, and the stress of the staff could be increased because it requires more time to cool the tube down for the next scan.

It seems advantageous to perform scanning of the cranium, in helical scan mode, continuously with that of the neck and trunk. This makes it possible to obtain a three-dimensional (3D) image in which the head and body are continuous (Fig. 28.1), which can be used for some forensic tasks, such as crime scene reconstruction [11]. However, this may cause a problem in that the image quality of the head is deteriorated as the head scan conditions need to be adjusted to that used for the trunk. At the very least, with regard to the head region, we should obtain a reconstructed image with a narrow field of view to improve imaging quality. However, helical artifacts arising from a helical scan of the skull cannot be improved by reconstruction alone. Although time consuming, we recommend adding a non-helical scan of the head by tilting the gantry along the orbitomeatal baseline (OM line) or anterior commissure–posterior commissure line (AC-PC line). Adding a non-helical scan not only removes the helical artifacts, but also allows scanning again with a dose setting appropriate for the brain (Fig. 28.2). Furthermore, adding a non-helical scan can change the direction of metal artifacts from teeth and lesions that are otherwise hidden may appear.

Of course, it is possible to scan the head and trunk separately. In a facility that allows over-

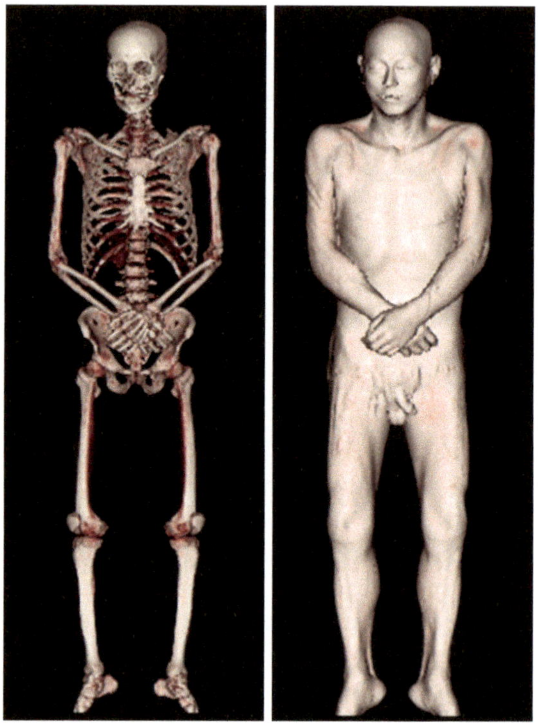

Fig. 28.1 Postmortem whole-body 3-dimensional (3D) images of the victim. These images can be used for various forensic tasks

coming of the barriers of postmortem rigidity and raises the arms routinely to reduce arm artifacts in trunk imaging, separate scans are typically taken. A point of caution when performing separate scans is that the neck area is often divided into half, and a part of the neck is sometimes not scanned. A number of findings related to the cause of death can be found in the neck region, which is therefore an important area for postmortem imaging. When separating the head and trunk, it is necessary to construct a scan protocol to ensure that evaluation of the neck will not be insufficient.

The evaluation of skull fracture is indispensable in the cranium region in forensic medicine. It is useful to create 3D images for evaluation of skull fractures [12]. For 3D reconstruction, it is desirable to reconstruct as thin slices as possible (Fig. 28.3). However, such thin images are not only burdensome to interpreters and software, but also increases the noise as the dose in each image is decreased (Fig. 28.2). It is recommended to use

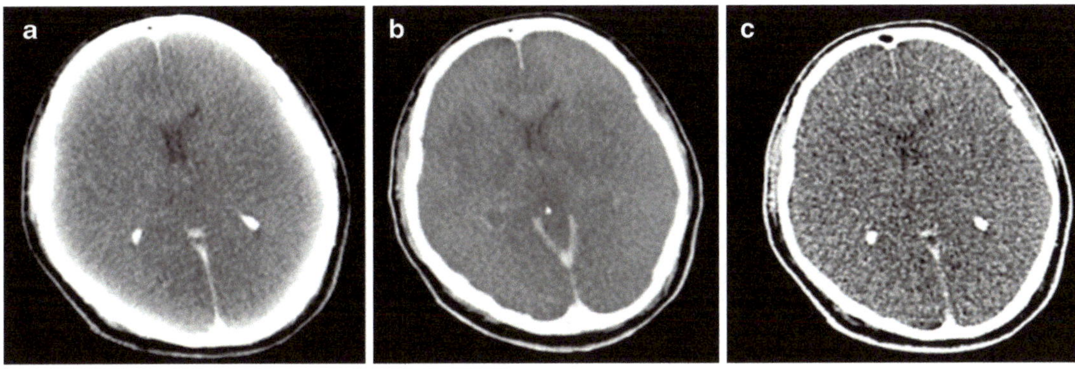

Fig. 28.2 Postmortem axial brain computed tomography images of the same subject, with similar section levels. (**a**) Helical scan mode, 5 mm slice thickness, 120 kV, 200 mA. Note the high-density area around the brain, suggesting a helical artifact from the skull. (**b**) Non-helical scan mode, 5 mm slice thickness, 120 kV, 270 mA. The helical artifact is removed and gray matter/white matter contrast is increased. (**c**) Helical scan mode, 0.625 mm slice thickness, 120 kV, 200 mA. The image becomes noisy and contrast is decreased compared to (**b**)

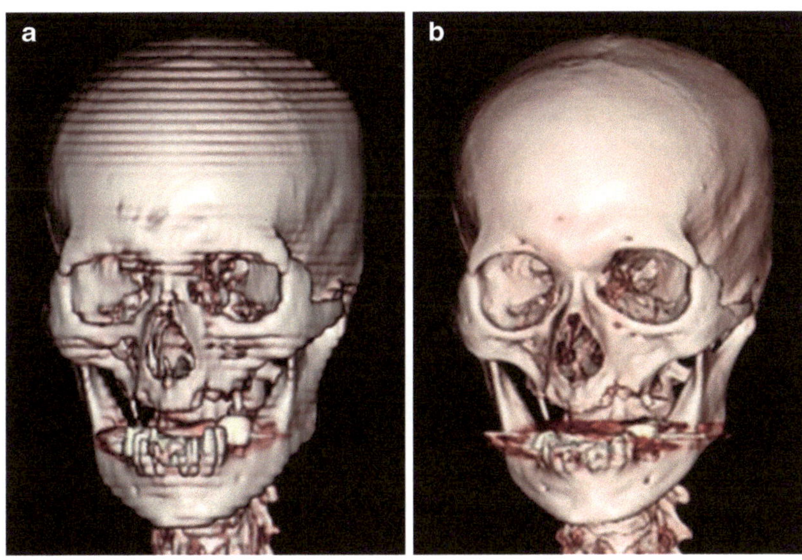

Fig. 28.3 3D images of the skull of the same subject, reconstructed from 5-mm-thick images (**a**) and 0.625-mm-thick images (**b**). As the slice is too thick, (**a**) shows steplike lines

thin-slice images only on CT consoles or workstations that create 3D images, and to produce reconstructed images of about 5 mm thickness, to reduce the load on interpreters and computers.

28.3 Postmortem Changes in Cranial Postmortem CT

Typical postmortem changes on postmortem CT of the cranium region include the following. For interpretation, it is necessary to differentiate between these "normal" postmortem changes and abnormal findings:

1. Decreased gray matter/white matter contrast
   In postmortem CT of the brain, the difference between CT values of the gray matter and white matter (GM/WM contrast) is lower than that on antemortem CT, and the images have a "flat" appearance (Fig. 28.4) [13, 14]. Takahashi et al. examined 41 patients who took antemortem brain CT images and CT images within 70 min after death [15]. After comparing both CT scans of the head, they reported that the CT value of the GM significantly decreased postmortem, and that the GM/WM contrast had decreased significantly. Although it was not statistically significant,

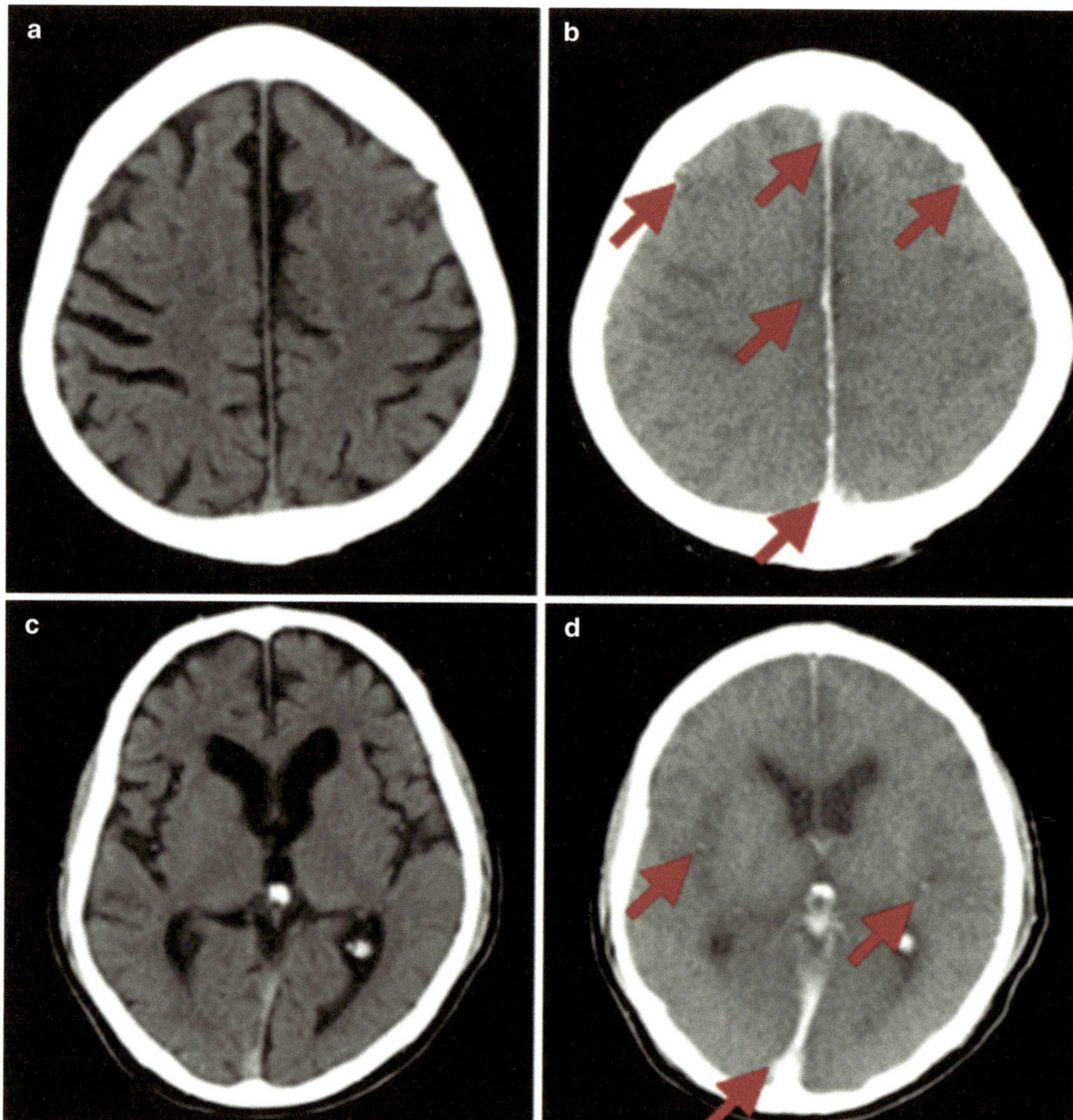

Fig. 28.4 Antemortem (**a**, **c**) and postmortem (**b**, **d**) brain computed tomography (CT) images at a similar section level of the same subject who died due to hanging. The decreased gray matter/white matter contrast and brain swelling postmortem can be observed. High densities of venous sinuses and cortical veins can also be seen on postmortem CT images, as shown by arrows

the CT value of the WM had increased postmortem. Shirota et al. examined 36 cases in which head CT was taken antemortem and again postmortem (within 20 h after death), and found a significant increase in CT value of the WM, as well as significantly decreased GM/WM contrast [16]. However, CT values of the GM also increased, in contrast to the findings of Takahashi et al. Nevertheless, these studies both showed that GM/WM contrast decreases from a relatively early postmortem period, due to an increase in the WM CT values and/or a decrease in the GM CT values. The cause of the increased WM densities remains unknown, but Shirota et al. speculated that postmortem venous congestion may play a role. Regardless, it is inappropriate to diagnose cerebral infarction or similar pathologies postmortem based only on observations of GM/WM contrast reduction in postmortem CT.

2. Brain swelling
   In postmortem CT of the cranium, the brain may be seen to swell (Fig. 28.4). Shirota et al. concluded that the brain swells on CT images as a postmortem change, based on observation of narrowing of the central sulcus and the ventricle from the same ante- and postmortem CT as described above [16]. On the other hand, according to the study by Takahashi et al., no significant narrowing was observed [15]. Shirota et al. assumed that the differences they observed may reflect differences in the conditions related to the deaths. Takahashi et al. dealt with sudden cardiac arrest cases, while Shirota et al. described instances in which blood pressure drops more gradually. Nonetheless, due to postmortem changes, swelling of the brain on the CT is observed postmortem, and caution is necessary when interpreting these findings.
3. Increased densities of the venous sinus or cortical veins
   In the blood vessels after death, sedimentation of erythrocytes and an increase in the hematocrit value occur, and this is more dominant on the side affected by gravity. This phenomenon is called hypostasis. In head postmortem CT, this phenomenon is observed as an increase in the CT value of the sagittal sinus, transverse sinus, sigmoid sinus, or cerebral cortical veins (Fig. 28.4). Takahashi et al. noted that, in comparisons of the antemortem CT and postmortem CT of the same patient, the densities of the dorsal side of the upper sagittal veins increased from an average of 42 HU antemortem to an average of 49 HU postmortem [17]. High absorption in the sinus makes it difficult to distinguish it from surrounding subdural hematoma (SDH). In addition, high absorption of brain surface veins is difficult to discriminate from subarachnoid hemorrhage (SAH) (Fig. 28.4).

   Similar to hypostasis, a pseudo SAH sign may pose a problem in postmortem CT [18]. This is not strictly a postmortem change, but is due to hypoxic encephalopathy or brain death, whether on postmortem CT or antemortem CT, where absorption of the subarachnoid space becomes as high as in SAH (Fig. 28.5). Compared to "true" SAH, the high densities in pseudo SAH tend to be symmetric and thinner, and are not complicated by intraventricular or parenchymal hemorrhage [19].
4. Intracranial gas
   If intracranial gas is found in the cerebrospinal fluid cavity on antemortem CT, it suggests a skull-base fracture. Intravascular gas in the head is also a fatal finding, suggestive of gas embolism. However, intracranial gas on postmortem CT is frequently observed even in

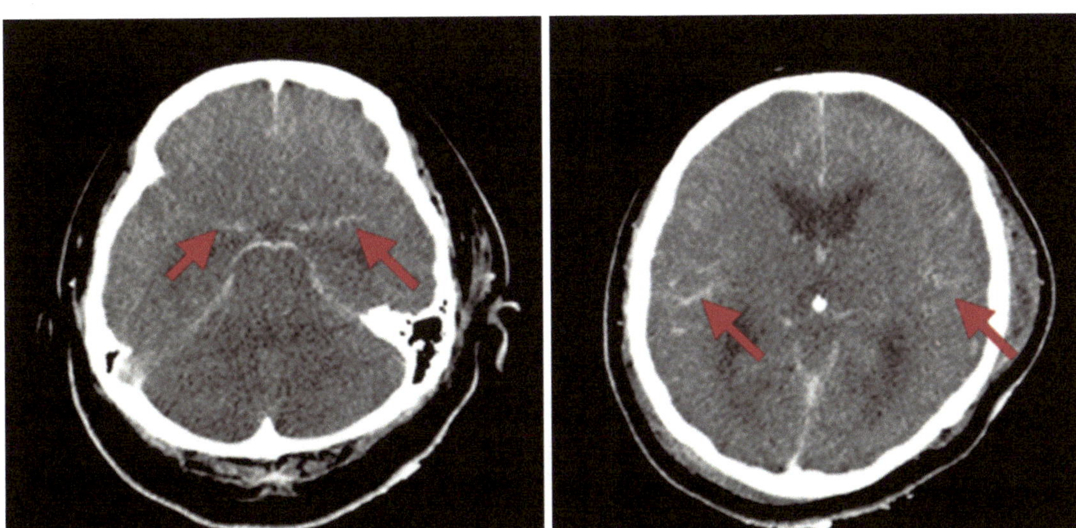

Fig. 28.5 Axial postmortem computed tomography images of the subject with hypoxic ischemic brain injuries. Relatively thin, bilateral high densities in the subarachnoid space can be observed, suggesting subarachnoid hemorrhage (SAH), but no such hemorrhage was found upon autopsy (pseudo-SAH)

cases where such trauma or gas embolism is not observed. In decomposed bodies, it is very common to observe gas inside and outside the brain. Typically, foamy gas is seen in the brain parenchyma and a gas-fluid level is formed between the liquefied brain and gas formed due to putrefaction (Fig. 28.6).

However, Shiotani et al. reported that intravascular gas in the cranium was seen in 29 of 404 cases even in postmortem CT performed within 2 h after death; in all these cases, resuscitation maneuvers were performed [20]. In addition, intravascular gas accumulations were observed (Fig. 28.7). It is therefore spec-

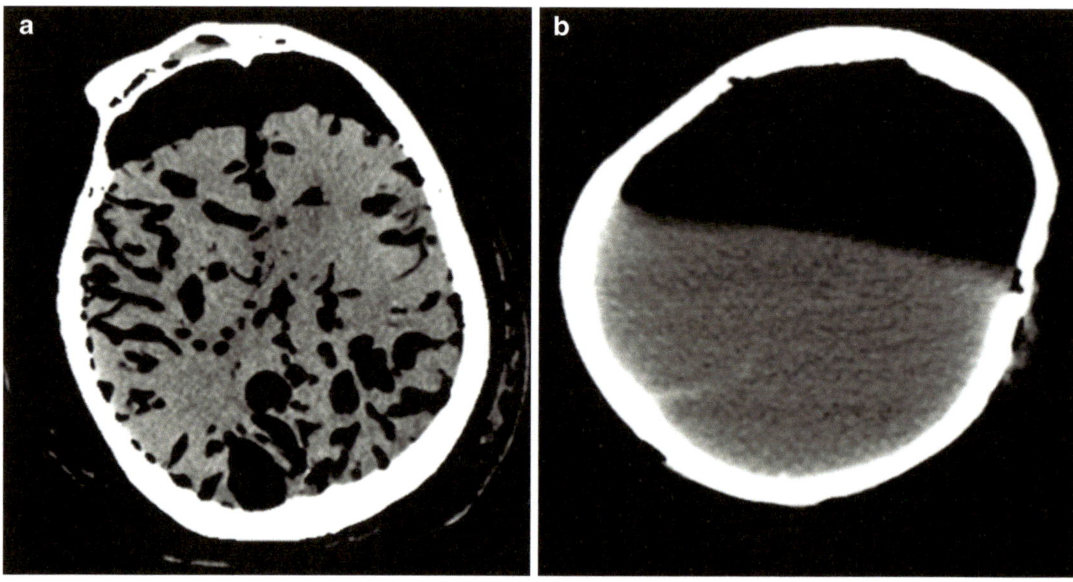

Fig. 28.6 Axial images of the two cases with severe decomposition. Parenchymal foamy gas formation (**a**) and gas-fluid level formation (**b**) can be observed. These are typical findings of the decomposed brain

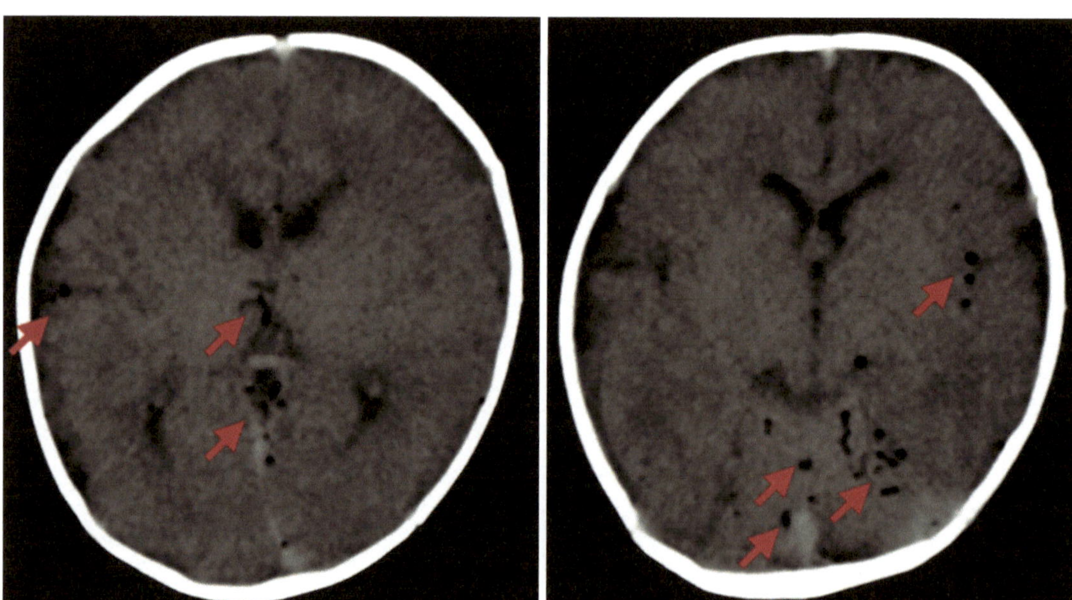

Fig. 28.7 Intravascular gas (arrows) found in computed tomography images obtained immediately after death. The patient was subjected to resuscitation efforts, which may have caused these gas accumulations

ulated that gas is aspirated into the right heart system from the lung due to compression during resuscitation efforts, and this gas may be carried to the cranium by the pumping effect.

28.4 Brain Postmortem CT for Support of Autopsy

By obtaining CT of the cranium prior to autopsy, CT can support autopsy findings in various respects, as already mentioned. Support for autopsy by postmortem CT includes detection of occult injuries, gas, and intracranial hemorrhage in putrefied bodies, each of which is described below. Although angiography is currently being researched, it is sometimes an important tool to search for bleeding sources in cases with difficult intracranial hemorrhagic lesions, which is also briefly described in this section.

1. Occult injuries
   It is important to perform head CT prior to dissection in order to find occult injuries. Particularly in the evaluation of gunshot wounds, CT holds many advantages [21]. In CT, it is possible to describe the appearances of internal fine bone fragments and metallic gunshot residue, which tend to be overlooked in autopsy (Fig. 28.8). In cases of burned bodies, it is difficult to assume gunshot wounds based on external examinations; CT is particularly useful for discovering gunshot wounds [22].

   In high-energy injury cases, the skull can be completely fragmented and pathologists commonly have great difficulty in describing such bursting fractures in detail. Autopsy pictures of such fractures can only be captured after destructive scalp peeling, which results in bone tips scattered on the autopsy table. CT can easily describe the fractures noninvasively, providing better information for forensic tasks (Fig. 28.9) [23].

   Maxillofacial fractures, including those of the orbital walls, paranasal-sinus walls, or nasal bones, are easily overlooked in autopsy. These are important as they are frequently related to assault, and can sometimes be fatal in and of themselves, due to airway obstruction. It is also worth noting a condition called flail mandible, in which tongue-base retraction occurs due to the

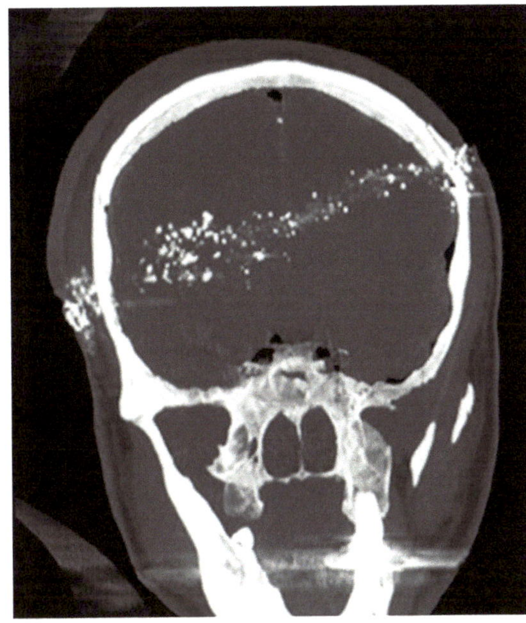

Fig. 28.8 Coronal postmortem computed tomography image of a gunshot victim. Distribution of the small metallic and bony fragments is apparent. These findings are difficult to describe using conventional autopsy

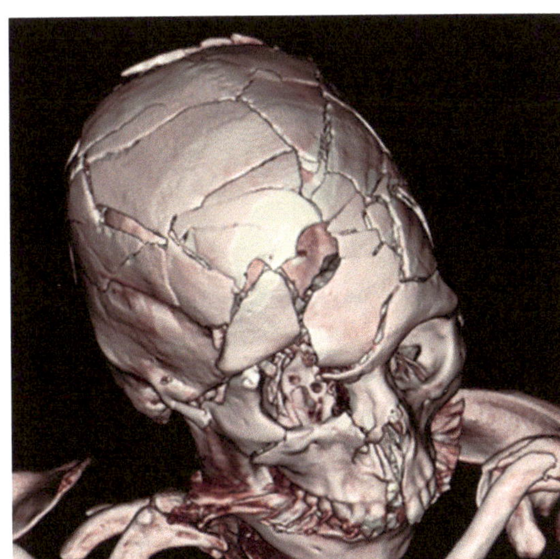

Fig. 28.9 Three-dimensional image of a bursting fracture of the skull in a high-energy injury case. When using an autopsy picture, it is more difficult to describe these types of bone fractures

fracture of a symphyseal fracture with a bilateral condylar fractures, which results in suffocation [24, 25].

Occipital condyle fracture is another type of damage that is easily overlooked in dissection. The occipital condyle is located at the lowest end of the occipital bone and forms the joint with the atlas. As the occipital condyle also provides the point of attachment for the alar ligament, avulsion fractures due to pulling of this ligament occur by excessive lateral bending, and a lethal occipito-atlanto dislocation/subluxation can occur (Fig. 28.10) [26].

When searching for these occult injuries, 3D images of the skull are indispensable. However, 3D images should not be used in isolation. In postmortem CT, intravascular gas can occur in the scalp and skull due to postmortem changes or trauma, but when viewed in 3D, these gases may appear fractured (Fig. 28.11). 3D images should always be evaluated along with the original images.

2. Gas detection
   CT clearly displays gas as a markedly low-density region. Pneumocephalus can be a good indicator of a skull-base fracture. CT can clearly detect embolized gas in cerebral gas embolism cases (Fig. 28.12) [27]. In some fatal diving accidents, massive amount of gas is detected in both the veins and arteries due to fatal decompression sickness and/or barotrauma. In such cases, the gas detected by CT, including cerebral vascular gas, can be a key to differentiating this condition from drowning [28, 29]. Of course, it should be considered that intracranial gas detected by CT may simply reflect postmortem changes.
3. Intracranial hemorrhage in highly decomposed bodies
   Although it is advantageous that various intracranial hemorrhagic lesions can be found in postmortem CT, fatal hemorrhagic lesions in fresh cadavers can be found by autopsy, even without CT, by skilled forensic pathologists.

On the other hand, even in a brain liquefied by putrefaction in a dead body, intracranial hemorrhagic lesions can still be recognized as high-density regions in CT images, which is a major advantage of postmortem CT [30, 31]. CT can sometimes allow evaluation of important anatomical structures even in a liquefied brain, and allows investigation of the origin of a hematoma (Fig. 28.13). Without CT, it would be possible to find a hematoma by efflux of the liquefied brain through the skull after opening, but it is

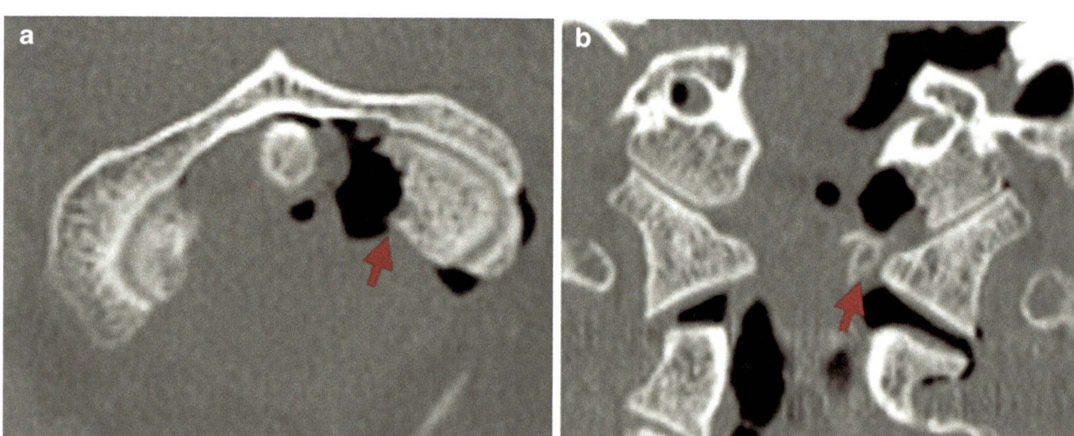

Fig. 28.10 (**a**) Axial and (**b**) coronal computed tomography of an occipital condyle fracture. A small bone tip (arrow) deviation into the spinal canal can be observed (**b**), suggesting fatal cervical cord injury. The detection of this fracture is difficult in autopsy

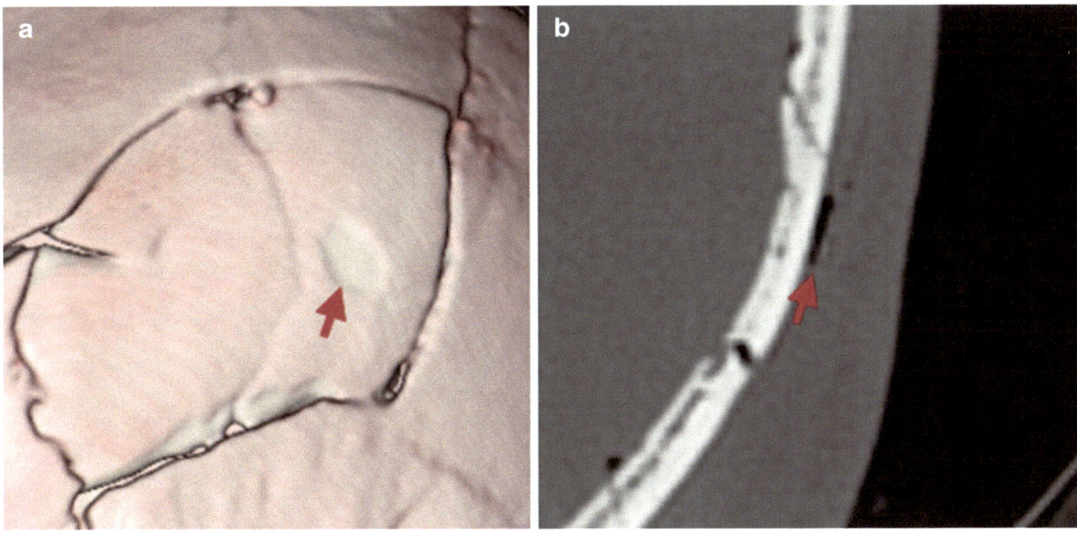

Fig. 28.11 Three-dimensional image of the skull (**a**) suggesting a patterned bony defect indicating a depression (arrow). However, the original axial computed tomography image (**b**) shows no bone fracture and subcutaneous gas

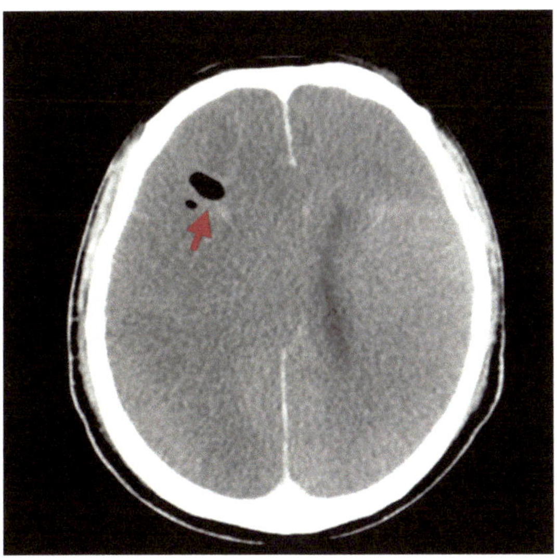

Fig. 28.12 Axial brain computed tomography image of a case with a fatal cerebral gas embolism. Intraparenchymal gas due to the gas embolism can be seen (arrow). Furthermore, there is cerebral low density in the right hemisphere and in the left anterior cerebrum due to infarction caused by gas emboli

extremely difficult to find the hematoma origin by autopsy.

4. Angiography for detection of bleeding sites

The detection of bleeding sites of intracranial hemorrhagic lesions is an important task in forensic medicine. In particular, in the case of SAH, it is important to search for a bleeding source in order to distinguish between traumatic vertebral artery rupture and pathological arterial rupture (dissection or aneurysm). However, once dissection has been performed, it is irreversible, and thus there is a risk for artificially damaging blood vessels and therefore failing to find the bleeding source.

Various postmortem whole-body angiography methods have been devised and further approaches are being researched [9, 32–35]. However, these studies are often performed for the purpose of verifying whether the cause of death can be determined without dissection. From a practical viewpoint for assisting dissection, selective angiography, which contrasts only the target vessel during dissection, may be sufficient [36–38]. Inokuchi et al. reported a contrast examination by inserting a catheter from the internal carotid artery and the vertebral artery, respectively, in cases of SAH. They reported that bleeding sites became clearer by using CT at multiple time phases after administration of a contrast agent (Fig. 28.14) [36].

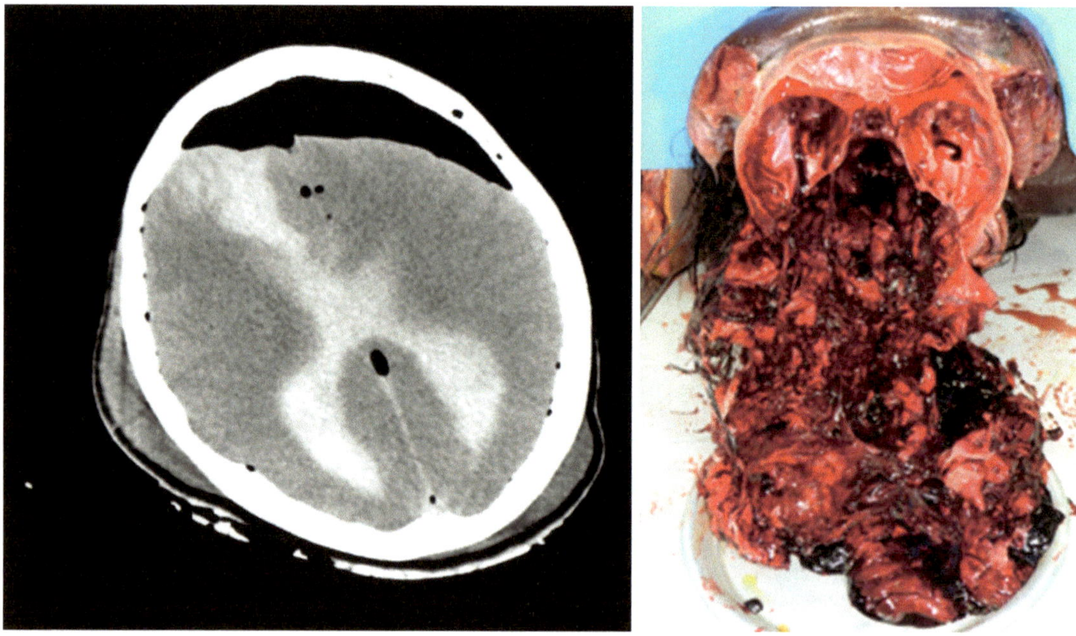

Fig. 28.13 Axial brain computed tomography (CT) image and the autopsy image of the intracerebral hematoma found in the putrefied brain. Even in the putrefied brain, CT indicated that the hematoma originated from the right anterior lobe with intraventricular hemorrhage, which is difficult to evaluate by autopsy

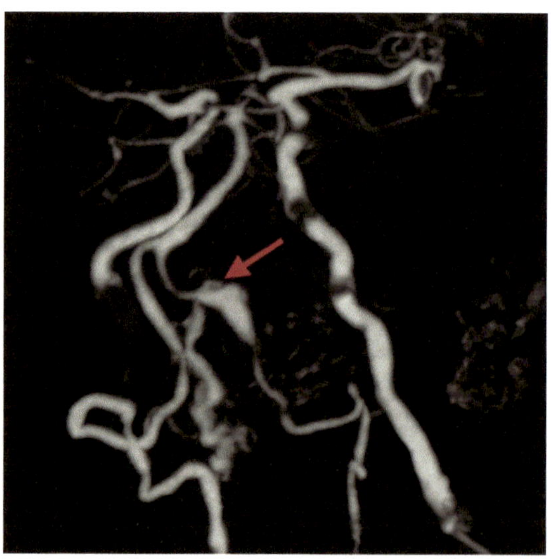

Fig. 28.14 Three-dimensional cerebral artery image produced by selective angiography in the case of vertebral artery aneurysm rupture. Dilatation of the vertebral artery and extravasation of the contrast media (arrow) are apparent using this method

28.5 Brain Postmortem CT for Autopsy "Triage"

As described in Sect. 28.1, it is controversial whether or not CT can be used as a substitute for autopsy. Without entering into the debate about the value of such "triage" by imaging, we will focus on the concerns of the person who has to decide whether the cause of death should be judged by postmortem CT for each pathological condition.

In postmortem CT of the head region, pathologic or traumatic fatal conditions, such as intracerebral hemorrhage (ICH), SAH, cerebral infarction, brain tumors, SDH, epidural hematoma (EDH), and cerebral contusion, can be detected [2, 3, 6, 7, 39]. Under ideal circumstances, it is certainly possible to judge the cause of death from these conditions, but there are caveats to consider.

Below, we describe a few representative pathologies that are frequently encountered from a forensic point of view; for more diverse, detailed findings of each of these, we recommend that neuroradiology textbooks be consulted.

1. Intracerebral hemorrhage
   The fundamental findings of ICH in CT are high absorption masses found in the brain parenchyma (Fig. 28.15). In the case of hypertensive ICH, the putamen, thalamus, cerebellum, and brainstem are preferred sites and are usually seen as single lesions. These features allow some level of distinction from traumatic ICH.

   In cases of small ICH, the victim may not die. To prove that ICH was fatal, it is important to determine from CT images whether cerebral herniation or intraventricular hemorrhage occurred simultaneously.

   Under plausible circumstances, such as cases in which an elderly person died with a well-witnessed history of hypertension, ICH on CT can definitely determine the cause of death [6]. However, all ICHs are not necessarily intrinsic. As described below, traumatic ICH occasionally forms a large single brain hematoma, mimicking hypertensive ICH. Moreover, ICH may be triggered by methamphetamine or cocaine, which can be thought of as a type of toxic death [40]. Even if ICH is observed on postmortem CT of an individual with an unknown cause of death, it is unwise to consider it as death by natural causes without adequate situational investigations and drug testing.

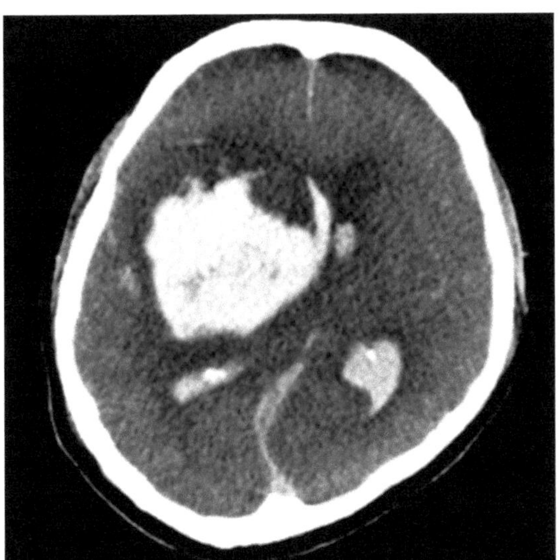

Fig. 28.15 Axial brain computed tomography (CT) image of the intracerebral hemorrhage. The center of the high-density mass is in the right basal ganglia area, compatible with typical hypertensive intracerebral hemorrhage. Complicating intraventricular hemorrhage and subfalcine herniation are also noted in this image

2. Traumatic ICH (brain contusion)
   Typical finding of intracerebral bleeding due to brain contusion is a "salt and pepper" appearance caused by a mixture of hemorrhage and edema occurring in typical contusion sites (e.g., the inferior surfaces of the frontal lobes and the temporal tips), whether it is a coup or contrecoup injury. In this case, diagnosis is easy (Fig. 28.16). However, it sometimes appears on CT as a single brain hemorrhage, as in the case shown in Fig. 28.17. In this case, it is very difficult to differentiate traumatic ICH from endogenous ICH. It is vital for interpreters to perform a careful search for possible merger fractures, or subcutaneous bleeding, suggestive of trauma.
3. Subarachnoid hemorrhage
   The fundamental findings of SAH are high-density areas in the cerebrospinal fluid cavities, such as the cerebral sulci, fissures, and cisterns. The distribution may distinguish between localized and diffuse SAH from CT findings (Fig. 28.18). In general, traumatic subarachnoid hemorrhage is often localized, accompanied by other traumatic findings including brain contusion, SDH, and skull fracture. Diffuse SAH is mostly intrinsic, such as cerebral aneurysmal rupture. However, in postmortem CT interpretation, diffuse SAH is always considered to be diagnosable as intrinsic, but this is a leap in logic and is not an evidence-based decision. Traumatic vertebral artery rupture or dissection is often encountered in forensics, and results in diffuse generalized SAH on CT [41]. This is a condition in which the vertebral artery is cut by excessive

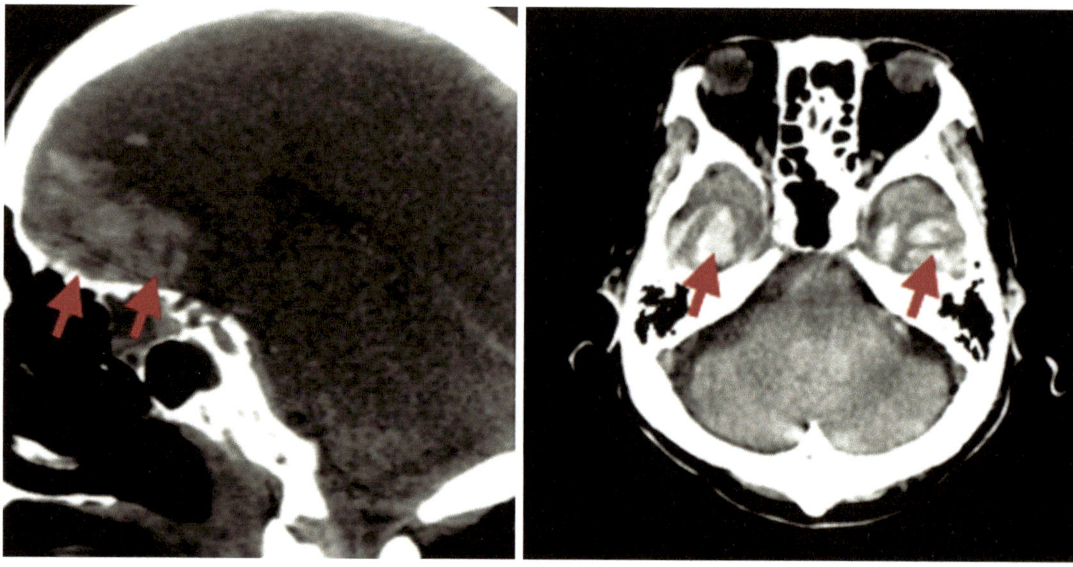

Fig. 28.16 Sagittal and axial brain computed tomography images showing mixed high- and low-density masses in the inferior part of the anterior lobe and the temporal tips, highly suggestive of brain contusion

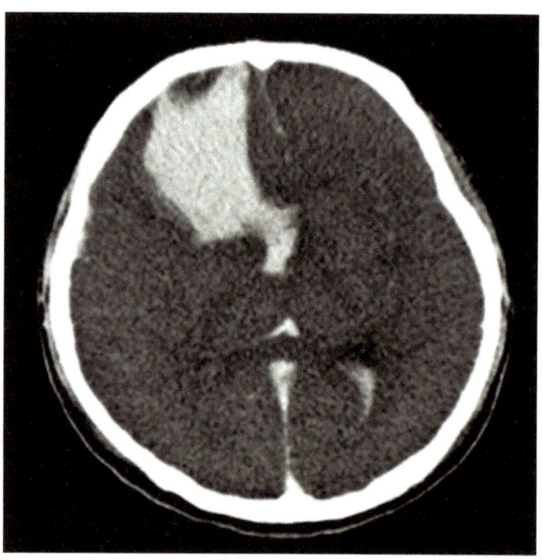

Fig. 28.17 Axial brain computed tomography image showing a right subcortical single hematoma, suggesting endogenous subcortical hemorrhage, without a "salt and pepper" appearance. However, this is actually a traumatic intracerebral hemorrhage caused by a fall, as revealed by autopsy

rotational force, such as when an individual is beaten in a drunken state, and in many cases immediate death is invoked. Accompanying trauma findings, such as brain contusion, subcutaneous bleeding, or skull fractures, are sometimes ambiguous on CT in this condition. For cadavers with diffuse SAH on postmortem CT, in which the situation surrounding death is unclear, interpreters must be careful to diagnose endogenous SAH based on CT findings.

4. Subdural hematoma

   Acute SDH (ASDH) is essentially recognized as crescent-shaped high-density areas between the skull and brain surface (Fig. 28.19). Frequently, the high-density regions can be mixed with low-density regions. Generally, hematomas spread beyond the skull suture line but generally do not across dural attachments. Evaluation of cerebral herniation is important for fatality assessments. ASDH is known to involve no lucid interval, so that consciousness is lost immediately after injury, but this is not always the case. If ASDH is found on CT, it is dangerous to presume that the place of death is the place of injury, without adequate information surrounding the death.

ASDH is considered to be mainly caused by rupture of bridging veins or cortical veins. This can occur due to nonimpact force, such

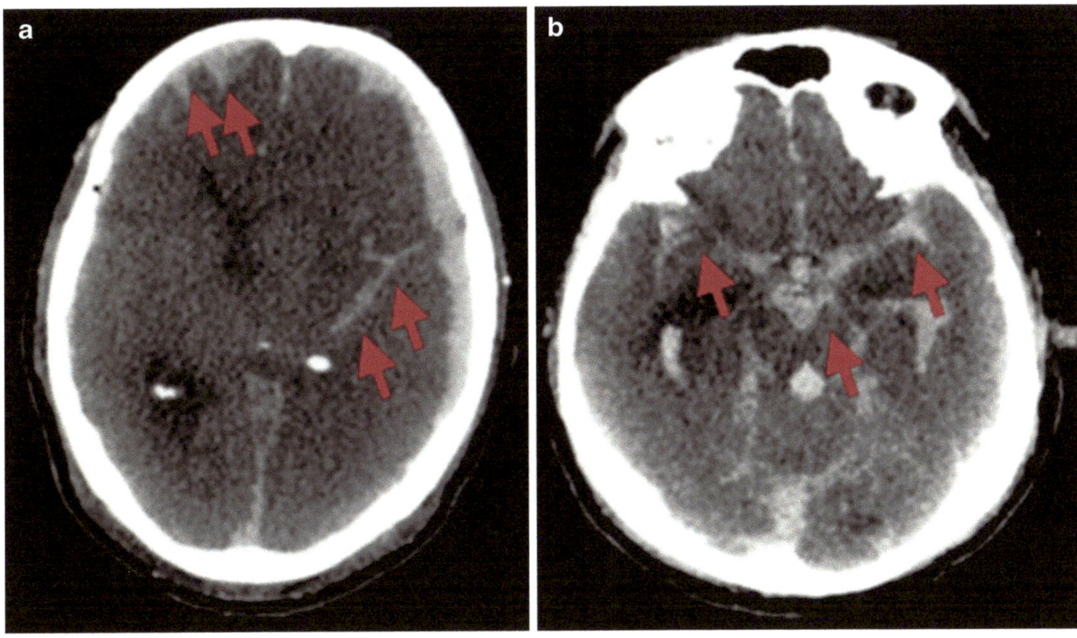

Fig. 28.18 Axial brain computed tomography images showing subarachnoid hemorrhage (SAH). In image (**a**), localized high-density areas can be found in the right anterior lobe sulci and left Sylvian fissure, which correspond to localized SAH. Left acute subdural hematoma is also found in this image. On the other hand, in image (**b**) high densities of the fissures or cisterns can be found bilaterally, corresponding to diffuse SAH

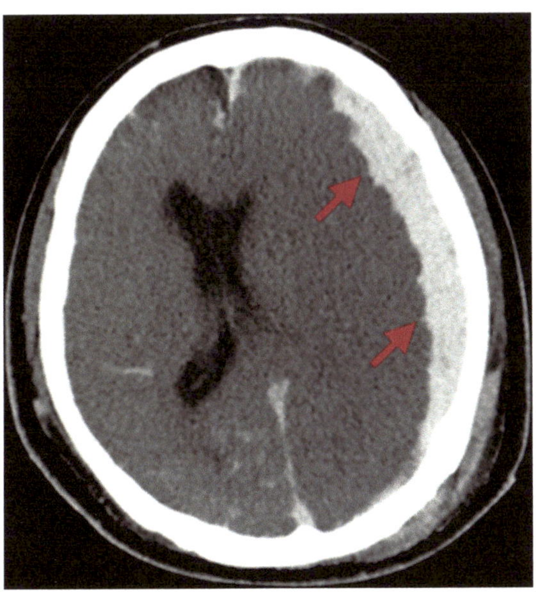

Fig. 28.19 Axial brain computed tomography image of the typical acute subdural hematoma. A crescent-shaped high-density area indicated by arrows is compatible with acute subdural hematoma complicated with localized subarachnoid hemorrhage and subfalcine herniation

as translational or deceleration–acceleration motion, and thus coarse head wounds or discoloration in external examinations are frequently negative. In such cases, skull fractures, brain contusions, and subcutaneous bleeding are also absent on CT. It is also dangerous to assume that ASDH has been intrinsically generated due to lack of other traumatic findings.

Chronic SDH (CSDH) may involve repeated rebleeding, and can sometimes result in cerebral herniation and death. In CSDH, one of the characteristics on CT is that the blood does not coagulate well, and a fluid-fluid level is caused by the hematocrit effect. Moreover, a thick film is formed between the hematoma and the arachnoid membrane, which can sometimes be confirmed by CT (Fig. 28.20).

CSDH can be seen as homogenous low-density areas on CT images. In this case, the differentiation from subdural hygroma is problematic, because the latter can form acutely after injury. A strict differentiation

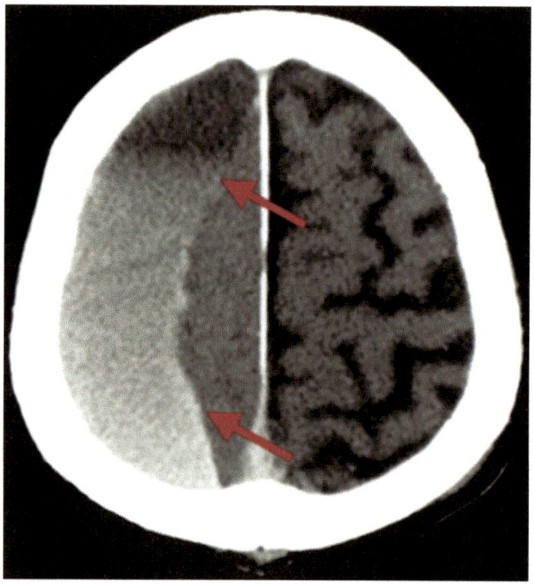

Fig. 28.20 Axial brain computed tomography image of a typical chronic subdural hematoma. Fluid-fluid level is formed inside the hematoma, suggesting hemorrhagic, less coagulated fluid in the cavity. Note the high-density linear lesion on the surface of the brain, suggesting that the membrane formed after injury (arrows)

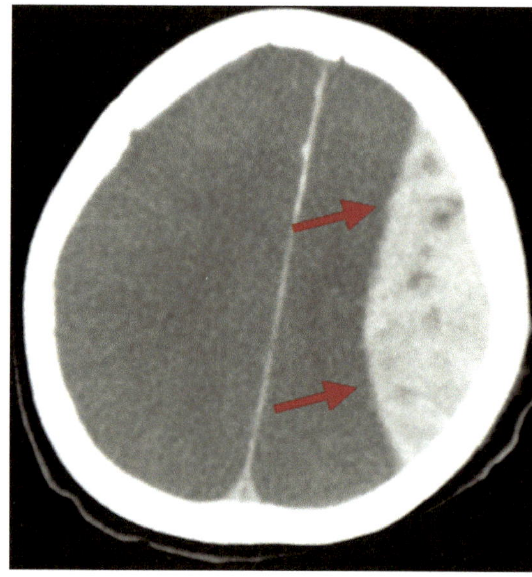

Fig. 28.21 Axial brain computed tomography image of a typical acute epidural hemorrhage. A convex lentiform high-density area can be seen in the left side (arrows)

between these conditions cannot be achieved with CT, and care must be taken when interpreting such cases.

5. Epidural hematoma
The basic observation of acute EDH on CT is convex, lentiform high-density areas between the skull and the brain surface (Fig. 28.21). In principle, this does not spread beyond the skull suture line. Unlike ASDH, most EDHs are due to direct external forces. Therefore, it is likely that there will be obvious trauma findings, including subcutaneous bleeding, or skull fractures, on the CT images, and it is unlikely that the interpreters will find difficulty in determining internal and external causes.
Discrimination from heat hematoma is a problem in forensic medicine. Heat hematoma or extradural burn, which is a postmortem change in a burned dead body, is reported to be crescent shaped rather than lentiform, and has lower densities than the typical traumatic EDH (Fig. 28.22) [42, 43].

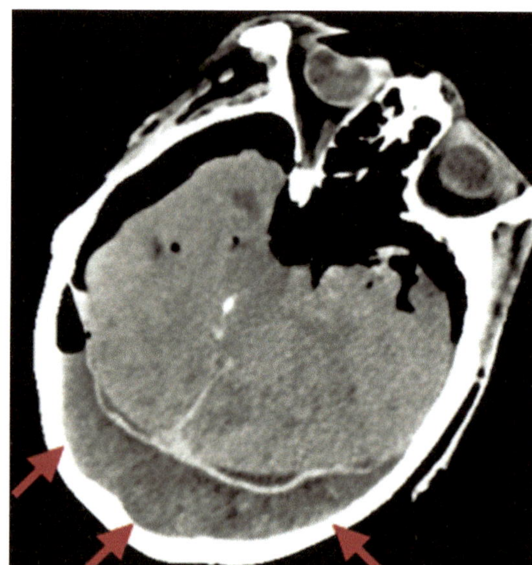

Fig. 28.22 Axial brain computed tomography (CT) image of the head of a burned cadaver. The brain and dura have shrunk and the epidural space has widened, with relatively lower density crescent-shaped fluid collection. This is a typical finding of heat hematoma on CT images

6. Cerebral herniation
CT findings of subfalcine herniation (corresponding to cingulate herniation) are quite common, and consist of a shift of the expected septum pellucidum, ipsilateral lateral ventricular compression, and contralateral lateral ventricular dilation. Herniation associated

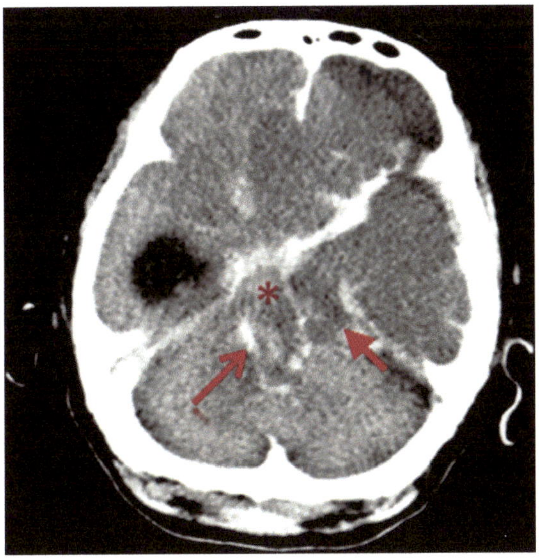

Fig. 28.23 Axial brain computed tomography image of a left descending transtentorial brain herniation. The median displacement of the left uncus (broad arrow), narrowing of the midbrain (asterisk), and Duret hemorrhage (narrow arrow) can be seen. The brain cistern around the midbrain is effacing and there is contralateral dilatation of the lateral ventricle

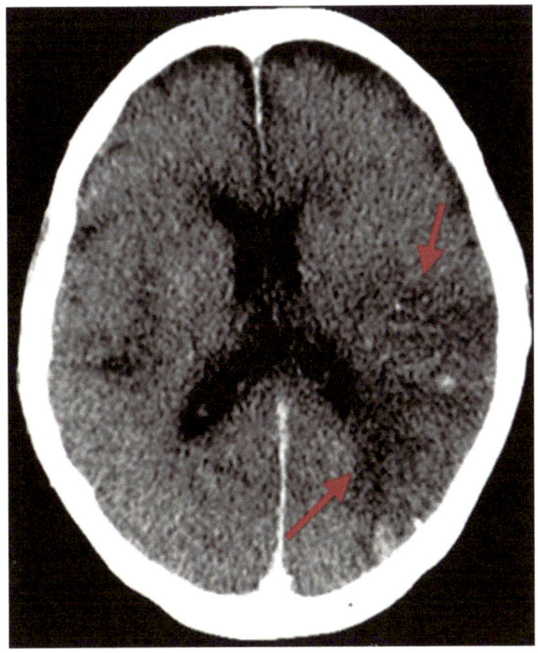

Fig. 28.24 Axial brain computed tomography image of the cerebral infarction. A gray and white matter low-density area can be seen in the middle cerebral artery territory. Inside the area, small high-density regions are also seen, corresponding to hemorrhagic infarction

with the posterior cranial fossa, which directly affects the brain stem, is more important for fatality assessments, and includes descending or ascending transtentorial herniation and tonsillar herniation. Unilateral descending transtentorial herniation (corresponding to uncal herniation) is most commonly seen in such cases. The representative findings are the medial displacement of the uncus or other surrounding cerebral structures, effacement of the cisterns around the midbrain, and deformation and hemorrhage of the midbrain (Fig. 28.23). Secondary bleeding due to cerebral herniation (i.e., Duret hemorrhage) is frequently encountered in cases of cerebral herniation. On CT, it is typically recognized as a longitudinal, linear-shaped high-density area in the midbrain or pons.

7. Cerebral infarction

   Acute cerebral infarction is essentially recognized as a low-density area consistent with the blood circulation on CT (Fig. 28.24). These low-density regions are seen both in the GM and WM, corresponding to cytotoxic edema. In cases of hemorrhagic infarction, it may be accompanied by high-density areas. These infarctions can be fatal when accompanied by cerebral herniation. However, even without obvious cerebral herniations, immobility due to paralysis, dehydration, starvation, hypothermia, or other environmental effects may converge and cause death. Cerebral infarction can be a complication of various conditions, including aortic dissection, malignant tumor, or trauma, including fat embolism. It is therefore important to assess the whole body by CT, and to make careful judgments.

28.6 Conclusion

In postmortem imaging, various cranial lesions and injuries that go unnoticed by external examination can be found, and if appropriate judgment criteria are established, combined with circumstance investigations and toxicological tests, it could change the approach to investigations of death and reduce the need for full autopsy. However, the approach has various difficulties, such as misinterpreting traumatic SAH as natural death. Thus, some care should be taken in embracing this approach unconditionally.

In postmortem CT, it is not possible to evaluate vascular conditions (vertebral artery dissection, venous thrombosis, and fat embolism), axonal injuries, meningitis, or encephalitis, which are all important in forensic evaluations. Needless to say, in clinical brain radiology, MRI, which provides better tissue contrast, can be widely implemented, and it is likely to be employed more widely in postmortem imaging in future. Postmortem changes and findings in brain MRI have been explored widely and are now being verified [2, 39, 44–48]. In future revisions of this chapter, the usefulness of MRI is likely to be reported more fully.

References

1. Donchin Y, Rivkind AI, Bar-Ziv J, Hiss J, Almog J, Dresher M (1994) Utility of postmortem computed tomography in trauma victims. J Trauma 37(4):552–555
2. Thali MJ, Yen K, Schweitzer W, Vock P, Boesch C, Ozdoba C, Schroth G, Ith M, Sonnenschein M, Doernhoefer T, Scheurer E, Plattner T, Dirnhofer R (2003) Virtopsy, a new imaging horizon in forensic pathology: virtual autopsy by postmortem multislice computed tomography (MSCT) and magnetic resonance imaging (MRI)—a feasibility study. J Forensic Sci 48(2):386–403
3. Leth PM (2009) Computerized tomography used as a routine procedure at postmortem investigations. Am J Forensic Med Pathol 30(3):219–222
4. Weustink AC, Hunink MGM, van Dijke CF, Renken NS, Krestin GP, Oosterhuis JW (2009) Minimally invasive autopsy: an alternative to conventional autopsy? Radiology 250(3):897–904
5. Roberts ISD, Benamore RE, Benbow EW, Lee SH, Harris JN, Jackson A, Mallett S, Patankar T, Peebles C, Roobottom C, Traill ZC (2012) Post-mortem imaging as an alternative to autopsy in the diagnosis of adult deaths: a validation study. Lancet 379(9811):136–142
6. Kasahara S, Makino Y, Hayakawa M, Yajima D, Ito H, Iwase H (2012) Diagnosable and non-diagnosable causes of death by postmortem computed tomography: a review of 339 forensic cases. Leg Med (Tokyo) 14(5):239–245
7. Proisy M, Marchand AJ, Loget P, Bouvet R, Roussey M, Pelé F, Rozel C, Treguier C, Darnault P, Bruneau B (2012) Whole-body post-mortem computed tomography compared with autopsy in the investigation of unexpected death in infants and children. Eur Radiol 23(6):1711–1719
8. Blanc-Louvry I, Thureau S, Duval C, Papin-Lefebvre F, Thiebot J, Dacher JN, Gricourt C, Touré E, Proust B (2013) Post-mortem computed tomography compared to forensic autopsy findings: a French experience. Eur Radiol 23(7):1829–1835
9. Rutty GN, Morgan B, Robinson C, Raj V, Pakkal M, Amoroso J, Visser T, Saunders S, Biggs M, Hollingbury F, McGregor A, West K, Richards C, Brown L, Harrison R, Hew R (2017) Diagnostic accuracy of post-mortem CT with targeted coronary angiography versus autopsy for coroner-requested post-mortem investigations: a prospective, masked, comparison study. Lancet 390(10090):145–154
10. Eriksson A, Gustafsson T, Höistad M, Hultcrantz M, Jacobson S, Mejare I, Persson A (2017) Diagnostic accuracy of postmortem imaging vs. autopsy—a systematic review. Eur J Radiol 89:249–269
11. Buck U, Naether S, Braun M, Bolliger S, Friederich H, Jackowski C, Aghayev E, Christe A, Vock P, Dirnhofer R, Thali MJ (2007) Application of 3D documentation and geometric reconstruction methods in traffic accident analysis: with high resolution surface scanning, radiological MSCT/MRI scanning and real data based animation. Forensic Sci Int 170(1):20–28
12. Ringl H, Schernthaner RE, Schueller G, Balassy C, Kienzl D, Botosaneanu A, Weber M, Czerny C, Hajdu S, Mang T, Herold CJ, Schima W (2010) The skull unfolded: a cranial CT visualization algorithm for fast and easy detection of skull fractures. Radiology 255(2):553–562
13. Levy AD, Harcke HT, Mallak CT (2010) Postmortem imaging: MDCT features of postmortem change and decomposition. Am J Forensic Med Pathol 31(1):12–17
14. Smith AB, Lattin GE Jr, Berran P, Harcke HT (2012) Common and expected postmortem CT observations involving the brain: mimics of antemortem pathology. Am J Neuroradiol 33(7):1387–1391
15. Takahashi N, Satou C, Higuchi T, Shiotani M, Maeda H, Hirose Y (2010) Quantitative analysis of brain edema and swelling on early postmortem computed tomography: comparison with antemortem computed tomography. Jpn J Radiol 28(5):349–354
16. Shirota G, Gonoi W, Ishida M, Okuma H, Shintani Y, Abe H, Takazawa Y, Ikemura M, Fukayama M (2015) Brain swelling and loss of gray and white matter differentiation in human postmortem cases by computed tomography. PLoS One 10(11):e0143848
17. Takahashi N, Satou C, Higuchi T, Shiotani M, Maeda H, Hirose Y (2010) Quantitative analysis of intracranial hypostasis: comparison of early postmortem and antemortem CT findings. AJR 195:W388–W393
18. Yuzawa H, Higano S, Mugikura S, Umetsu A, Murata T, Nakagawa A, Koyama A, Takahashi S (2008)

Pseudo-subarachnoid hemorrhage found in patients with postresuscitation encephalopathy: characteristics of CT findings and clinical importance. AJNR 29(8):1544–1549
19. Shirota G, Gonoi W, Ikemura M, Ishida M, Shintani Y, Abe H, Fukayama M, Higashida T, Okuma H, Abe O (2017) The pseudo-SAH sign: an imaging pitfall in postmortem computed tomography. Int J Legal Med 131(6):1647–1653
20. Shiotani S, Ueno Y, Atake S, Kohno M, Suzuki M, Kikuchi K, Hayakawa H (2010) Nontraumatic postmortem computed tomographic demonstration of cerebral gas embolism following cardiopulmonary resuscitation. Jpn J Radiol 28(1):1–7
21. Levy AD, Abbott RM, Mallak CT, Getz JM, Harcke HT, Champion HR, Pearse LA (2006) Virtual autopsy: preliminary experience in high-velocity gunshot wound victims. Radiology 240(2):522–528
22. Sano R, Hirasawa S, Kobayashi S, Shimada T, Awata S, Takei H, Otake H, Takahashi K, Takahashi Y, Kominato Y (2011) Use of postmortem computed tomography to reveal an intraoral gunshot injuries in a charred body. Leg Med (Tokyo) 13(6):286–288
23. Thomsen AH, Jurik AG, Uhrenholt L, Vesterby A (2009) An alternative approach to computerized tomography (CT) in forensic pathology. Forensic Sci Int 183(1–3):87–90
24. Gerlock AJ (1976) The flared mandible sign of the flail mandible. Radiology 119(2):299–300
25. Papadiochos I, Goutzanis L, Petsinis V (2017) Flail mandible and immediate airway management: traumatic detachment of mandibular lingual cortex results in obstructive dyspnea and severe odynophagia. J Craniofac Surg 28(5):1311–1314
26. Hanson JA, Deliganis AV, Baxter AB, Cohen WA, Linnau KF, Wilson AJ, Mann FA (2002) Radiologic and clinical spectrum of occipital condyle fractures: retrospective review of 107 consecutive fractures in 95 patients. AJR Am J Roentgenol 178(5):1261–1268
27. Pinho J, Amorim JM, Araújo JM, Vilaça H, Ribeiro M, Pereira J, Ferreira C (2016) Cerebral gas embolism associated with central venous catheter: systematic review. J Neurol Sci 362:160–164
28. Ozdoba C, Weis J, Plattner T, Dirnhofer R, Yen K (2005) Fatal scuba diving incident with massive gas embolism in cerebral and spinal arteries. Neuroradiology 47(6):411–416
29. Laurent P-E, Coulange M, Mancini J, Bartoli C, Desfeux J, Piercecchi-Marti M-D, Gorincour G (2014) Postmortem CT appearance of gas collections in fatal diving accidents. AJR 203(3):468–475
30. Motomura A, Makino Y, Ohdo Y, Inokuchi G, Yajima D, Hayakawa M, Iwase H (2013) Pre-autopsy computed tomography accurately detected cerebral hemorrhage in highly decomposed bodies: report of two cases. Forensic Sci Int 231(1–3):e33–e36
31. Sano R, Hirasawa S, Awata S, Kobayashi S, Shimada T, Takei H, Takahashi Y, Kominato Y (2013) Use of postmortem computed tomography to reveal acute subdural hematoma in a severely decomposed body with advanced skeletonization. Leg Med (Tokyo) 15(1):32–34
32. Grabherr S, Doenz F, Steger B, Dirnhofer R, Dominguez A, Sollberger B, Gygax E, Rizzo E, Chevallier C, Meuli R, Mangin P (2010) Multi-phase post-mortem CT angiography: development of a standardized protocol. Int J Legal Med 125(6):791–802
33. Ross SG, Thali MJ, Bolliger S, Germerott T, Ruder TD, Flach PM (2012) Sudden death after chest pain: feasibility of virtual autopsy with postmortem CT angiography and biopsy. Radiology 264(1):250–259
34. Roberts ISD, Benamore RE, Peebles C, Roobottom C, Traill ZC (2011) Technical report: diagnosis of coronary artery disease using minimally invasive autopsy: evaluation of a novel method of post-mortem coronary CT angiography. Clin Radiol 66(7):645–650
35. Iizuka K, Sakamoto N, Shiotani S, Komatsuzaki A (2013) Feasibility of resuscitation contrast-enhanced postmortem computed tomography using cardiopulmonary resuscitation technique with chest compression immediately after death. Springerplus 2:663
36. Inokuchi G, Yajima D, Hayakawa M, Motomura A, Chiba F, Torimitsu S, Makino Y (2014) Iwase. Postmortem dynamic cerebral angiography for detecting aneurysm and bleeding sites in cases of subarachnoid hemorrhage. Forensic Sci Med Pathol 10(4):487–495
37. Saunders SL, Morgan B, Raj V, Rutty GN (2010) Postmortem computed tomography angiography: past, present and future. Forensic Sci Med Pathol 7(3):271–277
38. Kuninaka H, Takahashi Y, Sano R, Takahashi K, Kubo R, Kominato Y, Takei H, Kobayashi S, Shimada T, Tokue H, Awata S (2016) Use of postmortem computed tomography angiography to detect vascular injuries accompanying skull base fracture. Leg Med (Tokyo) 23(C):55–58
39. Yen K, Lövblad K-O, Scheurer E, Ozdoba C, Thali MJ, Aghayev E, Jackowski C, Anon J, Frickey N, Zwygart K, Weis J, Dirnhofer R (2007) Post-mortem forensic neuroimaging: correlation of MSCT and MRI findings with autopsy results. Forensic Sci Int 173(1):21–35
40. Lappin JM, Darke S, Farrell M (2014) Stroke and methamphetamine use in young adults: a review. J Neurol Neurosurg Psychiatry 88(12):1079–1091
41. Ikegaya H, Yajima D, Iwase H (2008) Vertebral artery rupture in a sudden death case after mild trauma. Am J Forensic Med Pathol 29:276–278
42. Kawasumi Y, Usui A, Hosokai Y, Sato M, Funayama M (2013) Heat haematoma: post-mortem computed tomography findings. Clin Radiol 68(2):e95–e97
43. O'Donnell C, Woodford N (2008) Post-mortem radiology—a new sub-specialty? Clin Radiol 63(11):1189–1194
44. Van den Hauwe L, Parizel PM, Martin JJ, Cras P, De Deyn P, De Schepper AMA (1995) Postmortem MRI of the brain with neuropathological correlation. Neuroradiology 37(5):343–349

45. Ruder TD, Hatch GM, Siegenthaler L, Ampanozi G, Mathier S, Thali MJ, Weber OM (2012) The influence of body temperature on image contrast in post mortem MRI. Eur J Radiol 81(6):1366–1370
46. Ross S, Ebner L, Flach P, Brodhage R, Bolliger SA, Christe A, Thali MJ (2012) Postmortem whole-body MRI in traumatic causes of death. AJR 199(6):1186–1192
47. Tashiro K, Shiotani S, Kobayashi T, Kaga K, Saito H, Someya S, Miyamoto K, Hayakawa H (2015) Cerebral relaxation times from postmortem MR imaging of adults. MRMS 14(1):51–56
48. Adolphi NL (2016) An equation-free introduction to post-mortem MR image contrast and pulse sequence optimization. J Forensic Radiol Imaging 4(c):27–34

Bioethical Aspects of Postmortem Imaging

29

Luciano Sesta

29.1 Death and Autopsy in Current Medical-Cultural Context

As is well known, death has hardly ever been a mere "natural" event in human history. No doubt, death is as much a "cultural" event today as it was in times past. In the past, even death by old age was a "cultural" and not "natural" event, because it depended on, at the time, lack of available medical progress or adequate resources. What yesterday was "natural"—to die at 40–45—today is "unnatural"—thanks to medical, and therefore "cultural/artificial," progress. If in the past human beings died *only* because of accidents, wars, killing, diseases, old age, and so forth. In our technological civilization, in which there is an extraordinary possibility to prolong the life, death is more and more a result of a medical "letting die." The widespread fear of futile treatment is a very significant example of this. Indeed, there wouldn't be such fear if there was no risk to prolong life beyond its "natural" limits.

This general situation influences even the medical-legal profession to investigate causes of death. If death becomes an almost totally "artificial" fact, then to examine *how* and *why* somebody died should not be only in suspicious circumstances, but in all cases of death. Where death depends more and more on human power to prevent it or permit it, any circumstance tends to become "suspicious."[1] Part of the procedure's improvement to examine corpses, and therefore autopsy and postmortem imaging (PI), derives from this "medicalization" of life and death. The other part, instead, is due to the increasing circumstances in which it is necessary to investigate into suspicious death, for instance in migrant's corpses rescued from the sea.[2]

Given the above, it may be rather odd that in recent times autopsy has continued to decline.[3] There are cultural, scientific, medical-legal, psychological, and ethical reasons for this. The main one, it could be argued, is that while ethical and subjective reasons for autopsy are reducing, medical-legal and public reasons are increasing. Persistence in criminality creates persistence in legal needs and forensic work, as in the increas-

L. Sesta (✉)
Department for Health Promotion, Maternal and Child Care "G.D'Alessandro", University of Palermo, Palermo, Italy
e-mail: luciano.sesta@unipa.it

G. Lo Re et al. (eds.), *Radiology in Forensic Medicine*,
https://doi.org/10.1007/978-3-319-96737-0_29

[1] See Illich I (1974) *The Political Uses of Natural Death*, "Hastings Center Studies", Vol. 2 (1); 3–20.

[2] See Sesta L, Argo A (2017) *Identifying migrant's corpses: a really worthy duty?* forthcoming.

[3] Loughrey MB, McCluggage WG, Toner PG (2000) *The declining autopsy rate and clinicians' attitudes*, Ulst Med J; 69: 83–89.

ing suspicious deaths mentioned above. Furthermore, a large meta-analysis, which demonstrated that approximately one-third of death certificates are produced without autopsy, did not correctly identify the cause of death.[4] It should not be forgotten, however, that the higher our technological possibilities are, the more needs they will create. Accordingly, even if there might be fewer ethical reasons for an autopsy, needs to resort to it could be in any case increasing, especially if the used method was less invasive and so without exaggerated ethical complications. As is known, indeed, from the start of its history, autopsy—as well as removal of organs for transplantation—is considered by some people to be a sort of desecration of the body.[5]

29.2 Virtopsy as New Perspective

Another reason why autopsy rates are decreasing is the widespread use of advanced imaging techniques such as the computed tomography (CT) and magnetic resonance imaging (MRI).[6] These techniques can demonstrate findings that are not readily detected during the traditional autopsy, even if research shows that in specific cases autopsy remains superior to and more reliable than imaging.[7] Many studies demonstrate that, in some specific cases, PI is more accurate than traditional autopsy. For instance, Hayakawa et al. found that the cause of death, as demonstrated by IA, was different from that determined by superficial postmortem examination in 25% of cases.[8] Other studies show that PI can help to determine the etiology of sudden death due to nontraumatic causes in infants and children. Imaging autopsies in that study were able to point to the cause of death in 14 of 15 cases, when radiographic information was combined with premortem clinical and laboratory data.[9]

Postmortem imaging, or "virtopsy," is today being more and more considered as complementary or even as an alternative means of determining the cause of death.[10] Typically, in the history of medical science and techniques, a new procedure, that at the beginning was evaluated as "complementary," or "in addition to," then became "alternative," or "in place of." One day, perhaps, virtopsy will be the ordinary and only one procedure to investigate causes of death. However, the current common opinion is that more reliable findings are obtained when PI is combined with traditional autopsy.

As is known, autopsy can be defined as "the examination of a cadaver to determine or con-

[4]Stawicki PS, Aggrawal A, Dean AJ et al. (2008) *Postmortem use of advanced imaging techniques: Is autopsy going digital?* Scientist Vol. 2 (4): 17–26; Roulson J, Benbow EW, Hasleton PS (2005) *Discrepancies between clinical and autopsy diagnosis and the value of postmortem histology: a meta-analysis and review.* Histopathology; 47:551–559.

[5]See Quigley Ch (1996) *The Corpse. A History*, McFarland, Jefferson-London.

[6]Stawicki SP, Gracias VH, Schrag SP, Martin ND, Dean AJ, Hoey BA (2008) *The dead continue to teach the living: examining the role of computed tomography and magnetic resonance imaging in the setting of postmortem examinations.* J Surg Educ 2008; 65: 200–205. See also Ciaffi R, Gibelli D, Cattaneo C (2011) *Forensic radiology and personal identification of unidentified bodies: a review*, 116(6): 960–968.

[7]Jalalzadeh H, Giannakopoulos GF, Berger FH, Fronczek J, van de Goot FR, Reijnders UJ, Zuidema WP (2015) *Post-mortem imaging compared with autopsy in trauma victims - A systematic review*, Forensic Sci Int. 257: 29–48.

[8]Hayakawa M, Yamamoto S, Motani H, Yajima D, Sato Y, Iwase H (2006) *Does imaging technology overcome problems of conventional postmortem examination? A trial of computed tomography imaging for postmortem examination.* Int J Legal Med; 120: 24–26.

[9]Oyake Y, Aoki T, Shiotani S, Kohno M, Ohashi N, Akutsu H, Yamazaki K (2006) *Postmortem computed tomography for detecting causes of sudden death in infants and children: retrospective review of cases.* Radiat Med; 24:493–502. More generally, "La principale metodica radiologica applicata alle Scienze Forensi al giorno d'oggi risulta essere la multi-slice TC (CT-Virtopsy, MSCT-v), senza utilizzo di mezzi di contrasto; essa presenta numerosi vantaggi, quali la non-invasività, l'accuratezza, la riproducibilità, la rapidità di esecuzione e l'ampia possibilità di rielaborazione e ricostru- zione delle immagini (MPR, MIP, VR, etc) per la valutazione anche di organi specifici, della superficie cutanea o delle ossa" (Serraino S, Scopellitti L et al. *Ruolo dell'imaging TC nella valutazione post-mortem dei soggetti deceduti per caduta da altezze elevate: nostra esperienza*, "Il giornale italiano di Radiologia Medica", 2016, 3: 58–64, 58).

[10]Underwood J (2012) *Post-mortem imaging and autopsy: rivals or allies?* The Lancet, 379; 100–102 and Dirnhofer R, Jackowski C, Vock P, Potter K, Thali MJ (2006) *Virtopsy: minimally invasive, imaging guided virtual autopsy.* Radiographics; 26: 1305–1333.

firm the cause of death. Derived from the Greek words for 'self' (*autos*) and 'I will see' (*opsomei*)—'To see with one's own eyes'."[11] Similarly to other circumstances in the history of medicine, advances in the diagnosis and therapy field often cause a sort of distancing by the physician away from patient. This occurrence is more *ethically* significant than it appears. While in the traditional autopsy physicians examine corpses directly, in PI there is a technical process between physicians and corpses, creating difficulties both for their claim to see "with one's own eyes," typical of autopsy, and for the interpretation of the findings to inform relatives.

As a matter of fact, the replacement implemented by PI doesn't remove the physician's human view, but enhances it. In PI we are all yet to see, even if not with "our own eyes," but with scanners' "eyes." Certainly, in no way could a device "see" something, because it is always the physician—pathologist, radiologist, as well as the patient's primary physician—who really sees and transforms a simple "image" into a "diagnosis." As in other cases of use of technology in medicine, also in this case the personal skills of the individual physician are essential, and there is no technology, however sophisticated, that could replace such skills.

29.3 Postmortem Imaging and Principles of Biomedical Ethics

As Judge-Kronis et al. wrote, "Investigation after death should be viewed as a continuation of patient care and a professional service that can be offered to parents."[12] Such care and professional service and also social have consequences in terms of resource distribution and cost-benefit analysis. In medicine, as in other fields of social services, we cannot promote procedures, whose effectiveness and safety are not supported by scientific evidence.

We have seen that, in some specific cases, PI is as accurate as traditional autopsy, and sometimes more than that, but such criteria are not enough in themselves to establish in which circumstances we should provide PI rather than traditional autopsy. When either of these are available and unless the case has been requested by a judge, the choice will depend on the relatives' wishes. By and large, the relative's wishes should be respected, by having pity for the deceased and their loved ones. As often as not, it is not a problem for the rest of the society, except for situations in which relatives' wishes are clearly unreasonable. What is the criteria by which we can define a specific wish "unreasonable"?

A possible response can be found by referring to a well-known set of four principles, formulated by Tom Beachamp and James Childress in their influential book *Principles of Biomedical Ethics*,[13] and introduced for the first time into healthcare ethics by the so-called Belmont Report in 1978.[14] As is known, these principles are non-maleficence, beneficence, justice, and respect for autonomy. When it comes to postmortem examination, obviously, only some principles can be applied to the deceased, while others concern above all their relatives.

Corpses, and any parts thereof, should always be handled with moral awareness, in the knowledge

[11] Serraino S, Scopellitti L et al. (2016) *Ruolo dell'imaging TC nella valutazione post-mortem dei soggetti deceduti per caduta da altezze elevate: nostra esperienza*, "Il giornale italiano di Radiologia Medica" 3: 58–64; Thali MJ, Jackowski C, Oesterhelweg L, Ross SG, Dirnhofer R. (2007) *Virtopsy—The swiss virtual autopsy approach*, Legal Med; 9: 100–104 and Burton JL. *A bite into the history of the autopsy* (2005) Forensic Science, Medicine, and Pathology; 1: 277–284.

[12] Judge-Kronis L. et al. (2016) *Consent for paediatric and perinatal postmortem investigations: Implications of less invasive autopsy,* "Journal of Forensic Radiology and Imaging", 4: 7–11, 7.

[13] Beauchamp TL, Childress JF (2001), *Principles of Biomedical Ethics*, fifth ed. Oxford University Press, Oxford.

[14] The National Commission for the Protection of Human Subjects of Biomedical and Behavioral Sciences (1978), *The Belmont Report. Ethical Principles and Guidelines for the Protection of Human Subjects of Research*, Dhew Publication No. (OS) 78-0012, Washington.

that the feelings of other people, especially relatives, are involved.[15] What does non-maleficence mean before a bereaved family? Probably, to avoid every action, word, and advice that could hurt relatives' feelings, not only for the sake of such feelings in themselves, but also to respect the dignity of the deceased. Relatives' feelings are worthy, indeed, not because they are mere subjective feelings, but because they refer to death, namely something that has objectively a great prominence. Accordingly, in every postmortem medical action one should include, in the mentioned list of four principles, the principle of pity. Moreover, the principle of pity should be presented as a specific application of justice in cases of postmortem examination, that is, as the principle obliges to give to each their own.

What about beneficence? It is the positive side of the non-maleficence principle. It requires to do what is good according to medical standards and ethical respect for people. In a PI case, it means to do as much as possible, consistently with other values at stake, to guarantee what relatives need and the truth about the causes of death that they require.

Autonomy, which is the last principle, is a version of the wider human dignity. In general, it is against dignity to treat human beings as if they were unable to choose autonomously what is best for them. Even in this case, consistently with other values at stake, society and healthcare professionals have to allow individuals the right to choose what is best for them, by avoiding doing something without or against their consent. Autonomy, therefore, is a core principle in health care, because it prevents possible abuses of power, above all in medical situations where relatives are shocked, and especially vulnerable due to the death of their loved one. Such specific circumstances could impair or modify the capacity to express one's own autonomy or informed consent.

There are cases, furthermore, in which society and health professional have to intervene or not intervene, regardless of the autonomy of patients or their relatives. If a family requests a very expensive and not medically necessary PI, for instance, in no way could the principle of autonomy justify the intervention. When it comes to ethical reasons for our decisions and actions, we need to take into account not only individual rights, but also the interpersonal dimension of human life. If health resources are limited, then we need to distribute them in a right way, by weighing the different requirements. Every human being has equal dignity, even if everybody is not in the same circumstances as each other. Hence, more important than the notion of autonomy is the ground on which autonomy is based, namely human dignity and the corresponding duty of justice.

29.4 Noninvasive Examination and Pediatric Cases

To avoid that the human dignity principle appears too rhetoric or detached, one should point out its practical meaning. In this case, the human dignity principle and cost-benefit criteria imply—also when it comes to tragic grief experience—that the surrounding society has the right to interfere with relatives' decisions, resting on common good considerations and, if need be, appealing to duty to assign fairly limited resources.[16]

Ethical issues arise not only when someone asks for medical diagnosis or treatment, but also when someone rejects it. In this regard, there seems to be a crucial ethical issue that emerges especially in the pediatric population. Faced with sudden death, when the most perinatal and pediatric deaths do not fall within a jurisdiction, imaging autopsy might be offered as an alternative to traditional autopsy, especially when there

[15] Stawicki PS, Aggrawal A, Dean AJ et al. *Postmortem use of advanced imaging techniques: Is autopsy going digital?*: 19.

[16] About this topic, beyond postmortem examination, see the drammatic case of Child B in the United Kingdom, where it was denied experimental therapy for leukaemia, arguing that it was too expensive and of untested efficacy. See Ham C (1999) *Tragic choices in health care: lessons from the Child B case*, "British Medical Journal" 319: 1258–1261.

is parental unwillingness to give permission to perform it.[17]

Such unwillingness, however, could not concern only physical invasiveness of traditional autopsy, by involving a more specific ethical problem about human pity and knowledge of the truth. Undoubtedly, on the one hand "the decision to consent to autopsy is a personal choice, made by parents on behalf of their child in order to better understand the circumstances of their death, to answer specific questions or to improve the process for others."[18] On the other hand, when it comes to a child's death, as is known, the repression mechanism is very frequent as a form of defense. In a bereaved parent, the desire to not to know more often prevails than the desire to know. Where there are no legal requests or directives, the protection of relatives' feelings could be more important than the truth itself. Hence, we must recognize that there are circumstances where, from an ethical point of view, ignorance is better than knowledge. In this case, even what is *physically* noninvasive, as PI, could be *morally* invasive.

Further Reading

Beauchamp TL, Childress JF (2001) Principles of biomedical ethics, 5th edn. Oxford University Press, Oxford

Burton JL (2005) A bite into the history of the autopsy. Forensic Sci Med Pathol 1:277–284

Ciaffi R, Gibelli D, Cattaneo C (2011) Forensic radiology and personal identification of unidentified bodies: a review. Radiol Med 116(6):960–968

Dirnhofer R, Jackowski C, Vock P, Potter K, Thali MJ (2006) Virtopsy: minimally invasive, imaging guided virtual autopsy. Radiographics 26:1305–1333

Ham C (1999) Tragic choices in health care: lessons from the Child B case. Br Med J 319:1258–1261

Hayakawa M, Yamamoto S, Motani H, Yajima D, Sato Y, Iwase H (2006) Does imaging technology overcome problems of conventional postmortem examination? A trial of computed tomography imaging for postmortem examination. Int J Legal Med 120:24–26

Illich I (1974) The political uses of natural death. Hastings Center Stud 2(1):3–20

Jalalzadeh H, Giannakopoulos GF, Berger FH, Fronczek J, van de Goot FR, Reijnders UJ, Zuidema WP (2015) Post-mortem imaging compared with autopsy in trauma victims—a systematic review. Forensic Sci Int 257:29–48

Judge-Kronis L et al (2016) Consent for paediatric and perinatal postmortem investigations: implications of less invasive autopsy. J Forensic Radiol Imaging 4:7–11

Kumar P, Taxy J, Angst DB, Mangurten HH (1998) Autopsies in children: are they still useful? Arch Pediatr Adolesc Med 152:558–563

Loughrey MB, McCluggage WG, Toner PG (2000) The declining autopsy rate and clinicians' attitudes. Ulster Med J 69:83–89

Oyake Y, Aoki T, Shiotani S, Kohno M, Ohashi N, Akutsu H, Yamazaki K (2006) Postmortem computed tomography for detecting causes of sudden death in infants and children: retrospective review of cases. Radiat Med 24:493–502

Quigley CH (1996) The corpse. A history. McFarland, Jefferson-London

Roulson J, Benbow EW, Hasleton PS (2005) Discrepancies between clinical and autopsy diagnosis and the value of postmortem histology: a meta-analysis and review. Histopathology 47:551–559

Serraino S, Scopellitti L et al (2016) Ruolo dell'imaging TC nella valutazione post-mortem dei soggetti deceduti per caduta da altezze elevate: nostra esperienza. G Ital Radiol Med 3:58–64

Sesta L, Argo A (2018) Damnatio memoriae? Migranti, giustizia e medicina legale. Riv Ital Med Leg 2:869–879

Stawicki SP, Gracias VH, Schrag SP, Martin ND, Dean AJ, Hoey BA (2008) The dead continue to teach the living: examining the role of computed tomography and magnetic resonance imaging in the setting of postmortem examinations. J Surg Educ 65:200–205

Stawicki PS, Aggrawal A, Dean AJ et al (2008) Postmortem use of advanced imaging techniques: is autopsy going digital? Scientist 2(4):17–26

Thali MJ, Jackowski C, Oesterhelweg L, Ross SG, Dirnhofer R (2007) Virtopsy—the Swiss virtual autopsy approach. Legal Med 9:100–104

The National Commission for the Protection of Human Subjects of Biomedical and Behavioral Sciences (1978) The Belmont Report. Ethical Principles and Guidelines for the Protection of Human Subjects of Research, Dhew Publication No. (OS) 78-0012, Washington

Underwood J (2012) Post-mortem imaging and autopsy: rivals or allies? Lancet 379:100–102

[17]Kumar P, Taxy J, Angst DB, Mangurten HH (1998) *Autopsies in children: Are they still useful?* Arch Pediatr Adolesc Med 152:558–563.

[18]Judge-Kronis L. et al., 7.